Prentice Hall Health

Q&A review

for the Medical Assistant

Prentice Hall Health

Q&A review

for the Medical Assistant

Sixth Edition

Tom Palko, BA, MEd, MCS, MT(ASCP)
Director, Medical Assistant Program
Professor of Allied Health Sciences
Arkansas Tech University
Russellville, Arkansas

Hilda Palko, BS, MT(ASCP), CMA

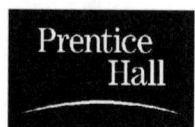

Prentice Hall
Upper Saddle River, NewJersey 07458

Library of Congress Cataloging-in-Publication Data
Palko, Tom.
    Prentice-Hall health Q&A review for the medical assistant
        p. cm.
    Fifth ed. published as: Appleton & Lange's review for the
    medical assistant. Includes bibliographical references.
    ISBN 0-13-088189-9
    1. Medical assistants—Examinations, questions, etc.
    2. Medical offices—Management—Examinations, questions, etc.
    3. Physicians' assistants—Examinations, questions, etc.
    I. Title: Health question and answer review for medical assisting.
II. Palko, Hilda. III. Palko, Tom. Appleton & Lange's review for
the medical assistant. IV. Title.

R728.8.P28 2000
610.73'7'076—dc21   00-061133

Publisher: Julie Alexander
Executive Editor: Greg Vis
Acquisitions Editors: Mark Cohen and Barbara Krawiec
Managing Development Editor: Marilyn Meserve
Director of Production and Manufacturing: Bruce Johnson
Managing Production Editor: Patrick Walsh
Production Editor: Tonia Grubb, York Production Services
Production Liaison: Danielle Newhouse
Manufacturing Manager: Ilene Sanford
Creative Director: Marianne Frasco
Cover Design Coordinator: Maria Guglielmo
Cover Designer: Janice Bielawa
Director of Marketing: Leslie Cavaliere
Marketing Coordinator: Cindy Frederick
Editorial Assistants: Melissa Kerian and Mary Ellen Ruitenberg
Interior Designer: Janice Bielawa
Composition: York Production Services
Printing and Binding: The Banta Company

Prentice-Hall International (UK) Limited, *London*
Prentice-Hall of Australia Pty. Limited, *Sydney*
Prentice-Hall Canada, Inc., *Toronto*
Prentice-Hall Hispanoamericana, S.A., *Mexico*
Prentice-Hall of India Private Limited, *New Delhi*
Prentice-Hall of Japan, Inc., *Tokyo*
Prentice-Hall Singapore Pte. Ltd.
Editora Prentice-Hall do Brasil Ltda., *Rio de Janeiro*

NOTICE:
The procedures described in this textbook are based on consultation with nursing authorities. The author and publisher have taken care to make certain that these procedures reflect currently accepted clinical practice; however, they cannot be considered absolute recommendations.

The material in this textbook contains the most current information available at the time of publication. However, federal, state and local guidelines concerning clinical practices, including without limitation, those governing infection control and universal precautions, change rapidly. The reader should note, therefore, that new regulations may require changes in some procedures.

It is the responsibility of the reader to familiarize himself or herself with the policies and procedures set by federal, state and local agencies, as well as the institution or agency where the reader is employed. The authors and the publishers of this textbook, and the supplements written to accompany it, disclaim any liability, loss or risk resulting directly or indirectly from the suggested procedures and theory, from any undetected errors, or from the reader's misunderstanding of the text. It is the reader's responsibility to stay informed of any new changes or recommendations made by any federal, state and local agency as well as by his or her employing health care institution or agency.

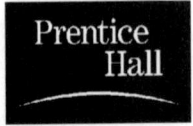

10 9 8 7 6 5 4 3 2
ISBN 0-13-088189-9

This book is dedicated to our three sons,
Mark, Carl, and James
who have always brought true joy to our lives.

Contents

Preface

The purpose of this sixth edition of Prentice Hall Health's *Q&A Review for the Medical Assistant* is to prepare the user to perform well on the Medical Assistant Certifying Examination (CMA or RMA) tests. The principle guides used throughout this revision have been the American Association of Medical Assistants (AAMA) Certification Examination Content Outline and the Registered Medical Assistant (RMA) Certification Examination Content Summary. The AAMA Certification Examination Content Outline is based on the AAMA Role Delineation Study, which is outlined on the Medical Assistant Role Delineation Chart (MARDC). The MARDC has defined the job entry-level skills and knowledge base that are necessary for a person to function effectively as a medical assistant in today's complex medical practice. Copies of the Medical Assistant Role Delineation Chart and the Registered Medical Assistant Certification Examination Content Summary are also included in this edition. The questions, answers, and rationales in this revised edition reflect the current knowledge, tasks, and procedures most often required of the medical assistant.

The book is divided into four major parts: General Information, Administrative Procedures, Clinical Procedures, and Practice Test. Both the CMA and RMA examinations cover the same first three areas.

Using this book should help you diagnose your strengths and weaknesses. This book is not meant to be a substitute for comprehensive medical assistant textbooks or for work experience. It is meant, as the title implies, to serve as a guide in the review process. A comprehensive review of any subject matter is a good way to locate your areas of strength as well as your areas of weakness. Areas of weakness may need to be corrected by referring to one or more of the current medical assisting books that are referenced in this edition (see page xxi). The comprehensive reference section of this edition should make it easier for you to locate any review materials needed. You will probably recognize several titles on this list that you used in your medical assistant program.

We are very grateful to the many individuals who provided assistance in the various areas of their expertise. We would like to give a special thanks to our contributors and reviewers. Their collective contributions have certainly strengthened the book. We would like to acknowledge the registered pharmacists, Gary Denton, PD, and Michael D. Smith, PD, for their contributions to the pharmacology section, and Lisa Marie Perks, AS, CMA, for her assistance in checking reference pages. We would also like to thank Mark Cohen and Barbara Krawiec, Acquisitions Editors; Robin Lazrus, Series Editor; and Melissa Kerian and Mary Ellen Ruitenberg, Editorial Assistants, for their help, support, and patience during the entire revision process.

We sincerely hope that this book helps many examination candidates in their certification endeavors. We would also appreciate comments from the users of this book.

Tom and Hilda Palko

Contributors

Melinda A. Wilkins, BS, MEd, RHIA
Director of Health Information
   Management Program
Arkansas Tech University
Russellville, Arkansas

Mark W. Palko, BFA, BS, MS
Formerly Assistant Director
Math Resource and Tutoring Center
University of Arkansas, Fayetteville
Fayetteville, Arkansas

Anitta L. Schwander, AS, CMA
Instructor, Medical Assistant
   Program
Arkansas Tech University
Russellville, Arkansas
and
Medical Records Department
St. Mary's Regional Medical Center
Russellville, Arkansas

Christina M. Merle, AS, BS, RHIA, CMA
Instructor, Health Information
   Management Program
Transcription Program Coordinator
Arkansas Tech University
Russellville, Arkansas

Reviewers

Barbara M. Dahl, CMA, CPC
Coordinator of Medical Assisting
 Program
Whatcom Community College
Bellingham, WA

Jean M. Dennerell, BS, CMA
Instructor and Coordinator of Medical
 Assisting Program
Jackson Community College
Jackson, MI

Sharon Paff, AS, RMA/AMT
Coordinator of Medical Assisting
 Program
Platt College
Rancho Cucamonga, CA

Introduction

NATIONAL MEDICAL ASSISTANT CERTIFICATION AGENCIES

The U.S. Department of Education recognizes two national certifying agencies for the medical assistant profession. These are the American Association of Medical Assistants (AAMA) and the Registry of Medical Assistants of the American Medical Technologists (RMA/AMT).

 ## CERTIFIED MEDICAL ASSISTANT EXAMINATION

The Certified Medical Assistant (CMA) examination is administered by the AAMA Certifying Board. The tests are given twice each year at locations throughout the United States, including testing centers in both Alaska and Hawaii. The CMA examinations are given each year on the last Friday in January and the last Saturday in June. The examination is based on the Medical Assistant Role Delineation Chart, which is located on the inside front cover of this book. A Candidate's Guide may be ordered, which includes information about the CMA examination, a bibliography of suggested study, and reference aids, as well as a 250-question sample examination with an answer key. This Candidate's Guide, a CMA Certification/Recertification Examination Application, or other general information about the test and who is eligible to sit for the exam may be obtained by writing: AAMA Certifying Board, 20 N. Wacker Drive, Suite 1575, Chicago, IL 60606-2903, or by calling 1-800-228-2262.

REGISTERED MEDICAL ASSISTANT EXAMINATION

The Registered Medical Assistant RMA/AMT examination is administered by the AMT. The tests are given three times each year at locations throughout the United States. The RMA examinations are administered on the second Saturday of March, June, and November. The examination is based on the Registered Medical Assistant Competency Areas Outline, which is developed by the RMA Education, Qualifications, and Standards Committee of the AMT. This RMA Competency Areas Outline is on the last page of this book. A Candidate Handbook for Registered Medical Assistant (RMA) Certification Examination and the Registered Medical Assistant Certification Examination Overview are available. These publications include general information about the examination as well as suggested study references and sample test questions. These publications as well as general information and an Application for Certification as an RMA/AMT can be obtained by writing: Registered Medical Assistants of American Medical Technologists, 710 Higgins Road, Park Ridge, IL 60068-5765, or by calling 1-800-275-1268.

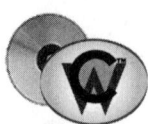 **COMPANION WEBSITE AND CD-ROM INFORMATION**

A CD-Rom is included in the back of this book that contains 900 questions. Of these 900 questions, 300 are unique to the CD while the remaining 600 are presented in the book. The 900 questions are divided into three tests. Each 300-question test is divided into three areas: General, Administrative, and Clinical with 100 questions in each area. The software was designed so that you can practice by categories or through simulated exams. Correct answers and comprehensive rationales follow all questions. You will receive immediate feedback to identify your strengths and weaknesses in each topic covered.

A "Basic Anatomy Review" is included with full-color art. This is an excellent resource for quick and easy review of basic anatomy and physiology as you prepare for this critical section of the exam.

An audio glossary, including 600 words and definitions (courtesy of Fremgen, *Essentials of Medical Assisting*), will help you review the definitions and practice pronunciations of the all-important terms you need to know.

You also have free access to the Online Companion Web Site at **www.prenhall.com/review**. For additional practice, information about the exam and links to related resources can be found when visiting this web site.

COMPANION STUDY GUIDE

Use this Question and Answer Review Book along with *Prentice Hall Health Outline Review for the Medical Assistant* by Marsha Hemby. With the easy-to-use outline format, you can quickly identify the important ideas, concepts, and facts you will need to know to prepare for the test. By combining quick content reviews with practice questions in print, on the CD, or on the web, you will increase your likelihood of success on the exam.

Study Skills and Test-Taking Strategies

Mark W. Palko

STRATEGIES FOR SUCCESS

For most people, standardized tests are among life's most stressful experiences: little better, if not worse, than a trip to the dentist's office. Unfortunately, these tests are almost unavoidable. Without satisfactory scores, you cannot graduate from high school, get into college, enter the military, or certify in most professions. Your test-taking skills can decide your future.

The stress curve (Figure 1) shows the effects of stress on test performance. The horizontal line (x-axis) represents the level of stress for a particular task, whereas the vertical line (y-axis) represents performance. The curve shows that when stress is too low or too high, the result is the same: low performance. Only when stress is balanced—not too high, not too low—can maximum performance be achieved.

FIGURE 1. Stress Curve

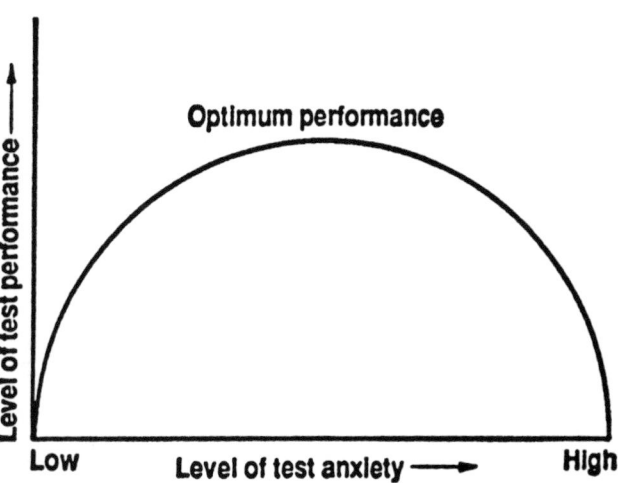

In simpler terms, this means that if you don't really care about a test, if it's not important to you, you won't do your best; but if you care too much—if it's too important to you—your results can be just as poor. Given the time and effort you've invested in this subject, it's obvious that you care enough. Your problem is keeping your anxiety level low enough so that it won't get in the way.

Knowing your subject is still the best way to reduce test anxiety. No amount of coaching can take the place of study. What test strategies can do is allow you to perform up to your potential to make a score that reflects the time you put in learning your subject. This book was designed to let you study for the CMA and RMA exams systematically and comprehensively. By reviewing the material in this book, you can establish the knowledge base you need for the exam and, by learning some test-taking fundamentals, you can get the most out of this knowledge when it counts.

 ## STUDY STRATEGIES

You've probably noticed that some people get more out of studying than others. These people spend the same amount of time studying but they learn more. These people have learned that how you study is just as important as how much you study. The following suggestions will get you studying on the right track.

I. Sample All Sections

This is probably the most important piece of information in this section. There are 13 chapters in this book, divided into three major subject area parts (General, Administrative, and Clinical). Do not spend an entire study session on one chapter, or even on one part. Every study session should include questions from all three subject areas.

II. Model Your Studying on the Test

If possible, try to cover 100 questions in each study session. You should probably do this by picking 10 chapters and doing 10 questions from each. When you skip over a chapter, as you go through your review the first time, make sure to hit it in the next session.

III. Keep Track of Your Work

Keep a record of which questions you have answered correctly and which ones you have missed in each of the three major sections of the book (General, Administrative, and Clinical). Make sure no question is skipped.

IV. Use a Dictionary

You cannot understand medical terms until you understand the other terms around them. Don't be afraid to look up unfamiliar words, particularly in questions you missed. You should have available a good English dictionary.

Prentice Hall Health Q&A Review for the Medical Assistant now has an audio glossary that allows you to hear as well as see many technical terms. Make sure to use this feature with terms you have trouble remembering.

TEST-TAKING STRATEGIES

I. Elimination

Good test performance is often determined, not by the ability to recognize the right answer, but by the ability to recognize the wrong ones. Eliminating wrong answers not only improves your score, it actually makes the test a more accurate measure of your knowledge. Guessing the right answer on a multiple-choice test can be compared to rolling a die (singular for dice). Eliminating the wrong answer (called a distracter) has the same effect as going to a die with one fewer sides. If you were to guess without eliminating any of the possible choices, you would have a one-in-four chance of getting the right answer. If you eliminated just one distracter, your odds would be 1 in 3. If you could eliminate two, your odds would be 1 in 2, a significant improvement. Of course, if you eliminate all of the distracters, you have a 100% probability of getting the right answer; but even eliminating just one or two distracters on each question should reduce the number of questions you miss by about one-third. That is the equivalent of going from a 64% to a 76%. Most multiple-choice tests are written to deliberately reward students who use elimination. Questions usually have one distracter that is obviously wrong, one distracter that is harder to eliminate, and one distracter that is very close to the correct answer. This gives a kind of partial credit based on your knowledge. If you know anything about the subject, you can eliminate the first distracter and improve your chances. If you know a little more, you can eliminate the second distracter and improve your chances even more. The more you know, the better you tend to do. Remember, the questions on the CMA and RMA examinations are of the best-answer type. This means that more than one answer may be considered correct, but only one answer is best.

Many books on test taking suggest complicated systems to eliminate bad answers and rank good ones, but to use elimination effectively, you need a procedure that is both quick and simple. The best way is probably to mark each choice as you read it with a large X if you think it is wrong, or a large check if you think it may be right. If you don't have an opinion, don't mark the question.

What you do next depends on how much time you have. Unless you are falling behind, you should go back and read the answers you have checked. Pick the one that seems best. If you did not put a check by any answer, pick the best choice from the unmarked answers. You DO NOT reread the answers you X'd out. Recognizing wrong answers is a skill. You can considerably improve your performance by following three simple rules:

- Always read all the responses before picking one.
- Always put an X through the worst response before trying to pick the best. (If you aren't certain of at least one wrong answer, then put an X through the one that sounds the worst.)
- Answer every question. (Remember, the CMA and RMA exams have no penalty for guessing.)

II. Time Management

Most students who take either examination will finish all the questions with time left over. For some, however, time will be a problem. Knowing when there is a problem and knowing what to do about it are the objectives of time management.

Keeping track of your progress is harder than it might first appear. Most of us have been surprised while taking a test by how little time was left. This experience is even more upsetting in the middle of a certifying examination. Even with your eye on the clock, calculating the time you have left is not always easy. On the CMA examination you have 4 hours to finish 300 questions. That gives you 48 seconds ($4/5$ minute) per question. In other words, you have to answer 75 questions per hour. On the RMA exam, you have 3 hours to complete 200 questions, which gives you 54 seconds per question. These numbers can be confusing under the best of circumstances (How long should it take to answer 12 questions?). You certainly do not want to deal with difficult calculations while taking a major examination, nor do you want to spend all of your time looking at the clock.

The sensible solution is to use round numbers and check your progress on a regular basis. Once an hour will usually be sufficient, but you may be more comfortable checking once every half hour. The choice is up to you.

On the CMA examination, try to do at least 40 questions every half hour or 80 every hour. On the RMA examination try to do at least 35 questions every half hour or 70 every hour.

There is one additional complication. Not all questions require equal time to work. It is quite possible to run across a string of difficult questions early in the test and fall behind, then make up the time with easy questions in the test. For this reason, being a few questions short of your goal after the first hour is not a cause for concern. However, if you have finished less than your goal at the halfway point, you are probably starting to fall behind and you need to start working faster.

If you do fall behind, what can you do to catch up? Often simply seeing that you are behind and trying to work faster will be enough to catch up. If that doesn't work, you have other options. Try to spend less time rereading the questions and answers (reading the question once is usually enough). If you have only checked one answer as likely to be right, put that choice down immediately: do not reconsider your answer.

Never skip (leave questions for later) if you are running seriously behind. Always mark your best choice before going on. (Skipping is covered in detail in Section III.)

The following is a rule of thumb even if you are not running behind. If an information question (one requiring you to recall a fact) has taken more than 1 or 2 minutes, make a mark beside it in the question book, put down your best answer or leave it for later, and go on. For a calculation problem (one requiring you to calculate some quantity) give yourself an extra minute or two. Very few of the questions on the RMA and CMA exams are calculation based.

A watch should always be in front of you, either on your wrist or on the table next to the test. Do not depend on the clock in the testing room. Looking up frequently will hurt your concentration.

III. Skipping

Though you should never leave a question blank when you hand in your test, there are situations where you might want to leave a question blank temporarily. In other words, you may want to skip it and come back when you have more time. Skipping can allow you to make the best possible use of your time during the test, or it can distract and slow you enough to cost you a good score.

Skipping around in the test can have two important advantages. First, skipping lets you decide in what order the questions will be asked, so that, should you run out of time, you'll only miss one or two 3-minute questions instead of five or ten 30-second questions. (Remember, an easy question counts just as much as a hard one.) This is particularly useful for questions involving any calculations. Second, skipping gives you a second chance at the question. Everyone has had the experience of trying to remember a name, then remembering the name after he or she stopped trying to remember. The same process sometimes works with test questions. A question that you stare at for a long time without progress might seem simple if you go on to other questions and come back 5 to 10 minutes later. There is also the possibility that another question will jog your memory. On professional tests, such as the medical assistant exams, this is fairly common.

There are also, however, strong arguments against skipping and going back. It takes time to go back and find the question you skipped. When you leave a question and come back to it, you have to start over and reread both the question and the responses. Add in the time spent deciding whether or not to skip the question, and you have spent a great deal of the time you were trying to save.

There are other problems. The secret of successful test taking is focusing the greatest possible amount of your attention and energy on answering the questions. Anything that distracts you hurts your test performance, and extensive skipping definitely distracts. It is hard to keep track of what questions remain to be answered, thus you run the risk of missing questions. It is nearly impossible to figure out how much time you have left per question. Skipping increases the chance of writing an answer in the wrong space on the answer sheet. This can lead to a string of numbers one line above their proper space. (Tips for avoiding this are included in The Check-on-Five Rule section.)

If you decide to answer certain questions out of order, the following rules may help you to decide whether or not to skip.

1. If one of the answers seems better than the rest, put it down and mark the question for future reference. Do not skip the question just because you are uncertain. You can always erase the answer if you change your mind.
2. If you can eliminate two of the possible answers, go ahead and guess, then mark the question for future reference. Do not skip.
3. Ask yourself, "Will more time really help me answer this question?" If your answer is "Probably not," go ahead and make your best guess, and mark the question for future reference. Do not skip.
4. Never skip a question during the last 30 minutes of the examination. Whenever you want to take a second look at a question (regardless of whether you left it blank), mark it clearly with a large slash or arrow next to the question and make a similar mark in the upper corner of the page of your test booklet. These marks have to be easy to see and quick to make. (Remember, you are doing this to save time.)

IV. The Check-on-Five Rule

Probably the most aggravating experience any test-taker has ever had was looking down at the answer sheet and realizing that the last 20 or 30 answers were all one line off. Because the question book and the answer sheet of a standardized test are separate, these mistakes are easy to make, particularly when you are leaving questions blank.

One way of preventing this problem is to pause before answering each question, read the number of the question, read the number on the answer sheet, and then write down your answer. With either 200 or 300 questions on the examination, checking each question could add 5 minutes to your time. More important, however, is the concentration lost. Failing to focus all of your attention on the test will usually result in a lower score.

You can avoid these problems by checking on every fifth question. In other words, check the number on the answer sheet whenever you get to a question number ending in 5 or 0. Do not check on the other four unless you have just skipped a question. Always check after skipping.

More than any other technique described in this book, the check-on-five rule should be pure, undiluted habit. Whether you are checking every fifth number or every single number, if you have to remind yourself to do it, you are diverting time and concentration from where it needs to go.

V. Practice

To master the skills of elimination and timing and be comfortable with the test, it is important that you practice as much as you can. When you answer the questions in the review book and the practice test, try to create conditions that closely resemble those of the actual exam. Find a quiet, well-lighted room, preferably with a long table. Bring a watch, set a reasonable time limit for yourself, and use materials similar to those you will use on the exam.

On every fifth question (those ending in 5 and 0), check to make sure you're putting the right answer in the right space. This will prevent time-consuming mistakes without breaking your concentration.

VI. About the Test

Both the CMA and the RMA exams are graded by a computerized device called an optiscanner. An optiscanner uses light sensors to determine which circles on the answer sheet have been filled in and which have been left blank. The computer marks a question incorrect if the wrong circle is filled in, if more than one circle is filled in, or if all the circles are left blank. To make sure that the scanner correctly reads your answer sheet, fill in the circles as completely as possible.

It should take about 2 to 3 seconds to correctly mark an answer. This should give you enough time to fill in the circle without going outside the line. If it takes you more than 5 seconds, you need to work faster.

Examples of Wrong and Right Ways to Mark Your Answer Sheet

WRONG   1   Ⓐ Ⓑ Ⓒ Ⓓ Ⓔ
circle not completely filled in

WRONG   2   Ⓐ ● Ⓒ ● Ⓔ
more than one circle filled in

WRONG   3   Ⓐ Ⓑ Ⓒ Ⓓ Ⓔ
no circle filled in

RIGHT   4   Ⓐ ● Ⓒ Ⓓ Ⓔ
circle completely filled in

SETTING UP A STUDY PLAN

In addition to studying this book, you'll probably want to review some textbooks on medical assisting. You can use books from classes you've taken, or you might want to obtain some of the books we have included in the References section. Either way, the following suggestions will help you get the most from your books.

You'll also want to go through the interactive tests and reference materials found on the CD-ROM that comes with this book. The repetition and instant feedback you'll get from this computerized practice will be a valuable part of your study plan, but remember: **The medical assistant test is still a paper and pencil test.**

In order to do your best, on your exam, most of your practice should be as similar as possible to the actual test. By going through this book in detail and using the CD-ROM as a supplement, you can work on the skills you will need the most.

You've often been told that you can't cram for a standardized test. This isn't entirely true. It is true that you can't condense years of study into a few weeks, but you can organize your review to learn and retain more. There are three plans of study presented here: the longest takes 6 months to 1 year; the shortest can take as little as a couple of weeks.

Plan One

Work through as many as possible of the texts and keep a reading journal. Use this book as a study guide. When you miss a question in this book, look up the appropriate reference in one of your texts.

The reading journal should be a small notebook that you can keep with the text at all times. Every time you read the text, briefly note the important points along with the page numbers where you found them. These notes should be as short as possible, sometimes as little as a single word, just enough to clearly indicate the part of the chapter you need to review. These notes should also be comprehensive, covering all the major points in your reading. Every other week, set aside some time to go through your journal and skim over those pages in the text. If you come across a cite you don't remember or understand, read it a second time. By the time you reach the end of the book, you will have mastered the entire contents.

Plan Two (Skim and Highlight)

If you don't have time for a comprehensive reading program, your best option is an organized review plan. In addition to completing this review book, take the best text you can find and divide it into segments short enough to skim over in a night's reading. While reading, go through the book with two distinct colors of highlighters. Reserve the brighter color for important terms and phrases. Save the other for important passages. Use your highlighter sparingly (mark 5% or less).

Plan Three (Twelve Facts)

If you find yourself with less than 2 weeks to prepare for the test, you can't possibly execute an adequate study or review plan, but you can give yourself a small head start in knowledge and confidence. First, study this review book as much as possible. Second, make a list of the 24 most important points from your studies, facts you know will be on the test. Read this list every night before you go to bed and at least once during the day. Two days before the test, narrow the list down to a dozen.

Of course, 12 facts won't make that much difference in your score, but they will help and, more important, they can prevent the sensation of going blank that often hits before the big test.

TAKING THE PRACTICE TESTS

One of the most important features in *Prentice Hall Health Q&A Review for the Medical Assistant* is the 300-question practice test with an answer key. This test will give you a chance to experience the exam before you actually have to take it, and it will also let you know how you're doing and where you need to do better. For best results we recommend you do the following: Take the practice test 2 to 3 weeks before you are scheduled to take the actual exam. Spend the next weeks targeting those areas in which you performed poorly.

You can also use this strategy with the CD-ROM. Keep track of the questions you miss and, after you've finished with the interactive test, find and review the sections that correspond to those trouble spots. Remember not to use interactive tests as a substitute for the paper and pencil version.

Make the experience of taking the practice test as close as possible to that of the actual exam. Take the tests at one sitting. Use the answer sheets labeled GENERAL QUESTIONS, ADMINISTRATIVE QUESTIONS, and CLINICAL QUESTIONS that can be found at the end of the PRACTICE TEST in this book. Mark your answer on these sheets. Fill in the circles on the answer sheets fully. Do not go over the time limit.

FINAL NOTES

Here are a few simple tips for the test day:

- Get a good night's sleep but don't overdo it. Too much sleep can be tiring.
- Eat a light meal before the test, enough to prevent hunger pangs during the test, but not enough to weigh you down. You might also want to take a small snack.
- Wear loose, comfortable clothes. It's a good idea to wear an extra layer that can be added or removed to adjust to an unusually warm or cold room.
- Make sure that you have your CMA (AAMA) or RMA (AMT) admission card and two forms of identification (one with a photo) when you arrive at the test site.
- Bring three no. 2 pencils, sharpened but not sharp enough to risk tearing the answer sheet. Double check the number on the pencils. The scanner that grades your test may not read no. $2^1/2$ lead pencils.
- Try to arrive a few minutes early. Never be late.

And a final reminder:

The CMA and RMA examinations are both pencil and paper tests. Therefore, it is important that you take some tests using a sample scantron sheet like the one included in the book.

References

Below is a list of reference sources pertaining to the material in the book. On the last line of each test item there appears an author's name(s) identifying the reference source and the page(s) where the information relating to the question and the correct answer may be found. For example, (*Fisher, p 80*) is a reference to the eighteenth book on the list, page 80.

Note: Some references are identified by numbers as well as authors. The reason for this is that two different textbooks were written by these same author(s). A # sign plus a number will appear each time these references are cited. Example: Bonewit-West #1, and Bonewit-West #2.

Abdelhak M. *Health Information: Management of a Strategic Resource.* Philadelphia: WB Saunders; 1996.

American Association of Medical Assistants (AAMA). *Health Care Law and Ethics.* Chicago: AAMA; 1996.

American Medical Association (AMA). *Current Procedural Terminology (CPT) 2000.* Chicago: AMA; 1999.

American Red Cross. *First Aid Responding to Emergencies.* 2nd ed. St. Louis: Mosby-Year Book; 1996.

Applegate A, Overton V. *The Elements of Medical Terminology.* Albany: Delmar Publishers; 1994.

Austrin M, Austrin H. *Learning Medical Terminology: A Worktext.* 9th ed. St. Louis: Mosby-Year Book; 1999.

Baptist C, Montgomery N, Stokes L, Vantrease MA. *Computers in the Medical Office.* Westerville, OH: Glencoe/McGraw-Hill; 1995.

Becklin K, Sunnarborg EM. *Medical Office Procedures.* 4th ed. Westerville, OH: Glencoe/McGraw-Hill; 1996.

Bonewit-West K. *Clinical Procedures for Medical Assistants.* 5th ed. Philadelphia: WB Saunders; 2000.

Bonewit-West K. *Computer Concepts and Applications for the Medical Office.* Philadelphia: WB Saunders; 1993.

Brooks ML, LaFleur DS. *Programmed Medical Language.* St. Louis: Mosby-Year Book; 1996.

Burdick Corporation. *Electrocardiography: A Better Way.* Milton, WI: Burdick Corporation; 1993.

Chabner D.-E. *The Language of Medicine.* 5th ed. Philadelphia: WB Saunders; 1996.

Dennerll JT. *Medical Terminology Made Easy.* 2nd ed. Albany: Delmar Publishers; 1998.

Dorland's Medical Dictionary. 28th ed. Philadelphia: WB Saunders; 1994.

Ehrlich A. *Medical Terminology for Health Professions.* 3rd ed. Albany: Delmar Publishers; 1997.

Estridge BH, Reynolds AP, Walters, NJ. *Basic Medical Laboratory Techniques.* 4th ed. Albany: Delmar Publishers; 2000.

Fisher JP. *Basic Medical Terminology.* 5th ed. Westerville, OH: Glencoe/McGraw-Hill; 1999.

Flight MR. *Law, Liability, and Ethics.* 3rd ed. Albany: Delmar Publishers; 1998.

Fordney MT. *Insurance Handbook for the Medical Office.* 6th ed. Philadelphia: WB Saunders; 1999.

Fordney MT, Follis JJ. *Administrative Medical Assisting.* 4th ed. Albany: Delmar Publishers; 1998.

Frew MA, Lane K, Frew DR. *Comprehensive Medical Assisting.* 3rd ed. Philadelphia: FA Davis; 1995.

Gauwitz DF, Bayt PM. *Administering Medications.* 4th ed. Westerville, OH: Glencoe/McGraw-Hill; 2000.

Gylys BA. *Computer Applications for the Medical Office.* 2nd ed. Philadelphia: FA Davis; 1997.

Gylys BA, Masters RM. *Medical Terminology Simplified: A Programmed Learning Approach by Body Systems.* 2nd ed. Philadelphia: FA Davis; 1998.

Hitner H, Nagle BT. *Basic Pharmacology.* 4th ed. Westerville, OH: Glencoe/McGraw-Hill; 1999.

Humphrey DD. *Contemporary Medical Office Procedures.* 2nd ed. Albany: Delmar Publishers; 1996.

Hurlbut PS. *PREP: Program Review and Exam Preparation—Medical Assistant.* Stamford, CN: Appleton & Lange; 1998.

Judson K, Hicks S. *Law and Ethics for Medical Careers.* 2nd ed. Westerville, OH: Glencoe/McGraw-Hill; 1999.

Keir L, Wise BA, Krebs SC. *Medical Assisting: Administrative and Clinical Competencies.* 4th ed. Albany: Delmar Publishers; 1998.

Kinn ME, Woods MA. *The Medical Assistant, Administrative and Clinical.* 8th ed. Philadelphia: WB Saunders; 1999.

Kizior RJ, Hodgson BB. *Saunders Drug Handbook for Health Professions 2000.* Philadelphia: WB Saunders; 2000.

Leonard PC. *Building a Medical Vocabulary.* 4th ed. Philadelphia: WB Saunders; 1997.

Lewis MA, Tamparo CD. *Medical Law, Ethics, and Bioethics for Ambulatory Care.* 4th ed. Philadelphia: FA Davis; 1998.

Memmler RL, Cohen DL, Wood D. *The Human Body in Health and Disease.* 8th ed. Philadelphia: JB Lippincott; 1996.

Miller BF, Keane CB. *Encyclopedia and Dictionary of Medicine, Nursing, and Allied Health.* 6th ed. Philadelphia: WB Saunders; 1997.

Milliken ME. *Understanding Human Behavior.* 6th ed. Albany: Delmar Publishers; 1998.

Newby C. *From Patient to Payment.* 2nd ed. Westerville, OH: Glencoe/McGraw-Hill; 1998.

Palko T, Palko H. *Medical Laboratory Procedures.* Westerville, OH: Glencoe/McGraw-Hill; 1999.

Physician's Desk Reference (PDR). 54th ed. Montvale, NJ: Medical Economics Co.; 2000.

Pickar GD. *Dosage Calculations.* 6th ed. Albany: Delmar Publishers; 1999.

Rice J. *Medical Terminology with Human Anatomy.* 4th ed. Norwalk, CT: Appleton & Lange; 1999.

Rice J. *Principles of Pharmacology for Medical Assisting.* Albany: 3rd ed. Delmar Publishers; 1999.

Robert HM. *The Scott, Foresman Robert's Rules of Order, Newly Revised.* Glenview, IL: Scott, Foresman; 1990.

Rowell JC. *Understanding Health Insurance: A Guide to Professional Billing.* 5th ed. Albany: Delmar Publishers; 2000.

Sanderson SM. *Computers in the Medical Office.* Westerville, OH: Glencoe/McGraw-Hill; 1999.

Scanlon VC, Sanders T. *Essentials of Anatomy and Physiology.* 3rd ed. Philadelphia: FA Davis; 1999.

Smith GL, Davis PE, Dennerll JT. *Medical Terminology: A Programmed Systems Approach.* 8th ed. Albany: Delmar Publishers; 1999.

Taber's Cyclopedic Medical Dictionary. 18th ed. Philadelphia: FA Davis; 1997.

Tamparo CD, Lewis MA. *Diseases of the Human Body.* 3rd ed. Philadelphia: FA Davis; 2000.

Tamparo CD, Lindh WQ. *Therapeutic Communications for Health Professions.* 2nd ed. Albany: Delmar Publishers; 2000.

Thibodeau GA., Patton KT. *Structure and Function of the Body.* 10th ed. St. Louis: Mosby-Year Book; 1997.

Thibodeau GA, Patton KT. *The Human Body in Health and Disease.* 2nd ed. St. Louis: Mosby-Year Book; 1997.

Tuttle-Yoder JA, Fraser-Nobbe SA. *STAT! Medical Office Emergency Manual.* Albany: Delmar Publishers; 1996.

United States Postal Services Consumer Guide to Extra Services. 1999.

United States Postal Service Rate Fold, Notice 123, January 10, 1999.

Wedding ME, Toenjes SA. *Medical Laboratory Procedures.* 2nd ed. Philadelphia: FA Davis Co.; 1998.

Willis MC. *Medical Terminology: The Language of Health Care.* Philadelphia: Williams & Wilkins; 1996.

Zakus SM. *Clinical Procedures for Medical Assistants.* 3rd ed. St. Louis: Mosby-Year Book; 1995.

General Information

CHAPTER

1 Medical Terminology and Basic Anatomy and Physiology

chapter objectives

Major areas of knowledge/content included in this chapter are:

I. Medical terminology

➤ basic structure including prefixes, suffixes, plurals, abbreviations, and symbols

➤ terms relating to physical descriptions, conditions, diseases, and surgical, diagnostic, and treatment procedures

➤ medical specialties and references

II. Anatomy and physiology

➤ body as a whole—vocabulary that describes anatomical planes, directions, divisions, and structures of the body

➤ body systems and their related conditions and diseases

➤ study hints

DIRECTIONS (Questions 1 through 364): Each of the numbered items or incomplete statements in this section is followed by answers or by completions of the statement. Select the ONE lettered answer or completion that is BEST in each case.

1. The word root pod- means
   A. ankle
   B. toes
   C. foot
   D. running
   E. children

   (Smith et al, p 412; Austrin and Austrin, p 24)

2. The suffix -phagia means
   A. false
   B. attracting
   C. eating
   D. drinking
   E. equaling

   (Brooks and LaFleur, p 221; Taber's, p 1459)

3. Onycho- is a combining form that means
   A. eardrum
   B. nail
   C. knuckle
   D. hair follicle
   E. formation of a tumor

   (Chabner, p 566; Fisher, p 55)

4. Coreo- is a combining form that means
   A. pupil
   B. cornea
   C. iris
   D. retina
   E. ciliary body

   (Brooks and LaFleur, p 178)

5. A combining form that means "umbilicus" or "navel" is
   A. kerato-
   B. omphalo-
   C. onycho-
   D. onco-
   E. oxy-

   (Austrin and Austrin, p 24; Taber's, p 1342)

6. Ex- is a prefix that means
   A. more than
   B. outside
   C. inside
   D. less than
   E. upon

   (Chabner, p 103)

7. "Antefebrile" means
   A. after fever
   B. during fever
   C. lack of fever
   D. against fever
   E. before fever

   (Smith et al, p 385; Taber's, p 116)

8. A word that means "suture of the region over the stomach" is
   A. epigastrorrhaphy
   B. episiorrhaphy
   C. colporrhaphy
   D. herniorrhaphy
   E. omentorrhaphy

   (Smith et al, p 350; Taber's, p 656)

9. An "antipyretic" is an agent that works against
   A. fever
   B. rash
   C. toothaches
   D. poison
   E. acne

   (Taber's, p 124)

10. A lateral curvature of the spine is a deformity called
    A. lordosis
    B. hemiplegia
    C. scoliosis
    D. kyphosis
    E. humpback
    (Miller and Keane, p 1457; Willis, p 134)

11. The side of the body containing the backbone is
    A. ventral
    B. posterior
    C. caudal
    D. anterior
    E. superior
    (Dennerll, p 34; Taber's, p 1531)

12. The cavity containing the heart and lungs is the
    A. abdominopelvic cavity
    B. dorsal cavity
    C. buccal cavity
    D. thoracic cavity
    E. transverse cavity
    (Smith et al, p 109; Miller-Keane, p 289)

13. A condition of the body that is abnormal and presents a group of clinical signs and laboratory findings is known as a/an
    A. inflammation
    B. illness
    C. disease
    D. immune disorder
    E. infection
    (Miller-Keane, p 465; Taber's, p 552)

14. A nerve that carries an impulse toward the brain is a/an
    A. efferent nerve
    B. afferent nerve
    C. synapse

D. neurotransmitter
E. receptor
(Applegate and Overton, p 160; Miller-Keane, p 1078)

15. Levels of organization of the body range from atomic to organismic. Which is the basic structural unit of the body?
    A. tissue
    B. organ system
    C. cell
    D. molecular
    E. electrolyte
    (Miller and Keane, p 290)

16. A word used to indicate the splitting open of a wound is
    A. dehiscence
    B. avulsion
    C. evisceration
    D. debridement
    E. homeostasis
    (Taber's, p 500)

17. The scar left by a healed wound is a
    A. cicatrix
    B. debridement
    C. collagen
    D. dehiscence
    E. fibroblast
    (Taber's, p 386)

18. A bluish discoloration of the skin is
    A. acrocyanosis
    B. acrodermatitis
    C. cyanoderma
    D. dermatosis
    E. leukoderma
    (Dennerll, p 45; Taber's, p 474)

19. Enlargement of the heart is
    A. cardialgia
    B. carditis
    C. tachycardia
    D. megalocardia
    E. bradycardia
    (Miller and Keane, p 977; Smith, p 36)

20. Low blood pressure is known as
    A. hypertension
    B. cyanosis
    C. bradycardia
    D. hypotension
    E. diastolic pressure
    (Leonard, p 124; Smith, p 62)

21. A herniation or projection of brain tissue from its natural cavity is
    A. encapsulation
    B. encephalasthenia
    C. an encephalocele
    D. an encephaloma
    E. encephalomalacia
    (Miller and Keane, p 525; Gylys and Masters, p 345)

22. A combining word meaning softening is
    A. arthro-
    B. chondro-
    C. dento-
    D. malac/o
    E. sclero-
    (Brooks and LaFleur, p 171; Smith et al, p 74)

23. A combining form meaning joint is
    A. arthro-
    B. chondro-
    C. malaco-
    D. costo-
    E. adeno-
    (Brooks and LaFleur, p 193; Dennerll, p 146; Gylys and Masters, p 333)

24. A combining form meaning development is
    A. -stomy
    B. -trophy
    C. -stasis
    D. -tomy
    E. -ptosis
    (Brooks and LaFleur, p 193; Dennerll, p 84)

25. A suffix meaning repair is
    A. myelo-
    B. -dactyly
    C. -dromy
    D. -plasty
    E. -plasia
    (Brooks and LaFleur, p 85; Smith et al, p 95)

26. A word that means "incision into the skull" is
    A. craniectomy
    B. cranioplasty
    C. craniotomy
    D. craniomalacia
    E. craniopathy
    (Brooks and LaFleur, p 86; Smith, p 75)

27. Swirling water baths are a form of
    A. thermotherapy
    B. hydrotherapy
    C. serotherapy
    D. hydrosudotherapy
    E. shock therapy
    (Leonard, p 406; Taber's, p 927)

28. The sticking together of tissues that are normally separated is referred to as
    A. aberrant
    B. addiction
    C. adduction
    D. adhesion
    E. abduction
    (Leonard, p 156; Miller-Keane, p 31)

29. A discharge from the nose is
    A. pyorrhea
    B. otorrhea
    C. otitis media
    D. hidrorrhea
    E. rhinorrhea

    (Smith et al, p 182; Willis, p 232)

30. Excision of the gallbladder is called a
    A. cholecystotomy
    B. cholecystectomy
    C. lithotomy
    D. lithotripsy
    E. cystostomy

    (Gylys and Masters, p 62; Taber's, p 372)

31. Inflammation of the middle ear is
    A. adenitis
    B. otitis media
    C. otalgia
    D. rhinitis
    E. cystitis

    (Chabner, p 616; Miller and Keane, p 1166)

32. A word that means "surgical tapping of the chest to remove fluids" is
    A. thoracectomy
    B. thoracodynia
    C. thoracocentesis
    D. thoracolysis
    E. thoracomyodynia

    (Chabner, p 71)

33. A disease of the periodontal area symptomized by the flow of pus is
    A. rhinorrhea
    B. otorrhea
    C. pyorrhea
    D. hidrorrhea
    E. pyrosis

    (Smith et al, p 128)

34. Pus-forming bacteria are also described as
    A. hematogenic
    B. oncogenic
    C. pyrogenic
    D. ankylogenic
    E. pyogenic

    (Smith et al, p 128)

35. A darkly pigmented malignant mole of the skin is a
    A. myofibroma
    B. hemangioma
    C. neurofibroma
    D. melanoma
    E. xanthoma

    (Leonard, p 88; Rice, p 71)

36. A collection of air in the chest cavity is
    A. pneumothorax
    B. pneumoderma
    C. thoracocentesis
    D. thoracotomy
    E. pneumonia

    (Fisher, p 126)

37. A hemorrhage of the bladder is
    A. ureterorrhaphy
    B. uretororrhagia
    C. cystorrhexis
    D. cystorrhagia
    E. cholerrhagia

    (Rice, p 333)

38. A word that means "suturing of the eyelids" is
    A. blepharorrhaphy
    B. ureterorrhaphy
    C. cystorrhaphy
    D. neurorrhaphy
    E. ophthalmoplasty

    (Fisher, p 158; Austrin and Austrin, p 328)

39. Making a new opening between the ureter and bladder is
    A. ureteroenterostomy
    B. ureteropyeloplasty
    C. ureteropyeloneostomy
    D. ureterocystoneostomy
    E. ureterocystostomy
    (Austrin and Austrin, p 223)

40. Enlargement of the kidney is
    A. nephrolysis
    B. nephropexy
    C. nephroptosis
    D. nephromegaly
    E. nephrolithiasis
    (Brooks and LaFleur, p 119; Gylys and Masters, p 88)

41. The part of the urinary tract that collects urine in the kidney is the
    A. ureter
    B. bladder
    C. urethra
    D. jejunum
    E. renal pelvis
    (Taber's, p 1431)

42. The term used to describe a prolapse of the uterus is
    A. ooblast
    B. hysteroptosis
    C. blepharoptosis
    D. oophoropexy
    E. nephroptosis
    (Taber's, p 956)

43. Destruction or breakdown of fat is called
    A. lipolysis
    B. hemolysis
    C. neurolysis
    D. myolysis
    E. angiolysis
    (Taber's, p 1118)

44. A word that means "inflammation of many joints" is
    A. polydactylism
    B. polyneuralgia
    C. polyarthritis
    D. polychondritis
    E. polyserositis
    (Taber's, p 1517)

45. A word that means "working together" is
    A. synergetic
    B. syndrome
    C. synarthrosis
    D. prodrome
    E. contusion
    (Chabner, pp 752, 759)

46. Macrodactylia means
    A. too many fingers or toes
    B. very large fingers or toes
    C. very small fingers or toes
    D. loss of large fingers or toes
    E. size and dexterity of fingers and toes
    (Taber's, p 1147)

47. Diathermy means
    A. oversensitivity to heat
    B. instrument for measuring heat
    C. pertaining to heat
    D. generating heat through tissues
    E. the science of heat production
    (Taber's, p 537)

48. A myelocele is a
    A. muscular tumor
    B. tumor of the kidney
    C. herniation of a nerve
    D. herniation of a muscle
    E. herniation of the spinal cord
    (Willis, p 276)

49. Surgical crushing of a nerve is
    A. neurolysis
    B. neuroplasty
    C. neuritis
    D. neurotrophy
    E. neurotripsy
    (Austrin and Austrin, p 300; Leonard, p 353)

50. Symptoms indicating an approaching disease are its
    A. prognosis
    B. diagnosis
    C. syndrome
    D. prodrome
    E. antefebrile
    (Chabner, p 105; Taber's, p 1567)

51. Macroglossia means
    A. large tongue
    B. large nose
    C. large ears
    D. small lips
    E. small tongue
    (Taber's, p 1148; Miller-Keane, p 951)

52. Inflammation of the gums is
    A. gingivoglossitis
    B. colitis
    C. myelitis
    D. gingivitis
    E. cheilitis
    (Chabner, p 140)

53. The condition in which an individual experiences an involuntary and unpredictable flow of urine is
    A. constipation
    B. incontinence
    C. dysuria
    D. urethral pressure
    E. anuria
    (Miller and Keane, p 818)

54. Tachy- is a prefix meaning
    A. slow
    B. fast
    C. rough
    D. soft
    E. smooth
    (Chabner, p 106)

55. A prefix meaning "slow" is
    A. brady-
    B. dys-
    C. sym-
    D. ad-
    E. ab-
    (Chabner, p 102)

56. Stomato- is a combining form meaning
    A. stomach
    B. small intestine
    C. large intestine
    D. mouth
    E. esophagus
    (Austrin and Austrin, p 24; Gylys and Masters, p 25)

57. Phas/o- is a combining form meaning
    A. paralysis
    B. irrigation
    C. development
    D. speech
    E. hearing
    (Austrin and Austrin, p 36)

58. As a suffix, -clysis means
    A. destruction
    B. irrigation
    C. paralysis
    D. rupture
    E. heat
    (Ehrlich, p 390)

59. Hepat/o- is a combining form meaning
    A. esophagus
    B. gallbladder
    C. liver
    D. jejunum
    E. colon
    (Brooks and LaFleur, p 150; Gylys and Masters, p 55)

60. A suffix meaning "crushing" is
    A. -orrhexis
    B. -tripsy
    C. -pexy
    D. -blast
    E. -ptosis
    (Rice, p 8)

61. Diplo- is a combining form that means
    A. tactful
    B. speech
    C. divided into quarters
    D. double
    E. through
    (Austrin and Austrin, p 38)

62. A combining form that means "lip" is
    A. entero-
    B. plaso-
    C. glosso-
    D. costo-
    E. cheilo-
    (Chabner, p 139)

63. Kinesio- is a combining form that means
    A. energy
    B. movement
    C. formation
    D. digestion
    E. seizure
    (Dennerll, p 170)

64. Litho- is a combining form that means
    A. destruction
    B. smooth
    C. rough
    D. irrigation
    E. stone
    (Chabner, p 142; Dennerll, p 316)

65. A combining form that means "pus" is
    A. py/o-
    B. pyel/o-
    C. pub/o-
    D. phil/o-
    E. pyr/o-
    (Brooks, p 90; Chabner, p 200)

66. Centesis is a word element meaning
    A. hundred
    B. middle
    C. calculus
    D. puncture
    E. toward a center
    (Smith et al, p 107)

67. Ot/o- is a combining form that means
    A. ear
    B. eye
    C. nose
    D. self
    E. discharge
    (Chabner, p 614; Gylys and Masters, p 433)

68. A prefix meaning "toward" is
    A. ab-
    B. ad-
    C. en-
    D. an-
    E. pro-
    (Chabner, p 101)

69. Dactylo- is a combining form that means
    A. spinal cord or bone marrow
    B. arms or legs
    C. fingers or toes
    D. skull or brain
    E. shoulders or neck
    (Willis, p 493)

70. The color blue may be expressed by the combining form
    A. melan/o-
    B. cyan/o-
    C. leuk/o-
    D. xanth/o-
    E. erythr/o-
    (Brooks and LaFleur, p 19; Chabner, p 359; Rice, p 230)

71. Men/o- is a combining form that means
    A. menses
    B. middle
    C. chin
    D. bone marrow
    E. measure
    (Gylys and Masters, p 195)

72. Xanth/o- is used in medical terms to represent the color
    A. red
    B. green
    C. brown
    D. black
    E. yellow
    (Brooks and Brooks, p 21)

73. Hidro- is a combining form that means
    A. water
    B. sweat
    C. blood
    D. vomitus
    E. bile
    (Willis, p 494)

74. The word that best describes the putting together of simpler compounds derived from nutrients into living organized materials usable by the body cells is
    A. calorie
    B. appetite
    C. metabolism
    D. anabolism
    E. catabolism
    (Frew et al, pp 512–513; Miller and Keane, p 76)

75. As a suffix, -emia refers to a condition of
    A. blood
    B. urine
    C. deficiency
    D. surplus
    E. discharge
    (Austrin and Austrin, p 15)

76. As a suffix, -stasis means
    A. without change
    B. dilatation
    C. paralysis
    D. twitching
    E. stoppage
    (Chabner, p 74; Smith et al, p 273)

77. Colp/o- is a combining form that means
    A. colon
    B. triple
    C. lip
    D. bile or gall
    E. vagina
    (Chabner, p 239)

78. Necr/o- is a combining form that refers to
    A. sleep
    B. drugs
    C. death
    D. pharynx
    E. kidney
    (Rice, p 12)

79. "Ectopic" is a term used to mean

A. pregnancy

B. tubal

C. misplaced

D. equal

E. dilatation

(Miller and Keane, p 501)

80. Home/o- is used in medical terms to mean

A. male

B. female

C. same

D. different

E. attraction

(Chabner, p 654)

81. Crypt/o- is a combining form that means

A. below

B. hidden

C. death

D. sleep

E. hernia

(Dennerll, p 182; Austrin and Austrin, p 38)

82. An oncologist is concerned with

A. eyes

B. bones and muscles

C. mental disorders

D. tumors

E. nature and causes of diseases

(Dennerll, p 93)

83. A word that means "prolapse of organs" is

A. blepharoptosis

B. oophoropexy

C. hysteropexy

D. visceroptosis

E. hysteroptosis

(Taber's, p 2090)

84. A medical term that means "blushing" is

A. cyanoderma

B. erythroderma

C. melanoderma

D. xanthoderma

E. leukoderma

(Gylys and Masters, p 153; Dennerll, p 45)

85. A word meaning "fever" is

A. pyrexia

B. pyrosis

C. pyrolysis

D. thermolysis

E. thermostasis

(Chabner, p 523; Taber's, p 1612)

86. A combining form that means "abdominal wall" is

A. latero-

B. viscero-

C. caudo-

D. ventro-

E. laparo-

(Smith et al, p 290)

87. An abnormal lack of appetite results in

A. amenorrhea

B. anhidrosis

C. metrorrhea

D. dysmenorrhea

E. anorexia

(Chabner, p 143; Taber's, p 113)

88. "Suprarenal" means

A. on the kidney

B. above the kidney

C. on the bladder

D. above the bladder

E. beyond the kidney

(Leonard, p 338)

89. The word "malaise" means
   A. discomfort and uneasiness
   B. heterosexual
   C. maladjusted
   D. malacia
   E. malabsorption
   (Taber's, p 1153)

90. A word that means "moving away from a midline" is
   A. abduction
   B. adduction
   C. circumduction
   D. kinetogenic
   E. transudate
   (Chabner, p 528; Taber's, p 5)

91. A word that means "self-destructing" is
   A. autodiagnosis
   B. autonomic
   C. autolysis
   D. otocleisis
   E. ototoxic
   (Taber's, p 179)

92. A word that means "turning forward" is
   A. antiversion
   B. retroversion
   C. anteversion
   D. anteromedian
   E. circumduction
   (Chabner, p 243; Taber's, p 116)

93. "Retrosternal" means
   A. under the sternum
   B. behind the sternum
   C. above the sternum
   D. beside the sternum
   E. in front of the sternum
   (Taber's, p 1676)

94. A word that means "inflammation of tissues near the vagina" is
   A. paracystitis
   B. paracolpitis
   C. perinephritis
   D. paranephritis
   E. vaginoscopy
   (Taber's, p 1403)

95. Low blood sugar is
   A. hyperglycemia
   B. hypoglycemia
   C. subluxation
   D. infrasonic
   E. hypocythemia
   (Chabner, p 660; Gylys and Masters, p 298)

96. The prefix con- means
   A. against
   B. with
   C. difficult
   D. painful
   E. false
   (Dennerll, p 299)

97. The prefix dis- means
   A. difficult or painful
   B. free of
   C. open
   D. against
   E. with
   (Dennerll, p 299)

98. The prefix epi- means
   A. upon
   B. through
   C. beside
   D. across
   E. against
   (Chabner, p 103)

99. Ankylo- is a combining form that means
    A. rough
    B. smooth
    C. stiff
    D. painful
    E. nervous
    (Austrin and Austrin, p 38)

100. Carpo- is a combining form referring to the bones of the
    A. knuckle
    B. wrist
    C. ankle
    D. pelvis
    E. skull
    (Dennerll, p 164)

101. Specific terms describe directional aspects of the body. Regardless of the patient's current position, these terms always describe the body in what position?
    A. anatomic position
    B. supine position
    C. lithotomy position
    D. dorsal position
    E. dorsosacral position
    (Austrin and Austrin, p 60; Memmler et al, p 5)

102. Dorsal is similar in meaning to
    A. posterior
    B. cranial
    C. anterior
    D. ventral
    E. sagittal
    (Memmler et al, p 5; Willis, p 125)

103. The body is divided into front and back by which of the following planes?
    A. transverse
    B. frontal
    C. sagittal
    D. midsagittal
    E. horizontal
    (Memmler et al, pp 6–7; Willis, p 125)

104. Those parts farthest from the midsagittal plane are
    A. anterior
    B. ventral
    C. dorsal
    D. lateral
    E. internal
    (Ehrlich, p 24; Memmler et al, p 5)

105. The opposite of cephalic is
    A. ventral
    B. dorsal
    C. caudal
    D. superior
    E. cranial
    (Memmler et al, p 5)

106. The opposite of ventral is
    A. anterior
    B. dorsal
    C. transverse
    D. cranial
    E. superior
    (Leonard, p 47; Memmler et al, p 5; Willis, p 125)

107. Caudal is synonymous with the term
    A. coronal
    B. inferior
    C. superior
    D. abdominal
    E. posterior
    (Memmler et al, p 5; Ehrlich, p 24)

108. A word meaning "near the surface" is
    A. intermediate
    B. superficial
    C. peripheral
    D. distal
    E. parietal
    (Taber's, p 1864; Chabner, p 47)

109. The body is divided into right and left sides by which of the following planes?
    A. sagittal
    B. coronal
    C. frontal
    D. transverse
    E. horizontal
    (Memmler et al, pp 6–7; Leonard, p 43)

110. A word meaning "between two other structures" is
    A. parietal
    B. proximal
    C. distal
    D. intermediate
    E. medial
    (Miller and Keane, p 843)

111. "Retinoid" means
    A. pertaining to the retina
    B. inflammation of the retina
    C. resembling the retina
    D. herniation of the retina
    E. softening of the retina
    (Miller and Keane, p 1409)

112. Surgical puncturing of the pleura is
    A. pleurocentesis
    B. pleurovisceral
    C. pleuroclysis
    D. pleurectomy
    E. pleuroscopy
    (Fisher, p 122; Leonard, p 157)

113. A bronchial hemorrhage is
    A. bronchorrhea
    B. bronchorrhagia
    C. bronchospasm
    D. bronchoplegia
    E. broncholithiasis
    (Gylys and Masters, p 247; Miller and Keane, p 240)

114. The word ending -al means
    A. pain
    B. pertaining to
    C. condition
    D. inflammation
    E. process of study
    (Gylys and Masters, p 7)

115. Pain in the trachea is
    A. trachealgia
    B. tracheitis
    C. trachelagra
    D. trachelopexy
    E. tracheomalacia
    (Dennerll, p 241; Taber's, p 1977)

116. "Thrombectomy" means
    A. incision into a clot
    B. excision of a clot
    C. incision into a vein
    D. excision of a vein
    E. excision of an artery
    (Gylys and Masters, p 399; Miller and Keane, p 1609)

117. The abbreviations of Hib, OPV, DPT, and Hep B-1 are types of
    A. vitamins
    B. vaccines
    C. antibiotics
    D. clinical laboratory instrument settings
    E. surgery terms
    (Kinn and Woods, pp 653–655)

118. Neo- means
    A. cancer
    B. night
    C. light
    D. vessel
    E. new
    (Fisher, p 245)

119. A vasorrhaphy is a suture of the
    A. urethra
    B. testes
    C. vas deferens
    D. ureters
    E. scrotum
    (Miller and Keane, p 1705)

120. A common word for "sternum" is
    A. pelvic girdle
    B. breastbone
    C. rib cage
    D. hip bone
    E. cooking gas
    (Chabner, p 507)

121. The acromion is located nearest to the
    A. head
    B. shoulder
    C. chest
    D. hips
    E. legs
    (Chabner, p 509)

122. Cycl/o- is a combining form for
    A. pupil
    B. cornea
    C. ciliary body
    D. iris
    E. tear duct
    (Taber's, p 475)

123. Plastic surgery of the pupil is
    A. keratoplasty
    B. otoplasty
    C. tympanoplasty
    D. ophthalmoplasty
    E. coreoplasty
    (Miller and Keane, p 380; Austrin and Austrin, p 328)

124. "Lacrimal" is a medical term that means pertaining to
    A. duct
    B. lymph
    C. tears
    D. nasal exudate
    E. ophthalmolith
    (Taber's, p 1067)

125. Inflammation of the cornea is
    A. iritis
    B. lymph
    C. retinitis
    D. corneitis
    E. scleroiritis
    (Taber's, p 444)

126. The hard outer covering of the eye is the
    A. iris
    B. pupil
    C. cornea
    D. sclera
    E. retina
    (Chabner, p 592)

127. The cornea is
    A. opaque
    B. transparent
    C. partly opaque and partly transparent
    D. opaque in darkness and transparent in light
    E. responsible for color vision
    (Taber's, p 443)

128. Rupture of the navel is
    A. omphalorrhexis
    B. omphaloplasty
    C. omphalocele
    D. onychomalacia
    E. onychomycosis
    (Leonard, p 247; Miller and Keane, p 1144)

129. Abnormally profuse menstruation is
    A. metrorrhagia
    B. menorrhagia
    C. menorrhea
    D. metrorrhea
    E. menorrhalgia
    (Miller and Keane, p 987; Ehrlich, p 327)

130. Rubeola is
    A. chickenpox
    B. measles
    C. whooping cough
    D. scarlet fever
    E. herpes simplex
    (Chabner, p 571)

131. "Suppuration" means
    A. formation of pus
    B. lack of adhesion
    C. abnormal dryness
    D. formation of urine
    E. formation of blood
    (Miller and Keane, p 1558)

132. A bruise is a/an
    A. alveolus
    B. alvius
    C. contusion
    D. clonic
    E. concussion
    (Taber's, p 439)

133. Spina bifida, cleft lip, talipes, and unde-scended testicle are all examples of
    A. musculoskeletal diseases
    B. subcutaneous hemorrhage
    C. complications of viral disease
    D. nervous system disorders
    E. congenital anomalies
    (Taber's, pp 397, 1803, 1902, 1927)

134. The ileum is the
    A. flank bone
    B. proximal portion of small intestine
    C. distal portion of small intestine
    D. large intestine
    E. hip bone
    (Rice, p 181)

135. Varicella is commonly called
    A. measles
    B. whooping cough
    C. chickenpox
    D. smallpox
    E. scarlet fever
    (Chabner, p 571)

136. Herpetic gingivostomatitis is a medical term for a condition commonly called
    A. bruise
    B. hives
    C. flat feet
    D. athlete's foot
    E. cold sore
    (Chabner, p 144)

137. Strabismus is a condition commonly referred to as
    A. farsightedness
    B. nearsightedness
    C. astigmatism
    D. squint (crossed eyes)
    E. blurred vision
    (Taber's, p 1841)

138. The medical term for "German measles" is
    A. rubella
    B. thromboangiitis obliterans
    C. singultus
    D. pediculosis
    E. ankyloglossia
    (Taber's, p 1697)

139. The lay term for "urticaria" is
    A. boil
    B. butterfly rash
    C. lice
    D. piles
    E. hives
    (Chabner, p 569; Taber's, p 2044)

140. The lay term for "epidemic parotitis" is
    A. trench mouth
    B. ringworm
    C. chickenpox
    D. mumps
    E. shingles
    (Miller and Keane, p 1026)

141. The medical term for "pinkeye" is
    A. conjunctivitis
    B. torticollis
    C. dementia praecox
    D. morbilli
    E. icterus
    (Taber's, pp 432, 1479)

142. "Pertussis" is the medical term for
    A. bed sore
    B. hay fever
    C. jaundice
    D. sleeping sickness
    E. whooping cough
    (Chabner, p 406)

143. A suffix that means "without opening" is
    A. -agra
    B. -atresia
    C. -facient
    D. -physis
    E. -pnea
    (Dennerll, p 58)

144. As a suffix, -algia means the same as
    A. -agra
    B. -desis

C. -dynia
    D. -pexy
    E. -plegia
    (Chabner, p 70)

145. A suffix meaning "disease" is
    A. -pathy
    B. -alis
    C. -esis
    D. -ode
    E. -some
    (Chabner, p 73; Dennerll, p 30)

146. The combining form -phren/o may refer to either the diaphragm or the
    A. pharynx
    B. larynx
    C. esophagus
    D. hearing
    E. mind
    (Austrin and Austrin, p 27)

147. As a suffix, -tome means
    A. injection
    B. cutting instrument
    C. to observe
    D. record
    E. shape
    (Austrin and Austrin, p 17)

148. A suffix that refers to the body is
    A. -ate
    B. -cytosis
    C. -pellent
    D. -pexy
    E. -some
    (Rice, p 522)

149. A suffix meaning "to turn or to change" is
    A. -cleisis
    B. -facient
    C. -ferent

D. -ious

E. -tropia

(Taber's, p 2005)

150. A suffix that means "to burst forth" is

A. -cele

B. -cleisis

C. -rrhage

D. -rrhea

E. -tocia

(Taber's, p 1697)

151. The finest gauge of suture material is referred to as

A. 0

B. 00

C. 11-0

D. 5

E. 1

(Kinn and Woods, p 1082)

152. A type of suture in which the surgeon ties each stitch separately is called

A. purse-string

B. interrupted

C. uninterrupted

D. blanket

E. mattress

(Miller and Keane, p 1562; Kinn and Woods, pp 1120–1122)

153. Movement that flexes the foot toward the sole is

A. retraction

B. inversion

C. extension

D. supination

E. plantar flexion

(Chabner, pp 528–529)

154. Ankle movement that turns the foot inward is

A. inversion

B. eversion

C. extension

D. retraction

E. hyperextension

(Rice, p 108)

155. Inflammation of bone and cartilage is

A. osteomyelitis

B. osteochondritis

C. osteoperiostitis

D. osteoarthritis

E. osteosynovitis

(Rice, p 122)

156. Gigantism, acromegaly, and dwarfism are caused by

A. rickets

B. disturbances of the endocrine system

C. tumors

D. disturbances of the lymph vascular system

E. anomalies of the spine

(Chabner, pp 661–662)

157. Of the following, an example of a malignant osteogenic tumor is

A. osteochondroma

B. osteoclastoma

C. osteosarcoma

D. xanthoma

E. osteofibroma

(Taber's, p 1370; Rice, p 123)

158. Abnormal hardness of bone is

A. osteosclerosis

B. osteoclastoma

C. exostosis

D. osteochondromatosis

E. otosclerosis

(Taber's, p 1370)

159. Inflammation of the joints is
    A. arthritis
    B. cretinism
    C. scoliosis
    D. syphilis
    E. arthrodesis
    (Gylys and Masters, p 333; Fisher, p 30)

160. The surgical breaking of bone is called
    A. osteoclasis
    B. osteosynthesis
    C. osteorrhaphy
    D. osteolysis
    E. osteoblast
    (Taber's, p 1365; Ehrlich, p 71)

161. The reconstruction or repair of bone is called
    A. osteosis
    B. osteoplasty
    C. otoplasty
    D. arthroplasty
    E. chondroplasty
    (Leonard, p 304; Miller and Keane, p 1158)

162. The excision of bone is called
    A. osteotomy
    B. osteoclasis
    C. otectomy
    D. ostectomy
    E. ototomy
    (Leonard, p 304; Miller and Keane, p 1158)

163. The slender, horseshoe-shaped bone below the mandible to which the tongue and other muscles are attached that may be felt just above the Adam's apple, or laryngeal prominence, is the
    A. ethmoid bone
    B. palatine bone
    C. sphenoid bone
    D. occipital bone
    E. hyoid bone
    (Memmler et al, p 92)

164. The bones that form the cheeks are called
    A. vomer
    B. maxillae
    C. zygomatic or malar bones
    D. hard palate
    E. temporal
    (Chabner, p 502; Memmler et al, p 92)

165. The number of cervical vertebrae is
    A. 1
    B. 5
    C. 7
    D. 9
    E. 12
    (Chabner, p 504)

166. The xiphoid process is part of the
    A. clavicle
    B. femur
    C. vertebrae
    D. sternum
    E. ulna
    (Chabner, pp 507, 511)

167. The bone on the outer or thumb side of the forearm is called the
    A. radius
    B. ulna
    C. humerus
    D. carpus
    E. scaphoid
    (Chabner, p 507)

168. The bones of the fingers are called
    A. navicular
    B. lunate
    C. hamate
    D. metacarpals
    E. phalanges
    (Brooks and LaFleur, pp 192–193; Memmler et al, p 97)

169. The longest and strongest bone in the skeleton is the
    A. fibula
    B. tibia
    C. humerus
    D. ulna
    E. femur

    (Chabner, p 508)

170. Aponeuroses are
    A. flattened tendons attaching muscles
    B. striated muscles
    C. smooth muscles
    D. bones of the lower extremities
    E. bones of the upper extremities

    (Taber's, p 135)

171. The muscle that compresses the cheeks and retracts the angles of the mouth is the
    A. inferior rectus
    B. superior oblique
    C. temporalis
    D. external pterygoid
    E. buccinator

    (Memmler et al, p 125)

172. What cell in the bone marrow gives rise to all types of blood cells?
    A. stem cell
    B. erythrocyte
    C. megakarocyte
    D. macrophage
    E. eosinophil

    (Scanlon and Sanders, pp 238–239)

173. The quickest way for the working medical assistant to know the set-ups and medications for complicated or seldom performed surgical procedures is
    A. prepare a written procedure manual
    B. remind your co-workers to help you
    C. memorize the set-ups
    D. keep a good medical assistance reference handy
    E. none of the above

    (Kinn and Woods, p 1111)

174. Phenylketonuria is an inherited disorder that if untreated will cause
    A. glaucoma
    B. high blood pressure
    C. mental retardation
    D. eczema
    E. hemoglobinopathy

    (Palko and Palko, p 161)

175. Muscles are named using a variety of methods. Which of the following is NOT a method used to name muscles?
    A. physician who first described the muscle
    B. location
    C. shape
    D. fiber direction
    E. origin and insertion

    (Memmler et al, p 122)

176. Which of the following is NOT a type of muscle tissue?
    A. clavicle
    B. smooth (visceral and nonstriated)
    C. cardiac (heart)
    D. skeletal (voluntary and striated)
    E. myocardium

    (Memmler et al, p 45)

177. The muscle that separates the thoracic and abdominal cavities is the
    A. psoas major
    B. psoas minor
    C. diaphragm
    D. serratus anterior
    E. epiglottis

    (Memmler et al, pp 26, 287; Taber's, pp 533–534)

178. The upper arm muscle named for its shape, often the site of injections, that abducts and rotates the arm is the
  A. biceps brachii
  B. triceps brachii
  C. deltoid
  D. flexor carpi ulnaris
  E. pronator quadratus
  (Thibodeau and Patton #2, pp 180, 182)

179. The biceps brachii muscle
  A. supinates the hand
  B. extends the little finger
  C. extends the index finger
  D. extends the wrist and abducts the hand
  E. flexes the arm and assists in supination
  (Scanlon and Sanders, pp 150–151)

180. Bursitis is caused by inflammation of the
  A. hipbone
  B. bursa
  C. scapula
  D. sciatic nerve
  E. spine
  (Memmler et al, p 105)

181. A chemical messenger that has a specific regulatory effect on target tissue(s) or organs is a/an
  A. hormone
  B. enzyme
  C. triglyceride
  D. DNA
  E. interferon
  (Memmler et al, pp 186–187)

182. A chronic disease characterized by muscular weakness and frequently affecting the face and throat is
  A. myodynia
  B. myalgia
  C. myeloplegia
  D. myosclerosis
  E. myasthenia gravis
  (Memmler et al, p 129)

183. An example of a condyloid joint that permits a variety of movements in different directions is
  A. elbow
  B. hip joint
  C. ankle joint
  D. adjacent vertebra
  E. finger and toe joints
  (Memmler et al, p 106)

184. Lumbar punctures are performed by inserting a fine needle between the L4 and L5 (the fourth and fifth lumbar vertebra) and withdrawing fluid from the subarachnoid space to
  A. obtain cerebrospinal fluid (CSF)
  B. determine CSF pressure
  C. detect a hemorrhage in the central nervous system (CNS)
  D. treat a CNS disorder
  E. perform any of the above
  (Scanlon and Sanders, p 174)

185. Paralysis of both arms and both legs is
  A. apoplexy
  B. quadriplegia
  C. quadripara
  D. hemiplegia
  E. paraplegia
  (Taber's, p 1654; Leonard, p 354)

186. A paralysis caused by a brain lesion, such as a tumor, or most commonly by a cerebral vascular accident (CVA) is
  A. quadriplegia
  B. hemiplegia
  C. paraplegia
  D. monoplegia
  E. Bell's palsy
  (Gylys and Masters, p 356; Austrin and Austrin, p 298)

187. Pain over the course of a nerve is
    A. polyneuritis
    B. neuralgia
    C. neurasthenia
    D. neurodermatitis
    E. neurectasia
    (Austrin and Austrin, p 298; Smith et al, p 253)

188. An irreversible coma is also known as
    A. severe concussion
    B. occlusion
    C. a contusion
    D. brain death
    E. embolism
    (Taber's, p 259)

189. The first cranial nerve (olfactory) is concerned with
    A. sense of taste
    B. sense of smell
    C. sense of hearing and equilibrium
    D. chief sensory nerve of face and head
    E. sense of sight
    (Memmler et al, pp 163–165)

190. The surgical joining of nerve ends is called
    A. neurorrhaphy
    B. neuroanastomosis
    C. ganglionectomy
    D. neurolysis
    E. neuroplasty
    (Taber's, p 1288)

191. Ménière's disease is
    A. a common form of neuralgia
    B. an auditory nerve disorder
    C. a psychosis of chronic agitated depression
    D. degenerative changes of peripheral nerves
    E. purposeless movements of various body parts
    (Chabner, pp 615–616)

192. An example of a superficial reflex is the
    A. plantar reflex
    B. patellar reflex
    C. ankle jerk
    D. triceps jerk
    E. masseter reflex
    (Miller and Keane, p 1385)

193. A disease that may cause change in the shapes of the valvular cusps of the heart and a consequent murmur is
    A. pericarditis
    B. myocarditis
    C. endocarditis
    D. cardiosymphysis
    E. valvulotomy
    (Memmler et al, p 227)

194. The red color of the blood derives from
    A. lymphocytes
    B. hemoglobin
    C. platelets
    D. basophils
    E. neutrophils
    (Memmler et al, p 204; Rice, p 269)

195. Although the volume of blood in the body varies, a male weighing 150 pounds will have an approximate blood volume of
    A. 7 liters
    B. 10 quarts
    C. 5 liters
    D. 12 liters
    E. 5 pints
    (Memmler et al, p 202; Scanlon and Sanders, pp 236–237)

196. The organ that serves as a reservoir for blood for use when the need arises is the
    A. spleen
    B. liver
    C. pancreas
    D. kidney
    E. gallbladder
    (Memmler et al, p 267)

197. The mitral valve is also called the
    A. bicuspid valve
    B. tricuspid valve
    C. semilunar valve
    D. pyloric valve
    E. coronary valve
    (Memmler et al, p 222)

198. The largest artery in the body is the
    A. carotid artery
    B. aorta
    C. pulmonary artery
    D. cerebral artery
    E. femoral artery
    (Memmler et al, p 238; Thibodeau and Patton #2, p 333)

199. The veins in the body that carry the highest concentration of oxygenated blood are the
    A. anterior veins of the heart
    B. venae vasorum
    C. supraorbital veins
    D. jugular veins
    E. pulmonary veins
    (Memmler et al, p 238; Thibodeau and Patton #2, pp 318–319)

200. From the right ventricle of the heart, blood is forced into the
    A. aorta
    B. pulmonary artery
    C. right atrium
    D. left atrium
    E. left ventricle
    (Thibodeau and Patton #1, p 336)

201. A localized area of ischemic necrosis in the heart muscle produced by an occlusion of the blood supply is called a/an
    A. angina pectoris
    B. neutropenia
    C. infarction
    D. purpura
    E. stroke
    (Memmler et al, pp 228–229; Thibodeau and Patton #2, pp 320–321, 335)

202. A stricture or narrowing of some portion of the aorta is
    A. aortolith
    B. aortomalacia
    C. aortoclasia
    D. coarctation of the aorta
    E. cardiac arrest
    (Memmler et al, p 228; Miller and Keane, p 344)

203. Greatly dilated veins in which pressure is elevated and blood flow is stagnant or reversed are called
    A. phleboclysis
    B. varicose veins
    C. vasa vasorum
    D. venosclerosis
    E. phleborrhexis
    (Memmler et al, p 256; Miller and Keane, p 1702)

204. The tissue that connects and supports body organs is
    A. muscle tissue
    B. nerve tissue
    C. epithelial tissue
    D. connective tissue
    E. visceral tissue
    (Chabner, p 33; Memmler et al, pp 40–42)

205. A cancer that arises from bone, bone marrow, lymphatic tissue, or adipose tissue is a
    A. carcinoma
    B. metastasis

C. sarcoma

D. adenoma

E. adenocarcinoma

(Memmler et al, p 49; Rice, p 559)

206. Leio- is a word component that means

A. connective

B. smooth

C. irritation

D. blood

E. lung

(Austrin and Austrin, p 39)

207. Obstruction of the valve orifice between the left atrium and left ventricle is called

A. aneurysm

B. mitral commissurotomy

C. mitral stenosis

D. infarct

E. pulmonic stenosis

(Chabner, p 366)

208. A localized dilatation of an artery is

A. mitral stenosis

B. infarct

C. aneurysm

D. enucleation

E. tularemia

(Taber's, pp 102–103; Austrin, p 155)

209. Closed heart massage is called

A. extracorporeal circulation

B. vascularization

C. cardioaccelerator

D. cardiolysis

E. cardiopulmonary resuscitation

(Chabner, p 413)

210. A hereditary disease in which patients bleed excessively is

A. Buerger's disease

B. hemophilia

C. Osler's disease

D. tetralogy of Fallot

E. angina pectoris

(Chabner, p 437)

211. A reduction of red cells per unit of circulating blood or reduced hemoglobin amount in each red cell or both is

A. anemia

B. apoplexy

C. atherosclerosis

D. Buerger's disease

E. enucleation

(Rice, p 266)

212. Rapid, random, ineffectual, and irregular heartbeats (350 or more/minute) are

A. flutter

B. fibrillation

C. ectopic rhythm

D. paroxysmal bradycardia

E. pancarditis

(Taber's, p 722)

213. Rheumatic heart disease (RHD) may develop until up to 20 years after the initial infection of

A. tuberculosis bacilli

B. syphilis spirochete

C. typhoid bacilli

D. streptococcus bacteria

E. diphtheria

(Chabner, p 366; Miller and Keane, pp 1414–1415)

214. Of the following, which is NOT a ductless gland?

A. thymus

B. sebaceous

C. adrenals

D. thyroid

E. gonads

(Memmler et al, p 40)

215. The glands that secrete a hormone that regulates the calcium content of the blood and bones are the
    A. pituitary glands
    B. adrenal glands
    C. parathyroid glands
    D. thymus glands
    E. pineal glands
    (Chabner, p 650)

216. Excessive thirst is
    A. polydipsia
    B. polyphagia
    C. polyuria
    D. polyhydruria
    E. polyphasia
    (Brooks and LaFleur, pp 589, 593; Willis, p 303)

217. Presence of sugar in the urine is
    A. glycopenia
    B. glycorrhea
    C. glycohemia
    D. glucohemia
    E. glucosuria
    (Taber's, p 807; Palko and Palko, p 137)

218. Failure of the testicles to descend into the scrotum is
    A. tetralogy of Fallot
    B. testosterone
    C. scotocele
    D. cryptorchidism
    E. orchidoptosis
    (Chabner, pp 281, 283; Willis, pp 430–431)

219. Hypofunction of the adrenal cortex leads to a syndrome called
    A. Cushing's syndrome
    B. Addison's disease
    C. Graves' disease
    D. myxedema
    E. SIDS
    (Chabner, p 659)

220. A rare abnormality of the pituitary gland that causes excessive growth, so that a child becomes an unusually tall adult is
    A. gigantism
    B. megalocephaly
    C. megalodactylia
    D. elephantiasis
    E. polytrophia
    (Miller and Keane, p 656; Willis, pp 306–307)

221. Another term for exophthalmic goiter is
    A. Paget's disease
    B. Graves' disease
    C. Bright's disease
    D. Pott's disease
    E. Raynaud's disease
    (Chabner, p 656; Willis, p 306)

222. Endemic goiter, cretinism, and myxedema are pathologic conditions due to
    A. hyperinsulinism
    B. hyperparathyroidism
    C. hyperthyroidism
    D. hypoparathyroidism
    E. hypothyroidism
    (Chabner, p 656; Willis, pp 308–309)

223. A disease characterized by a bronzing of the skin due to the deposition of an iron-containing pigment is called
    A. ochronosis
    B. porphyria
    C. xanthomatosis
    D. hemochromatosis
    E. alkalosis
    (Taber's, p 870)

224. A hormone produced in the testes is
    A. estrogen
    B. stilbestrol
    C. pituitrin
    D. adrenocorticotropin
    E. testosterone
    (Chabner, p 277; Willis, p 302)

225. An abnormally high concentration of sugar in the blood is
    A. hyperglycemia
    B. hyperglycosuria
    C. hyperlipemia
    D. hypoglycemia
    E. hypoxemia
    (Taber's, p 933)

226. Amyl- is a word component that means
    A. sugar
    B. carbohydrate
    C. fat
    D. starch
    E. protein
    (Miller and Keane, p 74)

227. Andro- is a word element that means
    A. rupture
    B. color
    C. male
    D. shield
    E. wing
    (Miller and Keane, p 74; Ehrlich, p 300)

228. The suffix -ptysis means
    A. prolapse
    B. pus
    C. irrigation
    D. puncture
    E. spitting
    (Taber's, p 1596)

229. The serous sac that encases the lung and is divided into two layers, visceral and parietal, is the
    A. pneumoretroperitoneum
    B. thorax
    C. pleura
    D. pneumoderma
    E. plantar
    (Memmler et al, p 290; Scanlon and Sanders, p 329)

230. The airway between the nasal chambers, the mouth, and the larynx is the
    A. pharynx
    B. nares
    C. trachea
    D. bronchi
    E. epiglottis
    (Taber's, p 1462)

231. The windpipe is the
    A. larynx
    B. pharynx
    C. esophagus
    D. nares
    E. trachea
    (Chabner, p 397)

232. The region between the lungs in the chest cavity is the
    A. diaphragm
    B. parietal pleura
    C. pectoralis major
    D. mediastinum
    E. scapula
    (Chabner, p 397; Willis, p 230)

233. A condition that includes obstruction of the larynx due to allergy, a foreign body, infection, or new growth and a barking cough, difficult breathing, spasms, and sometimes formation of a membrane is
    A. Cheyne-Stokes respiration
    B. pleurisy
    C. croup
    D. coryza
    E. epistaxis
    (Gylys and Masters, p 255; Taber's, p 463)

234. Detection of new growths arising within the bronchi may be made by use of
    A. bronchoscope
    B. bronchodilator
    C. bronchospirometry
    D. bronchiolectasis
    E. bronciectasis

    (Chabner, p 411; Gylys and Masters, p 234)

235. Myringitis, otitis media, and otorrhea are inflammatory conditions of the
    A. ear
    B. nose
    C. pharynx
    D. larynx
    E. bronchi

    (Taber's, pp 1262, 1372, 1373)

236. Tracheitis is usually accompanied by
    A. myringitis
    B. otitis media
    C. laryngitis and bronchitis
    D. pneumonia
    E. pneumonia and bronchitis

    (Taber's, p 1977)

237. Collapse of the lung so that the air sacs become smaller in size is known as
    A. atelectasis
    B. emphysema
    C. pneumoconiosis
    D. silicosis
    E. pleurisy

    (Chabner, p 406; Willis, p 233)

238. Overdistention of the air sacs of the lungs results in
    A. atelectasis
    B. emphysema
    C. pneumoconiosis
    D. silicosis
    E. siderosis

    (Chabner, p 406; Willis, p 233)

239. The large nodules in the walls of the pharynx are of three types: the adenoid tonsils, the palatine tonsils, and the lingual tonsils. They are composed of
    A. striated muscle
    B. lymph tissue
    C. mitral tissue
    D. epithelium
    E. integumentary

    (Scanlon and Sanders, pp 326–327)

240. A weak place in the diaphragm that allows a portion of an abdominal organ, such as the stomach, to protrude upward through the esophageal opening and into the thorax is a/an
    A. embolism
    B. infarction
    C. hiatal hernia
    D. strangulation
    E. rectocele

    (Memmler et al, p 308)

241. The most common lethal inherited disease in the Caucasian population, which occurs in a ratio of 1:2000, is
    A. Down syndrome
    B. Tay-Sachs disease
    C. sudden infant death syndrome (SIDS)
    D. cystic fibrosis
    E. sickle cell anemia

    (Memmler et al, p 396; Thibodeau and Patton, pp 30, 424, 570)

242. The surgical treatment for diaphragmatic hernia is
    A. hernioplasty
    B. herniorrhaphy
    C. herniotomy
    D. thoracostomy
    E. lobectomy

    (Miller and Keane, p 736)

243. Conditions resulting from pregnancy and parturition may be subject to surgery. Parturition refers to
    A. menopause
    B. menstruation
    C. perineum
    D. childbirth
    E. sterility
    (Chabner, pp 232, 238)

244. The part of the fetus that exists first at birth is called the
    A. protrusion
    B. prologue
    C. presentation
    D. anteversion
    E. preceptor
    (Chabner, p 243)

245. Change of position of the fetus in the womb is called
    A. version
    B. aversion
    C. anteversion
    D. ventilation
    E. ventriculation
    (Taber's, p 2125)

246. Cells obtained by chorionic villus sampling or amniocentesis are used for the purpose of
    A. detecting cancer
    B. diagnosing genetic fetal disorders
    C. testing spinal fluid
    D. confirming pregnancy
    E. detecting placenta previa
    (Damjanov, pp 126–127; Memmler et al, p 397)

247. Cystocele refers to
    A. hernial protrusion of urinary bladder
    B. hernial protrusion of gallbladder
    C. gallstone
    D. hernia of the uterus
    E. kidney stone
    (Taber's, p 480; Willis, p 455)

248. The major functions of fat in the body would include
    A. providing a source of energy
    B. carrying fat-soluble vitamins A and D
    C. supplying fatty acids essential for growth and life
    D. slowing down emptying of stomach, which increases satiety value of diet
    E. all of the above
    (Kinn and Woods, p 975)

249. Phimosis, redundant prepuce, and balanoposthitis are reasons for performing
    A. meatotomy
    B. orchioplasty
    C. orchiopexy
    D. circumcision
    E. orchidectomy
    (Taber's, p 391)

250. The presence of degenerative changes in the kidneys without the occurrence of inflammation is referred to as
    A. nephroptosis
    B. nephrolithiasis
    C. nephropexy
    D. nephroma
    E. nephrosis
    (Chabner, p 203; Willis, p 410)

251. Another term for baldness is
    A. alopecia
    B. hypertrichosis
    C. hypotrichosis
    D. trichocryptosis
    E. trichoclasia
    (Miller and Keane, p 60)

252. The surgical procedure for cleft lip repair is
    A. palatoplasty
    B. rhinoplasty
    C. glossoplasty
    D. cheiloplasty
    E. otoplasty
    (Taber's, p 361)

253. Face-lifting, or plastic surgery for the elimination of wrinkles from the skin, is
    A. blepharoplasty
    B. dermatoplasty
    C. dermatology
    D. rhytidectomy
    E. dermatitis
    (Miller and Keane, p 1420)

254. Excessive size of the ears is called
    A. otomycosis
    B. otodynia
    C. otoplasty
    D. macrotia
    E. microtia
    (Taber's, p 1149)

255. Incision of the eardrum and drainage of the middle ear is
    A. myringectomy
    B. otectomy
    C. tympanectomy
    D. osteotomy
    E. myringotomy
    (Brooks and LaFleur, pp 185–187; Chabner, p 616)

256. A term that relates to malignancies (cancer) is
    A. metastasis
    B. carcinoma
    C. sarcoma
    D. neoplastic
    E. all of the above
    (Thibodeau and Patton #2, pp 88–90)

257. A small discoloration of the skin, level with the surface, up to the size of a fingernail is a
    A. macule
    B. papule
    C. nodule
    D. vesicle
    E. pustule
    (Chabner, p 568)

258. The condition responsible for "oily skin" and "dandruff" is
    A. eczema
    B. hyperhidrosis
    C. seborrhea
    D. hypertrichosis
    E. hypotrichosis
    (Chabner, p 567)

259. Removal of the lacrimal (tear) sac is
    A. dacryocystectomy
    B. evisceration
    C. exenteration
    D. lacrimotomy
    E. dacryocystotomy
    (Taber's, p 486)

260. Removal of the eyeball is
    A. iridectomy
    B. enucleation
    C. sclerectomy
    D. myectomy
    E. discission
    (Taber's, p 653; Austrin and Austrin, p 328)

261. Hordeolum and chalazion are afflictions of the
    A. retina
    B. pupil
    C. eyelids
    D. cornea
    E. iris
    (Taber's, pp 356, 911)

262. The soft, jelly-like, transparent substance that fills the inner chamber of the eye is the
   A. retina
   B. aqueous humor
   C. cornea
   D. vitreous humor
   E. phacoemulsification
   (Chabner, pp 593, 597; Willis, pp 325–327)

263. A condition in which the curvature of the refracting surfaces of the eye is unequal is
   A. cataract
   B. astigmatism
   C. strabismus
   D. esotropia
   E. exotropia
   (Ehrlich, p 255)

264. The malleus is a bone of the
   A. nose
   B. ear
   C. eye
   D. thorax
   E. skull
   (Chabner, pp 610, 613; Rice, p 44)

265. The pinna is a part of the
   A. external ear
   B. internal ear
   C. tongue
   D. superior nasal conchae
   E. fingernail
   (Taber's, p 1512; Rice, p 440)

266. A defective condition of accommodation due to loss of elasticity of the ciliary body from increasing age is
   A. ametropia
   B. emmetropia
   C. hyperopia
   D. myopia
   E. presbyopia
   (Taber's, p 1553; Ehrlich, p 255)

267. Although there are 20 teeth in the first set of deciduous or milk teeth, the number of permanent teeth is
   A. 22
   B. 24
   C. 28
   D. 32
   E. 36
   (Memmler et al, p 304; Scanlon and Sanders, p 354)

268. The large blind pouch at the beginning of the large intestine is the
   A. jejunum
   B. ileum
   C. sigmoid colon
   D. vermiform appendix
   E. cecum
   (Chabner, pp 132, 135)

269. The large portal system in the body's blood circulation is in the
   A. pancreas
   B. prostate
   C. thyroid
   D. liver
   E. pituitary
   (Memmler et al, pp 313–314)

270. The reservoir for bile is the
   A. liver
   B. gallbladder
   C. pancreas
   D. duodenum
   E. spleen
   (Chabner, p 133; Memmler et al, p 314)

271. The basic structural unit of nerve tissue is called a
   A. neuroma
   B. neuron
   C. neurilemma
   D. neuraxis
   E. neuroceptor
   (Taber's, p 1292)

272. The person who is known as a universal donor has the type of blood called
    A. A
    B. B
    C. AB
    D. O
    E. Rh positive
    (Chabner, p 437)

273. The most important heat-regulating center in the body is the
    A. pituitary gland
    B. hypothalamus
    C. parathyroid gland
    D. thymus gland
    E. thermoreceptor
    (Chabner, pp 306–307)

274. Sweat glands are also known as
    A. temporal glands
    B. sublingual glands
    C. sudoriferous glands
    D. sentinel glands
    E. pyloric glands
    (Rice, p 66)

275. The delicate, spongy bone located between the eyes and forming a part of the cranial floor beneath the frontal lobes of the brain and the upper nasal cavities is the
    A. parietal bone
    B. temporal bone
    C. ethmoid bone
    D. sphenoid bone
    E. occipital bone
    (Taber's, p 678)

276. The soft spot in the skull of a young infant is called the
    A. foramen
    B. lumen
    C. occiput

D. sella turcica
    E. fontanel
    (Chabner, p 500)

277. Blood in the stools is called
    A. fecaluria
    B. fecolith
    C. melena
    D. hematemesis
    E. hematuresis
    (Taber's, p 1182)

278. The most common benign tumors of the digestive tract are
    A. fibromas
    B. granulomas
    C. fissures
    D. fistulas
    E. polyps
    (Miller and Keane, p 1282)

279. An outstanding symptom of liver disease and hemolytic blood disorders is
    A. rapid weight gain
    B. polydipsia
    C. erythema
    D. polyuria
    E. jaundice
    (Miller and Keane, p 866)

280. The end of a muscle that exerts the power and movement is called the
    A. action
    B. origin
    C. insertion
    D. fascia
    E. articulation
    (Taber's, p 1000)

281. The chief muscle of the calf of the leg is the
    A. sartorius
    B. quadriceps femoris

C. tibialis anterior

D. gastrocnemius

E. trapezius

(Memmler et al, pp 121–122)

282. The outermost, toughest, and most fibrous of the three membranes covering the brain and spinal cord is the

A. arachnoid membrane

B. pia mater

C. dura mater

D. dendrites

E. axons

(Chabner, pp 309–310)

283. Fatty tissue that is deposited in most parts of the body is called

A. adipose

B. areolar

C. retiform

D. mucoid

E. adenoid

(Chabner, pp 35, 50)

284. The mastoid process can be felt

A. on the breast

B. above the eye

C. on the elbow

D. at the side of the nose

E. behind the ear

(Chabner, pp 500, 510)

285. How many pairs of ribs are attached to the sternum anteriorly?

A. one

B. three

C. five

D. seven

E. nine

(Chabner, p 507)

286. A foramen is

A. an opening that allows a vessel or nerve to pass through or between bones

B. an air space in some skull bones

C. a depression in a bone surface

D. a spine on a bone

E. none of the above

(Memmler et al, p 90)

287. The largest bone of the foot is the

A. talus

B. navicular

C. calcaneus

D. cuboid

E. cuneiform

(Memmler et al, p 100; Scanlon and Sanders, p 117)

288. A joint in which one rounded extremity fits into a cavity in another bone, permitting movement in all directions, is called a

A. gliding or plane joint

B. condyloid joint

C. hinge joint

D. saddle joint

E. ball-and-socket joint

(Taber's, p 1036)

289. The elbow joint, the knee joint, and the finger joints are examples of

A. ball-and-socket joints

B. hinge joints

C. pivot joints

D. saddle joints

E. condyloid joints

(Memmler et al, p 106; Thibodeau and Patton #1, p 105)

290. A sudden loss of consciousness due to cerebral anoxia is
   A. petit mal
   B. vertigo
   C. anopsia
   D. syncope
   E. cephalalgia

   (Taber's, p 1883)

291. A collection of fluid in the pleural space is called
   A. caseation
   B. exudate
   C. ebullition
   D. effusion
   E. pleuroclysis

   (Miller and Keane, p 506)

292. Coryza is the scientific term for
   A. heat rash
   B. common cold
   C. grippe
   D. dandruff
   E. pinkeye

   (Taber's, pp 451–452)

293. A disorder that may occur during pregnancy and is manifested by high blood pressure, edema, proteinuria, renal dysfunction, and possibly coma is
   A. gravida
   B. kernicterus
   C. ectopic pregnancy
   D. puerperium
   E. eclampsia

   (Ehrlich, p 329)

294. Which of the following types of leukocytes (white blood cells) is increased in allergic conditions?
   A. neutrophil
   B. basophil
   C. monocyte
   D. lymphocyte
   E. eosinophil

   (Chabner, p 80; Ehrlich, p 112)

295. Which pair of veins returns blood from the head to the superior vena cava?
   A. saphenous
   B. jugular
   C. radial
   D. brachial
   E. subclavian

   (Memmler et al, pp 245–247)

296. Dysphagia means
   A. difficulty in swallowing
   B. impairment of ability to speak
   C. indigestion
   D. insatiable craving for food
   E. mental distress

   (Willis, p 370; Dennerll, p 132)

297. Which organ removes bilirubin from the blood, manufactures many of the plasma proteins, and is concerned with the production of clotting factors?
   A. gallbladder
   B. spleen
   C. liver
   D. pancreas
   E. kidney

   (Scanlon and Sanders, pp 370–372)

298. Which of the following is true of the lymphatic system?
   A. its terminal vessels empty lymph into the circulatory system
   B. it moves large molecules and fluid from the tissue spaces
   C. it moves fat-related nutrients from the digestive system to the circulatory system
   D. it plays a critical role in the immune system
   E. all of the above

   (Thibodeau and Patton #2, pp 355–360)

299. Aniso- is a word part that means
    A. black
    B. white
    C. equal
    D. unequal
    E. male

    (Brooks and LaFleur, p 652; Chabner, p 811)

300. Chromo- is a word part that means
    A. metal
    B. color
    C. gene
    D. tooth
    E. hair

    (Miller and Keane, p 323; Willis, p 496)

301. A mechanical soft diet is one that is modified by
    A. flavor
    B. levels of one or more nutrients
    C. feeding intervals
    D. consistency
    E. inclusion or exclusion of specific foods

    (Kinn and Woods, pp 983–984)

302. The diet modification that implies a bland diet is
    A. consistency
    B. bulk
    C. flavor
    D. feeding intervals
    E. caloric level

    (Kinn and Woods, p 984)

303. Allergies often are treated by means of a diet modified by
    A. consistency
    B. caloric level
    C. flavor
    D. feeding intervals
    E. inclusion or exclusion of specific foods

    (Kinn and Woods, p 984)

304. Night blindness, or the impairment of one's ability to adapt to darkness, may indicate a deficiency of
    A. vitamin A
    B. vitamin C
    C. vitamin D
    D. vitamin E
    E. vitamin K

    (Keir et al, p 723; Kinn and Woods, pp 978–979)

305. An area of specialization primarily concerned with diagnosing and treating diseases and disorders of the blood and blood-forming tissues is
    A. oncology
    B. ophthalmology
    C. neurology
    D. hematology
    E. gastroenterology

    (Keir et al, pp 18–20; Miller and Keane, p 713)

306. An area of specialization that diagnoses and treats diseases and disorders of the eye is
    A. orthopedics
    B. ophthalmology
    C. obstetrics
    D. oncology
    E. optometry

    (Keir et al, pp 18–20; Kinn and Woods, pp 45–47)

307. An area of specialization concerned primarily with diagnosing and treating diseases and disorders of the kidneys is
    A. nephrology
    B. neurology
    C. gynecology
    D. endocrinology
    E. dermatology

    (Keir et al, pp 18–20; Kinn and Woods, pp 45–47)

308. The medical specialty that diagnoses and treats pronounced emotional problems or mental illness that may have an organic cause is

A. podiatry

B. pathology

C. psychology

D. psychiatry

E. pediatrics

(Keir et al, pp 18–20; Kinn and Woods, pp 45–47)

309. A specialist that diagnoses and treats conditions of altered immunologic reactivity is a/an

A. anesthesiologist

B. allergist

C. cardiologist

D. endocrinologist

E. internal medicine specialist

(Keir et al, pp 18–20; Kinn and Woods, pp 45–47)

310. The integumentary system is the skin and performs all of the following functions for the body EXCEPT

A. protection

B. perception

C. temperature control

D. absorption

E. nitrogenous waste excretion

(Keir et al, pp 259–260)

311. Which of the following is NOT a disease or disorder of the integumentary system (skin)?

A. dermatitis

B. impetigo

C. nystagmus

D. psoriasis

E. urticaria

(Keir et al, pp 261–269)

312. The appendicular skeleton is made up of bones of all of the following EXCEPT the

A. arms

B. legs

C. skull

D. feet

E. pelvis

(Thibodeau and Patton #1, pp 87–100)

313. The skeleton has at least five basic functions for the body. Which of the following is NOT one of these functions?

A. the skeletal system lends support to the body

B. the skeletal system serves as a primary energy reservoir for the body

C. the skeletal system protects vital organs of the body

D. it serves as the point of attachment for skeletal muscles

E. the bones in the skeletal system are involved in the formation of blood cells, especially red blood cells

(Keir et al, pp 272–273)

314. The metabolic bone disease where proper storage of calcium does not occur in the bone is

A. osteomalacia

B. osteoarthritis

C. osteomyelitis

D. osteoporosis

E. osteitis deformans

(Keir et al, pp 282–283)

315. Smooth muscle activity is responsible for all of the following EXCEPT

A. breathing

B. moving food in the intestinal tract

C. moving bones

D. changing pupil size of the eye

E. dilating or constricting blood vessels

(Keir et al, pp 285–286)

316. The type of fracture that results in breaks that splinter with bone fragments embedded in surrounding tissue but does not break through the surface is called a/an

    A. simple or closed fracture
    B. compound fracture
    C. greenstick fracture
    D. comminuted fracture
    E. impacted fracture

    (Keir et al, pp 276–277)

317. A type of wavelike action by the smooth muscles that forces food through the intestine is called

    A. sphincters
    B. peristalsis
    C. fascia
    D. tendon
    E. aponeuroses

    (Keir et al, p 592)

318. The cartilage "lid" that closes to direct food down the esophagus is the

    A. trachea
    B. larynx
    C. septum
    D. epiglottis
    E. glottis

    (Scanlon and Sanders, p 328)

319. A type of respiratory or lung disease that results from inhaling inorganic dust over a prolonged period of time is

    A. pneumothorax
    B. pneumoconiosis
    C. pneumonia
    D. emphysema
    E. upper respiratory infection (URI)

    (Keir et al, p 303)

320. The smallest divisions of the trachea forming the air passageways (not air sacs) in the lungs are

    A. aveoli
    B. bronchi
    C. bronchioles
    D. bronchial artery
    E. pharynx

    (Kinn and Woods, pp 536–537)

321. The internal muscular wall that divides the heart into the right and left side is the

    A. endocardium
    B. mitral valve
    C. myocardium
    D. pericardium
    E. septum

    (Keir et al, pp 308–309)

322. The part of the circulatory system that collects and returns blood from the lower part of the body to the right atrium is the

    A. inferior vena cava
    B. pulmonary vein
    C. subclavian vein
    D. superior vena cava
    E. femoral vein

    (Keir et al, pp 314–315)

323. A condition of the circulatory system in which the artery wall weakens and balloons out is called an

    A. aneurysm
    B. angina
    C. arrhythmia
    D. arteriosclerosis
    E. atherosclerosis

    (Keir et al, pp 322–323)

324. A condition in the lumen of the arteries having deposits and accumulation of fatty materials is
    A. aneurysm
    B. angina
    C. arrhythmia
    D. arteriosclerosis
    E. atherosclerosis
    (Keir et al, pp 324–325)

325. The anatomic structure that is NOT part of the small intestine or support of the small intestine is the
    A. duodenum
    B. jejunum
    C. cecum
    D. mesentery
    E. ileum
    (Keir et al, p 360)

326. The vermiform appendix is a small projection that extends from the
    A. descending colon
    B. cecum
    C. sigmoid colon
    D. ileum
    E. transverse colon
    (Keir et al, p 360)

327. A disease that results in autodigestion (digestion of self) is
    A. paralytic ileus
    B. pancreatitis
    C. cirrhosis
    D. acute cholecystitis
    E. diverticulitis
    (Keir et al, pp 370–371)

328. The anatomic structure that is the functional unit of the kidney is the
    A. nephron
    B. ureter
    C. bladder

D. urethra
E. renal pelvis
(Memmler et al, pp 340–344)

329. The anatomic structure of the urinary tract responsible for carrying urine from the bladder to the outside of the body is the
    A. nephron
    B. ureter
    C. bladder
    D. urethra
    E. renal pelvis
    (Memmler et al, p 350)

330. A kidney disease that is inherited and produces grapelike, fluid-filled sacs or cysts in the collecting tubules of the cortex of the kidney is
    A. pyelonephritis
    B. glomerulonephritis
    C. polycystic kidney disease
    D. cystitis
    E. renal calculus
    (Memmler et al, p 352)

331. A urinary tract disease that causes inflammation of the bladder is
    A. pyelonephritis
    B. glomerulonephritis
    C. polycystic kidney disease
    D. cystitis
    E. renal calculus
    (Leonard, p 239)

332. An organ in the body that functions both as an exocrine and an endocrine gland is the
    A. pituitary
    B. pancreas
    C. parathyroid
    D. pineal
    E. adrenal
    (Memmler et al, p 315)

333. The endocrine gland considered to be the "master gland" of the body is the
    A. thymus
    B. parathyroid
    C. testes
    D. ovaries
    E. pituitary
    (Memmler et al, pp 186–189)

334. The endocrine gland that is located in the neck and requires iodine for normal function is the
    A. pituitary gland
    B. thymus gland
    C. thyroid gland
    D. islands of Langerhans
    E. thalamus
    (Memmler et al, pp 189–191)

335. Cretinism causes the body to be short and stocky. Another name for this condition is
    A. hyperparathyroidism
    B. hypothyroidism
    C. hyperthyroidism
    D. hypoparathyroidism
    E. Cushing's syndrome
    (Memmler et al, p 190)

336. The disease diabetes insipidus is caused by insufficient secretion of vasopressin (also known as antidiuretic hormone, ADH). ADH is produced by the
    A. parathyroid gland
    B. thyroid gland
    C. pancreas gland
    D. pituitary gland
    E. adrenal gland
    (Memmler et al, p 189)

337. The sex of a child is determined by
    A. the mother
    B. the mother 1 month after conception
    C. the father 1 month before conception
    D. both parents
    E. the father at conception
    (Memmler et al, p 394; Scanlon and Sanders, pp 460–461)

338. A sexually transmitted disease (STD) caused by a protozoal infestation of the vagina, urethra, or prostate is
    A. gonorrhea
    B. herpes
    C. candida
    D. syphilis
    E. trichomoniasis
    (Keir, pp 426–427)

339. The cerebrum is the largest part of the mature brain. Which of the following is NOT part of the cerebrum?
    A. frontal lobe
    B. parietal lobe
    C. cerebellar hemisphere
    D. temporal lobe
    E. occipital lobe
    (Scanlon and Sanders, pp 167–172)

340. The junction between two nerve (neuron) endings that permits the transmission of nerve impulses to continue is the
    A. gap
    B. synapse
    C. connectors
    D. receptors
    E. sensors
    (Scanlon and Sanders, pp 154–157)

341. Any diffuse pain occurring in different portions of the head is a
    A. cerebral contusion
    B. headache
    C. cerebral concussion
    D. brain abscess
    E. stroke
    (Taber's, pp 843–845)

342. A disease that is characterized by severe muscle rigidity, a peculiar gait, and a progressive tremor is
    A. Parkinson's disease
    B. Alzheimer's disease
    C. Bell's palsy
    D. cerebral palsy
    E. meningitis
    (Damjanov, pp 513–514; Thibodeau and Patton #2, pp 209, 215)

343. Infections of the central nervous system (CNS) can be caused by almost any bacteria or virus. When an inflammation of the meninges results, it is
    A. neck and back stiffness
    B. a headache
    C. a fever
    D. a sensory disturbance
    E. meningitis
    (Taber's, p 1192; Thibodeau and Patton #2, pp 221–222)

344. Chemicals and drugs may affect the nervous system by acting as depressants or stimulants. Which of the following substances is NOT classified as a depressant?
    A. barbiturates
    B. alcohol
    C. amphetamines
    D. Librium
    E. Valium
    (Miller and Keane, p 65; Taber's, p 84)

345. A brain disease with seizure disorders associated with abnormal electrical impulses from the neurons of the brain is
    A. Bell's palsy
    B. encephalitis
    C. Parkinson's disease
    D. epilepsy
    E. brain abscess
    (Thibodeau and Patton #2, pp 216–218)

346. Presenile dementia was a term previously used to describe a chronic organic brain syndrome with death of neurons in the cerebral cortex and their replacement by microscopic "plaques." This disease is now known as
    A. Alzheimer's disease
    B. multiple sclerosis
    C. Parkinson's disease
    D. Bell's palsy
    E. peripheral neuritis
    (Scanlon and Sanders, p 171; Tamparo and Lewis, pp 236–237; Thibodeau and Patton #2, p 216)

347. The tough, white, fibrous tissue that covers the outside of the eye is the
    A. conjunctiva
    B. sclera
    C. choroid
    D. cornea
    E. retina
    (Scanlon and Sanders, pp 190–193)

348. The structure of the eye that contains muscles controlling the shape of the lens for near and far vision is the
    A. vitreous humor
    B. aqueous humor
    C. retina
    D. ciliary body
    E. pupil
    (Keir et al, p 248)

349. Refractive errors are defects in visual acuity. The eye has lost its ability of effectively focusing light on the surface of the retina. Which of the following is a refractive error?
    A. hyperopia (farsightedness)
    B. astigmatism
    C. presbyopia (irregular curvature of lens)
    D. myopia (nearsightedness)
    E. all of the above
    (Scanlon and Sanders, pp 194–195)

350. A condition of the eye with excessive intraocular pressure that can damage the retina and optic nerve, often causing blindness, is

A. glaucoma

B. cataract

C. retinal detachment

D. astigmatism

E. corneal ulcers

(Scanlon and Sanders, p 194)

351. An inherited disorder of the ear that forms spongy bone, especially around the oval window, and results in immobilization of the stapes is

A. otitis media

B. otitis externa

C. impacted cerumen

D. otosclerosis

E. Ménière's disease

(Thibodeau and Patton #2, pp 254–256)

352. An accumulation of fluid within the middle ear is called

A. otitis externa

B. otitis media

C. otosclerosis

D. Ménière's disease

E. swimmer's ear

(Thibodeau and Patton #2, p 255)

353. The abbreviations CC, FH, and HEENT are common terms used for

A. laboratory tests

B. surgical procedures

C. patient histories

D. emergency situations

E. x-ray

(Kinn and Woods, p 211)

354. Correct spelling is very important in medical documents because the difference of a letter or two may change the meaning of the word and, consequently, the report. Which of the following resources can be used to verify spelling?

A. medical dictionary

B. computer dictionary with added list of troublesome words

C. English dictionary

D. *Physician's Desk Reference*

E. all of the above

(Kinn and Woods, pp 143–144)

355. Which of the following is a general term describing any inflammation of the integumentary system (skin)?

A. dermatitis

B. impetigo

C. dermatosis

D. psoriasis

E. urticaria

(Brooks and LaFleur, pp 22-23; Thibodeau and Patton #2, pp 120–122)

356. The diseases of genital warts, gonorrhea, Hepatitis B, trichomoniasis, and AIDS are

A. degenerative diseases

B. autoimmune diseases

C. sexually transmitted diseases (STDs)

D. inherited diseases

E. salmonella infections

(Thibodeau and Patton #2, pp 529–530)

357. The abbreviation meaning "four times a day" is

A. qid

B. qd

C. q2h

D. qs

E. qsuff

(Willis, p 499)

358. The abbreviation for "twice a day" is
    A. bid
    B. hs
    C. tid
    D. ac
    E. od
    (Willis, p 498)

359. AS pertains to the
    A. left ear
    B. right eye
    C. nose
    D. arm
    E. right leg
    (Willis, p 498)

360. The symbol s̄ means
    A. saline
    B. single
    C. water
    D. without
    E. pulse
    (Willis, p 499)

361. The abbreviation for "repeat once if urgently needed" or "if necessary" is
    A. rept
    B. rre
    C. qv
    D. +R
    E. SOS
    (Chabner, p 840)

362. CA or Ca is an abbreviation for
    A. costovertebral angle
    B. cerebrovascular accident
    C. cancer
    D. college ability test
    E. caffeine
    (Chabner, p 836)

363. Abnormally white skin is
    A. leukemia
    B. leukocyte
    C. leukoderma
    D. cyanoderma
    E. xanthoderma
    (Chabner, p 569; Miller and Keane, p 913)

364. Blueness of the extremities is
    A. acrocyanosis
    B. acromegaly
    C. cyanoderma
    D. cyanosis
    E. acrodermatitis
    (Taber's, p 28)

Forming plurals in medical terminology is more involved than in standard English. Many medical terms originated from Greek or Latin and follow the rules of these languages. Some words (e.g., virus, viruses) are changed to the plural form using English rules. Therefore, medical terms must be considered individually, and a medical dictionary should be used until the singular/plural forms are learned (and added to the computer speller).

The following list contains a partial listing of the rules.

1. For singular words ending in -a, keep the -a and add -e for the plural form.
2. For singular words ending in -ax, drop the -ax and add -aces for the plural form.
3. For singular words ending in -ex, drop the -ex and add -ices for the plural form.
4. For singular words ending in -ix, drop the -ix and add -ices for the plural form.
5. For singular words ending in -is, drop the -is and add -es for the plural form.
6. For singular words ending in -ma, drop the -ma and add -mata for the plural form.
7. For singular words ending in -on, drop the -on and add -a for the plural form.

8. For singular words ending in -um, drop the -um and add -a for the plural form.

9. For singular words ending in -us, drop the -us and add -i for the plural form.

10. For singular words ending in -y, drop the -y and add -ies for the plural form.

11. For singular words ending in -anx, drop the -anx and add -anges for the plural form.

DIRECTIONS (Questions 365 through 386): For the following words, indicate which singular/plural ending from the answer key best applies and note its number as your answer. Also write the correct plural or singular form in the blank space provided.

Questions 365 through 386. Change the singular term to the plural term.

365. _____ bursa

366. _____ metastasis

367. _____ thorax

368. _____ diverticulum

369. _____ nucleus

370. _____ phalanx

371. _____ ovum

372. _____ sarcoma

373. _____ apex

374. _____ ganglion

375. _____ cervix

376. _____ biopsy

Questions 377 through 386. Provide the singular form of the plural medical term.

377. _____ prostheses

378. _____ ova

379. _____ nuclei

380. _____ vertebrae

381. _____ spermatozoa

382. _____ bacteria

383. _____ arteries

384. _____ diagnoses

385. _____ corneae

386. _____ lumina

DIRECTIONS (Questions 387 through 401): Each of the numbered items or incomplete statements in this section is followed by answers or by completions of the statement. Select the ONE lettered answer or completion that is BEST in each case.

---

387. Which word element(s) describes structures or conditions in the oral area?
   A. cheilos
   B. glossa
   C. stoma
   D. lingua
   E. all of the above
   (Willis, p 497)

388. Medical terms relating to the digestive system often are constructed according to the sequence in which food passes through the system. Which of the following sequences is/are correct?
    A. mouth, pharynx, stomach, jejunum, ileum, cecum, sigmoid colon, rectum
    B. ileum, jejunum, cecum, sigmoid colon, rectum
    C. mouth, ileum, pharynx, stomach, cecum, sigmoid colon, rectum
    D. sigmoid colon, descending colon, transverse colon, ascending colon, rectum
    E. mouth, cecum, ileum, jejunum, rectum
    (Chabner, p 134)

389. Muscle weakness on one side of the body is
    A. hemiataxia
    B. hemiplegia
    C. hemidiaphoresis
    D. hemiparesis
    E. none of the above
    (Miller and Keane, p 717)

390. Pus in the pleural cavity is
    A. pyorrhea
    B. pyothorax
    C. pleural effusion
    D. pyopneumothorax
    E. none of the above
    (Rice, p 304)

391. A disease characterized by extensive bone destruction could be described by the medical term
    A. osteitis deformans
    B. osteometry
    C. mastectomy
    D. osteoma
    E. all of the above
    (Memmler et al, p 93; Taber's, p 1364)

392. Creating a new connection between segments of an organ is called
    A. diastasis
    B. cystostomy
    C. tenodesis
    D. anastomosis
    E. a Papanicolaou smear
    (Rice, p 238)

393. An abnormal accumulation of fluid in the peritoneal cavity is
    A. edema
    B. intussusception
    C. melena
    D. ascites
    E. all of the above
    (Rice, p 192)

394. Which of the following organs are part of the endocrine system?
    A. pancreas
    B. thyroid gland
    C. ovaries and testes
    D. adrenal gland
    E. all of the above
    (Thibodeau and Patton #1, pp 51–52)

395. A suffix meaning "condition or state of" is
    A. -sis
    B. -esis
    C. -osis
    D. -ia
    E. all of the above
    (Willis, p 496)

396. Organs in the abdominal cavity include the
    A. intestines
    B. stomach
    C. gallbladder
    D. pancreas
    E. all of the above
    (Thibodeau and Patton #1, p 8)

397. Which of the following are common medical abbreviations?
    A. DPT
    B. BP
    C. F
    D. CPR
    E. all of the above
    (Keir et al, pp 770–772)

398. Which of the following can result from improper use of a laser light?
    A. burn
    B. fire
    C. inhalation of plume
    D. electrical hazards related to high-wattage equipment
    E. all of the above
    (Keir et al, pp 92–96)

399. A surgical opening into a fallopian tube is a/an
    A. oophorectomy
    B. oophorotomy
    C. salpingectomy
    D. salpingostomy
    E. hysterectomy
    (Miller and Keane, p 1437)

400. Which of the following specific body regions is found in the appendicular portion of the body's skeleton?
    A. thoracic region
    B. patella
    C. vertebral column
    D. cranium
    E. none of the above
    (Keir, pp 270–271; Thibodeau and Patton #1, pp 87, 94–99)

401. The term "stat" means
    A. immediately
    B. a verbal order

    C. a placebo
    D. a signature
    E. surgery
    (Frew et al, p 560)

STUDY HINTS

1. Read the Test-Taking Strategies section in the front of this book and follow its directions to maximize your study. Also refer to the CD accompanying this book for glossary terms, anatomy illustrations, and sample tests. Study the illustrations to learn the major body structures.

2. Acquire a personal medical library for personal reference as well as for review for this examination. Begin with a medical dictionary. Look up the medical terms that you do not understand. You also will need a medical assisting textbook.

3. Medical science is much easier to learn if you understand the vocabulary. In turn, medical terminology is easier to master when broken into smaller parts. Instead of just memorizing the terms, divide them into smaller parts. Sort the word components into categories. Then review the different categories by easy methods such as creating flash cards and studying them in your spare time, recording the word forms on audiotape and playing them back, or having someone review the terms with you. A medical terminology textbook will make reviewing medical terms easier.

   Read complex medical terms from *right* to *left*. Example: Cardi/o/megaly, reading from right to left, means enlargement of the heart. Prefixes are to the left and suffixes to the right of the word.

   Following is a brief list of some of the most common medical terminology word parts. A medical dictionary or textbook should be consulted for a more complete list.

PREFIXES

Size

macr/o- = large

mega-, megalo- = very large; also 1 million

micro- = very small; also one-millionth

mini- = small

Quantity

a-, an- = without

diplo- = double

hemi-, semi- = half

hyper- = greater than normal

hypo- = less than normal

nulli- = none

penia- = deficiency

super- = excessive

ultra- = excessive or beyond

Numbers

mono-, uni- = one

bi- = two or twice

centi- = one hundredth (0.01)

di- = two or twice

poly- = many

tetra-, quadri- = four

tri- = three

Directions

ab- = from

ad- = to

anter/o- = toward the front, ventral

cephal/o- = toward the head

crani/o- = skull

epi- = on, upon

infer/o- = below

later/o- = nearer the side farther from the midline

medi/o- = middle or nearer middle

peri- = around

post- = behind or after

poster/o- = toward the back, dorsal

pre- = before or ahead of

proxim/o- = nearest point of attachment

retro- = backward

sub- = below, under

supra- = location above or over

trans- = across

ventr/o- = belly side; in humans same as ventral

Colors

albin/o- = white

chlor/o- = green

chrom/o- = color

cyan/o- = blue

erythr/o- = red

leuk/o- = white

melan/o- = black

rub- = red

xanth/o- = yellow

Surgical Suffixes

-centesis = puncture

-clasis = surgical fracture of a bone

-ectomy = excision (removal)

-lysis = destruction

-pexy = fixation

-plasty = repair

-scope = instrument for viewing or with a light

-scopy = visual examination

-stomy = forming an artificial opening

-tome = cutting instrument

-tomy = incision

-tripsy = crushing

Suffixes Describing Diagnosis and Symptoms

-algia = pain

-dynia = pain

-ia = condition

-iac = one who suffers from a condition

-iasis = condition

-ism = resembling

-itis = inflammation

-lysis = destruction or decomposition

-oid = resembling

-osis = condition

-ous = pertaining to

-pathy = disease

-stasis = stopping, controlling

Prefixes-Suffixes for Diagnosis and Symptoms

a-, an- = absent, deficient

-cele = hernia

dis- = free of, to undo

dys- = bad, difficult or painful

-ectasis = dilation or stretching

-edema = swelling

-emesis = vomiting

-lepsy = seizure

-malacia = abnormal softness

-oma = tumor

-ptosis = sagging, dropping

-rrhagia = hemorrhage

-rrhea = discharge or flow

-rrhexis = rupture

-sclerosis = hardening

-stasis = stopping, controlling

Parts of the Body

card-, cardi/o- = heart

cephalo- = head

cervi- = neck

-cyte = cell

dactyl- = fingers, sometimes toes

denti- = tooth

derm- = skin

-emia = blood

gastr- = stomach

genito- = organs of reproduction

gyn-, gyneco- = woman

hem-, hemat/o- = blood

hepato- = liver

mast-, mast/o- = breast

my-, myo- = muscle

neph-, nephr/o- = kidney

ophthalm- = eye

osteo- = bone

ot-, oto- = ear

rhin-, rhin/o- = nose

thoraco- = chest

MEDICATION ABBREVIATIONS

General

$\bar{a}$	before
aq	water
$\bar{c}$-	with
gtt	drop
noct	night
NPO	nothing by mouth
p-	after
p.r.n.	when necessary
q	every
Rx	to take
$\bar{s}$	without

Frequency

a.c.	before meals
b.i.d.	twice a day
h	hour
h. s.	at bed time (hour of sleep)
min.	minute
p.c.	after meals
q. h.	every hour
q.12h	every 12 hours
q.2h	every 2 hours
q.3h	every 3 hours
q.4h	every 4 hours
q.d.	once a day, every day
q.i.d.	four times a day
q.o.d.	every other day
t.i.d.	three times a day

Route of Administration

A.D.	right ear
A.U.	both ears
ID	intradermal
IM	intramuscular
O.D.	right eye
O.S.	left eye
O.U.	both eyes
p.o.	by mouth
SC	subcutaneous
SL	sublingual

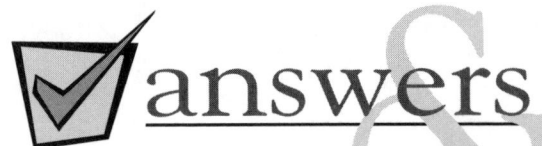

answers & rationales

1.

C. Pod- and also ped- means pertaining to the foot or feet. The term podagra (pod-, foot; -agra, excessive pain) is used to describe the effect of gouty arthritis on the big toe, a joint often affected by gout. A podiatrist is a health professional who is responsible for the condition of the feet.

2.

C. The suffix -phagia and the combining form phag/o- mean eating or ingestion. Phagocytic white cells phagocytize (engulf or ingest) microorganisms and foreign matter.

3.

B. Onycho- is a combining form that means nail, fingernail, or toenail (e.g., onychophagia means biting of the nails). Onychopathy (-pathy = disease) is any disease of the nails.

4.

A. Coreo- is a combining form that means pupil, the opening in the center of the iris of the eye. A coreometer is an instrument for measuring the diameter of the pupil. Coreoplasty is any plastic (repair) operation on the pupil.

5.

B. Omphalo- is a combining form that means umbilicus or navel. An omphalocele is a congenital hernia of the navel. Other terms regarding the navel are omphalitis (inflammation of the navel), omphaloncus (umbilical tumor or swelling), omphalorrhagia (umbilical hemorrhage), and omphalorrhexis (rupture of the navel).

6.

B. Ex- means "outside of, away from, beyond the scope of," or "in addition" (e.g., "Excise" [ex-, out; -cis/e, cut], reading from suffix forward, means to cut out or remove surgically). (Warning: Several combined word forms contain ex- as an integral part of the spelling, and it has no separate meaning in this context.)

7.

E. Antefebrile means "before fever." The prefix ante- means before, and -febrile refers to fever. Postfebrile means after fever.

8.

A. Epigastrorrhaphy is the suture of an abdominal wound in the region of the stomach (epi-, upon; gastr/o-, stomach; -rrhaphy, suture). All the possible answer choices contain the suffix -rrhaphy and describe suture of various body areas.

9.

A. An antipyretic is an agent that works against fever. Examples of antipyretics are cold packs, aspirin, and quinine. The word is dissected as anti- (against) and -pyretic (concerning fever).

10.

C. A lateral (sideways) curvature of the spine is a deformity called scoliosis. If present at birth, it is congenital scoliosis; otherwise, it is acquired. Lordosis (swayback) is another abnormality of the back where there is an abnormal anterior convexity of the spine. Kyphosis is commonly known as humpback or hunchback.

11.

B. Posterior (sometimes referred to as dorsal) means directed toward or situated at the back. The opposite term is anterior (ventral), which describes the abdominal location. The caudal area (the sacral vertebra region) is posterior to the abdomen because it is on the back or dorsal side.

12.

D. The thoracic cavity contains the heart and lungs. The combining form of the word, thorac/o-, means "chest." The abdomino-pelvic cavity contains the major organs of digestion, and the pelvic area of the cavity contains the organs of the reproductive and excretory systems. The dorsal cavity contains both the cranial and spinal cavities. The buccal cavity is the mouth.

13.

C. A disease (meaning literally dis-ease, lack of ease) defines a medical entity that can be described as a disorder of the body that has a definite group of symptoms and laboratory findings that distinguish it from other states of the body. A disease should be distinguished from the illness that describes the condition of a person who has a disease. For example: One person with the disease diabetes mellitus, IDDM, type I, may have the disease under control with only slightly elevated blood glucose, while another person with the same disease may have very high blood glucose. The disease diabetes mellitus is caused by insufficient production of insulin by the pancreas, which causes definite body symptoms such as a disturbed carbohydrate metabolism. The high level of blood glucose and also the spillage of glucose into the urine provide laboratory findings relevant to diabetes mellitus.

The word form path- (and path/o-) is a combining form that means disease or suffering. It is used with many other word forms to describe disease conditions. For example: A pathogen is a disease generator, and a pathologist is a physician specializing in the study of disease. The vocabulary of disease is varied, covering all disorders of the body that can be described. Terms describing disease are sometimes taken from many sources (e.g., names are derived from medical researchers, history, and different languages). However, standardized medical terminology originating from Latin and Greek is also used to describe the causes or symptoms of disease.

Diseases are categorized in various ways, such as by cause (e.g., infectious, genetic, environmental, occupational) or by the organ system(s) affected (e.g., lung, kidney, liver, bone, blood).

A number of word forms describe the symptoms and diagnosis of disease. Among these are the suffixes -osis, which means condition, process, or status, and -itis, which indicates infection. Several terms describe the severity of the disease (e.g., acute means severe but usually lasting a short time; chronic means less severe but continuous or recurring over long periods; subacute means intermediate, or between acute and chronic).

14.

B. Afferent nerves carry impulses toward the brain. The term afferent means conducting toward the center of a structure (Latin: af-, toward; -ferre, to bear). Efferent means conducting away from the center; therefore, efferent nerves carry impulses away from the brain and spinal cord. Afferent and efferent nerves are part of the peripheral (outside) nervous system, which connects to the brain or spinal cord.

15.

C. The cell is the basic living structural unit of the body from which tissues, organs, and organ systems are built. Tissues are formed from cells, organs from tissues, and systems from organs. Together, the organ systems form the organism. Organismic refers to the whole body and the complete organism. Cytology is the study of cells (cyt/o-, cell).

Some authorities treat the atom as the simplest structural unit of the body even though it is not living because it is the basic chemistry unit. Atoms are organized into molecular structures, which in turn are organized into cells, and so on.

16.

A. The separation of all the layers of a wound or an incision is called dehiscence. Avulsion can result from a small piece of flesh being torn away or a whole structure (as an arm). Evisceration is the spilling out of the contents as a result of dehiscence or the removal of contents from a cavity. Debridement is the removal of foreign material and dead or damaged tissue, especially in a wound. These complex terms are used when it is important to exactly describe the condition of the wound for the purpose of treatment.

17.

A. A cicatrix, or scar, is composed of epithelium, fibrous tissue, and blood cells. Collagen is a fibrous, insoluble protein found in connective tissue, including skin, bone, ligaments, and cartilage.

18.

C. Cyanoderma is a bluish discoloration of the skin. The word is formed from the combining form, or root, cyan/o-, meaning blue, and the combining form or root, -derma, meaning skin. In medical terminology, when two words, or a prefix and suffix, are combined to form a medical term, the vowel, o, is used between them if the second word begins with a consonant. This makes the term easier to pronounce. Many medical terms consist of a combination of words.

The color of body structures may provide important diagnostic information. Note in the study hints (pp. 45–47) that color is denoted by a variety of prefixes in medical terminology.

19.

D. Megalocardia (or cardiomegaly) is enlargement of the heart. The root cardi- means heart and megal/-o- means great size. Note that the term was constructed from the name of a body structure (the heart) and its condition, in this case, its size. All the answer selections are combinations of the root cardi- and describe the heart or its functions. Note that only one term, megalocardia, among the possible choices used the vowel, o, in the combined word form. Size is indicated in medical prefixes (e.g., the prefixes micro- and mini- mean small; megalo- means very large and macro- means large).

20.

D. Hypotension is low blood pressure (hypo- means low, -tension refers to pressure). The term hyper- (high) tension refers to high blood pressure.

Regarding the other answers: Bradycardia is an abnormally slow pulse rate. Cyanosis is a bluish discoloration of the skin due to lack of oxygen. Diastolic pressure exerts the least amount of pressure and systolic pressure the maximum pressure on the arterial walls during recording of the blood pressure.

21.

C. An encephalocele is a herniation (protrusion) of brain or neural tissue from its natural cavity through a defect in the skull. The prefix en- (within) and the root word cephal/o- (head) attached to the suffix -cele (hernia) is read from the suffix forward to mean, literally, hernia within the head. Since the suffix -oma means tumor, the term encephaloma means a tumor of the brain, and encephalosthenia means weakness (asthenia) of the head. Encapsulation is enclosure in a sheath or capsule not normal to the part.

22.

D. Malacia is a combining word meaning softening. Osteomalacia is a condition of the bones where they are not as rigid as they should be and the person may have rickets as a result. Also listed in the possible answer choices are other combining forms: arthr/o- = joint; chondr/o- = cartilage; dent/o- = tooth; and scler/o- = hard.

23.

A. Arthro- is the combining form for joint and can be combined with suffixes describing surgery or condition. Arthrocentesis is a term meaning a surgical procedure performed on a joint (-centesis, surgical puncture of a joint cavity with aspiration of fluid). Other combining forms are chondr/o- (cartilage), cost/o- (rib), and aden/o- (gland). Lists of medical combining forms and their definitions can be found in numerous sources, such as textbooks and medical dictionaries. Note that they are more easily learned by category.

24.

B. A combining form meaning development (growth) is -trophy (or -troph/o-) (e.g., atrophy means an absence of growth or a wasting away). Dystrophy (as in muscular dystrophy) means a bad kind of growth. The combining form -stasis means controlling, -stomy means new mouth, -tomy means incision or cutting, and -ptosis means drooping or sagging as in visceroptosis.

25.

D. A combining form meaning formation or plastic repair is -plasty (e.g., cranioplasty is a plastic (repair) operation on the skull). Other combining forms listed are myel/o- meaning spinal cord or bone marrow, -dactyly meaning fingers or toes, -dromy meaning running, and -plasia meaning development or growth.

26.

C. Craniotomy is an incision into the skull. Note that all possible selections contained the combining form, crani-, meaning cranium or skull. All had suffixes that described a condition or procedure relating to the cranium. Craniectomy means excision of a segment of the skull, cranioplasty means any plastic (molding) surgery on the skull, craniomalacia means abnormal softening of the skull, and craniopathy means a disease of the skull.

27.

B. Hydrotherapy is the use of water in treating disease, either internal or external. Swirling water baths are a form of hydrotherapy (hydro-, water; -therapy, treatment). Note that all the selections contain the word therapy. (Therapeutic meaning "to practice a healing art" is a word containing the combining form, therap-.) The prefixes of the answer selections indicated the type of therapy (thermo = heat; sero = serum; shock uses electricity). Hydrosudotherapy is treatment by both sweating (sudo- = sweat) and water (hydro-).

28.

D. Adhesion (adhes-, stick together, cling to) is the term that describes the sticking and healing together of tissues. It comes from the same root word as adhesive, adherent, and adhere. The prefix ad- meaning "to" is the opposite of the prefix ab- meaning "from" as in abduction.

29.

E. When a discharge from the sinuses takes place through the nose, the term used is rhinorrhea. The word rhinorrhea (rhin/o-, nose; -rrhea, flow, discharge) means discharge from the nose. Otorrhea means discharge from the ear (ot/o-, hearing or ear). Note the suffix -rrhea is used with different prefixes to denote different medical disorders where flowing is a symptom and results in a discharge.

30.

B. Excision of the gallbladder is termed cholecystectomy, meaning literally gallbladder removal. The other surgical procedure commonly performed on the gallbladder is cholecystostomy (meaning literally gallbladder incision), in which an incision is made for the purpose of drainage.

31.

B. Otitis media is inflammation of the middle ear and occurs most frequently in infants and young children. The condition may be acute or chronic and often accompanies or follows a respiratory infection. Otitis media is dissected into the following word forms: ot/o-, ear; -itis, inflammation; and -media, middle. Note that possible selections including the -itis suffix include rhinitis (inflammation of the nose) and cystitis (inflammation of the bladder). The suffix, -itis, is one of the most common in medical terminology and is attached to many terms describing a body structure to indicate inflammation or infection.

32.

C. Thoracocentesis is a word meaning surgical tapping of the chest to remove fluids. The term is also spelled thoracentesis. The word, thoracocentesis, is a combined word form: thorac/o-, chest; -centesis, surgical puncture to remove fluid. The other terms are combined words containing the word form thorac/o-, which refers to the chest. Therefore, together they pertain to either a procedure or a condition of the chest.

Note that the suffix -centesis describes a surgical procedure. Refer to the study hints for other suffixes that describe surgery.

33.

C. Pyorrhea is a disease symptomized by the flow of pus and often refers to infections of the periodontal area. It is a combined word form that dissects into py/o- (pus) and -rrhea (flow or discharge). The prefix pyo- is used with many other medical word forms to denote pus formation in different body structures.

34.

E. The term pyogenic means pus forming (pyo- = pus; -genic = producing or forming). The term most commonly refers to bacteria that are phagocytized by white blood cells, resulting in pus that forms boils. Foreign bodies in the body may also cause pus. A similar term is "purulent," which means forming or containing pus. The other answer terms also have the suffix, -genic, which means to produce or form. Hematogenic is blood forming, oncogenic means tumor forming, ankylogenic means adhesion forming, and pyrogenic means fever producing.

35.

D. A melanoma is a darkly pigmented cancer, as indicated by analysis of the combined word form naming it. Melan/o- is a combining form for black, and -oma is tumor. Therefore, the name signifies a black, cancerous tumor. The other possible answer choices all contain the suffix -oma, signifying some type of tumor, and describe various tumor types.

36.

A. Accumulation of air or gas in the pleural, or chest, cavity, resulting in a collapse of the lung on the affected side, is called pneumothorax. The term is a combined word form. Pneum/o- means air, and -thorax means chest.

37.

D. Cystorrhagia is a hemorrhage of the bladder, as indicated by the word components in the combined word form of the term. Cyst/o- means bladder; -rrhagia means hemorrhage. These individual word forms may combine with other word forms to describe other conditions of the bladder (cyst/o-) or hemorrhages of other tissues (-rrhagia).

38.

A. Blepharorrhaphy means the suturing of the eyelids. The term is a combined word form dissected into blephar/o- meaning eyelid and -rrhaphy meaning suture. Each of these word forms can be combined individually with other word forms to describe other conditions.

39.

E. Making a new opening between the ureter and bladder is ureterocystostomy. The term is dissected into the following parts: ureter/o- meaning ureter, cyst/o- meaning bladder, and -stomy meaning formation of an opening. These word forms can be combined individually with other word forms to create other medical terms to describe other conditions and procedures.

40.

D. Enlargement of the kidney is nephromegaly. The term is dissected into nephr/o- meaning kidney and -megaly meaning enlargement. Note that all the other answer choices begin with the combining form, nephr/o-, followed by another combining form or word that describes a condition of the kidney. These other suffixes may be used with other organ names to describe other conditions (e.g., acromegaly: acro-, extremities; -megaly, enlargement).

41.

E. The renal pelvis serves as a collecting funnel for the urine in each kidney, and the urine is then passed through the two ureters into the bladder and stored until urination. The renal pelvis is the expanded proximal end of the ureter (nearest the kidney) that lies within the renal sinus of the kidney and receives the urine through the major calyces.

42.

B. A prolapse of the uterus is called hysteroptosis. The term is dissected as follows: hyster/o-, uterus, and -ptosis, sagging. Prolapse is a falling or dropping down of an organ or internal part, such as the uterus or rectum. Note in the possible answers that several of the terms contain the word form -ptosis, indicating sagging of the indicated organ.

43.

A. Lipolysis is the splitting up of, or the destruction or breakdown of, fat. The term dissects into the following combined word form: lip/o- means fat and -lysis means process of destroying. Note that the suffix -lysis was in all of the possible answer choices and denotes destruction of the tissue denoted in the attached word form.

44.

C. Polyarthritis is the inflammation of many joints. The term dissects as follows: poly- means many, arthr- means joint, and -itis means inflammation. Note that the prefix poly- describes a number. See the study hints for other number designations.

45.

A. Synergetic is a term meaning "working together." It is dissected as follows: syn- means joined together, -erg/e means work, and -tic means pertaining to.

46.

B. Abnormal largeness of the fingers or toes is called macrodactylia. The term is dissected as follows: macro- means large, -dactyl means digits (fingers or toes), and -ia denotes condition. Note that more than one medical term can have similar but more precise meanings (e.g., phalanges are the bones of the fingers and toes).

47.

D. Diathermy means generating heat through tissues. Diathermy involves the use of high-frequency electric current for therapeutic or surgical purposes. It requires special care in its use, since severe burns may occur from improper usage.

48.

E. A myelocele is a herniation (protrusion) of the spinal cord through a defect in the vertebral column. The term is dissected as follows: myel/o- refers to either the spinal cord or bone marrow; -cele means hernia. Note that a word form with very similar spelling, my/o-, means muscle and can be confusing.

49.

E. The surgical crushing of a nerve is neurotripsy. The term dissects as follows: neur/o- = nerve; -tripsy = surgical crushing. Note that all the possible answer choices had the word form, neur/o- or neur- with various other terms attached to indicate different procedures or conditions.

50.

D. Prodrome is a term used to indicate symptoms of an approaching disease. The term dissects into the word forms: pro- = before and -drome = running (as in the disease running its course). Contrast the term prodrome with the term syndrome, which dissects into word parts that mean "running together" and defines a set of symptoms describing a current disorder.

51.

A. The medical term for a large tongue (a congenital disorder) is macroglossia. The term dissects as follows: macro- means large, -gloss- means tongue, and -ia means condition. The term for an abnormally small tongue is microglossia.

52.

D. Gingivitis indicates inflammation of the gums. The term dissects as follows: gingiv- means gums, -itis means inflammation.

53.

B. Incontinence occurs when the excretory functions cannot be controlled. Incontinence may refer to either urinary or bowel function. Urinary incontinence can be divided into several types, such as: functional, which is due to impairment of physical or cognitive functioning; stress incontinence as in sneezing or coughing; and total incontinence. Enuresis is a similar term which refers to bed wetting.

54.

B. Tachy- is a prefix meaning fast or rapid and is used to describe a rapid heart rate in the word "tachycardia." Contrast this word with the word bradycardia, meaning an abnormally slow pulse.

55.

A. Brady- is a prefix meaning slow, the opposite of tachy-, meaning fast. Bradycardia is an abnormally slow pulse, and tachycardia is an abnormally fast pulse. Note the word form, card- = heart and the suffix, -ia = condition of.

56.

D. Stomato- is a combining form meaning mouth. This may be confused with the ordinary English usage for stomach. Stomach in medical terminology is the combining form gastr- as in the words gastric and gastroenteritis.

57.

D. A combining form for speech is phas/o-. Aphasia, for example, describes a person who is speechless; tachyphasia means abnormally fast speech.

58.

B. As a suffix, -clysis means irrigation. It is also used to mean the infusion of fluid into tissue or a body cavity, such as an enema (e.g., cystoclysis is irrigation of the bladder). The suffix -clysis has a very similar spelling to -lysis (destruction) but a very different meaning. Therefore, caution should be taken to distinguish between them.

59.

C. Hepat/o- is a combining form meaning liver. Hepatitis is inflammation of the liver. Hepatotherapy is treatment of liver disease. Note in the examples given that the /o- is added between the combining forms when the second word form does not start with a vowel but is omitted if the suffix begins with a vowel. This creates an easier flowing pronunciation of the words.

60.

B. A suffix meaning crushing is -tripsy. Neurotripsy is the surgical crushing of a nerve. Vasotripsy is the surgical crushing of a blood vessel. Lithotripsy is the crushing of a kidney or bladder calculus or stone.

61.

D. Diplo- means double and is found in the word meaning double vision, diplopia. Another example is Diplococcus, a genus of gram-positive bacteria that occur in pairs.

62.

E. Cheilo- is a combining form that means lip. Cheilorrhaphy is the repair of a cleft lip. Cheilophagia is the habit of biting one's own lip (-phagia, to eat). Cheiloplasty is plastic surgery of the lips. Cheilosis is the dry scaling and breaking open of the lips and angles of the mouth, possibly due to riboflavin deficiency. Cheilotomy is an incision of the lips.

63.

B. Kinesio- is a combining form that means movement. Kinesioneurosis is a function disorder marked by tics and spasms. Kinesiotherapy is therapeutic exercise. Kinesiology is the study of the movement of body parts.

64.

E. Litho- means stone or calculus. Lithotripsy makes use of this word component to describe the crushing of calculi in the bladder or urethra. Lithonephritis is inflammation of the kidney due to a calculus (stone). A lithoscope is an instrument for examining calculi in the bladder.

65.

A. Py/o- is a combining form that means pus. Some examples using this combining form are pyogenic (pus forming) and pyocele (a collection of pus). Note the similar word forms that may be confusing in the other possible answer choices: pyel/o-, renal pelvis; pub/o-, pubis; phil/o-, attraction; and pyr/o-, fire or fever.

66.

D. Centesis is a word element meaning puncture. Combined with other word roots, it describes the puncture of organs and tissues to aspirate fluid. Cardiocentesis is surgical puncture of the heart, and thoracocentesis is the surgical puncture of the chest cavity to aspirate fluid.

67.

A. Ot/o- is a combining form meaning ear. One example is otoencephalitis, meaning inflammation of the brain due to extension from an inflamed middle ear. An otologist is a specialist in otology, the branch of medicine dealing with the ear and its anatomy, physiology, and pathology. An otoscope is a lighted instrument used to examine the ear.

68.

B. Ad- means toward. Do not confuse this prefix (ad-) with the prefix (ab-), meaning the opposite or away from. Examples of the prefix ad- are adrenal (added to the kidney), indicating location of the adrenal glands, and adhesive meaning to stick or adhere to. The term adduction means to draw toward the middle, whereas the term abduction means to draw away from the middle.

69.

C. Dactylo- is a combining form that means fingers or toes. Examples are the words dactylitis (inflammation of fingers or toes) and dactylospasm (cramp or twitching of the fingers or toes). A related term is phalanx (pl. phalanges), which is a bone of a toe or finger.

70.

B. The color blue is expressed by the combining form cyan/o-. Cyanosis is an abnormal bluish discoloration of the skin and indicates a lack of adequate oxygen. Other terms denoting color are melan/o-, black; leuk/o-, white; xanth/o-, yellow; and erythr/o-, red.

71.

A. Men/o- is a combining form that means menses, menstruation, or month. The term "menopause" denotes the permanent cessation of menstruation. Menorrhagia is excessive bleeding during the menstrual period. Menorrhea is normal menstruation.

72.

E. Xanth/o- is yellow. Examples are the terms xanthoderma from xanth/o- meaning yellow and -derm/a meaning skin (a yellow coloration of the skin) and xanthochromia derived from the word forms xanth/o- meaning yellow and -chromia meaning color (any yellow discoloration of the skin or spinal fluid).

73.

B. Hidro- is a combining form that means sweat (e.g., hyperhidrosis is excessive sweating). Do not confuse this word form hidr/o-, meaning sweat (perspiration), with the similar word form, hydr/o-, meaning water.

74.

D. Anabolism is the constructive putting together phase of metabolism. (The term, anabole, means building up; -ism means condition.) In an anabolistic reaction in the body, simple compounds derived from nutrients are converted into complex, organized matter usable by the body cells. Catabolism is the breaking down phase of metabolism by the cells that releases energy (Gr. katabole = casting down; -ism = condition). Metabolism is defined as the sum total of all the chemical reactions of the body. Anabolism and catabolism are the two stages of metabolism.

75.

A. The suffix -emia refers to blood. Examples are leukemia, a progressive malignant disease of the blood-forming organs involving the leukocytes of the blood, and polycythemia, an increase in the total mass of the blood. Anemia literally means lack of blood; however, the term has come to have a more precise meaning relating to the ability of the blood to supply oxygen to tissue through the red blood cells and hemoglobin.

76.

E. Stasis means stoppage, as a stoppage of the flow of blood or other body fluid or of intestinal contents. Hemostasis (hem/o-, blood; -stasis, stoppage) is the checking of the flow of blood or interruption of blood flow through any vessel. Enterostasis (enter/o-, intestine; -stasis, stoppage) is the stopping of food in its passage through the intestine.

77.

E. Colp/o- means vagina (e.g., colp/o/scope, a speculum for examining the vagina and cervix by means of a magnifying lens; colp/o/rrhaphy, suture of the vagina). The word form vagin- (meaning sheath) also is used to create words pertaining to the vagina as in vaginitis meaning inflammation of the vagina.

78.

C. Necr/o- is a combining form referring to death. Examples of words using the word form necr/o- are necropsy, another term for autopsy, and necrosis, meaning death of tissue.

79.

C. Ectopic means misplaced. The term is often used in connection with an ectopic pregnancy, in which the fertilized ovum becomes implanted outside the uterus, commonly in the fallopian tube. An ectopic heartbeat is irregular or abnormal.

80.

C. Home/o- and homo- mean the same. The opposite of homo- is hetero-, which means different. Examples are homozygous, meaning having two genes of the same kind for the same trait, and heterozygous, meaning having two genes of different kinds for the same trait. A blue-eyed person is homozygous for blue eyes.

Another important term using the word form, homeo-, is homeostasis (homeo- = same; -stasis = standing). The body maintains homeostasis, or equilibrium, to stay healthy in the face of external and internal change. The body accomplishes this by the processes of feedback and regulation by the hormonal and other body systems.

81.

B. Crypt/o- means hidden. Cryptopodia is swelling of the lower leg and foot, covering all but the sole. Cryptorchidism is the state of hidden (undescended) testicles, the result of the failure of the testicle(s) to descend from their fetal position in the abdomen near the kidneys.

82.

D. An oncologist is concerned with neoplasms, or new growths (tumors), especially with cancerous tissue. Tumors are either benign (nonmalignant with controlled growth) or malignant (cancerous) with growth that is uncontrolled and progressive. "Neoplasm" (meaning new form) is sometimes used interchangeably with the term cancer.

83.

D. The prolapse or downward displacement of the viscera or organs is called visceroptosis. Another term for the same definition is splanchnoptosis. (Splanchna is a Greek term for the intestine or viscera.)

84.

B. A medical term that means blushing is erythroderma (erythro/o-, red; -derma, skin). The other selections all include the word form -derma and have descriptive word forms attached that denote other colors.

85.

A. Pyrexia means fever. Synonyms are fever and febrile. Pyretic and pyrectic are terms meaning "pertaining to fever."

86.

E. A combining form that means "abdominal wall" is laparo-, hence the term, laparotomy, meaning a surgical opening of the abdomen or an abdominal operation. The term laparorrhaphy means suture of the abdominal wall. A laparoscope is used to examine the peritoneal cavity.

87.

E. Anorexia is a sustained loss of appetite and is seen in malaise, illnesses, drug addiction, alcoholic excesses, and other conditions.

88.

B. Suprarenal means "above the kidney" (supra-, above; -renal, kidney). Suprarenal gland is a synonym meaning the same as adrenal gland.

89.

A. Malaise (from French) means discomfort, uneasiness, or indisposition, often indicative of infection. (Note: Not all medical terms are derived from combining word forms of Greek or Latin. There are exceptions.)

90.

A. Abduction means "moving away" from a midline, whereas adduction means "moving toward" a midline. An abductor muscle draws a part away from the median plane of the body or axial line of an extremity. Abduction of a limb in physical therapy is the movement away from the axis or median plane.

91.

C. A word that means "self-destructing" is autolysis (auto-, self; -lysis, destruction). The prefix auto- is a very common one meaning self and is used in both medical terms and everyday English. Lysis is used as an independent word and as a suffix, in both cases meaning destruction.

92.

C. Anteversion means the "turning forward" or tipping of an organ as a whole, without bending. Note the very similar spelling and, therefore, the possibility of confusing the prefix ante- with anti- which means against. The word version used alone means turning and, with modifying terms, describes the different positions a fetus is turned during delivery for a better presentation at birth. The term retro means turning backwards.

93.

B. Retrosternal means "behind the sternum." The prefix retro- means behind (e.g., retrolingual means behind the tongue). Retroflexion is the bending of an organ so that its top is bent backward; often used to describe the backward bending of the uterus upon the cervix.

94.

B. A word that means "inflammation of tissues near the vagina" is paracolpitis. Pericolpitis has the same meaning. Analysis of word form: para- = beyond; colp- = vagina; and -itis = inflammation.

95.

B. Low blood sugar is hypoglycemia, meaning that there is an abnormally low level of glucose in the blood (hypo- = low; glyc/o- = glucose; -emia = condition of blood). The condition may result from varying causes, and specific treatment depends on the primary cause. The prefix hypo- means low; the prefix hyper- has the opposite meaning, high.

96.

B. Con- means with. Other prefixes that also mean with include com-, sym-, and syn-. A prefix with a very similar spelling but with an opposite meaning is contra-, meaning "against."

97.

B. Dis- means free of, reversal, or separation. (Example: disintegration) Dys- means painful or difficult. (Example: dysmenorrhea is painful menstruation.) Do not confuse the two similar spellings.

98.

A. The prefix epi- means on or upon. The epidermis is the outermost, nonvascular layer of the skin. An epizoon is an external animal parasite.

99.

C. Ankylo- means stiff. It may also mean bent, crooked, in the form of a loop, or adhesion. Ankylodactylia means adhesion of the fingers or toes to one another. Ankylosis is a term meaning the immobility of a joint.

100.

B. Carpo- is a combining form meaning wrist. The term carp/o/phalangeal pertains to the carpus (wrist joint) and phalanges (fingers). Carpal tunnel syndrome, an occupational disease affecting the wrist, is caused by stress or overuse.

101.

A. The anatomic position is assumed when a person stands upright facing the viewer with arms at the sides, palms forward. The body planes and positions are always described as if the patient were in the anatomic position, although the patient is examined in various positions. This avoids the uncertainty and error that would occur if the planes and directions were not related to one position.

102.

A. Dorsal and posterior are terms that refer to locations nearer the back. The terms ventral and anterior indicate locations near the belly surface or front of the body. The frontal plane divides the back from the front of the body.

Locations on or in the body may be described in many ways. The designation depends on what term the doctor believes is best. In addition to planes, location may be described in the following ways: regions (e.g., abdominal region); distance from the patient's head (e.g., cranial, cephalic); distance from the tail (e.g., sacral vertebra); nearness to the surface (e.g., superficial); distance from the centerline of the body or organ (e.g., lateral); distance from point of reference or attachment (e.g., proximal or distal); above (superior) or below (inferior); and front (ventral) or back (dorsal).

103.

B. The frontal plane divides the body from head to feet into front (ventral) and back (dorsal) sections. It is sometimes called the "coronal plane." The body is divided by three chief imaginary planes for purposes of identifying locations: the frontal plane (front from back), the transverse plane (top from bottom), and the sagittal plane (left from right). (Actually, the CT scan and other devices may image the body into many different planes (slices) for the purpose of diagnosis or treatment.)

104.

D. Lateral means to the side of a body or structure. Therefore, lateral parts are farthest from the midsagittal plane, which splits the body down the center, top to bottom, into the left and right portions. The little toe is lateral to the big toe because it is farther from the midsagittal plane (middle) of the body.

105.

C. Caudal means "away from the head," whereas cephalic or cephalad mean "pertains to the head" (cranial refers to the skull). A similar term, superior, pertains to a structure that is higher than an inferior (lower) structure in the anatomic position of the body, the position always used for reference. Therefore, the organs nearer the head (e.g., thyroid) are superior in position to those (e.g., intestines) nearer the caudal

region. These regions may be divided by transverse (horizontal) planes.

106.

B. Dorsal refers to the back of the body, whereas ventral refers to the front of the body or belly surface. These two regions are divided by the frontal (coronal) plane. Anterior also refers to the ventral area, whereas posterior refers to the dorsal area.

107.

B. Inferior means below or lower. Therefore, in humans the caudal location (near the tail-sacral region of spine) is inferior or lower, and superior locations are above or in a higher position. The abdominal region is anterior to the spine, which is posterior to the abdominal region. (A reminder: These terms are based on the anatomic position of the body.)

108.

B. Superficial means at or near the surface (e.g., a superficial vein). The term peripheral has a similar meaning "outer part of a surface or a body or away from the center" (e.g., peripheral nervous system).

109.

A. Sagittal planes divide the body vertically into left and right portions. The midsagittal plane divides the body into equal right and left halves. This contrasts with the frontal (coronal or vertical) plane, dividing the body into front and back regions, and the transverse plane, which divides the body horizontally into top and bottom cross-sections. These are imaginary planes along which a body could be cut.

110.

D. Intermediate means "between two other structures or extremes," after the beginning and before the end. It is a combined word (inter + mediate). The term medial, from Latin, means "pertaining to the middle." This term is an example of how many complex medical terms are constructed from smaller, simpler "root words." The meaning of the large word is readily apparent when it is divided into its simpler roots.

111.

C. Retinoid means "resembling the retina." The retina is the third coat of the eyeball. The first coat is the cornea, a clear transparent layer on the front of the eyeball, and the second coat is the choroid, which contains blood vessels. The retina contains rods and cones, which are specialized cells sensitive to light.

112.

A. Pleurocentesis is the surgical puncture and drainage of the pleural cavity. The word is dissected as pleur/o-, (pleura), a serous membrane that enfolds the lungs, and -centesis, surgical puncture to remove fluid. Note that all the possible answer choices had the combined word form pleur- and, therefore, are concerned in some way with the pleura.

113.

B. A bronchial hemorrhage is bronchorrhagia. The word is dissected as bronch/o-, bronchus, or bronchial tube, and -rrhagia, bursting forth or hemorrhage. The similar suffix, -rrhea, means to flow.

114.

B. The word ending -al, or pertaining to, makes a term an adjective. Venal and arterial are the descriptive (adjective) forms of the words vein and artery. The word ending -ous makes a term an adjective, as in mucous (noun, mucus). The suffix -ic is combined with words to form adjectives that indicate some characteristic (e.g., acidic means having the quality of an acid; basic has the quality of a base).

115.

A. Pain in the trachea is trachealgia (trache-, trachea; -algia, suffering, pain). All possible answer choices had the combined word form trache- and, therefore, described the trachea in some manner.

116.

B. Thrombectomy means excision of a clot. The word dissects into thromb-, clot, and -ectomy, surgical removal.

117.

B. The abbreviations of Hib, OPV, DPT, and Hep B-1 refer to types of childhood vaccinations. Hib is short for Hemophilus influenzae type b; OPV stands for polio vaccine; DPT for the combined vaccine of diphtheria, tetanus, and pertussis (whooping cough) while Hep B-1 is for Hepatitis B. In addition to these, MMR stands for measles, mumps, and Rubella. Var is the vaccine for Varicella zoster (chickenpox).

118.

E. Neo- means new and is a combined word form found in many terms (e.g., neonate [newborn] and neoplasm [a new and abnormal formation of tissue that serves no useful function but grows at the expense of the healthy organism]). All cancers are neoplasms.

119.

C. A vasorrhaphy is the suture of the vas deferens, the excretory ducts of the testes. The word is dissected as vas/o-, vessel or duct, in this case vas deferens, and -rrhaphy, surgical suture.

120.

B. The sternum is commonly called the breastbone. It is a plate of bone forming the middle of the anterior wall of the thorax and joins with the first seven ribs. It has three parts, the manubrium, the body, and the xiphoid process.

121.

B. The acromion is located nearest to the shoulder. It is the lateral extension of the spine of the scapula (shoulder blade), forming the highest point on the shoulder. It overhangs the glenoid cavity, which articulates with the humerus to form the shoulder joint.

122.

C. Cycl/o- is a combining form for ciliary body (cycl/o-, circle, the shape of the ciliary body). An example of its use is cyclochoroiditis (inflammation of the ciliary body and the choroid). The ciliary body is the organ connecting the choroid and iris in the eye and is made up of the ciliary muscle and the ciliary processes. It alters the shape of the lens during the process of accommodation.

123.

E. Plastic surgery of the pupil is coreoplasty (core/o-, pupil; -plasty, plastic repair of). Plastic surgery in general is concerned with restoration, correction, or improvement of the shape and appearance of body structures that are defective, damaged, or misshapen.

124.

C. Lacrimal is a medical term that means "pertaining to tears." The lacrimal gland, located in the optical orbit, superior and lateral to the eyeball, secretes tears. The lacrimal bone is at the inner side of the orbital cavity.

125.

D. Inflammation of the cornea is corneitis. Keratitis also means inflammation of the cornea. The word corneitis is dissected as corn/e- = cornea and -itis = inflammation. Inflammation of the iris is iritis; of the retina, retinitis; of the sclera and iris, scleroiritis; and of the conjunctiva, conjunctivitis. Pinkeye is a contagious form of conjunctivitis often seen in physicians' offices.

126.

D. The sclera is a tough, white covering of approximately the posterior five-sixths of the eyeball, continuous anteriorly with the cornea. The Greek word element scler/o- means "hard." Scleritis is inflammation of the sclera.

127.

B. The cornea is the transparent, anterior covering of the eye, protecting the eye from foreign bodies, bacterial infection, and viral infection. Any corneal injury or infection should receive prompt treatment to avoid ulceration and loss of vision.

128.

A. Omphalorrhexis is rupture of the navel or umbilicus. It is a combined word form: omphal/o- (navel) and -rrhexis (rupture). Note that two other choices contained prefixes with similar spellings but different meanings. Combining the prefix, omphal/o- with various suffixes gives the names of various medical terms concerning the navel. Similarly, the prefix, onych/o- combined with different suffixes gives terms describing the nails.

129.

B. Abnormally profuse menstruation is menorrhagia. Among the causes of menorrhagia are pelvic inflammatory disease, uterine tumors, and abnormal conditions of pregnancy. The prefix, men/o-, refers to month. The prefix, metr/o-, refers to uterine tissue. The term metrorrhagia refers to uterine bleeding that occurs at completely irregular intervals and is sometimes prolonged.

130.

B. Rubeola is measles, a highly communicable viral disease characterized by a maculopapular eruption over the entire body, along with fever, symptoms of respiratory tract infection, and spots on the buccal mucosa. Because of public apathy toward the measles vaccine, measles epidemics still occur.

131.

A. Suppuration means the formation or discharge of pus. Two other terms meaning the formation of pus are pyogenesis and purulence.

132.

C. A bruise is a contusion, an injury to tissues without breakage of the skin. In a contusion, blood from the broken vessels accumulates in surrounding tissues, producing pain, swelling, and tenderness. A word with a similar spelling, concussion, is an injury resulting from impact with an object; a cerebral concussion is loss of consciousness due to a blow to the head.

133.

E. Congenital anomalies are physical or mental abnormalities existing at birth. They include a very wide range of disorders. Spina bifida is an incomplete development of the spine. Cleft lip is a split or nonsymmetrical development of the lip. Cleft palate has a gap along the center of the roof (palate) of the mouth due to a failure of the bones to fuse. Talipes may describe clubfoot and other various deformities of the foot and ankle. Undescended testicles are the result of one or both testes (testicles) failing to move from the abdominal cavity where they developed to the scrotum outside. This move normally occurs in late pregnancy.

134.

C. The ileum is the distal portion of the small intestine (between the jejunum and the cecum). The spelling of this term is similar and often confused with ilium, the lateral flaring portion of the hipbone.

135.

C. Varicella is commonly called chickenpox. It is caused by a herpes virus, which also may cause shingles (herpes zoster) at a later time in life. When the virus that lies dormant in the body's nerve cells emerges due to an apparent lowering of the immune defenses, the nerve endings are attacked. Shingles may be a very painful disease.

136.

E. Herpetic gingivostomatitis is a combined word form for cold sores meaning a herpes virus infection (-itis) of the gums (gingiv/o-) and the mouth (stomat-). The herpes group of viruses includes a large number of viruses that cause a number of diseases in humans, including herpes genitalis, shingles, infectious mononucleosis, and chickenpox.

137.

D. Strabismus is a condition commonly referred to as squint or crossed eyes. The various forms of strabismus are spoken of as tropias (growth), their direction being indicated by the appropriate prefix (e.g., esotropia [toward the other eye], exotropia [away from the other eye], hypertropia [upward deviation], and hypotropia [downward deviation]).

138.

A. Rubella is the medical term for German measles, also called 3-day measles. The disease is caused by a virus. The disease, most common in children 3 to 12 years of age, is usually mild, but it may cause various developmental abnormalities in fetuses of mothers who contract it during pregnancy.

139.

E. Hives is a transient vascular reaction of the skin to various causes, such as allergic reactions to food or drugs, infection, or emotional stress. Slightly elevated patches (wheals) that are redder or paler than the surrounding skin appear and may be further classified according to the causes or appearance.

140.

D. Mumps is the contagious, epidemic form of parotitis caused by the mumps virus. Parotitis is a combined word form meaning inflammation (-itis) of the parotid glands (salivary glands), located on the face in front of and slightly lower than each ear.

141.

A. The medical term for pinkeye is conjunctivitis, an inflammation of the thin membrane that covers the eyeball and lines the eyelid. It may be caused by bacteria, viruses, chemicals, or allergies. The infectious form is highly contagious and should be handled with extreme care to prevent its spread.

142.

E. Pertussis is whooping cough, an infectious disease of the respiratory tract causing peculiar bouts of coughing, ending in a prolonged whooping respiration. Because it is a serious disease, immunization is given in the DPT shots in infancy and with booster shots before entering school.

143.

B. Atresia means "without opening." Examples of atresia that are congenital in origin are found with an imperforation (abnormal closure) of the anus or esophagus, or with aortic or tricuspid atresia.

144.

C. Both -algia and -dynia mean pain. Examples are neuralgia (pain of the nerves) and cephalodynia (headache).

145.

A. A suffix meaning "disease" is -pathy. This suffix has frequent usage, being combined with many prefixes to describe diseases of various structures (e.g., adenopathy, enlargement [due to disease] of glands, especially of the lymph nodes).

146.

E. The combining form -phren/o may refer either to the diaphragm or to the mind. An example referring to the mind is schizophrenia, a broad term encompassing a large number of mental disorders. The word form schiz/o- means split or fissure. Phren/o- has the "o" dropped and -ia meaning condition is added to coin the term schizophrenia, meaning condition of a split mind or personality. An example using the diaphragm is the phrenic nerve, a motor nerve to the diaphragm with sensory fibers to the pericardium. In this case, the combining form phren- has the suffix -ic added to it (-ic is a suffix meaning "pertaining to").

147.

B. As a suffix, -tome means cutting instrument (e.g., microtomes, machines that slice sections of tissue for microscopic viewing). (Do not confuse the suffix -tome with the complete word, tome, which means an important book or one of a set of books.)

148.

E. A suffix that refers to the body is -some. The term psychosomatic is a combined word form meaning pertaining to mind and body. Psychosomatic medicine stresses the importance of mind-body interrelationships in all illnesses and their treatments.

149.

E. The suffix -tropia means "to turn" or "to react." Ectropion means eversion, or turning outward, such as the eyelid; entropion means inversion, or turning inward. Strabismus, a condition in which the eyes do not focus together, is termed heterotropia and further subdivided into -tropias, such as crossed eyes (esotropia).

150.

C. A suffix that means "to burst forth" is -rrhage. Examples of usage are in the words hemorrhage, meaning to bleed, and menorrhagia, meaning excessive bleeding at the time of a menstrual period in terms of either days or blood or both.

151.

C. The gauge (diameter) of the suture material varies from extremely fine (11-0) designated by zeros to very coarse designated by whole numbers. The sizes most often used in clinics vary from 2-0 (00) to 6-0 (000000). The 2-0 may also be written as 00. The 6-0, called six aught, might be written as 000000 although this is cumbersome. (Aught is another word for zero.) Six aught (6-0) is very fine.

Whole numbers such as 1, 2, 3, and 4 designate large diameter thread, which is coarser. From fine to coarse, the sizes commonly used in clinics would be arranged from 6-0 (six aught) very fine to 0 (one aught) medium to 4 (a whole number), which is very coarse. Sutures come in a variety of materials such as silk, cotton, catgut (actually from sheep's intestines), synthetic collagen, polyester, stainless steel, and so on. Each material has its advantage. The most important classification is absorbable versus nonabsorbable. (Catgut is absorbable.) A curved, cutting-edged atraumatic needle is most often used for suturing. The atraumatic (swaged) needle does not have an eye but is purchased continuous with the suture thread. It is generally preferred because there is no double thread thickness and therefore less tissue damage. The size of suture material is standardized by the United States Pharmacopeia. The finer the thread, the less scarring.

152.

B. The type of suture in which the surgeon ties each stitch separately is called interrupted. This interrupted stitch is used most often in the doctor's office because it offers less trauma to the tissue and is easier to remove. The uninterrupted stitch, as its name denotes, is continuous. The apposition suture is superficial and used to make an exact approximation of the cutaneous edges of the wound. The buried suture is deep in the tissues and not visible from the surface. The purse-string stitch is used to close a circular wound by drawing it together in the middle in the way that a purse string would. The blanket and mattress stitches are other types. There are many types of stitches, each best suited for a particular purpose.

___

153.

E. Plantar flexion is movement that flexes the foot toward the sole (underpart of foot) so that the forepart of the foot is lower than the ankle. The word plantar concerns the sole of the foot. Goniometers are instruments that measure joint motion and angles.

___

154.

A. Ankle movement that turns the foot inward is inversion. Eversion is ankle movement that turns the foot outward. Range of motion (ROM) exercises are important to therapy that helps restore full ROM after an injury to a joint. See the medical dictionary references for exercises for other joints.

___

155.

B. Inflammation of bone and cartilage is osteochondritis. Osteochondritis is a combined word form meaning inflammation (-itis) of the bone (oste/o-) and cartilage (chondr/o-).

___

156.

B. Gigantism, acromegaly, and dwarfism are caused by disturbances of the pituitary gland, which is part of the endocrine system. Gigantism is due to a high level of growth hormone produced by the pituitary gland before puberty; acromegaly is caused by a high level of growth hormone produced after puberty. Pituitary dwarfism is caused by a low level of growth hormone before puberty.

___

157.

C. Osteosarcoma is an example of a malignant osteogenic tumor (oste/o-, bone; -sarcoma, cancer arising from connective tissue, such as muscle or bone).

___

158.

A. Osteosclerosis is abnormal hardness of bone. This is a combined word form: oste/o- = bone; -sclerosis =

hardness). Both of these combining word forms are used with a variety of other combining forms to describe various disabilities and diseases.

___

159.

A. Arthritis, meaning literally the inflammation of the joints, is the principal group of diseases of the joints (arthr-, joint; -itis, inflammation). Arthritis is subdivided into different diseases (e.g., gouty arthritis, osteoarthritis, rheumatoid arthritis, gonorrheal arthritis). The cause of some forms of arthritis is not understood.

___

160.

A. The surgical fracture of bone to remedy a deformity is called osteoclasis (oste/o-, bone; -clasis, breaking). A similar term, osteotomy (oste/o-, bone; -tomy, incision) is the surgical cutting through of a bone.

___

161.

B. Osteoplasty (oste/o-, bone; -plasty, form) is the reconstruction or repair of bone by plastic surgery or grafting. Either of these word forms may be combined with a variety of other word forms to create other medical terms.

___

162.

D. The surgical excision of a bone or a portion of one is called ostectomy. The combined word form is oste-, bone; -ectomy, excision).

___

163.

E. The hyoid bone is a horseshoe-shaped bone situated at the base of the tongue, just above the thyroid cartilage, between the lower jaw and larynx. It supports the tongue, and certain muscles that help in moving the tongue and swallowing are attached to it.

___

164.

C. The zygomatic or malar bones form the prominence of the cheeks. They also form the lateral walls and floors of the orbits (for the eyes).

165.

C. There are seven cervical vertebrae, which form the neck and are labeled as C1 through C7 (C, cervical). There are twelve thoracic (chest) vertebrae, which form the outward curve of the back and are numbered T1 through T12 or sometimes as the dorsal vertebrae numbered D1 through D12. Below the thoracic vertebrae are five vertebrae known as the lumbar (back) vertebrae, the largest and strongest of the vertebrae, forming the inward curve of the spine, numbered L1 through L5. The sacrum, below the lumbar vertebrae, is a triangular bone, and last is the coccyx, also known as the tailbone.

166.

D. The xiphoid process is connected with the lower end of the body of the sternum (breastbone), which is the long flat bone in the middle of the front of the rib cage. The sternum, ribs, and thoracic vertebrae make up the rib cage, which encloses the thoracic cavity containing the lungs and heart.

167.

A. The bone on the outer or thumb side of the forearm is called the radius. (Remember the anatomic position, in which the thumbs are held outward.) The other, larger bone of the forearm is the ulna.

168.

E. The bones of the fingers are called phalanges, as are the bones of the toes (singular, phalanx). The phalanges of the fingers (three in each finger, the proximal, middle, and distal phalanx, and two in the thumb) are joined to the metacarpals of the hand.

169.

E. The femur is the longest and strongest bone in the skeleton. At its proximal end, it has a rounded head that fits into a depression (socket) in the hipbone to form the acetabulum joint. The femur, of necessity, is very strong, since the pressure of the entire body is transferred to it in standing or walking.

170.

A. Aponeuroses are flattened tendons attaching muscles. They serve as specialized tendons to fasten muscles to bone or sometimes as fascia to hold muscles together.

171.

E. The buccinator muscle compresses the cheeks and retracts the angles of the mouth. There are seven different muscles that perform movement around the mouth region. They are activated by facial nerve CN VII (cranial nerve VII).

172.

A. The stem cells within the bone marrow constantly undergo mitosis to produce all types of blood cells, both red and white. The stem cells' offspring differentiate into the following: red cells (erythrocytes) that contain hemoglobin and transport oxygen; thrombocytes (platelets) which promote clotting; and different types of white cells (basophils, neutrophils, eosinophils, lymphocytes, monocytes, and macrophages).

173.

A. The easiest way to know each surgical set-up when needed for a patient is to develop a procedure manual that includes all anticipated procedures including the complicated and seldom performed ones. In turn, the needed information should be transferred to 5″ x 8″ cards that are color coded for each physician. The instructions, medications, instruments used, and so on should be listed. The information should be kept current. The universal blood and body-fluid precautions should be listed for each procedure. These include personal protection barriers (masks, gloves, etc.), how the used equipment should be cleaned, and how waste is disposed of.

174.

C. Phenylketonuria (PKU) is an inherited disorder caused by defective recessive genes. Mental retardation results if it is not treated by limiting the dietary intake of phenylalanine during childhood. (PKU adults tolerate a reasonable amount of phenylalanine.) PKU must be detected in early infancy to prevent mental retardation. Therefore, Phenistix (Ames Company), a urine reagent strip, is used to monitor infant urine for this disorder. A blood test also exists for screening newborns and infants.

175.

A. The muscles are not named after persons. They are named for qualities that describe them, such as (1) location (e.g., orbicularis [circular] oris [mouth] is the circular muscle that surrounds the mouth); (2) shape (e.g., deltoid means shaped like the Greek letter delta; it forms the shoulder cap); (3) fiber direction (e.g., transversus abdominis is the transverse abdominal muscle); and (4) origin and insertion (e.g., sternoclei-domastoid originates from the sternum and clavicle and inserts into the mastoid process of the temporal bone).

176.

A. The clavicles are commonly known as the collar-bones. Referring to the other answer choices, the three types of muscle tissue are the voluntary striated skele-tal muscles, which permit us to move about; the *non-striated, involuntary, smooth muscles* found in internal organs and hollow spaces such as blood vessels; and the *cardiac muscle of the heart* with involuntary, rhyth-mic, and automatic contractions.

Each muscle receives its own nerve impulse allow-ing many varied motions. The nerve impulse signals a change of chemical energy to the mechanical energy of a muscle contraction. The fuel used is glycogen and also free fatty acids. For skeletal muscles to move, they must have attachments to the bone, by means of ten-dons or aponeuroses; to other muscles; or to the skin. Skeletal muscles act as levers in opposing groups (movers and antagonists) to perform different move-ments. Terms often used to describe body motion are flexion (bending) and extension (straightening); abduction (moving away from the body's midline) and adduction (moving toward the body's midline); rota-tion as in shaking your head "no"; forearm motions of supination (rotation to the position of the hand palms up) and pronation (rotation to the position of palms down); and foot motions of dorsiflexion (curling toes upward) and plantar flexion (standing on your toes).

177.

C. The diaphragm is a strong, dome-shaped muscle that separates the thoracic and abdominal cavities. Its contraction expands the thoracic cavity and compresses the abdominopelvic cavity thus allowing breathing. Innervation is by the phrenic nerves. Hiccups are involuntary spasms of the diaphragm.

178.

C. The deltoid (named for the triangular Greek letter Delta) muscle abducts the arm. It is assisted by the supraspinatus, subscapularis, and teres major in mov-ing the arm. It, like the other muscles attached to the skeleton, is a striated muscle so named because of the light and dark bands in the muscle fibers that create a striped (striated) appearance.

The deltoid muscle in the upper arm and the glu-teus maximus in the buttocks are the large muscle sites most commonly used to give intramuscular injections. The vastus lateralis muscle of the upper thigh is also being used.

179.

E. The biceps brachii is a muscle that flexes the fore-arm and assists in supination. It originates on the scapula (shoulder blade), and insertion is to the radius (lower arm bone). It is innervated by the radial nerve. The term "biceps" (meaning two heads) indicates it has two tendons that attach it at its origin.

180.

B. Bursitis is the painful inflammation of one or more bursa. Bursa are closed, fluid-filled sacs associated with freely movable joints. The knee has a suprapatel-lar bursa, a prepatellar bursa, and an infrapatellar bursa. Bursitis can be caused by irritation due to exces-sive friction, trauma, calcification of joints, and infec-tion. It is often named for the occupation causing the irritation, such as "housemaid's knee" or "student's elbow" (from hours of leaning on it while studying).

Olecranon bursitis is located near the elbow. The olecranon forms the prominent point of the elbow. Ischial bursitis affects the hips of workers such as truck drivers who must sit a great deal in their jobs. Subdeltoid bursitis is in the shoulder region.

181.

A. Hormones are chemical messengers that have a precise regulatory effect on certain target cells, tissues, or organs in the body. Principally, hormones consist of amino acid compounds but in the case of steroids are derived from lipids (fats). A homeostatic balance of hormones is maintained by a negative feedback mech-anism. The hormone gland tends to overproduce, and the target cells become more active and signal more strongly to the hormone secretor to curtail production of the hormone. This often creates a rhythmic effect (e.g., the adrenal gland tends to have a 24-hour cycle; the menstrual cycle is a monthly one).

The endocrine system's hormone production and the nervous system control and coordinate the systems of the body. The nervous system acts rapidly and the hormonal system more slowly. The nervous system controls the pituitary gland, the master gland of the body, which in turn controls the other endocrine glands such as the thyroid, gonads, and adrenal glands. The anterior pituitary gland releases growth hormone; thyroid stimulating hormone; prolactin (milk stimulator); FSH (promotes activity of ovaries or testes); ADH (antidiuretic hormone); and oxytocin (uterine contraction, milk produced in mammary glands).

The glands stimulated by the pituitary hormones and their secretions in turn are as follows: thyroid–thyroxine and triodothyronine to increase metabolic rate and calcitonin—decreases blood calcium; parathyroids–parathyroid hormone to regulate calcium in blood and bones; adrenal cortex–glucocorticoids—metabolism of fats, carbohydrates, and proteins and sex hormones to influence secondary sexual characteristics; pancreatic islets–insulin and glucogon to regulate blood sugar levels; testes–testosterone—development of secondary sexual characteristics and maturation of sperm cells; and ovaries–estrogens and progesterone, which aid in fertilization and maintaining pregnancy as well as promoting secondary sexual characteristics. Other hormone-producing tissues are not listed due to lack of space.

A number of disorders are related to the endocrine gland system and to overproduction or deficiency of hormones. Hormones are the treatment for a number of diseases (for example, diabetes mellitus, which results from a deficiency of insulin); hypothyroidism and cretinism, which result from a deficiency of thyroxine production; and hyperthyroidism, which results from an overproduction of thyroxine. Growth hormone treats a deficiency in short children. Epinephrine is used to treat asthma, anaphylaxis, and shock. Oxytocin may be used after delivery because it causes contraction of uterine muscle helping to control postpartum hemorrhage.

182.

E. Myasthenia gravis is a chronic disease characterized by muscular weakness. Muscles affected frequently are those of the face, eyelids, larynx, and throat, producing the "hatchet-face" appearance. It is an autoimmune disease caused by a chemical deficiency in the myoneural region (where muscles receive control from nerves) and is sometimes reversed by drug therapy. Another group of inherited (genetic) diseases that also affects muscles is muscular dystrophy. The term means "wasting (nongrowth) of muscles," and most forms are eventually fatal. The most common form is inherited from a defect on the X (sex) chromosome and affects males. The "floppy baby syndrome" describes another inherited group (progressive muscular atrophies) of muscle diseases.

The musculoskeletal disorders have a weakness of the muscles that results in a skeletal disorder. Talipes (flat feet or fallen arches) are due to a weakness of the muscles supporting the feet. Scoliosis is believed to be caused in part by muscles that do not support the spine properly.

183.

E. The joints of the fingers and toes between the phalanges and metacarpals are examples of condyloid (ellipsoidal) joints. The ovoid condyle of one bone fits into the elliptical cavity of another. (A condyle is a rounded projection on a bone, usually part of a joint.) These joints permit a variety of movements in different directions. Joints are classified according to the type of movement they permit. The jaw is also a condyloid joint as is the wrist joint. Other types of joints are the ball and socket in the shoulder and hip joints; the hinge joints in the elbow and knee joints; the gliding joints in the vertebral column; and the saddle joint found only in the base of the thumb. A pivot joint is in the atlas and axis of the neck vertebra.

All of the previously mentioned joints are synovial joints (except the gliding joints) so called because they are lined with a synovial membrane. In contrast, the joints between the vertebra, only slightly movable, are cartilaginous.

184.

E. All these choices may be the purpose of a spinal tap. A sample of cerebrospinal fluid (CSF) can yield valuable information about infections within the CNS. It is sometimes important to measure the pressure of the CSF and give treatment to lower it if it is critically high. The spinal tap lumbar puncture is made between L4 and L5 to prevent damage to the spinal cord. The spinal cord ends between the first and second lumbar vertebra.

185.

B. Paralysis of both arms and legs is called quadriplegia (quadr-, four; -plegia, paralysis or palsy) and affects all four extremities. Paraplegia affects the lower extremities (in this instance, the prefix para- = pair). Hemiplegia affects either the right or left half of the body (hemi-, half).

186.

B. Hemiplegia is paralysis of either the right or left half of the body and occurs on the side opposite the brain damage. The most frequent cause is a cerebrovascular accident (CVA) caused by a cerebral thrombosis, cerebral embolism, or cerebral hemorrhage.

187.

B. Neuralgia is a term indicating pain over the course of a nerve. The combined word form is neur-, nerve and -algia, pain. Neurasthenia is nerve weakness or exhaustion. The two word forms, neur- and -algia, are combined independently with other word forms to create medical terms describing other conditions.

188.

D. Brain death exists when there is a flat encephalogram (signifying no brain activity), no spontaneous movement or breathing, and no response to stimuli. The term irreversible coma implies that there is no recovery and, therefore, brain death.

189.

B. The olfactory nerve is concerned with the sense of smell and is designated as cranial nerve one (CN I). Actually there is a forest of tiny olfactory nerves lumped together as CN I, the only cranial nerves attached to the cerebrum. The rest of the cranial nerves are attached to the brainstem, not to the spinal cord as are the other body nerves.

190.

B. The joining of nerve ends is called neuroanastomosis. This is a combined word form (neur/o-, nerve; anastomosis, new surgical connection between segments of an organ).

191.

B. Ménière's disease is an intracranial nerve disorder and may lead to progressive deafness. It is specifically a disorder of the labyrinth of the inner ear. A primary symptom is severe vertigo (an inappropriate sense of motion, such as spinning and rolling). Another symptom is "hearing" unusual sounds, such as tinnitus (ringing sound in ears).

192.

A. The plantar reflex, stroking of the plantar surface (bottom) of the foot, is an example of a superficial reflex, which is elicited by stroking the skin. A normal response is plantar flexion (bending the foot downward) except in babies and adults with certain neurologic disorders, who have a Babinski reflex of flexing the big toe and fanning the other toes.

193.

C. Endocarditis is an inflammation of the endocardium (inside lining) of the heart. It is sometimes caused by bacterial diseases, such as streptococcal infection (scarlet fever, rheumatic fever) or syphilis. It may cause lasting damage by changing the shape of the valves of the heart.

194.

B. The red pigment in hemoglobin, the oxygen carrier of the red cells, gives blood its color. The color varies from bright red in the arteries when the red blood cells are well oxygenated to dark red in the veins when the red blood cell oxygen concentration is low. The skin appears bluish when the body is deprived of oxygen, a condition called cyanosis. Cyanosis results from a prolonged oxygen deficiency (hypoxia).

195.

C. An average-size person will have an approximate blood volume of 5 liters. Blood transfusions are measured in cubic centimeters (cc) or milliliters (mL), which are equivalent to cc's, although common usage speaks incorrectly of pints of blood. About 55% of the blood is straw-colored liquid plasma, 45% is red cells, and less than 1% is white cells. Another small component is platelets (cellular fragments of thrombocytes), which aid in clotting.

196.

A. The spleen (a saclike mass of lymphatic tissue) serves as a reservoir for blood. Other functions of the spleen include the destruction of damaged red cells and the formation of lymphocytes by the lymphoid tissue in the spleen. The spleen is not essential for life and occasionally is removed surgically for medical reasons (splenectomy).

197.

A. The mitral valve and the bicuspid valve are two names for the same valve. This valve is located on the left side of the heart and has two flaps, or cusps. It regulates the flow of blood from the left atrium into the left ventricle.

198.

B. The largest artery in the body is the aorta. It extends from the left ventricle, arches to the left over the heart, creating the aortic arch, and descends medially downward through the trunk of the body. Above the diaphragm, it is the thoracic aorta; below the diaphragm, it becomes the abdominal aorta.

199.

E. The pulmonary veins are the only veins in the body that carry oxygenated blood. They carry blood from the capillaries of the lungs where CO_2 was released and oxygen acquired to the left atrium of the heart. The other veins carry carbon dioxide back from other parts of the body to the heart.

200.

B. From the right ventricle of the heart, blood is forced into the pulmonary trunk, which gives rise to the left and right pulmonary arteries. From there, the blood enters the lungs, giving up deoxygenated blood from the heart to the lung capillaries. The oxygenated blood then enters venules and goes on to the large pulmonary veins that empty into the left atrium.

201.

C. An infarction is a localized area of ischemic necrosis (ischemic, deficiency in blood supply; necrosis, localized tissue death).

202.

D. A stricture or narrowing, usually severe, of some portion of the aorta is called coarctation of the aorta. Surgical treatment (anastomosis) consists of removing the constriction and rejoining the remaining segments of the aorta (ana-, apart; -stomosis, new opening).

203.

B. Varicose veins are greatly dilated veins in which pressure is elevated and blood flow is stagnant or reversed. This is due to damaged valves that do not prevent the backflow of blood. Hemorrhoids (piles) are a type of varicose veins. The surgical procedure for treating varicose veins is vein stripping. A medical term for varicose veins is varix (singular) or varices (plural).

204.

D. Connective tissue, which includes osseous (bone) and adipose (fat) tissue, connects and supports the body. Tissue is a type of cells grouped together and specialized to carry on a certain function. Muscle tissue produces movement, nerve tissue carries impulses to and from the brain, and epithelial tissue provides a covering (skin) for the body and linings for the blood vessels, urinary tract, intestines, and other organs.

205.

C. A sarcoma is a malignant neoplasm (cancer) of supportive and connective tissue (sarc/o-, flesh; -oma, growth). The sarcoma cells are spread by the bloodstream and often form secondary growths in the lungs.

Other cancers include the following types. Carcinomas, the most common type of cancer, are neoplasms of the epithelial tissue that tend to metastasize (spread) to other parts of the body by means of the lymphatic system. They commonly occur in the skin, mouth, lung, breast, stomach, colon, prostate, and uterus. Adenocarcinomas are malignant (cancerous) tumors of the glands (aden/o-, gland). Lymphomas occur in the lymphatic tissue. Melanomas occur in birthmarks or moles.

The most common methods of diagnosing cancer include biopsies of tissue for microscopic examination; ultrasound to distinguish various kinds of tissue; CT (computed tomography) to produce pictures of the body; MRI (magnetic resonance imaging) to show alterations in soft tissue; and certain specific laboratory tests.

Treatment of cancers includes radiation therapy with x-ray or radiation seeds within the tumor and chemotherapy such as the use of antineoplastic agents (drugs and drug combinations). Lasers have also been used to kill specific masses of cells while limiting the amount of bleeding.

206.

B. Leio- means smooth. A leiomyoma, for example, is a myoma (tumor formed of muscular tissue) of non-striated muscle fibers. Fibroid tumors of the uterus are a type of leiomyoma.

207.

C. Obstruction of the valve orifice between the left atrium and left ventricle is called mitral stenosis, or Lutembacher's syndrome. There is also aortic stenosis. (Stenosis is an abnormal closing.) Heart murmurs are the rushing, gushing sound produced when the valves do not completely block the circulation.

208.

C. A localized dilatation of an artery is an aneurysm (ballooning). An aneurysmectomy removes the aneurysm, which may be due to atherosclerosis (ather/o-, plaque; -sclerosis, hardening) or some other weakness of the arterial wall.

209.

E. Closed heart massage is called cardiac pulmonary resuscitation, cardiopulmonary resuscitation, or CPR. There are three basic steps: (1) open airway by tilting head, (2) restore breathing by mouth-to-mouth respirations, and (3) restore circulation by external chest compression.

210.

B. A hereditary disease in which patients bleed excessively is hemophilia. The most prevalent form of hemophilia is limited to males and is transmitted through the mother to the next generation, since it is caused by a recessive gene on the X chromosome. Treatment consists of supplying the missing plasma clotting factor by transfusion.

A nonhereditary cause of excessive bleeding may be a low platelet count or an out-of-control heparin or coumarin medication prescribed for patients with a high probability of recurring blood clots (thrombi). Clinical laboratory tests are used in the diagnosis and monitoring of these disorders.

211.

A. A reduction either of red cells per unit of circulating blood or of hemoglobin or both is anemia. The oxygen-carrying ability of the blood is reduced by lowered amounts of hemoglobin, whether due to a reduction in number of red cells (which contain hemoglobin) or because each red cell has a lower than normal amount of hemoglobin. There are numerous causes (and types) of anemia: hemorrhaging, iron-deficiency anemia from a poor diet, some inherited anemias such as sickle cell, and some resulting from medications or chemicals, such as chloramphenicol and benzene.

212.

B. Fibrillation is the condition of rapid heartbeats (350 or more/min) characterized by uncoordinated contractions because small regions of the myocardium (middle muscular layer of the heart) contract independently of the other areas. Ventricular fibrillation is especially serious and may cause death in a few minutes. Treatment is defibrillation by applying a strong electric shock to the myocardium through the chest wall to restore a normal cardiac rhythm.

213.

D. Rheumatic heart disease results from a streptococcal infection that is usually a "strep throat." Beta-hemolytic, type A streptococcus is pathogenic and is further subdivided into various strains. It is most important that initial streptococcal infections receive treatment, since up to 3% of untreated streptococcal infections subsequently develop symptoms of rheumatic fever. The other pathogens listed in the answer choices also have been implicated in infections of the heart.

214.

B. The sebaceous gland is an exocrine gland (with a duct) that secretes an oily, colorless, and odorless fluid (sebum) through the hair follicles. Sebaceous cysts (steatomas) may occur when the duct becomes clogged and may require surgical removal (steatoma is a combined word form: steat-, fat; -oma, mass or tumor).

Other exocrine glands (glands with ducts) are the lacrimal glands, which produce tears, and the glands that produce digestive juices. They deliver their secretions and are effective in only a limited area (unlike the endocrine glands whose hormones secrete through the blood and affect target cells far away from their source).

215.

C. The parathyroid glands secrete a hormone (parathormone) that regulates the calcium content of the blood and bones. If there is a decrease in blood calcium (which may occur in pregnancy, rickets, or a dietary deficiency), the parathyroid glands secrete more parathormone to cause calcium to enter the blood from the bones. Conversely when the calcium level in the blood rises from an excess of calcium in the diet, the parathormone level drops.

216.

A. Polydipsia is excessive thirst. It occurs in many diseases, including diabetes insipidus and diabetes mellitus.

217.

E. The presence of sugar (glucose) in the urine is glucosuria or glycosuria. If the renal plasma threshold is reached, there will be more glucose than the kidneys' active transport mechanism can remove from the filtrate, and some glucose will remain and be excreted in the urine.

218.

D. Cryptorchidism (crypt-, hidden; -orchidism, testicle), also called cryptorchism, is a failure of the testicles to descend into the scrotum. Normally, the testes leave the abdomen before birth and descend outside the body cavity to the scrotal sac. If they do not descend by age 7 years, the surgical procedure orchipexy (orchi/o-, testicle; -pexy, fixation) places the testes in the scrotum.

219.

B. Hypofunction of the adrenal cortex leads to a syndrome called Addison's disease. Daily cortisone administration and intake of salts is the treatment. Some symptoms are melanin pigmentation of the skin, hypoglycemia, weakness, and weight loss. Cushing's syndrome, however, is caused by hyperfunction of the adrenal cortex. Some of its symptoms are a moon face, central obesity, and impaired carbohydrate tolerance, among other findings. Graves' disease is another name for hyperthyroidism where the thyroid gland is overactive while myxedema results from an underactive thyroid gland. SIDS is an acronym for sudden infant death syndrome.

220.

A. Gigantism is a rare abnormality of the pituitary gland that causes excessive growth in a child so that the child becomes an unusually tall adult. In adults, the abnormality results in acromegaly, with a characteristic appearance of enlarged face, jaws, hands, and feet.

221.

B. Another term for exophthalmic goiter is Graves' disease. A goiter (enlargement of the thyroid) is a symptom of Graves' disease, as is exophthalmos, a protrusion of the eyeballs, occurring because of the swelling of tissue behind the eyeball. Excessive thyroid hormone is produced, speeding up the body's metabolism.

222.

E. Goiter, cretinism, and myxedema are pathologic conditions due to hypothyroidism (low production of thyroid hormones). Cretinism occurs in infancy and childhood, myxedema in adulthood. Endemic goiter (due to a lack of the nutrient, iodine) is a hypertrophy (growth), sometimes very large, of the thyroid resulting from the thyroid's working very hard to produce hormones.

223.

D. Hemochromatosis is a disease characterized by a bronzing of the skin due to the deposition of an iron-containing pigment and generally occurs in men older than age 40.

224.

E. Testosterone is a hormone produced in the testes whose chief function is to stimulate the development of the male reproductive organs, including the prostate, and secondary male characteristics. It also encourages growth of bone and muscle.

225.

A. Hyperglycemia is an abnormally high concentration of sugar in the blood (hyper-, above or excessive; glyc-, glucose; -emia, blood condition). It occurs as a symptom of diabetes mellitus. A laboratory test for blood glucose is used to diagnose hyperglycemia. The opposite condition, hypoglycemia (hypo-, under), is an abnormally low level of glucose in the blood. It may result from an overdose of insulin given to regulate hyperglycemia.

226.

D. Amyl- is a word component that means starch. The enzyme amylase (amyl-, starch; -ase, enzyme), as its name implies, converts starch to glycogen and sugars. Produced in the salivary glands of the mouth and the pancreas, it begins the digestive process.

227.

C. Andro- is a word element meaning male or masculine. Androgens are, therefore, hormones that produce male characteristics (andro/o-, male; -gen, create). Testosterone produced in the testes (as its name implies) is the most important androgen.

228.

E. The suffix -ptysis means spitting. Hemoptysis, for example, is the coughing and spitting of blood (hem/o-, blood; -ptysis, spitting).

229.

C. The pleura is the serous sac that encases the lung and is divided into two layers, the visceral and parietal. Pleuritis is an inflammation of the pleural lining, which results in the abnormal accumulation of fluid between the two layers of the pleura (the visceral and parietal pleura), which ordinarily has only a small amount of lubricating fluid.

230.

A. The pharynx is the airway between the nasal chambers, the mouth, and the larynx. Its three regions are the nasopharynx, the oropharynx (oris, mouth), and the laryngopharynx. It is lined with a mucous membrane that resists mechanical abrasion and pathogenic invasion.

231.

E. The windpipe is the trachea, a vertical tube 4 1/2 inches long by 1 inch in diameter. It is kept open by about twenty C-shaped rings of cartilage separated by connective tissue. It is flexible on the backside, which is adjacent to the esophagus.

232.

D. The mediastinum divides the chest into two compartments containing the left and right lung. The heart, esophagus, and thymus gland are located within the mediastinum.

233.

C. Croup is a narrowing of the air passage in the larynx and may be caused by infection, allergy, a foreign body, or a new growth. It is generally a childhood disease and has a characteristic cough and suffocating breathing symptoms. A treatment for croup is humidification of the air using steam or a vaporizer.

234.

A. Detection of new growths arising within the bronchi may be made by using a bronchoscope, an endoscope designed for passage through the trachea. Specimens for laboratory analysis can be obtained by aspiration of bronchial secretions or by inserting fluid and retrieving it (bronchial washing). Bronchial brushing (a biopsy by forceps or a brush) also can be obtained.

235.

A. Myringitis, otitis media, and otopyorrhea are inflammatory conditions of the ear. Myringitis is an inflammation of the myringa (tympanic membrane). Otitis media is an inflammation of the middle ear. Otopyorrhea is a discharge of pus from the ear (oto- = ear; pyo- = pus; -rrhea = flow).

236.

C. Tracheitis is usually accompanied by laryngitis, bronchitis, or both. The word laryngotracheobronchitis means inflammation of the larynx, trachea, and bronchi.

237.

A. Collapse of the lung so that the air sacs become smaller in size is known as atelectasis. All or part of the lung may be involved. Common causes include blockage of a bronchus or smaller bronchial tube or air leakage into the chest cavity from a chest wound. Treatment may involve therapy to remove the underlying cause (tumor, excess secretions, or foreign matter), respiratory therapy, antibiotics to combat infection, and, in extreme cases, a lobectomy (lobe excision).

238.

B. Emphysema is the overdistention of the air sacs of the lungs. Eventually, there is a loss of elasticity in the lung tissue, which makes breathing difficult. Chronic bronchitis is a usual symptom. The heart must work harder because of the dyspnea (difficult breathing) and hypoxemia (low blood oxygen supply). Eventually, cor pulmonale (enlargement of the right ventricle of the heart due to a disorder of the lung) occurs.

239.

B. The pharyngeal lymph nodules that circle the pharynx are known as tonsils and represent a first line of defense against pathogenic invasion of the pharyngeal tissues. Tonsillitis is a recurring infection of the tonsils that may cause them to swell, creating high fever, and making swallowing and breathing difficult. It is generally caused by strep or staph bacteria or possibly a virus.

Tonsillectomy is removal of the tonsils located to the sides of the soft palate. Tonsiladenoidectomy is the removal of the lateral tonsils and the lymph tissue on the upper wall of the pharynx known as adenoids.

240.

C. A hiatal hernia is a weakness in the diaphragm that allows the protrusion of abdominal organs through the esophageal hiatus (opening) into the thoracic cavity. It may result from congenital factors or from an injury that weakens the diaphragm. There are different types of hernias, such as umbilical hernia, inguinal hernia, and cystocele, which often are named to designate the organ or area affected.

241.

D. Cystic fibrosis has the highest lethal rate of inherited disease among Caucasians. It is a disorder of the exocrine glands that secrete into ducts or onto a body surface and is characterized by production of very thick, sticky mucus. The symptoms include chronic respiratory infections and pancreatic insufficiency, which affects digestion.

242.

B. A hernia of the diaphragm is treated surgically by herniorrhaphy. The term herniorrhaphy refers to a suturing of the hernia. The term hernioplasty refers to the repair of a larger hernia with reconstruction. Surgical repair may become necessary if the hernia becomes strangulated, cutting off blood supply to the protruding organ with the likelihood that the tissue will become gangrenous. Heartburn, difficulty in swallowing, and ulceration may occur with diaphragmatic hernias.

243.

D. Parturition refers to childbirth, the expulsion or delivery of the fetus from the body of the maternal organism. The arrival of the newborn infant outside the body of the mother represents the delivery. Cesarean section is parturition by surgically removing the child from the uterus.

244.

C. The part of the body of the fetus that is in advance at birth is called presentation. Normal presentation is cephalic presentation (head first). In a breech presentation, the buttocks or legs of the fetus enter the birth canal first.

245.

A. The change of position of the fetus in the womb is called version. The term is used particularly to refer to the manual turning of the fetus in delivery. The fetus is manipulated into a more favorable birth position.

246.

B. Chorionic villa sampling and amniocentesis are two methods used to obtain cells for the study of chromosomal and genetic disorders in developing fetuses. The cells can be analyzed for almost 200 congenital conditions, such as spina bifida, anencephaly, Down syndrome, and abnormal hemoglobin synthesis. Ultrasonograms (pictures of the fetus obtained by ultrasound) can be used to diagnose malformations of the fetus, as well as abnormal development and positioning of the placenta. Analysis of the mother's blood for high levels of certain substances can reveal fetal disorders such as congenital kidney malformations and anencephaly (congenital absence of the brain and cranium).

Some fetal disorders can be prevented. Among these are AIDS transmission to the fetus from the mother; fetal alcohol syndrome resulting from consumption of alcohol during pregnancy; and defects from the rubella measles virus. Prospective parents, in particular, should be counseled to practice a healthy lifestyle and refrain from unsafe sex practices and substance abuse.

247.

A. Cystocele refers to hernial protrusion of the urinary bladder (e.g., herniation of the urinary bladder into the vagina). Injury during childbirth may cause a cystocele. A synonym is vesicocele (vesic/o-, bladder; -cele, protrusion).

248.

E. The major functions of fat in the body include providing a source of energy, transporting proteins and fat-soluble vitamins A and D, and supplying fatty acids essential for growth and life. Fat also causes the stomach to empty more slowly, which gives a person a longer feeling of satisfaction from food. Fats are also known as lipids.

Cholesterol is a lipid commonly found in saturated fats but is also an essential compound manufactured in our body. Research has implicated high levels of cholesterol, especially the low-density cholesterol, as indicators of heart disease. The circulating lipids in our body may be divided into three categories according to the weight of the molecule—HDL (high-density lipid), LDL (low-density lipid), and VLDL (very low-density lipids). A high level of high-density lipoprotein (HDL) is healthier, while a high level of low-density lipoprotein (LDL) may indicate approaching heart disease. Levels of HDL and LDL can be changed through diet.

It is also believed that consuming unsaturated fats that are in the forms of vegetable oils is healthier than eating saturated, solid fats, such as coconut fat, solid shortening, and animal lard. Most animal fat also contains a high level of dietary cholesterol.

249.

D. Circumcision of the penis may be done for phimosis, redundant prepuce, and balanoposthitis. However, most circumcision is done at the request of parents and not because of medical indications.

250.

E. Nephrosis is any disease of the kidneys in which there is malfunction of the kidney tissue without inflammation, but particularly those diseases involving degenerative lesions of the renal tubules.

251.

A. Alopecia is a term describing the occurrence of baldness. Alopecia areata has well-defined bald patches. Alopecia universalis is the total loss of hair on all parts of the body (alopec/o-, baldness; -ia, condition).

252.

D. The surgical procedure for cleft lip (harelip) is cheiloplasty (cheilo-, lip; -plasty, surgical repair). Palatoplasty is surgical repair of the cleft palate. Cleft palate results from the bones of the palate failing to fuse together during early fetal development. Cleft lip (cheiloschisis) occurs when the overlying skin and tissue fail to fuse (cheil/o-, lip; -schisis, splitting).

253.

D. Rhytidectomy or rhytidoplasty is performed to eliminate wrinkles from the skin (rhytid/o-, wrinkle; -ectomy, excision; -plasty, repair). This is also known as a face-lift. Following are explanations of the other answer choices: Dermatoplasty is a replacement of lost skin. Dermatology is the medical specialty that diagnoses and treats skin disease (dermat/o- = skin; -ology = study of). Dermatitis is an inflammation of the skin (dermat- = skin; -itis = inflammation). Blepharoplasty is plastic surgery of the eyelid (blephar/o- = eyelid; -plasty = surgical repair).

254.

D. Abnormal enlargement of the pinna (plural = pinnae) of the ear is called macrotia (macro- = large; -ot- = ear; -ia = condition). In contrast, microtia refers to abnormally small ears (micro- = small; -ot-, ear; -ia, condition). The pinna is the outside auricle or flap of the ear.

Following is an explanation of the other answer choices. Otomycosis is a fungal infection of the ear (ot/o- = ear; myc/o- = fungus; -osis = condition). Otodynia is pain in the ear (oto- = ear; -dynia = condition of pain). Otoplasty is surgical (plastic) repair of the outer ear (oto- = ear; -plasty = surgical repair).

Other relevant terms: otopyorrhea, a flow of pus from the ear (py/o- = pus; -rrhea = flow); oto/rhino/laryng/ology, the branch of medicine dealing with disease of the ear, nose, and throat (sometimes shortened to otolaryngology); and otoscopy, examination of the ear with an otoscope (-scope = light).

255.

E. Incision of the eardrum (tympanic membrane) and drainage of the middle ear is myringotomy (myring/o-, eardrum; -tomy, cutting). Otitis media (inflammation of the middle ear with accumulation of serum) may require myringotomy and placement of tympanostomy tubes in the eardrum to allow drainage of the middle ear. Myringoplasty is the surgical repair of the eardrum. Tympanoplasty is the surgical reconstruction of the eardrum (tympanic membrane).

256.

E. All of the terms (metastasis, carcinoma, sarcoma, and neoplastic) relate to malignancies. Metastasis is the process by which cancer cells break away from the original growth and travel through the blood and lymph vessels to other parts of the body and grow. Carcinomas are cancers that arise from epithelial tissues. Sarcomas are cancers that arise from connective tissue, muscle, or bone. Cancer cells are neoplastic (neo- = new; -plastic = form) because unlike ordinary body cells they are large, divide quickly, and serve no useful purpose.

257.

A. A macule is a small discoloration of the skin, level with the surface, up to the size of a fingernail. A papule is elevated, and a nodule is larger than a papule. A vesicle, also elevated, is about the size of a papule but contains clear fluid, and a pustule is a vesicle that contains pus. These precise terms enable the medical professional to give more exact descriptions of skin disorders.

258.

C. Seborrhea, the excessive secretion of the sebaceous glands, is responsible for oily skin and dandruff. It is also responsible for a susceptibility to the formation of blackheads, eczema-like lesions, and pimples (sebo-, sebum; -rrhea, flow). Acne, common among teenagers, is usually associated with seborrhea.

259.

A. Excision or removal of the lacrimal sac is called dacryocystectomy (dacry/o-, tear; cyst, sac; -ectomy, excision). The lacrimal sac is part of the lacrimal apparatus that continually lubricates the eye by secreting tears in the lacrimal gland and carrying them away via the lacrimal ducts and sac to the nasal cavity.

260.

B. Enucleation is the removal of an organ or other mass intact, without rupture, from its supporting tissues. A diseased eyeball is an organ that may be enucleated, as might a diseased uterus. The term also may be used to describe cataract removal and surgical removal of tumors.

261.

C. Hordeolum and chalazion are afflictions of the eyelids. A hordeolum is a stye generally caused by staphylococci invading a sebaceous gland in the eyelid. A chalazion is a small, hard mass on the eyelid, the result of the enlargement of a sebaceous gland. Drooping of the upper eyelid is blepharoptosis (sometimes referred to simply as ptosis).

262.

D. Vitreous humor is the fluid filling the vitreous chamber behind the lens and in front of the retina, the rods and cones. The aqueous humor fills the aqueous chamber between the cornea and the lens. The term humor describes any body fluid or semi-fluid, whereas the term vitreous indicates a glasslike, clear quality. Vitrectomy is the surgical procedure of removing diseased vitreous humor and replacing it with a clear solution. Eventually, the body replaces the solution with a healthy vitreous humor.

263.

B. Astigmatism is a condition in which the curvature of the refracting surfaces is unequal. In astigmatism, there is a defect and deviation from spherical curvature in either the surface of the lens or the cornea. It is treated by corrective lens, as are farsightedness (hyperopia) and nearsightedness (myopia).

264.

B. The malleus, so named because of its hammer-like shape, is a bone of the middle ear attached to the eardrum. It, along with the incus (anvil) and stapes (stirrup), form a bridge to transmit and intensify vibrations from the tympanic membrane (eardrum) to the inner ear. Inflammation of the middle ear is otitis media.

265.

A. The external ear is composed of the pinna, or auricle, and the external auditory meatus (canal). The auricle of the ear intensifies hearing by collecting sound waves and directing them into the auditory meatus. The ear is commonly classified into the external, middle, and inner parts. Otitis externa is inflammation of the outer ear.

266.

E. Presbyopia is a condition of defective accommodation (focusing of lens on retina) due to aging of the individual in which distant objects are seen distinctly but near objects are indistinct. Emmetropia is the ideal accommodation in which parallel rays are focused on the retina. Ametropia is a failure to focus parallel rays of light on the retina and includes both hyperopia (farsightedness) and myopia (nearsightedness).

267.

D. The second set of teeth, or the permanent teeth, includes sixteen in each jaw, or a total of thirty-two permanent teeth. Arranged from the midline, they are the central incisor, lateral incisor, cuspid, first and second bicuspid, and first, second, and third molar.

268.

E. The large blind pouch at the beginning of the large intestine is the cecum. The ileocecal valve (between the ileum and cecum) controls the movements of food from the small intestine to the cecum. The vermiform appendix is attached to the cecum. Appendicitis is an inflammation of the appendix. An appendectomy is the surgical removal of the appendix.

269.

D. The largest portal system in the blood circulation of the body is in the liver. The veins that carry blood from the spleen, stomach, pancreas, and intestines empty their blood into the liver by way of the hepatic (liver) portal vein. There, the vein branches eventually into sinusoids that allow liver cells to contact the blood. In this way, waste materials are removed and nutrients are processed, stored, and released as needed before being carried into the general circulation.

The liver is the largest gland in the body and ordinarily weighs from 42 to 56 ounces. It has multifunctions in the metabolism of proteins, carbohydrates, and fats, the most vital being that of protein metabolism. It is necessary for survival.

Jaundice, a yellowing of skin and tissue, is due to an increase in blood bilirubin and is a symptom of liver disease. A blood test for the bilirubin level is, therefore, one of the battery of liver function tests. The liver is prone to damage from infection such as viruses, drugs, and toxins such as alcohol. Inflammation of the liver is hepatitis (hepat/o- = liver; -itis = inflammation). Viruses that attack the liver are named A through E. Hepatitis B, C, and D are diseases transmitted by body fluids, such as blood, for which there is no specific treatment. However, there are vaccines available for Hepatitis A and B. Hepatitis A is transmitted in fecal matter and by contaminated food and water. Cirrhosis of the liver, where the liver cells are replaced by scar tissue, is most commonly caused by alcohol. Liver cancer may occur especially when cancers from the intestine or some other abdominal organ travels through the veins to the liver.

270.

B. The gallbladder is the reservoir for bile produced by the liver before it is released into the duodenum of the small intestine. It is about 3 to 4 inches in length, 1 inch wide, and pear shaped. Gallstones (cholelithiasis) may form in the gallbladder if there is inflammation (cholecystitis) and may necessitate removal of the gallbladder (cholecystectomy). Bile (gall), the secretion of the liver stored in the gallbladder, assists in emulsifying fats during digestion. Helpful word forms to remember: chol/e-, bile or gall; cyst-, bladder; -itis, inflammation; lith-, stone; -iasis, condition; and -ectomy, surgical removal.

271.

B. The basic structural unit of nerve tissue is the neuron, which consists of a nerve cell body plus small branches or fibers that send messages (axons) or receive messages (dendrites). Nerve cells are highly specialized body cells and react to certain changes in their surroundings by sending impulses to other nerve cells, muscles, or glands. The brain, spinal cord, and nerves are all composed of nerve tissue.

Three types of neurons are (1) sensory (afferent) neurons carrying messages to the spinal cord or brain; (2) motor neurons carrying messages away from the brain or spinal cord to muscles or glands; and (3) associative neurons that carry messages between other neurons. The synaptic cleft (synapse) is a space between neurons that is bridged from axon to dendrite by chemicals called neurotransmitters.

The complete nervous system can be subdivided into categories. The central nervous system consists of the brain and spinal cord. The peripheral (peripheral means at the edge) nervous system is outside the brain and spinal cord; it in turn is divided into the voluntary system and the autonomic system. The voluntary system, with both sensory and motor neurons, carries messages to and from the brain and controls voluntary muscles. The autonomic nervous system carries messages to involuntary muscles and glands.

Nervous system disorders are due to degenerative disease, injuries, and inflammation. Symptoms may be pain, paralysis, loss of sensation or sensory malfunction, or convulsive seizures. Parkinson's disease, multiple sclerosis, and myasthenia gravis are degenerative diseases.

272.

D. Persons with type O blood are universal donors, meaning that they may safely give blood in an emergency to anyone without creating an ABO blood reaction. This is true because there are no A or B antigens on the red blood cells of the O type person. However, the universal donor must also be Rh negative if the recipient is Rh negative. In reality, the same blood type is preferred if it is available, and every blood donation must be cross-matched with the recipient's blood to ensure compatibility.

The ABO and the Rh blood group systems are two independent group systems that are clinically important because the human body will produce antibodies to the blood antigens present in some of the types. The Rh blood group involves only two types of individuals— those Rh positive and those Rh negative. Rh positive antigens (actually three separate antigens) occur on the red cells of Rh positive individuals and Rh negative individuals have none of the Rh antigens. Within this blood group system, Rh negative individuals develop antibodies to the Rh positive antigen after an initial exposure. An incompatibility will also develop if a pregnant Rh negative woman is exposed through tears in body tissue to the antigens of her Rh positive fetus. Her antibodies will react against the fetus producing a disease called erythroblastosis fetalis. Hemolytic disease of the newborn (HDN), the same disorder affecting the newborn, is caused by Rh incompatibility and sometimes by incompatibility between the mother and fetus ABO blood types. (Erythroblastosis fetalis is a medical term: erythro- = red; blast = immature cell; -osis = condition; fetalis = condition of fetus.)

The major symptoms of this disabling and often fatal disease are immature red cells, jaundice, a very high blood bilirubin, and possibly mental retardation if not treated. These symptoms are due to the destruction of the fetus's red cells by the maternal antibodies.

Blood typing and tests for this condition are often performed in medical offices treating obstetric patients. Fortunately, Rh disease is largely preventable if susceptible mothers receive the Rh immune globulin after giving birth to an Rh positive infant.

273.

B. The hypothalamus is the most important heat-regulating center. Located at the base of the brain, it aids in regulating many functions of the body, such as sleep, appetite, water and electrolyte balance, blood pressure, and heart rate.

274.

C. Sweat glands are known as sudoriferous glands, each of which has an excretory tube that extends to the skin surface and opens at a pore.

275.

C. The ethmoid bone is the delicate, spongy bone located between the eyes and contains the ethmoid sinuses. (One type of sinus is a cavity within a bone.) The ethmoid bone forms a part of the cranial floor beneath the frontal lobes of the brain and the upper nasal cavities. The term ethmoid means sievelike (ethm-, sieve; -oid, resembles).

276.

E. The soft spot in the skull of a young infant is called a fontanel. The anterior fontanel usually does not close until the child is about 18 months old. The term fontanel means little fountain and refers to the pulse of blood vessels that can be felt under the skin in those areas. The infant's skull must be given protection against injury to the fontanel.

277.

C. Melena is the medical term indicating black, tarry stools, the appearance being due to the presence of digested blood. Hemoccult is a test for occult (hidden) blood in the stools. Occasionally, stools are black from food pigments. Blood in the stools is a serious symptom because it indicates hemorrhaging within the digestive system. This, in turn, may indicate a bleeding ulcer or cancer.

The digestive system is prone to several disorders. Among the more common are gastritis, an inflammation of the stomach; gastroenteritis, a cause of diarrhea among infants; and peptic ulcers in the stomach (gastric) or intestine (duodenal). Crohn's disease, diverticulitis, colitis, and irritable bowel syndrome are also common and may cause constipation or diarrhea. Carcinoma can occur in any part of the intestinal tract.

Organs connected to the digestive system such as the pancreas or liver can also suffer inflammation and infections.

278.

E. Polyps are the most common benign tumors of the digestive tract, and they are common in the colon but rare in the small bowel. Two types are pedunculated polyps and sessile polyps. Colonic polyposis is the growth of polyps from the mucous membrane of the colon.

279.

E. An outstanding symptom of hepatitis is jaundice, a yellowish discoloration of the skin and eyes due to a higher than normal amount of bilirubin (bile pigments) circulating in the blood. These bile pigments, the products of red blood cell breakdown, would normally be excreted by a healthy liver through the gallbladder into the intestines. Hepatitis is an inflammation of the liver and may be due to a number of causes such as viruses, bacteria, and chemical agents.

280.

C. The end of a muscle that exerts the power and movement is called its insertion. The fixed attachment of a muscle is known as its origin, and the actual movement of the muscle is its action. Near the point of insertion, a muscle narrows and is connected to the bone by a tendon.

281.

D. The chief muscle of the calf of the leg is the gastrocnemius, which ends near the heel in the Achilles tendon (the largest tendon in the body). The Achilles tendon may be torn during athletic activities and require surgical treatment. The gastrocnemius is a powerful flexor that helps push the body forward when a person walks or runs.

282.

C. The outermost, toughest, and most fibrous of the three membranes covering the brain and spinal cord is the dura mater (dura means durable). The second layer is the arachnoid membrane, and the third thin, delicate inner layer is the pia mater. Meninges is a collective term for the three membranes. Meningitis is inflammation of the meninges due to infectious agents such as bacteria or viruses.

283.

A. Adipose tissue is fatty tissue deposited in most parts of the body. Adipose tissue provides an energy reserve, cushions delicate organs, and insulates against heat loss through the skin. Women have a higher percentage of adipose tissue than men. (The combining form is adip/o-, fat.)

284.

E. The mastoid process can be felt behind the ear—the conical projection from the portion of the temporal bone lying behind the ear. Infections may travel from the middle ear to the mastoid process and then possibly to the nearby membranes that surround the brain.

285.

D. The upper seven pairs of ribs are attached to the sternum anteriorly. The lower five pairs of ribs contain the eighth, ninth, and tenth, which are attached indirectly to the sternum by means of the attachment of their costal (rib) cartilages to the cartilage of the rib above, and the last two pairs of ribs, which are unattached in front, making a total of twelve pairs of ribs.

286.

A. A foramen is an opening through or between bones that permit a vessel or nerve to pass through. There are several foramina in the human body. One of these is the foramen magnum at the base of the brain where the spinal cord communicates with the brain. The foramen ovale in the heart of the fetus between the right and left atrium permits the fetal circulation to bypass the lungs until birth. The obturator foramen, the largest foramen in the skeleton, is an opening between the pubic bone and the ischium, which is filled in with membrane. At its upper part, the obturator vessels and nerves pass from the pelvis into the thigh.

287.

C. The largest bone of the foot is the calcaneum (also called calcaneus). It is the heel bone, which helps support the body's weight and serves as an attachment for the foot muscles.

288.

E. A joint in which one rounded extremity fits into a cavity in another bone, permitting movement in all directions, is called a ball-and-socket joint. This type of joint permits a wider range of motion than any other type. Examples are the shoulder and hip joints.

289.

B. The elbow and knee joints are examples of hinge joints. The phalanges (finger and toe bones) also have hinge joints. This type of joint permits movement in only one plane (as do the hinges of a door).

290.

D. The sudden loss of consciousness due to transient cerebral hypoxia is syncope. Fainting is an example of syncope. Cerebral hypoxia means that there is a temporary lowering of the oxygen supply to the brain.

291.

D. Effusion is a collection of fluid in the pleural space. Empyema is pus in the pleural cavity, and hemothorax (hemo- = blood; -thorax = -chest) is blood in the pleural cavity.

292.

B. Coryza is the technical name for the common cold. It may also mean a profuse discharge from the mucous membrane of the nose. Allergic coryza is hay fever. Other terms that describe the common cold are "upper respiratory infection" and "acute nasopharyngitis." (Coryza is derived from Gr. catarrh—to flow).

293.

E. Eclampsia, also called toxemia, is a serious disorder of pregnancy accounting for 20% of maternal deaths and a large number of neonatal (newborn) deaths. The symptoms of high blood pressure, edema, and proteinuria can be detected during prenatal visits to the physician.

294.

E. Eosinophils, so named because the cytoplasmic granules absorb the reddish eosin stain, are granular leukocytes found in large number in allergic conditions. The various kinds of leukocytes that were listed in the answer selections serve several different functions in the immunity system of the body and have either granular or agranular cytoplasm. Eosinophils, neutrophils, and basophils are granulocytes, whereas lymphocytes and monocytes are agranulocytes.

295.

B. The jugular veins return blood through the neck to the superior vena cava from the head. The carotid arteries transport blood to the head. Regarding the other answer choices: The paired saphenous veins of the leg, the longest veins of the body, run from the foot up through the thigh. The subclavian vein (also paired), as its name indicates, drains the area underneath the clavicle (collarbone). The brachial veins are in the upper arms. The radial artery serves the forearm and wrist.

Veins may develop several disorders. Phlebitis is the inflammation of a vein that may become complicated by a thrombus (clot) and then become *thrombophlebitis*. An *embolus* may break loose from the clot and travel through the bloodstream until it reaches the lungs or brain causing death or a cerebrovascular accident. Veins may become *varicose* (varices = plural; varix = singular, from L. meaning twisted vein). *Hemorrhoids* are varicose veins that occur in the rectum. *Statis dermatitis* results from a stoppage in normal blood flow through the veins of the legs possibly due to valves that no longer close completely. The skin becomes inflamed and scaly, fissures (cracks) form, and ulcers follow.

296.

A. Dysphagia means difficulty in swallowing (dys-, difficult; -phagia, swallowing). Swallowing (deglutition) involves a set of complex reflexes triggered by the mouth, tongue, and pharynx. Swallowing has three phases, the buccal (mouth), pharyngeal, and esophageal phases.

297.

C. The liver removes bilirubin from the blood, manufactures most of the plasma proteins, and is involved with the production of prothrombin and fibrinogen. More than 200 functions have been assigned to the liver, including modifying waste materials and toxic substances, secreting bile, forming urea, acting on fats, and storing and distributing glycogen, fat, vitamins, and iron. As a result, any serious damage to the liver is a threat to life.

298.

E. All of the statements are true. Lymph is the fluid that moves protein molecules and other cellular substances. The lymph system allows one-way movement of the lymph toward the circulatory system. It also moves fat-related nutrients from the digestive system to the circulatory system. The lymphatic system contains lymph nodes that filter foreign agents from the lymph fluid, and also specialized lymphatic organs, the spleen and thymus.

Lymphedema is the swelling of tissue because lymph fluid has accumulated there due to blockage of the lymph vessels. *Lymphangitis* is the inflammation of the lymph vessels, possibly from an infection that may spread into the bloodstream and cause *septicemia* (blood poisoning). The lymph nodes may be the site of cancer that has migrated there through the lymph fluid. The lymph nodes may also develop lymphomas, which are most often malignant.

The *thymus*, a specialized lymphatic tissue organ, early in childhood produces *T-lymphocytes* that are essential to the immune system. A ring of lymphoid tissue, called the *tonsils*, is located around the back of the mouth and throat and serves the purpose of filtering bacteria that invade the area. The largest lymphoid organ, the spleen, is in the upper left quadrant of the abdomen. It filters worn-out blood cells and bacteria from the blood and recycles the iron from old hemoglobin. Enlargement of the spleen is known as *splenomegaly*. The surgical removal of the spleen is a *splenectomy*.

299.

D. Anis/o- is a word form that means unequal (e.g., anisocytosis means the presence in the blood of erythrocytes showing abnormal variations in size). Anisocoria is inequality in the size of the pupils of the eyes (anis/o-, unequal; cor-, pupil; -ia, condition).

300.

B. Chromo- means color. A chromocyte is a cell with color or pigment. Hemochromatosis (hemo-, blood; -chromat-, color; -osis, abnormal condition) is a condition with excessive deposits of iron throughout the body and a bronze coloration of the skin. This condition generally occurs in males older than 40 and may cause serious problems, such as an enlarged liver and cardiac failure.

301.

D. A mechanical soft diet is an example of a diet modified by consistency. A soft diet is used when a person has chewing difficulties. The food may have strong flavor and spices, but it must be chopped, ground, or pureed.

302.

C. A bland diet or liberal bland diet is restricted in flavor and usually is used with patients who have gastrointestinal problems, such as ulcers.

303.

E. The inclusion or exclusion of specific foods is a way of modifying a diet for patients suffering with different allergies. The treatment of allergies may be by two different methods. One method removes only one or two foods that are suspected of causing an allergy. The Rowe method starts with only a few hypoallergenic foods, and single food groups are slowly added to the diet.

304.

A. The impairment of a person's ability to adapt to darkness is a symptom of vitamin A deficiency. Vitamin A is required for healthy skin and mucous membranes in the nose, throat, eyes, gastrointestinal tract, and genitourinary tract. Carotene is converted to vitamin A by the body. Vitamins are essential for normal metabolism and are regulators of metabolic processors acting as coenzymes. Vitamin A deficiency disorders include nightblindness, reduced resistance to infection, and impaired growth and development in children.

Vitamin B complex is a group of vitamins, thiamine (B1), riboflavin (B2), niacin (nicotinic acid), pyridoxine (B6), biotin, folic acid, and cyanocobalin (B12). They affect growth and the nervous and endocrine systems, and are important in the metabolism of carbohydrates.

Vitamin C (ascorbic acid) is contained in fresh citrus fruits and other fresh fruits and vegetables. It is easily destroyed by heat. Deficiency disorders include scurvy, defective teeth, gum disease, and injury to bones, cells, and blood vessels.

Vitamin D aids in the building of bones and the use of calcium and phosphorus in the body. Deficiency disorders are imperfect skeletal formation, rickets, cavities in teeth, and bone diseases.

Vitamin E is an essential vitamin but its exact biochemical reaction in the body is unknown.

Vitamin K aids in the clotting of blood and is necessary for the formation of prothrombin. It is manufactured by bacteria in the human intestinal tract and also occurs in foods such as alfalfa and fishmeal. Prolonged bleeding occurs as a result of a deficiency of Vitamin K.

305.

D. Hematology is the area of specialization that diagnoses and treats diseases and disorders of the blood and blood-forming tissue. Diseases diagnosed and treated by hematologists include anemias and leukemias. Anemias are diseases that cause a reduction in the number of circulating red blood cells or in the quantity of hemoglobin. Leukemias are malignant diseases of the blood-forming organs.

306.

B. Ophthalmology is the medical specialty area that diagnoses and treats diseases and disorders of the eye. Ophthalmologists are medical doctors with a residency in ophthalmology. An optometrist is not a physician and only measures the accuracy of vision for corrective eyeglasses. Two common eye diseases treated by ophthalmologists are cataracts (opacity or clouding of lens) and glaucoma (accumulating fluid pressure within the eye).

307.

A. Nephrology is the area of specialization that is concerned primarily with diagnosing and treating diseases and disorders of the kidney. The principal functional units of the kidney are the 1 million nephrons in each kidney. Urologists are concerned with not just the kidney but the whole urinary system in females and the genitourinary system of males.

308.

D. Psychiatry is the specialization that diagnoses and treats pronounced manifestations of emotional problems or mental illness that may have an organic causative factor. Psychiatrists are medical doctors who prescribe medications, in contrast to psychologists, who are not physicians and cannot prescribe medication but do evaluate and counsel emotional problems.

309.

B. The area of specialization that diagnoses and treats conditions of altered immunological reactivity (allergic reactions) is allergy. The practitioner is called an allergist. Allergic reactions are hypersensitive reactions to some nonself material. Hypersensitivity reactions may result from drugs, foods, pollens, and so on.

An immunologist is the specialist that treats diseases of the immune system. The immune system protects the body against outside invaders and cancer cell mutations. Both cell-mediated and humoral (noncellular) immunity are studied. The white cells recognize foreign proteins (antigens), send signals to other white cells, and produce antibodies. The plasma of the blood contains complement fixation that binds to antigens altered by antibodies. Other body fluids also contain antibodies. The best-known disease of the immune system is AIDS caused by the HIV virus.

Diagnostic tests of the immune system generally involve antibodies and include (1) the complement-fixation test for the presence of a particular antibody; (2) the antibody titer, which measures the amount of antibody in the blood; and (3) the fluorescent antibody test.

310.

E. The integumentary system is not responsible for nitrogenous waste excretion. The nitrogenous waste in our bodies is excreted in the form of urea through the kidney and excretory system. The skin does excrete water, which is a metabolic product of carbohydrate and fat (lipid) metabolism.

311.

C. Nystagmus is an eye disease that causes repetitive, involuntary movement of the eye. (The term nystagmus means "to nod" in Greek, referring to the involuntary movements.) The other terms describe disorders of the skin; dermatitis is any form of skin inflammation, and impetigo is a contagious, superficial skin infection caused by streptococcus or staphylococcus. Urticaria, more commonly known as hives, is an inflammatory reaction to allergens, such as drugs, foods, insect stings, or airborne agents, and psoriasis is a chronic disease of the skin of unknown cause, with silvery, yellow-white scales.

312.

C. The skull is not a part of the appendicular skeleton; it is part of the axial skeleton. The appendicular skeleton includes the bones of the arms, hands, legs, feet, shoulders, and pelvis. The bones that form the axial skeleton are the spinal column, skull, and rib cage.

313.

B. The skeletal system is not a primary energy reservoir for the body. It is the body's store for calcium. Calcium is very essential for muscle contraction and in the blood-clotting process. The bones of the skeleton also store phosphorus and lesser amounts of magnesium, sodium, potassium, and carbonate ions.

314.

D. Osteoporosis is a metabolic bone disorder especially common in older women that is characterized by the loss of calcium and phosphate from the bone. Osteo-myelitis is an infection of the bone characterized by inflammation and edema. Osteomalacia is a defective mineralization of the bone caused by insufficient body storage or ineffective use of vitamin D. It is called rickets in children.

315.

C. Smooth muscles are not responsible for the movement of bones. This is the function of skeletal muscles, which are called voluntary muscles. Smooth muscles are known as involuntary muscles because they function without conscious direct control. The autonomic nervous system controls smooth muscle action.

316.

D. The type of fracture where the bone breaks and splinters with bone fragments embedded in surrounding tissue but does not come through the skin is a comminuted fracture. The compound or open fracture is one where the bone protrudes through the skin. An impacted fracture is one in which the bone is broken, with one end forced into the interior of the other.

317.

B. Peristalsis is the type of wavelike action, by the smooth muscles, that forces food through the intestine. Sphincters are smooth muscles that are donut-shaped and pinch shut to control materials in the digestive system and in blood vessels. Fascia, tendons, and aponeuroses are all connective tissues associated with voluntary muscles of the skeletal system.

318.

D. The cartilage "lid," called the epiglottis, covers the trachea (windpipe) when we swallow. The opening to the larynx (voicebox) located at the top of the trachea is called the glottis. The prefix epi- means on top of.

319.

B. Pneumoconiosis is a respiratory or lung disease that is the result of inhaling dust particles over a prolonged period. One kind is silicosis caused by silica sand dust. Others are asbestosis, caused by asbestos fiber, and anthracosis (black lung disease), caused by accumulation of carbon dust in the lungs. URI (upper respiratory infection) refers to symptoms associated with the common cold.

320.

C. The smallest divisions of the trachea forming air passageways in the lungs are bronchioles. Each bronchiole ends in a grapelike cluster of microscopic air sacs called an alveolus. The alveoli (plural) have surrounding capillaries that absorb oxygen and release carbon dioxide to the outside (gas exchange).

321.

E. The internal muscular wall that divides the heart into the right and left sides is the septum. The heart is lined internally with endothelial tissue called endocardium. The outside covering of the heart is the pericardium. The valve between the right atrium and right ventricle is the bicuspid or mitral valve.

322.

A. The inferior vena cava collects blood from the lower body regions and returns it to the right atrium of the heart. The blood from the head, chest, and arms is returned to the heart by way of the superior vena cava. The pulmonary vein returns oxygenated blood from the lungs to the left atrium.

323.

A. A condition of the circulatory system in which the artery wall weakens, resulting in ballooning, is known as an aneurysm. Common types of aneurysms include abdominal, thoracic, and peripheral artery aneurysms. Angina is a heart condition causing severe chest pain that radiates down the inner surface of the left arm.

324.

E. A condition in the lumen of the large and medium arteries in which fatty materials (cholesterol, lipids) are deposited and accumulate is known as atherosclerosis. In atherosclerosis, the arteries affected are major and supply vital tissue. Arteriosclerosis is a "hardening" of the small arteries and arterioles, which results in loss of elasticity of the walls.

325.

C. The anatomic structure that is not a part of the small intestine or its support is the cecum. The three sections of the small intestine are the duodenum, jejunum, and ileum. The mesentery is a fan-shaped fold of tissue that suspends the jejunum and ileum in the abdominal cavity. The cecum is the first section of the large intestine.

326.

B. The vermiform appendix is a small projection that extends from the cecum. The cecum is the small, pouchlike segment of the colon, the first part of the large intestine. The ileum is the last segment of the small intestine.

327.

B. A disease that results in autodigestion is pancreatitis, either acute or chronic. The pancreatic enzymes normally produced and then secreted directly into the duodenum via the pancreatic duct remain because of inflammation in the duct and digest the pancreatic tissue. This causes varying degrees of edema, swelling, tissue necrosis, and hemorrhaging.

328.

A. The anatomic structure that is the functional unit of the kidney is the nephron. The parts of the nephron include the glomerulus, Bowman's capsule, proximal and distal convoluted tubules, Henle's loop, and collecting tubules. The nephron is responsible for filtration of the blood and reabsorption of materials back into the blood.

329.

D. The urethra is the anatomic structure of the urinary tract that carries urine from the bladder to the outside of the body. The ureters are the tubes that carry urine from the pelvis of the kidneys to the bladder. The renal pelvis is the collecting chamber of all the collecting tubules of the nephrons.

330.

C. Polycystic kidney disease is an inherited disorder that produces grapelike, fluid-filled sacs or cysts in the collecting tubules of the cortex of the kidney (poly- = many; cyst = sac; -ic = pertains to). The disease will lead to kidney failure, uremia, and eventual death. Dialysis treatments can help to prolong life.

331.

D. Cystitis is a urinary tract disease that causes inflammation of the bladder. Inflammation of the urethra is urethritis. Cystitis is more common in women due to the short distance from the outside to their bladder. The inflammation is generally caused by contamination with *Escherichia coli* from the rectum and may result from improper cleansing following defecation. Glomerulonephritis is an inflammation of the glomerulus of the nephron. An understanding of the medical terms that describe the urinary system and general disease processes will "decode" the meaning of words such as cystitis and polycystic kidney disease. (The word cystitis is created by combining the word form for bladder with the word form for inflammation.)

332.

B. The pancreas tissue of the body functions both as an exocrine gland and an endocrine gland. The pancreas produces digestive juices that are secreted by way of the pancreatic duct into the duodenum of the small intestine. The pancreas also is an endocrine gland that secretes insulin directly into the bloodstream. Insulin is produced in the islands of Langerhans in the pancreas.

333.

E. The endocrine gland considered to be the "master gland" of the body is the pituitary gland. Divided into an anterior and posterior lobe, it is called the "master gland" because it controls the secretions of other endocrine glands, including the adrenal cortex, thyroid, and the gonads (testes and ovaries). Secretions of the anterior lobe include the hormones, growth hormone, thyroid-stimulating hormone (TSH), ACTH, prolactin, and the gonadotropins, FSH and LH. The posterior lobe secretes antidiuretic hormone (ADH) and oxytocin.

Tumors of the pituitary may cause *gigantism*, a very tall stature resulting from a childhood tumor, or *acromegaly*, with wide, heavy bones of the face, hands, and feet resulting from a tumor developed in adulthood. Underactivity and a deficiency of other endocrine glands may develop if the tumor destroys the ability of the pituitary to produce certain secretions.

334.

C. The endocrine gland located in the neck and requiring iodine for normal function is the thyroid gland. When the thyroid gland does not produce enough thyroxin, the anterior pituitary produces more thyroid-stimulating hormone (TSH), causing the thyroid to increase in size so more thyroxin can be produced. An enlargement of the thyroid gland (hyperplasia) is a goiter.

335.

B. Another name for cretinism is hypothyroidism. When it appears as a congenital condition, individuals are cretins. Infants with this condition must be treated promptly with administration of thyroid extract. Cretins are short, stocky persons who usually suffer mental deficiencies due to lack of thyroid hormones. Myxedema is adult hypothyroidism. An excessive level of thyroid hormones produces the disorder of hyperthyroidism or Graves' disease.

336.

D. The disease diabetes insipidus is caused by the insufficient secretion of vasopressin (ADH) which is produced by the posterior lobe of the pituitary gland. The distal tubules of the nephrons of the kidneys lose the ability to concentrate urine. This results in polyuria. This disease commonly affects more males than females. This condition should not be confused with the two types of diabetes mellitus (insulin-dependent, or IDDM, and noninsulin-dependent, or NIDDM). Diabetes mellitus results from either insufficient insulin production or a deficiency in utilization of insulin.

337.

E. The sex of a child is determined by the father at the time of conception. Females only produce gametes (eggs) that have an X chromosome. Males produce gametes (sperm) that have either an X or a Y chromosome. A zygote that is XX (one X from each parent) develops into a female. A zygote that is XY (an X from the mother and a Y from the father) will develop into a male. Klinefelter's syndrome is a chromosomal abnormality where males have two XX chromosomes from their mother and a Y chromosome from their father. Down syndrome is another chromosomal abnormality with an extra chromosome.

338.

E. An STD caused by a protozoal infestation of the vagina, urethra, or prostate is trichomoniasis. The protozoan is *Trichomonas vaginalis*. The diagnosis of trichomoniasis is made by a microscopic examination of vaginal or urethral discharge or urine, where the organism is seen and identified.

339.

C. The cerebellar hemisphere (cerebellum) is not part of the cerebrum. The cerebellum is one of the major portions of the brain. The others are the cerebrum, the hypothalamus and thalamus, and the brain stem (includes the medulla, pons, and midbrain). All are interconnected and function together. The cerebellum functions as a center for the control and coordination of skeletal muscles. The cerebrum is the largest part of the brain with right and left hemispheres. It controls voluntary movement, sensation, learning, and memory. The brainstem regulates the heart, respiration, blood pressure, and reflex centers.

340.

B. The junction between two nerve (neuron) endings that permits the transmission of nerve impulses to continue is the synapse. Transmission of nerve impulses across the synapse is made possible by chemicals called neurotransmitter substances. Among these are acetylcholine (ACh) and norepinephrine.

341.

B. Any diffuse pain occurring in different portions of the head would best describe a headache. The cause of a headache is irritation of one or more of the pain-sensitive structures or tissues in the head and neck. Usually, a headache signals nothing more serious than fatigue or tension unless it is chronic or severe.

342.

A. Parkinson's disease is characterized by severe muscle rigidity, a peculiar gait, drooling, and a progressive tremor. The onset of the disease is slow and insidious. The body tends to bend forward with the head bowed. The excitatory transmitter, dopamine, is deficient and the drug, levodopa, may be used to help relieve symptoms.

343.

E. Meningitis, an inflammation of the meninges, is produced by many infectious agents such as bacteria and viruses. Headache, neck and back stiffness, and fever occur, as well as some neurological symptoms for which the physician will test.

344.

C. Amphetamines are stimulants that have structures similar to the excitatory transmitter, norepinephrine. Librium and Valium are tranquilizers. Alcohol is a depressant that can cause death if consumed in large amounts in a short period of time because of its depressive effect on the brain functions.

345.

D. Epilepsy is a brain disorder resulting in seizures that are associated with abnormal electrical impulses from the neurons of the brain. The neurons within the brain discharge in a random, intense manner. This abnormality may occur in a small section of the brain or in several areas of the brain all at once. The prognosis is good with proper drug therapy. Diagnosis and evaluation of epilepsy and other seizure disorders are made with the electroencephalogram, a graphic representation of brain activity.

346.

A. Alzheimer's disease formerly was called presenile dementia. It is due to atrophy of the frontal and occipital (back) lobes of the cerebrum. The disease involves progressive, irreversible loss of memory, deterioration of intellectual functions, disorientation, and speech disturbances. It generally begins after the age of 65.

347.

B. The tough, white, fibrous tissue that covers the outside of the eye is the sclera. The choroid is the covering under the sclera, and it is supplied with blood vessels that serve the tissue of the eye. The cornea is a transparent covering in front of the pupil that causes refraction of light.

348.

D. The structure of the eye that contains muscles controlling the shape of the lens for near and far vision is the ciliary (circular) body. The ciliary body contains ciliary muscles. Regarding other answer choices: The fovea is a very special region of the retina where there are only cone cells. Vision is most acute in this area. The vitreous humor is the tissue fluid of the eyeball; aqueous humor is the tissue fluid in the anterior part of the eye between the lens and the cornea. Glaucoma is an abnormally high increase in the pressure of the aqueous humor that in turn creates pressure on the lens, vitreous humor, and retina. If the pressure is not controlled with medications, blindness may eventually result.

Cataracts are a clouding of the lens of the eye that mostly affect the elderly. The clouding or opacity blurs vision. Laser surgery is used to remove the clouded lens. Contact or glass lenses are used to replace the refractive ability of the original eye lens.

349.

E. All the answer choices are types of refractive error in vision. Refraction is the bending of light as it goes through structures. In the eye, it enters through the cornea, passes through the aqueous humor, lens, and vitrous humor, finally contacting the retina. Only the lens can adjust and change the angle of light. A lens with irregular curvature, opaque fluid, or a long or short eyeball will affect the refraction of the light and the image our brain sees. Hyperopia is commonly referred to as farsightedness. Myopia is commonly known as nearsightedness. Astigmatism occurs when an irregular curvature of the cornea or lens causes the light to be scattered and blurred. Another refractive error (presbyopia) occurs in older persons when the lens loses its elasticity and ability to thicken as needed for near vision, resulting in farsightedness. Note the terms that can be dissected into word forms (e.g., presby- = elder; -opia, condition of vision).

Color-blindness is an inherited defect in vision, not a refractive error that causes people with the genetic defect to not distinguish certain colors. There is a red/green color-blindness that is linked to the X gene and is more common in men. Total color-blindness is very rare.

350.

A. Glaucoma is a group of eye diseases that results in excessive intraocular pressure that can cause damage to the retina and optic nerve, often causing blindness. This pressure build-up occurs because more fluid, known as aqueous humor, is produced than can be drained from the eye. The condition affects mostly people older than 40, more women than men, and can be in one eye or both. Congenital glaucoma in newborns due to a congenital defect is also known as hydrophthalmos.

351.

D. Otosclerosis is an inherited condition of the ear that is caused by the formation of spongy bone, especially around the oval windows, resulting in immobilization of the stapes. Otosclerosis (oto- = ear, -sclerosis = hardening) causes tinnitus and then chronic, progressive deafness. A gradual hearing loss, in both ears, to low tones or soft sounds is the first symptom. Cranial nerve VIII connects the ear to the brain.

352.

B. An accumulation of fluid within the middle ear is called otitis media. This condition may be caused by either a serous or a suppurative process. The serous form is caused by the secretion from the membranes lining the inner ear. The suppurative form is produced by pus-producing bacteria. The prognosis of the condition is good if it is treated properly. Chronic otitis media may cause hearing loss due to scarring.

353.

C. The abbreviations listed are terms used in patient histories and physical examinations. CC means chief complaint, FH means family history, and HEENT is the abbreviation for head, ears, eyes, nose, throat. Obviously, these abbreviations are time savers and great conveniences for medical personnel, but the possibility of error should be kept in mind.

354.

E. All of these may be used depending on the situation. A medical dictionary, a computer, an English dictionary, and a *Physician's Desk Reference* should be a part of the medical office library, available when needed. An electronic dictionary to which terms may be added is a great convenience, whether it is attached to a word-processing program or is a separate device. A card index of frequently used terms in the practice is useful. An index of drugs is also useful.

355.

A. Dermatitis is any form of skin inflammation. Referring to the other answer choices: Impetigo is a contagious, superficial, skin infection caused by streptococcus or staphylococcus. The term dermatosis refers to any skin condition, not necessarily with inflammation. Psoriasis is a chronic disease of the skin with silvery, yellow-white scales. Urticaria, more commonly known as hives, is an inflammatory reaction to allergens, such as drugs, foods, and so on.

356.

C. The leading communicable disease problem of today is the spread of STDs (sexually transmitted diseases). These include acquired immunodeficiency syndrome (HIV leading to AIDS), Hepatitis B and C, gonorrhea, syphilis, herpes simplex 1 and 2, chlamydia, and genital warts. They are spread primarily by sexual contact and, in the case of AIDS and Hepatitis B and C, by body fluids and blood. Bacteria, protozoa, and viruses are all causative agents.

357.

A. The abbreviation meaning "four times a day" is qid (quater in die). It may be written with or without periods and also in capital letters (QID). However, current usage favors dropping the periods. The abbreviation qd means every day, q2h means every 2 hours, and qs means of sufficient quantity.

358.

A. The abbreviation for twice a day is bid. The abbreviation hs means at bedtime, tid means three times a day, and ac means before meals. The abbreviations most commonly used in a medical office should be posted in a convenient place for reference when deciphering notes.

359.

A. AS pertains to the left ear (auris sinistra). The abbreviation AD means right ear.

360.

D. The symbol "s" with a bar over it, s̄, means without, as contrasted to the symbol for with, c with a bar over it, c̄.

361.

E. The abbreviation for "if necessary" is SOS or sos.

362.

C. CA or Ca means carcinoma or cancer.

363.

C. Leukoderma is a combined word form meaning white skin (leuk/o-, white; -derma, skin). The other possible answer choices when the words are dissected are as follows: xanth/o/derma is yellow skin, cyan/o/derma is blue skin, leuk/o/cyte is white cell (meaning white blood cell), and leuk/emia literally means white blood, but describes any cancer of the blood-producing tissues.

364.

A. Acrocyanosis is a blueness of the extremities and may be associated with lack of oxygen getting to the hands and feet. This is a combined word (acro-, extremity; cyano, blue; -o/sis, abnormal condition). Note that complex medical terms are read right to left from the suffix back to the first part of the word.

365. **(1)** bursae

366. **(5)** metastases

367. **(2)** thoraces

368. **(8)** diverticula

369. **(9)** nuclei

370. **(11)** phalanges

371. **(8)** ova

372. **(6)** sarcomata

373. **(3)** apices

374. **(7)** ganglia

375. **(4)** cervices

376. **(10)** biopsies

377. **(5)** prosthesis

378. **(8)** ovum

379. **(9)** nucleus

380. **(1)** vertebra

381. **(7)** spermatozoon

382. **(8)** bacterium

383. **(10)** artery

384. **(5)** diagnosis

385. **(1)** cornea

386. **(12)** lumen

387.

E. All the terms described are structures or conditions in the oral area. Glossa is Greek for tongue, and lingua is Latin for tongue. Other terms describing the oral area are stoma (mouth), bucca (cheek), and cheilos (lip). These are root words that are combined with various prefixes and suffixes to describe conditions in the oral region. Buccal administration of medication is placing medicine in the cheek, where blood-rich membranes absorb it quickly. Sublingual administration of medicine is placing medicine (such as digitalis, a quick-acting heart medication) under the tongue.

388.

A. Food takes the following pathway through the digestive tract: oral cavity, pharynx, esophagus, stomach, duodenum, jejunum, ileum, cecum, ascending colon, transverse colon, descending colon, sigmoid colon, rectum, anus. Digestion first occurs in the mouth, where the enzyme amylase acts on the food, and continues through the large intestine, where water and vitamins are absorbed.

389.

D. Muscle weakness on one side of the body is hemiparesis. The term hemiparesis is dissected as follows: hemi-, half; -paresis, incomplete paralysis. All the possible answer choices were terms that included the prefix hemi- (half). Ataxia means failure of muscular coordination; therefore, hemiataxia is ataxia on one side of the body. Hemidiaphoresis is sweating on only one side of the body. Hemiplegia is paralysis of one side (probably caused by a brain tumor or CVA).

390.

B. Empyema of the pleura (accumulation of pus in a body cavity, especially the pleural cavity) and pyothorax (py/o-, pus; -thorax, chest) are two terms that mean "pus in the pleural cavity." This condition is treated with antibiotics and rest. Thoracentesis may be performed to identify the microorganism responsible.

391.

A. Osteitis deformans is used to refer to a slowly progressive disease of the elderly in which there is extensive bone destruction. The term osteitis (oste-, bone; -itis, inflammation) denotes inflammation of the bone, and deformans denotes deformity. The cause of the disease is unknown.

Referring to the other answer choices: osteometry refers to the measurement of bones. Osteoma is a benign bone tumor (-oma = tumor).

392.

D. Creating a new connection between segments of an organ (e.g., two parts of an intestine after removing a diseased portion) is known as anastomosis. Reading from right to left the meaning of the term is -osis, increased or abnormal; stom/a-, mouth; ana-, of each.

After removal of the colon, an ileorectal anastomosis joins the ileum and the rectum.

393.

D. An abnormal accumulation of fluid in the peritoneal (abdominal) cavity is ascites. It is also sometimes called dropsy and can result from tumors, infections, heart failure, or cirrhosis of the liver.

394.

E. Aside from these organs, the pancreas, thyroid gland, ovaries and testes, and adrenal gland, others that are part of the endocrine system include the pituitary gland, parathyroid glands, pineal gland, and thymus gland. They share the common characteristic of releasing hormones directly into the bloodstream (not through a duct).

395.

E. All these suffixes are used to mean "condition or state of."

396.

E. All the organs listed and also the liver are located in the abdominal cavity. The abdominal cavity and the thoracic cavity (containing the heart and lungs) are the two ventral cavities. These cavities are partitioned by the diaphragm and are not continuous like the dorsal cavities of the spine and brain.

397.

E. All the abbreviations are common medical abbreviations. DPT = Diphtheria, pertussis, and tetanus immunization; BP = blood pressure; F = female; CPR = cardiopulmonary respiration. The context in which an abbreviation is used is probably the best clue to its meaning. A standardized list of abbreviations should be agreed upon by the staff and adhered to in recording patient data.

398.

E. Dangers of the laser include burns, fire, possible inhalation of plume (smoke) as well as electrical hazards related to high-wattage equipment. Laser light is useful as a surgical tool because it destroys (burns) tissue. If it is improperly handled it can also destroy unintended tissue and harm the patient, physician, and the medical assistant. Protective goggles should be worn by the patient and all members of the operative team.

399.

D. A salpingostomy is a surgical opening into a fallopian tube for surgical restoration of the tube or for drainage purposes because it has been occluded (closed up). The term dissects into the following combined word forms: salping/o-, tube (in this case a fallopian tube); -stomy, formation of an opening. Salpingectomy is the excision (removal) of a fallopian tube. Hysterectomy is the removal of the uterus (hyster-, uterus; -ectomy, excision). An oophorectomy is removal of one or both ovaries (oophor/, ovary). An oophorotomy is incision (surgical opening) of an ovary.

400.

B. The patella (kneecap) is part of the appendicular skeleton. The word, appendicular, means attached to a larger, major part. Our extremities (arms and legs) along with the shoulders and hips comprise our appendicular skeleton. Our torso (spinal column, rib cage, neck [cervical vertebra] and head [skull] comprise our axial skeleton.

The axial and appendicular portions of the body are also divided into general body regions for the purpose of locating wounds, surgical sites, and so on. Some regions are the thoracic area (chest), the dorsal area (back), the buttock, and the groin.

Another method of locating areas is by using palpable bony landmarks, which can serve as reference points for other structures. These landmarks, such as the iliac crest and anterior superior iliac spine, can be touched and identified through the skin.

401.

A. The term "stat" means "immediately." It is used during emergencies and other situations where a procedure or action is needed immediately before other scheduled events. In such situations a voice order may be given for medication by the physician. It should be verified immediately by the medical assistant to ensure accuracy and then, as soon as possible, written in the patient's record with a VO (verbal order) notation.

2 Medical Law and Ethics

chapter objectives

Major areas of knowledge/content included in this chapter are:

I. The medical code of ethics as

➤ a moral obligation

➤ basis for standards of medical practice

II. Legal guidelines for

➤ licensing of medical professionals

➤ patient rights and records; patient abandonment; charges of assault and battery; slander and libel; practicing within scope of medical training, etc.

III. Results of noncompliance with federal and state laws:

➤ license revocation

➤ malpractice suits

➤ criminal penalties

IV. Regulatory agencies

➤ required reports such as public health, OSHA, CLIA '88, and DEA

➤ OSHA concerns for public and employee safety

➤ nondiscriminatory practices

➤ DEA guidelines for controlled substances

DIRECTIONS (Questions 402 through 476): Each of the numbered items or incomplete statements in this section is followed by answers or by completions of the statement. Select the ONE lettered answer or completion that is BEST in each case.

402. The main purpose of filing reports of certain communicable diseases to government agencies is to
  A. facilitate statistical analyses of diseases
  B. protect the health of the community
  C. determine the need for educational programs
  D. determine priorities for research funding
  E. determine geographic requirements for medical care

  (AAMA, pp 151–152; Frew et al, p 560; Lewis and Tamparo, p 92)

403. Important dates to remember in the medical practice office are the due dates for license renewals, narcotics registration, and insurance premiums. A good way to remember these upcoming dates is to
  A. associate the name of the month with the payment due
  B. ask a co-worker to help remember the dates
  C. maintain a tickler or time schedule file
  D. put notices on an office bulletin board
  E. insert a notation in the appointment book

  (Frew et al, p 97; Lewis and Tamparo, pp 72–73)

404. Which of the following statements pertaining to medical jurisprudence is FALSE?
  A. the patient has the right to assume that a physician possesses the required knowledge
  B. a physician is obligated to keep informed as to the best modern methods of diagnosis and treatment
  C. the majority of malpractice claims are merited
  D. a physician serving on active duty with the armed forces may be guilty of malpractice
  E. malpractice may be the basis for revoking a physician's license

  (Flight, p 105)

405. The Truth in Lending Act (Regulation Z of the Consumer Protection Act of 1968), when applied to medical offices, deals with collection of patients' payments. Which statement is FALSE?
  A. the agreement must be in writing
  B. finance charges must be specified
  C. it is often applied to arrangements for surgery, orthodontia, and prenatal/delivery care
  D. it forbids a finance charge
  E. unilateral payment plans by the patient are not covered

  (Lewis and Tamparo, pp 136–137)

406. When a patient receives care under Worker's Compensation from his or her regular physician, the medical assistant should
  A. keep two medical records
  B. bill the patient for the deductible
  C. file a bill with the insurance carrier every 2 weeks
  D. file a claim within 5 days
  E. bill the patient for unpaid portion

  (Frew et al, pp 297–300)

407. In a Worker's Compensation case, the medical assistant should
    A. bill the patient for the deductible
    B. file a bill with the insurance carrier every 2 weeks
    C. send no bill to the patient
    D. bill the patient for the unpaid portion
    E. bill the carrier in one lump sum
    (Frew et al, p 297)

408. Complete information regarding the filing of reports and taxes from the employee's earnings and employer's tax contributions can be found in
    A. *Physician's Desk Reference*
    B. *Medical Office Handbook*
    C. *IRS Income Tax Guide*
    D. *IRS Circular E Employer's Tax Guide*
    E. *Federal Tax Deposits*
    (Frew et al, pp 276–277)

409. Physicians who administer narcotics are required to register with the
    A. Federal Trade Commission
    B. Internal Revenue Service
    C. Occupational Safety and Health Review Commission
    D. Drug Enforcement Agency
    E. General Services Administration
    (AAMA, pp 159–160; Lewis and Tamparo, p 60)

410. Which of the following statements pertaining to medical jurisprudence is FALSE?
    A. a physician's carrier of malpractice insurance will provide for an attorney and pay court costs in the event of a lawsuit
    B. it is absolutely necessary to obtain a patient's consent, either oral or written, prior to an operation
    C. many of the suits against physicians arise from x-ray therapy
    D. if a patient is a minor, the consent of his or her parent will suffice for an operation

    E. as a general rule, a physician's records are subject to subpoena
    (Flight, p 188; Lewis and Tamparo, p 126)

411. A physician who regularly dispenses drugs is required to keep records of drugs and must take an inventory
    A. every 6 months
    B. once a year
    C. every 18 months
    D. every 2 years
    E. when requested by the federal agency
    (AAMA, p 159; Lewis and Tamparo, p 60)

412. A physician who dispenses nonnarcotic or narcotic drugs listed in the Schedule of the Controlled Substances Act must keep records of such drugs for a period of
    A. his or her own discretion
    B. 1 year
    C. 2 years
    D. 6 years
    E. 7 years
    (Frew et al, p 551; Lewis and Tamparo, p 60)

413. A common requirement for licensing physicians by endorsement in a given state is that they have passed an examination titled
    A. American Medical Association Test
    B. National Board of Medical Examinations
    C. United States Medical Licensing Examination
    D. National Medical Association Examinations
    E. Educational Testing Service
    (Lewis and Tamparo, pp 72–73)

414. Medical practice acts are
    A. resolutions of the American Medical Association
    B. recommendations passed by local medical societies
    C. state statutes
    D. basic tenets of the National Medical Association

E. endorsements passed by the Board of Medical Examiners

(AAMA, pp 14–15; Flight, p 16)

415. The performing of an act that is wholly wrongful and unlawful is called
   A. feasance
   B. malfeasance
   C. misfeasance
   D. nonfeasance
   E. negligence

(Frew et al, p 895; Kinn and Woods, p 63)

416. The branch of moral science that deals with the duties of a professional toward colleagues and patients or clients is
   A. civil law
   B. organic law
   C. statute law
   D. ethics
   E. prudence

(Frew et al, p 29; Kinn et al, p 51)

417. Which one of the following statements pertaining to medical law is FALSE?
   A. there is no significant legal difference between performing acts on the doctor's orders and performing them under his or her supervision
   B. a patient who willfully or negligently fails to follow a physician's instructions is barred from recovering damages in court
   C. in most cases, it is difficult for a claimant to sustain a malpractice suit against a physician after ten years
   D. a physician is generally required to report to a local police department all injuries and deaths resulting from violence
   E. conspiracy is very closely related to being an accessory before the fact, the difference being one of degree rather than kind

(Flight, p 5; Abdelhak, p 388)

418. A private or civil wrongdoing or injury is a/an
   A. assault
   B. battery
   C. felony
   D. misdemeanor
   E. tort

(Flight, p 28; Lewis and Tamparo, pp 72, 79–80)

419. The giving of drugs in some type of bottle, box, or other container to a patient is called
   A. administering
   B. deposition
   C. dispensing
   D. diagnosing
   E. prescribing

(Lewis and Tamparo, p 52)

420. A contract, to be enforceable in law, must meet all of the following criteria, EXCEPT
   A. mutual consent
   B. any two parties
   C. no mistake or fraud (legal subject matter)
   D. offer and acceptance (meeting of the minds)
   E. valid consideration

(AAMA, pp 25–26; Lewis and Tamparo, p 77)

421. In the Patient's Bill of Rights approved in 1973 by the American Hospital Association, patients are to be guaranteed all of the following EXCEPT
   A. receive considerate and respectful care
   B. receive a refund of all fees if any complications arise
   C. receive complete current information concerning their diagnosis, treatment, and prognosis
   D. receive information necessary to give informed consent prior to the start of any procedure and/or treatment
   E. none of the above

(Judson and Hicks, p 67)

422. When the medical assistant interviews for employment, the interviewer will ask questions. Which is an illegal question topic?
    A. religious affiliation
    B. prior employment
    C. grade point
    D. references
    E. your weaknesses
    (AAMA, pp 189–190; Frew et al, p 910)

423. In the implied contract with the patient, the physician is not bound contractually to any of the following EXCEPT
    A. possess the ordinary degree of skill and learning commonly held by reputable physicians in the same general line of practice in the same or similar locality
    B. accept employment from anyone who solicits his or her services
    C. affect a recovery with every patient
    D. make a correct diagnosis
    E. be familiar with various reactions of patients to anesthetics or drugs
    (AAMA, pp 26–27; Lewis and Tamparo, pp 75)

424. The general law of negligence is expressed by the term
    A. litigation
    B. locum tenens
    C. non compos mentis
    D. res ipsa loquitur
    E. respondeat superior
    (AAMA, pp 96–97; Flight, p 93)

425. Spoken statements, as opposed to written statements, that tend to damage an individual's reputation are called
    A. assault
    B. battery
    C. felony
    D. libel
    E. slander
    (Frew et al, p 3)

426. In the application of the doctrine of res ipsa loquitur, the burden of proving innocence is on the
    A. patient
    B. physician
    C. nurse
    D. medical assistant
    E. hospital
    (AAMA, pp 96–97; Lewis and Tamparo, p 81)

427. A physician is bound contractually to
    A. guarantee success for any treatment or operation
    B. display infallibility of judgment
    C. restore the patient to the same condition as before treatment
    D. be free from mistakes of judgment in difficult cases
    E. advise patients against needless or unwise surgery
    (Frew et al, p 34; Kinn and Woods, p 68)

428. Which one of the following is a reason for revoking a physician's license?
    A. professional conduct
    B. ethical advertising
    C. reporting a communicable disease to the U.S. Health Department
    D. failing to prescribe drugs for known addicts and police characters
    E. betraying professional secrets
    (AAMA, pp 17–18; Kinn and Woods, p 65)

429. Of the following, which is NOT a reason for the revocation of physicians' licenses?
    A. drug addiction
    B. fraud in application
    C. alcoholism
    D. failing to accept a person as a patient
    E. mental illness
    (AAMA, p 30; Kinn et al, p 65)

430. The license that a physician obtains to practice medicine is issued by
    A. the American Medical Association
    B. the county medical society
    C. a licensing board in each state
    D. the Association of American Medical Colleges
    E. the U.S. Department of Health and Human Services

    (AAMA, pp 13–16; Kinn and Woods, p 64)

431. If a third party agrees to pay a patient's medical bills, the agreement must be
    A. in writing
    B. witnessed by two other people
    C. drawn up by an attorney or insurance company
    D. carried out within 1 year
    E. authorized by the physician in charge

    (Frew et al, p 32; Judson and Hicks, p 61)

432. Statutes protecting physicians from liability for damages as a result of rendering emergency care are called
    A. medical practice acts
    B. Good Samaritan acts
    C. emergency care statutes
    D. statutes of frauds
    E. statutes of limitation

    (Kinn and Woods, p 72)

433. The term describing the failure of a physician to perform his or her duty, resulting in definite injury to a patient, is
    A. assault
    B. battery
    C. feasance
    D. litigation
    E. malpractice

    (Kinn and Woods, pp 67–68)

434. A case involving infections resulting from broken glassware, needles, or unsterilized instruments would imply the application of which of the following doctrines?
    A. respondeat superior
    B. res ipsa loquitur
    C. res judicata
    D. locum tenens
    E. proximate cause

    (Flight, p 93; Lewis and Tamparo, pp 81–82)

435. What facility would provide surgery on an outpatient basis?
    A. an ambulatory surgery facility
    B. a nursing care facility
    C. a geriatric facility
    D. an ancillary care facility
    E. none of the above

    (Abdelhek, pp 15–16)

436. Which of the following statements is NOT a valid guideline of consent for release of patient information?
    A. The patient may not rescind an authorization for release of information once it is signed.
    B. Authorizations should include basic patient information, such as name, address, and date of birth for positive identification.
    C. Authorizations should be signed by the patient or applicable guardian.
    D. Information to be released, including specific treatment dates, should be detailed in the authorization.
    E. Patient's consent must be written.

    (Judson and Hicks, p 119)

437. A physician who treats or operates on a patient without having authority to do so commits
    A. assault and battery
    B. misdemeanor
    C. fraud
    D. tort
    E. conspiracy

    (AAMA, pp 118–119; Kinn and Woods, pp 63, 71)

438. When a dispute between a physician and a patient is settled by a third person's decision, which they both agree to accept, the process is called
    A. arbitration
    B. litigation
    C. informed consent
    D. expert witness
    E. none of the above

    (*Judson and Hicks, pp 90–92*)

439. The purpose of the statute of limitations is to
    A. fix a maximum sum that may be collected in damages from physicians in malpractice suits
    B. fix a period of time or a deadline for initiating legal action
    C. set limitations on the practice of specialties by physicians
    D. prescribe the limits of the duties of medical assistants and other paraprofessionals
    E. set the maximum fees that a physician may charge for specified services

    (*Frew et al, pp 36–37; Kinn and Woods, pp 209, 297*)

440. If it is necessary to make corrections in a medical record, the proper technique is to
    A. obliterate the error and write in the correction
    B. draw a line through the error and write in the correction
    C. use an eraser to make a neat correction
    D. use correction fluid
    E. use Ko-Rec-Type

    (*Kinn and Woods, p 2199*)

441. In which of the following situations is informed consent required?
    A. an adult who is to undergo elective surgery
    B. a patient who expresses a desire to remain ignorant of the risks

    C. an adult being treated in an emergency situation
    D. a minor being treated in an emergency situation
    E. an unconscious person without relatives

    (*Frew et al, pp 34–35; Judson and Hicks, p 120*)

442. Informed consent should include which of the following?
    A. the procedure and method
    B. risks and expected results
    C. alternative procedures and their risks
    D. results from no treatment
    E. all of the above

    (*Frew et al, pp 34–35; Lewis and Tamparo, pp 95–98*)

443. Artificial insemination by husband (AIH) is a procedure that
    A. uses a donor's serum
    B. uses the husband's semen
    C. poses many legal problems
    D. constitutes adultery on the part of the woman involved
    E. renders a child illegitimate

    (*Flight, p 235; Judson and Hicks, p 179*)

444. Which one of the following statements is true with reference to the Uniform Anatomical Gift Act?
    A. the act establishes statutory standards for determining the time of death of the donor
    B. the physician who determines the time of death may remove any part of the dead body
    C. the act does not apply to the present donation of an organ by a living donor
    D. even though a donor authorizes a gift to be made after death, a survivor has the right to bar a gift
    E. the act does not specify the persons or institutions that may be recipients of the gifts

    (*Flight, p 255; Frew et al, p 47*)

445. There is an implied contract between patient and physician for the physician to do all of the following EXCEPT

   A. perform to the best of his or her ability whether there is a fee or not

   B. continue services after being discharged by the patient if harm might otherwise come to the patient

   C. consider the established customary treatment of the profession in similar cases

   D. furnish proper and complete instructions to each patient

   E. abstain from performing experiments on a patient without the patient's complete understanding and approval

   (Kinn and Woods, pp 66–67; Judson and Hicks, p 68)

446. In health care facilities where the physicians and patient or patient's family cannot agree on prolonging the patient's life, the decision may be made by

   A. the church

   B. a panel of physicians

   C. the hospital board

   D. the courts of law

   E. the patient or patient's family

   (Lewis and Tamparo, pp 235–237)

447. Which of the following procedures do NOT require written (express) consent?

   A. proposed major surgery or invasive treatments

   B. prescribing of experimental drugs

   C. use of unusual procedures that have high risk

   D. confinement to a hospital

   E. removal of broken glass from foot

   (Kinn and Woods, p 72; Lewis and Tamparo, pp 110–111)

448. With regard to advertising, which one of the following is definitely NOT an acceptable ethical or professional practice?

   A. establishing a reputation for professional ability and fidelity

   B. follow-up announcements to patients

   C. announcement of the opening of a physician's office

   D. telephone listing

   E. testimonials of patients

   (AAMA, pp 235–236; Kinn and Woods, pp 55–56)

449. Macroallocation deals with

   A. euthanasia

   B. collection of overdue patient debts

   C. legal requirements

   D. amount and distribution of funds for medical resources

   E. benefit and cost analysis of geriatric care

   (Lewis and Tamparo, pp 169–170)

450. Which types of business structure used in medical practices will protect an individual practitioner from obligations of personal loss?

   A. sole proprietorship

   B. partnership

   C. corporation

   D. all of the above

   E. none of the above

   (Flight, pp 138–139; Frew et al, p 233)

451. Which of the following types of patients generally requires the consent of another person before the physician may begin treatment?

   A. unconscious person who needs emergency treatment

   B. married minor

   C. married adult woman

   D. 14-year-old boy

   E. adult patient who refuses proper treatment

   (Kinn and Woods, p 72)

452. Rules of conduct that govern the relationship between physicians are a part of
    A. medical ethics
    B. medical etiquette
    C. medical law
    D. professional cooperation
    E. human relations
    (Kinn and Woods, p 55)

453. In a physician-patient contract, the consideration is a term for
    A. keeping an appointment
    B. agreeing to have medical treatment
    C. submission of insurance forms
    D. following physician's instructions for follow-up care
    E. paying the fee
    (AAMA, p 26; Flight, p 72)

454. Euthanasia is a bioethical issue defined as
    A. causing or allowing death for a person with an incurable disease
    B. code red, code blue, or code 9
    C. eugenics
    D. chorionic villas sampling
    E. the practice of using surrogate mothers
    (Judson and Hicks, p 224)

455. What type of medical practice is an artificial entity with a legal and business status independent of its shareholders or employees and can often offer its employees an attractive package of fringe benefits, including pension and profit-sharing plans, medical expense reimbursement, and insurance packages?
    A. sole proprietorship
    B. group practice
    C. professional corporation
    D. associate practice
    E. partnership
    (Flight, pp 138–139; Kinn and Woods, p 42)

456. When a medical assistant observes actions or signs that arouse suspicion of child abuse or neglect, what should be the next step?
    A. advise the doctor privately of the suspicion
    B. notify the health department
    C. notify the police
    D. wait for further confirmation
    E. scold the patient
    (AAMA, pp 135–138; Judson and Hicks, p 140)

457. Which one of the following is ethical?
    A. a physician accepts a gift of a compact refrigerator from a drug distributor for prescribing certain drugs for patients
    B. a physician bills a patient for respiratory services provided by a lay organization
    C. a physician may not ask another surgeon to perform surgery on a patient without the patient's knowledge of the substitution
    D. a physician directs his or her medical assistant to send out bills that are not itemized to the patient
    E. a physician accepts a contingent fee
    (AAMA, pp 27–28; Kinn and Woods, p 58)

458. The sharing between two or more physicians of a patient's fee that has been given by a patient to reimburse one physician alone is called
    A. fee-splitting
    B. an ethical procedure
    C. compensatory medical service
    D. contract practice
    E. profit sharing
    (Frew et al, p 43; Kinn and Woods, p 56)

459. The primary responsibility of a physician is the
    A. furtherance of medical knowledge and research

B. welfare of his or her patients

C. treatment of communicable diseases

D. continual assessment of medical problems in the community

E. holding of regular office hours

(Frew et al, p 2)

460. Which of the following statements is a poor practice?

A. when a patient's care must be discussed and privacy is not protected, use the patient's name to prevent misunderstanding

B. medical personnel should not browse through records they do not need to access

C. sensitive confidential documents should be shredded or incinerated

D. fax machines, computers, and printers in medical facilities should have privacy

E. the physician has an obligation to society as a whole, as well as to the patient as an individual

(AAMA, pp 51–57)

461. "That which, in a natural and continuous sequence, unbroken by any efficient intervening cause, produces an injury, and without which the result would not have occurred" is the definition of

A. proximate cause

B. due process

C. assault

D. contributory negligence

E. res ipsa loquitur

(Flight, p 96)

462. Birth certificates are

A. state records

B. city records

C. federal records

D. patients' records

E. county records

(Lewis and Tamparo, p 93)

463. Which of the following is NOT one of the four Ds of negligence?

A. duty owed by physician to patient

B. dereliction of duty by physician to patient

C. determination of negligence to patient

D. direct cause of the patient's injuries due to physician's breach of duty

E. damages to the patient resulting from breach of duty

(Kinn et al, p 68; Lewis and Tamparo, p 81)

464. A way for a physician to terminate his or her services to a patient could be any of the following EXCEPT

A. need for further treatment ends

B. patient dismisses the physician

C. physician withdraws from the case

D. physician abandons the case

E. physician notifies the patient in writing that he or she wishes to end the obligation

(AAMA, pp 34–36; Kinn and Woods, pp 66–67)

465. In a legal sense, the relationship between the physician and patient could be best described as

A. social

B. contractual

C. expressed

D. an attorney

E. a committee from the county medical society

(AAMA, pp 25–26; Kinn and Woods, p 58)

466. Certificate of Need programs seek to help control health care costs by

A. preventing duplication of equipment and services

B. identifying indigent persons

C. providing supplies at reduced prices

D. allocating health care workers to specific institutions

E. none of the above

(Abdelhak, p 517)

467. Which of the following bioethical issues concern conception, pregnancy, birth, or birth control?

A. sterilization

B. genetic screening

C. rights of the fetus

D. rights of a newborn

E. all of the above

(Flight, pp 233–243)

468. An Employment Eligibility Verification Form 1-9 is issued by the Department of Justice, Immigration, and Naturalization to ensure that workers

A. meet required status as national citizens or authorized aliens

B. contribute to a retirement fund

C. are drug free

D. have met income tax stipulations

E. none of the above

(Keir et al, p 199)

469. Several federal laws protect workers from discrimination or workplace hazards. Which of the following regulates hiring and employment practices for persons with disabilities?

A. ADA

B. FADA

C. ERISA

D. OSHA

E. FLSA

(AAMA, pp 187–188; Flight, pp 151–153)

470. The majority of states have passed legislation concerning elder abuse. The laws generally name a health care professional as the person who should report the abuse. The laws address abuse to persons

A. 55 years and older

B. 60 years and older

C. 65 years and older

D. 70 years and older

E. 75 years and older

(Lewis and Tamparo, p 102)

471. The federal Privacy Act of 1974 covers programs under federal jurisdiction and establishes the rights of individuals to review their records. The Privacy Act requires a statement of

A. authority for the request

B. principal purpose of the request

C. routine use of the information

D. effect on individual if information is not provided

E. all of the above

(Abdelhek, p 371)

472. Exceptions are made with regard to maintaining the confidentiality of patients' records when releasing information

A. in Worker's Compensation cases

B. when the patient is suing parties who must protect themselves

C. when the patient's records are subpoenaed

D. when required by law to protect public health

E. all of the above

(Abdelhek, pp 373–383)

473. The file of an employee that contains information regarding promotions, pay increases, performance evaluations, training, disciplinary actions, and letters of recommendations would be considered

A. public property

B. confidential

C. of no legal value

D. of no value to the employee

E. none of the above

(Frew et al, p 113)

474. Medical facilities are required to account for controlled substances to the Drug Enforcement Agency (DEA) of the U.S. government. Since the medical office may be an attractive target for the addict or thief, which of the following actions should be taken?
   A. prescription blanks should never be left where they could be taken by unauthorized persons
   B. the key to the drug cabinet should be kept in a concealed, safe place
   C. doors, windows, and drug cabinets should be equipped with suitable locks
   D. cash, drugs, and other valuables should be placed where they are concealed in a safe place
   E. all of the above

   (Judson and Hicks, pp 142–143)

475. Which of the following practices with patient records helps prove in court that good medical practices were followed?
   A. a delay in filing
   B. incomplete files
   C. records are not legible
   D. records are neat, legible, and complete
   E. records have been altered or fabricated

   (AAMA, pp 172–175; Flight, pp 188–194)

476. The Patient's Self-Determination Act, which includes "Advance Directives," is intended to make sure all adult patients know
   A. their right to choose a physician
   B. their right to confidentiality
   C. their right to see their itemized medical charges
   D. their right to control their health care decisions
   E. none of the above

   (Abdelhek, p 110; Judson and Hicks, p 185)

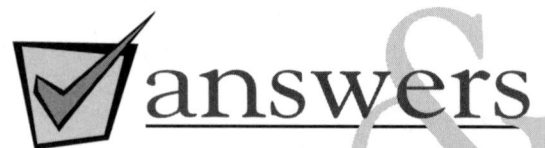

answers & rationales

402.

B. The purpose of filing reports of designated communicable diseases to government agencies is to protect the health of the community. The local health department will supply the information and forms needed for filing. These reports are used in formulating quarantine laws and instituting appropriate preventive measures. Forms and reference information about filing these reports should be kept convenient. Failure to file a report about a case as required by law could result in either criminal prosecution or a civil lawsuit.

403.

C. A tickler file should be maintained in a box or rotary file with a list of important dates and the specific tasks to be performed at that time. Important renewals should not be left to memory. Detailed descriptions of these tasks and examples of each procedure should be maintained in the office's procedural manual. Established patterns must be maintained for drug inventory and record keeping. A standard operating procedure (SOP) manual is usually maintained to enable a medical office to operate efficiently. The manual's first major division is often a checklist of tasks arranged according to a time schedule (daily, weekly, monthly, and annually). Other sections may include the topics of business office procedures, quality assurance, Occupational Safety and Health Administration (OSHA) guidelines, controlled substance regulations, and clinical procedures.

404.

C. The majority of malpractice claims are often without merit. Unfortunately, almost any physician is vulnerable to damage to his or her reputation even when the suit is groundless. Patient or patient/family anger, which may be due to many causes, is believed to be the predominant cause of malpractice suits. Therefore, the medical assistant is a valuable asset to the physician in maintaining a friendly, comfortable atmosphere for the patient in the medical office, as well as preventing negligence.

405.

D. A finance charge is both legal and ethical, although few physicians charge a separate fee. The Truth in Lending Act requires that when a bill is to be paid in more than four installments, the agreement between the patient and medical office must be in writing and must specify the finance charge. However, if a patient, alone, decides to create his or her own installment plan, the act does not apply. Situations requiring application of the Truth in Lending Act most often include very large medical bills that are not completely covered by insurance.

406.

A. Two medical records and two financial ledger cards must be kept of a regular patient's illnesses, one of each that contains only information related to the treatment of the work-related illness or injury. The compensation laws require that any medical records concerning compensation cases contain only information about the work-related injury or illness. In this way, the privacy of the patient's medical records is safeguarded.

407.

C. The patient is not billed for any unpaid portion of the Worker's Compensation account. (However, if the claim is rejected, the patient may be responsible for the bill. The patient may appeal a rejection to the Worker's Compensation Appeal Board.) There is no deductible; the physician agrees to accept the compensation carrier's approved fees for services as payment in full. Carefully itemized and coded bills should be filed with the compensation carrier every 30 days until the bill is paid.

408.

D. *The IRS Circular E Employer's Tax Guide* gives complete tax information about filing the needed forms and deposits. The payment for federal income taxes, employee FICA taxes, employer FICA taxes, and unemployment taxes must be made periodically by depositing the proper amount in a federal depositary institution, probably a nearby bank. FICA taxes, commonly referred to as social security, support Old Age, Survivors, and Disability Insurance (OASDI) and Medicare programs.

409.

D. Physicians who administer narcotics are required to register with the Drug Enforcement Agency (DEA). The registration number, assigned by the DEA, must appear on each prescription for a controlled or narcotic substance. Each medical office must have its own registration number that is renewed annually. Any change in medical office address must be reported to the DEA. A physician who regularly dispenses (gives out) controlled substances must keep a record of drugs dispensed and submit a written inventory of the office drug supply every two years to the DEA. The current records of the inventory are subject to inspection by the DEA at any time.

410.

E. As a general rule, a physician's records are not subject to subpoena, and all information obtained from patients is regarded as secret and confidential, with this confidentiality protected by law. There are some exceptions. In the physician's office, the best rule to follow, unless instructed otherwise, is to refuse to disclose information about a patient. Written authorization should be obtained from the patient before releasing information for standard requests from third parties, such as insurance companies.

411.

D. A physician who is required by law to keep records of drugs dispensed must take an inventory every two years. Dangerous drugs controlled by the federal government include narcotics. These are divided into five separate classes (schedules) ranging from the most dangerous to those with least potential for abuse. They are written as roman numerals (I, II, III, IV, V) with Schedule I drugs (LSD, etc.) having the highest potential for abuse but no accepted medical use. Separate records are required for Schedule II drugs (the most dangerous or addictive that have a medical use) and must be submitted every two years to the Drug Enforcement Agency (DEA) at the time of re-registration. Records for all drugs dispensed must be available for DEA inspection on request.

412.

C. A physician who dispenses or administers controlled substances "that is, who gives regulated drugs to patients from his or her office stock" must, if the drug is listed in the Schedule of the Controlled Substances Act, keep records of these drugs for a period of two years. The records must include the patient's name, address, date of administration, medication and quantity, method of dispensing, and reason (indication) for giving the drug. Physicians are not required to keep these detailed records of prescribed drugs because, in this case, the pharmacy that dispenses the drugs keeps the detailed records. Note the difference in the terms "dispense or administer" and "prescribe."

413.

C. Although states differ in their licensing requirements, a common requirement for a physician to be licensed by endorsement is the successful completion of the United States Medical Licensing Examination by the National Board of Medical Examiners. Not all physicians need to be licensed by the state in which they work. Exemptions include physicians engaged strictly in research, and those employed with the U.S. Public Health Service, the VA facilities, and the armed forces.

414.

C. Medical practice acts are state statutes that regulate the licensing of physicians. They generally define medical practice, list the qualification necessary for a license, list reasons for revoking a license, and create a state board to administer the statutes.

415.

B. The performing of an act that is wholly wrong and unlawful is called malfeasance, a type of malpractice. Malpractice acts are subdivided into several categories depending on the particular circumstances of the alleged act. A malfeasance malpractice claim charges that the physician wrongfully treated a patient, thus committing a wrongful act. In contrast, a nonfeasance malpractice claim alleges that proper treatment was delayed or not attempted. A misfeasance claim alleges a correct procedure was performed incorrectly.

416.

D. Ethics is the branch of moral science that defines the duties of a professional toward colleagues and patients or clients. The medical profession has several codes of ethics, including those for the conduct of physicians, nurses, and medical assistants and those defining the limits of biomedical research. Medical etiquette defines the polite manners and customs with which medical professionals treat their colleagues.

417.

A. There is a significant legal difference between performing acts on the doctor's orders and performing them under his or her supervision. The doctrine of respondeat superior ('let the master answer') extends the legal responsibility of the physician to his or her employee. However, medical assistants who are negligent may be sued. The medical assistant should know the bounds of his or her professional capabilities and stay within them.

418.

E. A private or civil wrongdoing or injury, as distinguished from a crime, is a tort. It is tried in a civil court as a lawsuit and the compensation sought is usually either monetary or involving restoration of rights. Many malpractice suits seek payment due to a personal injustice even though there is no claim of a crime that could be prosecuted by the state.

419.

C. The giving of drugs in some type of container to a patient is called dispensing. Dispensing also includes such acts as labeling, mixing, compounding, and transferring from bulk storage. Under the Controlled Substances Act, the administering of controlled substances is also considered to be the dispensing of a drug. Prescribing a drug involves issuing a drug order to a patient to be filled by a pharmacist or supplier.

420.

B. The parties to a contract must be adults of a sound mind that are capable of contracting under the law. Infants, minors, and incompetent adults cannot enter into valid, binding contracts and, therefore, must be represented by a competent adult when entering into the patient-physician contract except with certain teenage minors in some states. For instance, a teenager who is married is generally considered to be an adult.

421.

B. Complications will arise from time to time in the treatment of patients. It is unrealistic to assume that every course of treatment will be perfect. Many factors are out of the health care provider's realm. Therefore, there is no guaranteed refund of fees. However, in addition to the listed statements, the American Hospital Association further endorses that every patient has a right to: (*) refuse treatment to the extent permitted by law; (*) receive every consideration of privacy; (*) be assured of confidentiality; (*) obtain reasonable responses to requests for services; (*) obtain information about his or her health care; (*) know whether treatment is experimental; (*) expect reasonable continuity of care; (*) examine his or her bill and have it explained; (*) know which hospital rules and regulations apply to patient conduct.

422.

A. There are certain areas that cannot be legally questioned during an employment interview. Therefore, the applicant may decline to answer them. Among them are place of employment of spouse or relatives, birthplace, religion, maiden name, marital status, and children. The interviewer will be assessing such job skills as confidence, assertiveness, and interpersonal skills. You should anticipate questions regarding your views of the medical assisting profession, your ambitions, your future plans, your administrative and clinical skills, and your strengths and weaknesses. You should also prepare your own list of questions to ask the interviewer. A plan of action to find the right job, analysis of job factors to determine the best job offer, and perseverance are tools you should use to find the professional employment best suited to you.

423.

A. Physicians imply when entering into the patient-physician contract that they possess the ordinary degree of skill and learning commonly held by other reputable physicians in the same type of practice in the same or similar locality. Since it is not humanly possible to guarantee a cure, given the many variables in human biology, no express promise of a cure should be made by physicians or their agents (employees).

An implied contract is inferred by the law, and this is the type of contract that commonly exists between physician and patients. Every state stipulates in its Statute of Frauds which contracts must be written, but no state requires that a physician-patient contract be written out.

424.

D. The general law of negligence is expressed by the term *res ipsa loquitur*. This law applies whenever a patient is injured in a situation entirely under the control of the physician; e.g., an instrument or towel is left in the body cavity after surgery, the patient is burned, or unsterilized instruments are used causing an infection. A judge makes the decision, before the trial and after weighing the evidence, about whether to try the case under this doctrine. It is to the patient's advantage for a case to be tried under this doctrine. The burden of proof shifts to the medical worker who then must prove that the fault was not his or hers. If a malpractice case is not tried under this general law of negligence, then the patient must prove that the doctor was at fault.

425.

E. Spoken statements that are untrue and damage an individual's reputation are slander. Written statements that are untrue or damage an individual's reputation constitute libel. Thoughtless remarks about other doctors and loose talk in and out of the office should be avoided, since it may constitute slander. A slip of the tongue, a flash of temper, or misplaced joking could

invite a lawsuit. Furthermore, such activity is unprofessional for a medical assistant who should be a trustworthy team member in the medical office as well as a competent clinical or office worker.

426.

B. The physician has the burden of proving innocence when the doctrine of *res ipsa loquitur* ("the thing speaks for itself") applies. Ordinarily, the complaining party (patient) in a malpractice suit has the responsibility of proving negligence. However, when the injury is an obvious result of negligence, the medical worker involved must prove he or she is not negligent.

427.

E. A physician is bound contractually to inform patients of the risks of needless or unwise surgery. Informed consent is the right of a patient to know beforehand the effects and dangers of a particular treatment. In the case of major surgery or risky procedures, a written statement should be signed by the patient indicating he or she understands the procedures and its risks and gives permission. Only the physician is capable of explaining the risks of major surgery; it is beyond the scope of a medical assistant. The physician must advise against needless or unwise surgery because of the obligations he or she has assumed in the patient-physician contract for providing reasonable patient care. Therefore, he or she is legally responsible for making certain that the patient understands the terms of consent and is not confused by the medical terminology.

428.

E. Betrayal of professional secrets is unprofessional conduct and, therefore, one of several reasons for revocation of a physician's license. The duty to keep patient confidences also is a responsibility of the medical assistant as an employee of the physician. Other reasons for the license revocation are conviction of a crime and personal or professional incapacity, such as drug abuse or physical incapacity. The physician has a right to legally appeal the revocation of the license. Gross failure to keep accurate narcotic records is a crime in which allied health personnel, as well as the physician, may have liability.

429.

D. A physician is not bound contractually to accept employment from all who may solicit his or her services. The physician may choose whom to treat, but once the treatment and the patient-physician contract are entered into, the physician may not abandon the patient and can terminate the contract only through legally acceptable methods. As an extension of the right to choose their patients, physicians may also specialize, open offices where they choose, and set their own office hours.

There are, however, limitations to whom the physician may choose to treat. For instance, physicians on hospital staffs who are taking their turn at call for the emergency room service cannot refuse to treat emergency patients brought to that hospital. Participation in government programs such as Medicaid also limits the choice of who can be treated or refused treatment.

430.

C. A licensing board in each state issues the license for the physician to practice medicine either after a candidate has passed the initial examination (with the National Board of Medical Examiners) or by reciprocal agreement with another state. The physician may then obtain a license by either reciprocity (from another state's licensure) or by endorsement (meeting the state's own requirements).

431.

A. The agreement must be in writing, signed by the third party, and witnessed. Otherwise, the physician may have no legal right to require payment from the third party if that party refuses. This added precaution of a written agreement is taken because third-party payment cases are more prone to misunderstanding about payment. There is no implied contract between the doctor and the third party as is ordinarily the case between the doctor and his or her patient.

432.

B. Good Samaritan acts are state statutes that disallow the creation of a patient-physician contract in the giving of emergency care. This encourages health professionals to assist at the scene of accidents and disasters because they are not liable to be sued unless there is gross negligence. Health professionals should know their specific state's Good Samaritan law as these laws vary from state to state.

433.

E. Malpractice has two essential elements: failure of the physician to perform his or her duty and definite injury to the patient as a result. There are three basic types of malpractice claims: (1) malfeasance (claim of incorrect treatment), (2) misfeasance (claim that treatment was incorrectly performed), and (3) nonfeasance (claim that proper treatment was delayed or not attempted).

434.

B. The doctrine of res ipsa loquitur applies where the negligence is obvious and the result was such that it could not have happened without someone being negligent. A professional responsibility, therefore, falls on the medical assistant to anticipate accidents and negligence and check both before and after treatments to be certain that no negligence is possible.

435.

A. Ambulatory surgical facilities provide outpatient surgery to patients either as a satellite or hospital-based facility or an independent facility. They are often operated for profit and owned by physicians or investor-owned companies. Ambulatory surgery is a fast-growing segment of health care. In 1992, more than one half of the total surgeries performed by hospitals were outpatient surgeries. In addition to these hospital-based surgeries, physicians' offices and other ambulatory settings were the sites of many other surgeries.

436.

A. Patients may rescind their requests at any time after authorizations to release information have been signed. Additionally authorizations should be in writing to avoid any subsequent problems or misunderstandings. The authorization is normally kept in the patient's medical record to serve as a source on what information has been sent and to whom it was sent.

437.

A. Assault and battery is committed when a physician treats or operates on a patient without the authority to do so. Such a physician may be prosecuted criminally or held civilly liable depending on the particular circumstances. This type of charge can be an unintentional or intentional tort, either of which are handled as lawsuits in civil court, or it may be a criminal offense prosecuted by the state in a criminal court of law. It can be as benign as the act of giving necessary or effective treatment to a patient who refused it (a patient has the right to refuse treatment), or it may be as severe as a criminal act of sexual assault or physical attack.

438.

A. Arbitration is the process whereby two parties settle a dispute by agreeing to abide by the decision of a neutral third party. Usually the third party is selected by both the physician and client. However, in some cases, the third party may be preselected. The arbitrators make the decision on the basis of established rules and laws. Once the decision is made, there is no appeal except to have a court decide whether the decision was binding on both parties. The advantages of arbitration are that the process is less expensive and more private and time saving than taking the case to court. Regarding the other possible answer choices, litigation is the legal process of filing or contesting a lawsuit in court. Expert witnesses are persons who are trained in medicine; they define in medical lawsuits what the professional standard of care is in a community by which the defendant in a lawsuit should be judged.

439.

B. The purpose of a statute of limitation is to fix a period of time or a deadline for initiating legal action. Generally, the statute of limitations applying to malpractice begins to apply from the date of appearance of symptoms rather than from the date that the injury was caused. The law varies from state to state but the deadline for taking legal action is generally between three and seven years. Exceptions are minors who may have their limitation period extended to adulthood and legally insane patients whose period of limitation begins only after the period of insanity has ended. Another statute of limitations applies to payment of debts. The physician is limited in debt collection by the time period of debt collection defined in the statute of limitations concerning debts.

440.

B. The proper way to correct an error in a medical record is to draw a single line through the error, then write in the correction, initial it, date it, and provide an explanation if warranted. The medical record serves as a legal document of medical treatment as well as a medical history that aids in treatment. Therefore, erasure is not permitted.

441.

A. An adult or other capable person has a right to control what happens to his or her body. Only if the patient voluntarily refuses the explanation or is being treated in an emergency situation is the right of informed consent waived. The guardians and parents of minors have the right of informed consent where the bodies of their children are involved. An exception occurs when a court order has been issued to administer treatment. In this case, the right to withhold consent is overruled by the court.

442.

E. All of the above should be explained to the patient in language that is easy to understand. Individual states determine the exact scope of their informed consent laws. The decision of what course to follow should be the patient's alone. Written consent forms must be signed by the patient. This form should be understandable and broad enough to cover contemplated procedures but specific enough to create informed consent. The form should have an expiration date.

443.

B. AIH is a procedure that uses the husband's semen. AID uses the semen of another man. Both husband and wife should sign written consent forms for artificial insemination whether the sperm is donated by the husband (AIH, artificial insemination by husband) or by an unrelated donor (AID, artificial insemination by donor). Many legal and ethical questions surround the realm of artificial insemination, particularly in the case of outside donors. Many states have no laws governing AIH and AID, and rely on physicians to act prudently and protect themselves and their patients in the process. All other available avenues to fertility should first be exhausted before accepting a donor outside the marriage. The donor, if outside the marriage, should have a sperm analysis, a genetic history, and extensive testing for AIDS and other diseases. The identity of both outside donor and recipient must be protected. The recipient should have counseling to be certain that AID is really desired.

444.

C. The Uniform Anatomical Gift Act applies only to donations of organs after death. Although a relative does not have the legal power to bar the donation of an organ that has been authorized before the donor's death, most physicians and hospitals would not insist on the transplant.

445.

B. A physician is not bound contractually to continue his or her services after being discharged by the patient or by some responsible person, even if harm should come to the patient. However, a physician should protect him- or herself by obtaining a signed statement of the facts from the patient or by sending a letter to the patient confirming the discharge.

446.

D. The decision is likely to be made in the courts of law when there is disagreement that cannot be resolved concerning extreme measures to prolong life. The court will consider the wishes of the patient or the patient's family, but many circumstances influence decisions. Age, availability of resources, religion, whether a patient is comatose, and the patient's wishes all may be considered.

447.

E. Minor surgical procedures, such as removal of warts or splinters from the body, are exceptions to the rule for surgery. Minor procedures generally include an oral explanation by the physician and an oral acceptance of the procedure by the patient.

448.

E. Although standards for advertising have become more liberal over the past years, any advertising must be ethical and of high standard. The advertising method may include general information relevant to selecting a doctor's services such as educational background, payment options and plans, and location of office. All advertising must comply with federal regulations. Testimonials of patients are unacceptable because they are difficult, if not impossible, to substantiate or measure by any objective means.

449.

D. Macroallocation concerns how much can be expended for medical resources as well as how these resources can be distributed on a larger level by Congress, state legislatures, health organizations, health insurance companies, and so on. Public Law 93-641 (National Health Planning and Resources Development Act) enacted by Congress in 1974 addresses allocation of medical resources through national health goals and priorities.

450.

C. Only the corporate business structure will protect the individual against personal responsibility for business losses. The most an individual investor may lose is the amount of the original investment in the corporation. A corporation is formed by filing a certificate of incorporation in the state where the organization has its main place of business. This certificate is also called a corporate charter. The charter describes all of the pertinent information about the organization including the purpose, method of finance, the name, the number of directors, addresses, and so forth. An individual may also form a corporation. A sole proprietorship also known as a private practice involves only one person. The two reasons why a person would choose this type of business structure are (1) he or she wants to "run the whole show," and (2) all of the financial rewards from the practice belong to the owner and are not shared. Debts or liability incurred in the course of the business are not limited to the amount of capital invested in the business. A partnership is formed between two or more people. A partnership requires that an agreement be executed and a document identified as a "certificate of doing business as partners" filed in the county clerk's office. Debts of the partnership are not limited to monies invested by partners in the business. Personal assets of each partner are liable.

451.

D. Minors and mentally incompetent persons require the consent of a guardian for medical treatment except in an emergency. However, the state laws in which the practice is located should be explored. Various states have established statutory exceptions regarding older minors in cases of pregnancy, communicable diseases, emancipated minors, counseling for drug and alcohol problems, and so on. Generally, minors with the right to consent, unless there is a statutory exception, also have the right to protection of their confidences, even from parents.

452.

B. Traditional protocol of the medical profession extends privileges to other members of the profession. Each office has its own policies, which the medical assistant should learn and adhere to. Generally, doctors who visit another doctor are ushered in as soon as the doctor is free, ahead of patients (although this should be explained to the waiting patients). Telephone calls from one doctor to another are put through immediately. The fees for treating other physicians and their immediate family members often are waived.

453.

E. In a medical contract, the patient's obligation is to pay for the services received. The patient's part of the agreement includes liability for payment of services (consideration means exchange of something of value) and willingness to follow the advice of the doctor. Most physician-patient relationships are implied contracts.

454.

A. Euthanasia is defined as willfully causing or allowing death to prevent suffering by a patient with a terminal illness. There are two classes of euthanasia, passive and active. An example of passive euthanasia would be when a person who is near death from an incurable cancer is allowed to die without intervention. Active euthanasia would occur if a patient were actively assisted in his or her death by enabling him or her to use a fatal dose of medicine. Regarding other possible answer choices, code red, code blue, or code 9 is medical jargon for a life or death emergency. Chorionic villas sampling is a means of genetic testing whereby a sample of the chorion that contains the same genetic makeup as the fetus is studied for possible genetic defects. The term "surrogate" means substitute and refers to a woman who allows her body to be used to carry a fetus through pregnancy for another couple.

455.

C. A professional corporation offers many advantages not found in other types of business arrangements for medical practice. Another advantage of the corporate entity is its stability—employees are liable only for their own acts, and the corporation does not dissolve with the death or absence of a shareholder or employee. In an unincorporated solo practice or in a partnership practice, the death or discontinuance of practice by a physician necessitates a new agreement.

456.

A. The doctor should be privately advised of the facts. (In most ambulatory facilities, the doctor is the authorized reporter of suspected abuse.) If the doctor agrees that the symptoms do indeed indicate child abuse or neglect, an investigation will be requested. Because states for the most part regulate the laws concerning abuse, the law and, therefore, actions to be taken vary from state to state. Some designate medical assistants, day care workers, and preschool workers, as well as doctors, to report abuse. The medical office SOP manual should outline what is expected of the employees in such situations.

Abuse involves physical, sexual, or emotional injury. Neglect is failure to provide the basic needs of life such as food, shelter, love, supervision, and medical care. The report of suspected abuse should be made to the proper authorities before the abused child (or elderly person and, in some states, spouse) is returned to the suspected abusers. This helps prevent further abuse. Elderly and dependent adults, and spouses may also be observed as victims of abuse. Elderly people are generally classified as those persons 60 or older, depending on the individual state laws. Dependent adults have disabilities, mental or physical, and are unable to protect their own rights.

457.

C. The patient has a right to choose his or her own physician, including the surgeon, and is permitted to agree or disagree with the substitution of a physician. "Ghost surgery" substitutes another surgeon without the patient's knowledge or consent. If a clinic has a policy of rotating the group of doctors in the office or of being on call so that the doctor of choice is not always available, the patient should be informed of this on the first office visit. The patient may then choose to accept or reject this course of action.

458.

A. The sharing by two or more physicians of a fee that has been given by a patient supposedly as reimbursement for one physician alone is called fee-splitting. Giving or receiving a commission also is an example of fee-splitting. The American Medical Association condemns this practice.

459.

B. The primary responsibility of a physician is the welfare of his or her patients. The American Medical Association's Principle I states that a physician shall be dedicated to providing competent medical service with compassion and respect for human dignity.

460.

A. The patient's name should not be used when it may divulge sensitive information or help other patients or unintended participants to identify the patient's illness due to the doctor's specialty. The patient's right to confidentiality must be protected with a general office policy that is part of the daily work schedule. The following guidelines apply: Telephone inquiries should be relayed to other workers in writing to prevent being overheard. Inquiries from well-meaning friends and relatives must be politely but firmly refused or referred to the doctor. Records from office machines, such as computers and fax machines, must be protected from unauthorized persons. Confidential documents must be disposed of in some manner that protects confidentiality. Office workers must not snoop into unauthorized files.

There are, however, limited exceptions to the rule of confidentiality. The welfare of society as a whole is deemed more important than the confidentiality of one individual. Therefore, certain acts such as births and deaths are public knowledge—certain diseases must be reported to the appropriate government agency—criminal acts such as abuse of elderly persons, children, and, in some states, spouses, must be reported to the appropriate government authorities. Courts may subpoena records in certain legal circumstances. Patients can give permission for exceptions of confidentiality in instances such as employment exams and insurance reports.

461.

A. Proximate cause is the legal definition of the action that is the cause of a malpractice suit. Proximate cause is that which, in a natural and continuous sequence, unbroken by an efficient intervening cause, produces an injury, and without which the result would not have occurred.

462.

A. Birth certificates are state records. State laws require that certain disclosures must be made, such as births, deaths, venereal and certain communicable and occupational diseases, suspected child abuse, and violent injuries. These reports are considered necessary for the public's welfare.

463.

C. Although determination of negligence to the patient is the overall goal of the litigation, medical negligence has been broken down into four aspects that are related to one another and are known as the four Ds of negligence. It must be proved that the physician had a duty to the patient, that he or she was derelict and failed to perform the duty in the manner of a competent physician in the same community under similar circumstances, that this dereliction of duty was the direct cause of the patient's injuries, and that damages resulted to the patient because of the dereliction of the physician's duty to the patient.

464.

D. A physician cannot arbitrarily disengage from the contract with a patient by abandoning a case. Several situations may result in the physician being charged with abandonment. Some of these are to abruptly, without notice, discontinue treatment of a patient who requires additional care; fail to see the patient as often as required; incorrectly advise the patient that no further treatment is needed; or fail to arrange for and provide a qualified substitute physician when he or she must be absent. The physician may withdraw from a patient's case while treatment is still needed only under certain circumstances, such as noncooperation of the patient. Even then he or she should notify the patient in advance in writing by certified mail with a receipt requested. Otherwise, the physician is subject to liability for abandonment.

465.

B. The relationship between physician and patient is a contractual one. There are four characteristics of a valid contract: (1) assent (offer and acceptance), (2) legal subject matter (not illegal), (3) legal capacity (must be competent individuals entering into contract), and (4) consideration (benefits passed between the parties). The patient-physician contract generally is an implied one (not a written one). Note that different texts may use slightly different terminology to describe these four characteristics.

466.

A. Certificate of Need programs are authorized by the state to control health care costs by preventing duplication of expensive equipment and services. The institution applying must verify that there is a local need for the new facility or services being proposed or the purchase of equipment.

467.

E. All of these bioethical issues are currently debated. Sterilization by different methods includes vasectomy (removing a portion of the vas deferens) and tubal ligation. Genetic screening may involve taking a history of the parents and also submitting fetal tissue to tests for genetic disorders such as Down syndrome, hemophilia, sickle cell anemia, and Tay-Sachs disease. Fetal rights concern issues such as the individuality of the fetus. The rights of the newborn especially concern newborns with severe or life-threatening disabilities.

468.

A. An Employment Eligibility Verification Form I-9 is issued by the Department of Justice, Immigration, and Naturalization to ensure that workers meet citizenship or authorized alien status in the United States. By law the prospective client must fill out this form before being officially hired. An employee's salary cannot be lawfully paid if a Form I-9 is not on file.

469.

A. The Americans with Disabilities Act (ADA) of 1990 covers both physical and mental disabilities in the workplace. The conditions covered in this act range from infection with the AIDS virus to cancer and mental retardation. It excludes homosexuality and active illegal drug use. Listed as follows are a number of other federal regulations that prevent discrimination or provide greater safety in the workplace. The Fair Labor Standards Act (FLSA), administered by the U.S. Department of Labor establishes a federal minimum wage, regulates the employment of children, and mandates extra pay for overtime work. The Federal Age Discrimination Act (FADA) protects older workers from age discrimination. The Employee Retirement Income Security Act (ERISA) protects and regulates pensions. The Occupational Safety and Health Act (OSHA) establishes rules and regulations to prevent injuries and promote job safety, and is now in effect in hospitals, clinics, and other health care delivery facilities. OSHA is authorized to enforce its standards by investigating complaints, and inspecting health facilities and records. Right-to-know laws, administered by OSHA, apply to hazardous materials. The content of toxic chemicals, corrosive irritants, flammable materials, and carcinogens must be available to workers exposed to these materials through Material Safety Data Sheets (MSDS). OSHA also requires universal precautions to guard against exposure to blood-borne pathogens. Universal precautions are discussed further in Chapter 10 (Laboratory Procedures). The Medical Waste Tracking Act mandates the disposal of medical waste.

470.

B. The elder abuse laws in most states refer to abuse of people 60 years and older. In some states it is a requirement to report suspected elder abuse. The definition of elder abuse is physical abuse not caused by accident. Some laws also address the issues of trust, neglect, and abandonment.

471.

E. All answers are correct. Patients in federal treatment programs that are covered have the right to the answer to several questions when asked for information. For instance, the authority the medical personnel has for requesting the information, the purpose of the request, the routine use of the information, and the effect a refusal to give the requested information will have on his or her treatment all require a statement to the patient when being treated in a program under federal jurisdiction. Forms related to the privacy act are used when claims are made to Civilian Health and Medical Program of the Uniformed Services (CHAMPUS) and the Social Security program.

472.

E. Confidentiality is waived in the following situations: when the physician examines a patient at the request of a third party who is paying the bill (the patient has given his or her approval by submitting to the examination); when the patient sues someone, such as an employer or attending physician (released only on a subpoena unless authorized by the patient); when the courts of law subpoena the medical record; and when public welfare, as determined by law, requires reporting of designated diseases.

473.

B. Employee records are confidential because the information that they contain is important to the employee. Information such as promotions, pay increases, performance evaluations, training, and disciplinary actions should not be available to other employees who might resent or misuse the information.

A record also important to employees is the personnel policy statement generally contained in the procedures manual. This detailed written description covers general topics such as job definitions and descriptions, and job compensation and benefits. It informs workers of their rights and responsibilities and, therefore, helps guarantee that job responsibilities and rewards are not left to chance with one employee favored over another.

474.

E. All of the choices are good precautions against crime. A general office policy should be in effect to prevent crime and make the medical office less attractive to drug addicts and criminals. Theft should be guarded against by keeping prescription pads, drugs, and valuables, such as cash, checks, and keys, out of sight except during actual use. A survey of the premises can be used to devise a plan to prevent theft and assess the need for additional protection, such as an electric security system for after hours.

475.

D. Records must be neat, legible, timely, and complete to serve both as legal documents in cases of disputes and as valuable histories of patient illness and treatment. If an investigation of the medical record reveals alterations, gaps in charting, or unreadable material, the record-keeping procedure would be subject to question. The record-keeping procedure would also be in question if it showed that information had been concealed or lost (which may happen when charting is not done on time). Alteration of the medical record is the modification of the content, while fabricating records is making up details for the purpose of deception.

476.

D. The Patient's Self-Determination Act is intended to ensure that all adult patients know their health care rights and understand "advance directives." Advance directives express a person's wishes concerning future health care in the event that the person becomes incapacitated and unable to make an informed decision regarding his or her health care.

3 Professional Communications and Human Relations

chapter objectives

Major areas of knowledge/content included in this chapter are:

I. Standards for ethical, therapeutic professional behavior; recognition of medical assisting role as agent of physician, and a member of a medical team and professional organization

➤ enhancing role of physician/employer in a therapeutic manner

➤ professional handling of difficult work situations such as angry patients, coworker conflicts, and sexual harassment

➤ understanding and coping with the basic motivations of all persons and especially patients of different ages and/or special needs

➤ maintaining a therapeutic role toward grief and the stages of dying

II. Therapeutic interaction including the basics of verbal and nonverbal communication, good articulation, and courtesies

➤ using interviewing techniques to obtain excellent patient data

➤ telephone techniques

➤ communicating with patients of different ages/needs/ethnic backgrounds

DIRECTIONS (Questions 477 through 499): Each of the numbered items or incomplete statements in this section is followed by answers or by completions of the statement. Select the ONE lettered answer or completion that is BEST in each case.

477. When the medical assistant restates, reflects, focuses, or seeks clarification of the patient's communication, he or she is _____ the patient's contribution.
    A. refuting
    B. acknowledging
    C. misdirecting
    D. delegating
    E. none of the above
    (Tamparo and Lindh, pp 36-37; Drafke, pp 33–34)

478. CMAs and RMAs are members of which profession?
    A. accounting
    B. teaching
    C. medical assisting
    D. secretarial
    E. nursing
    (Kinn and Woods, pp 10–11)

479. A regular patient has asked to be referred to a dermatologist. The medical assistant should
    A. give the name and phone number of one dermatologist
    B. follow the policy of her physician/employer
    C. not give the names of any dermatologists in spite of the physician's permission
    D. give the patient an appointment with the physician/employer so he or she can recommend a dermatologist
    E. find out exactly what is wrong with the patient and have the physician-employer return the call
    (Kinn and Woods, p 114)

480. Which of the following describes the professional medical assistant?
    A. a multi-skilled person
    B. works under the supervision of a physician
    C. communicates well
    D. adheres to ethical and legal standards of medical practice
    E. all of the above
    (Kinn and Woods, pp 4–9; Keir et al, pp 30–34)

481. Which one of the following situations is illegal?
    A. office is well ventilated
    B. chairs are comfortable
    C. background music is played for relaxation and to muffle the sounds of voices
    D. dressing areas are provided for patients
    E. the clinic has no wheelchair entrance
    (Keir et al, pp 57–58)

482. The best way for a medical assistant to greet an established patient entering the office for an appointment would be
    A. "Hello."
    B. "Your name, please."
    C. "You're Mrs . . . ?"
    D. "Good morning, Mrs. Jones."
    E. "You must be the 9:30 appointment. Please sit down and make yourself comfortable."
    (Kinn and Woods, pp 84–88)

483. The attitude of the medical assistant might be characterized best as
    A. calculating
    B. businesslike
    C. empathetic
    D. distant
    E. condescending
    (Keir et al, pp 30–33)

484. Questions in an interview that begin with "do," "is," or "not" and are generally answered with "yes," "no," or a short answer are what type?
    A. open-ended questions
    B. closed questions
    C. indirect statements
    D. pedantic
    E. redundant
    (Tamparo and Lindh, pp 53–54)

485. Which of the following is part of verbal communication?
    A. clothing
    B. attitude
    C. facial expression and eye contact
    D. gestures
    E. articulation
    (Kier et al, pp 85–88)

486. The best initial response to an angry or aggressive patient is
    A. ignore the behavior
    B. tell the angry patient to stop the unacceptable behavior
    C. threaten the patient
    D. be patient, listen, and later document the incident
    E. report the incident to the supervisor
    (Lewis and Tamparo, pp 150–153)

487. A physician expects the medical assistant to ask patients to pay at the time of their visits. When a patient passes the desk after seeing the physician, the medical assistant might say
    A. "The bill for today is $24, Mrs. Jones."
    B. "Do you have enough insurance to cover today's appointment?"
    C. "Do you want us to add this bill to your account?"
    D. "Will you need some time to pay for today's visit?"
    E. "Would you like to have us bill you, Mrs. Jones?"
    (Kinn and Woods, p 283)

488. After seeing the physician, a patient stops at the desk of the medical assistant for a new appointment. When the medical assistant speaks with the patient, she says
    A. "Are you to come back?"
    B. "Mrs. Doe, will Tuesday or Thursday the 6th or 8th at 10 A.M. be satisfactory?"
    C. "May I help you?"
    D. "Do you need another appointment?"
    E. "Has the doctor finished with you?"
    (Kinn and Woods, p 129)

489. A physician's appointments are running behind the scheduled appointment times because she had to perform an unexpected surgery at the hospital. An appropriate statement to each waiting patient by a medical assistant would be to say
    A. "The doctor will see you soon."
    B. "Please be patient and take your turn."
    C. "I am sorry that there will be a delay of about a half hour before the doctor can see you. She had to perform an unexpected surgery this morning at the hospital."
    D. "You are very lucky to have an appointment with Dr. Doe. She is very busy, and the reason you have to wait is that she had to perform an emergency surgery at the hospital this morning."
    E. "It's going to be quite awhile before the doctor can see you. Please make yourself comfortable."
    (Kinn and Woods, p 133)

490. Which of the following should a medical assistant avoid?
    A. eliciting patients' symptoms during phone conversations to judge the urgency of the complaints and to determine when the physician should see the patients
    B. letting the doctor know when patients do not keep appointments
    C. protecting children from electric shocks by covering unused wall outlets with safety plates
    D. discarding drugs that have passed their expiration date
    E. letting the doctor know all of his patients' complaints
    (Kinn and Woods, pp 131–132)

491. The first and most important means of marketing a medical practice is
    A. send newsletters to patients
    B. advertise in the community
    C. treat the patient well
    D. keep a highly visible profile
    E. send holiday remembrances
    (Kinn and Woods, pp 379–380)

492. The best way to end most sexual harassment on the job is
    A. ignore the suggestions
    B. promptly express displeasure and establish limits
    C. threaten the harasser
    D. report the harassment to another person
    E. none of the above
    (Milliken, pp 170–171; Tamparo and Lindh, pp 197–200)

493. To assist a visually impaired or totally blind patient, the medical assistant should
    A. provide a convenient appointment when public transportation is used
    B. tell the patient ahead of time what the next action is going to be
    C. allow the blind patient and the sighted caretaker, if present, to work as a team
    D. speak to the patient in a direct and distinct manner and tell them about approaching obstacles and sharp corners
    E. all of the above
    (Hurlbutt, pp 57–58)

494. Which of the following changes are often found in the elderly?
    A. failing senses such as eyesight, hearing, and smell
    B. weakened memory
    C. susceptibility to accidental hypothermia
    D. muscles that have become smaller and stringier
    E. all of the above
    (Kinn and Woods, pp 766–780)

495. When making a collection telephone call, the medical assistant should
    A. call between 8 A.M. and 9 P.M.
    B. not show hostility
    C. adopt an optimistic tone
    D. presume that the patient is going to pay
    E. all of the above
    (Kinn and Woods, p 293)

496. The most important attributes sought in a medical assistant include the following EXCEPT
    A. accuracy
    B. sensitivity and pleasant disposition
    C. codependency
    D. flexible efficiency
    E. self-control
    (Tamparo and Lindh, pp 17; Keir et al, pp 30–33)

497. When children who are patients ask questions, the medical assistant should
    A. give the answers to the parents
    B. ignore the children
    C. take time to give short, honest answers
    D. tell the child not to talk
    E. divert their attention
    (Tamparo and Lindh, pp 128–129)

498. Which is the most basic of Maslow's hierarchy of needs?
    A. physiologic needs such as food
    B. need for knowledge
    C. status and self-esteem
    D. self-actualization
    E. safety needs
    (Tamparo and Lindh, pp 119–121)

499. A patient has been diagnosed with a life-threatening or terminal illness and retorts that the diagnosis is "absurd." Which stage of accepting death is this patient in?
    A. denial
    B. anger
    C. bargaining
    D. depression
    E. acceptance
    (Tamparo and Lindh, pp 239–240; Keir et al, p 94)

STUDY PLAN

Apply these important principles of professionalism and human relations.

- **Medical assisting is a profession of persons who assist physicians in the healing arts.**
- **Medical assistant organizations work under a physician's supervision.**
- **Recognized professional organizations are the *American Association of Medical Assistants* and *Registered Medical Assistants of American Medical Technologists*.**
- **Individuals in a profession are responsible for their own actions and promote patient welfare as an agent of the physician.**

- **Professional codes of ethics protect patients' rights**, and **define work relationships**.
- **Licensure** consists of either **certification or registry** and is gained by professional education and passing a qualifying exam. It protects professional medical assistants' identity and right to practice the profession.
- **Medical assistants** should support each other as health care team members with positive personality traits and therapeutic communication.
- **Positive personality traits** promote therapeutic responses in the patient and efficient interaction with co-workers. Negative traits retard therapeutic responses and create difficulties in the workplace.
- **Therapeutic communication is mastered through study and practice.** All communication, including therapeutic, consists of (1) **verbal and** (2) **nonverbal communication.**
- **Patient interviews** must have a structure that permits (1) **needs identification,** (2) **exchange of useful information,** and (3) **problem resolution.**
- **A therapeutic manner requires knowledge of human psychology. Common barriers** between patients and medical assistants, which must be overcome, are (1) **emotional needs and disabilities of the patient** include denial, fear, depression, anger, suicidal tendencies, drug dependency; (2) **cultural differences** between different ethnic groups; (3) **language barriers**—illiteracy or different languages; (4) **physical disabilities**—immobility, deafness, blindness, frailty, incompetency; (5) **needs of specific age groups**—children, adolescents, adults, the different sexes, the elderly; (6) **needs relating to disadvantaged groups**—the abused, racial and ethnic minorities, AIDS patients; (7) **needs relating to specific diseases**—cancer, chronic diseases, etc.; and (8) **bias and subtle discrimination** by society and health care worker.

HELPFUL PSYCHOLOGICAL CONCEPTS RELATING TO HEALTH ISSUES

Human Needs—Abraham Maslow's Hierarchy of Needs

Level 5 (highest level)	Self-actualization—full development of one's potential
Level 4	Esteem and recognition of worth
Level 3	Love, affection, and belongingness needs
Level 2	Safety needs
Level 1	Most basic of needs—survival (food, clothing, shelter)

Death and Grief—Elizabeth Kubler-Ross's Five Stages of Grief and Loss

First	Denial
	Anger
	Bargaining
	Depression
Last	Acceptance

(Note that not all patients go through all five stages or experience them in the order given.)

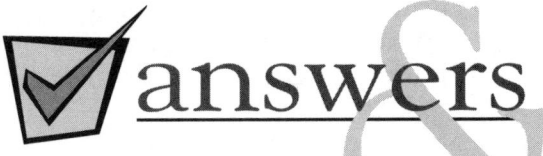

answers & rationales

477.

B. The patient's contribution in interviews and other communications is acknowledged by listening and then using communicative interactions. Focusing on important statements, restating or repeating statements, and seeking clarification are techniques that provide recognition and acknowledgment. Patience and courtesy are extremely important. At times the patient may need to restate your directions to confirm that they were understood correctly. At other times you will need to repeat or restate the patient's message to ensure accurate communication.

478.

C. CMAs and RMAs are medical assistants trained to assist physicians. They are certified or registered after receiving professional education and passing a professional entry examination. The CMA certification is maintained by the American Association of Medical Assistants and the RMA registry is maintained by the American Medical Technologists professional organization. The purposes of maintaining these organizations is to further the profession of medical assisting by (1) defining the goals, standards, and ethics of the profession, (2) providing a means to demonstrate expertise in the profession and a distinction from novices who might appropriate the title of medical assistant, (3) providing continuing education to update professional knowledge with CEUs (continuing education units) courses, (4) providing an organization that monitors current events and advises the profession, (5) providing communication between members of the profession, and (6) providing bargaining power for the profession as a whole.

A person can be a member of more than one profession. For example an instructor who is either a CMA or RMA belongs to both the medical assisting and teaching professions.

479.

B. The physician-employer's policy regarding the referral of regular patients should be followed. It is usually preferable to give the patient the names of three or more specialists so that a choice is provided. Following the conversation, the medical assistant should make a note in the patient's chart or record.

480.

E. All of the choices are considered characteristics of a good medical assistant. Both the AAMA (American Association of Medical Assistants) and RMA/AMT (Registry of Medical Assistants of the American Medical Technologists) organizations stress the need of medical assistants to continually strive to improve their knowledge and skills as professional health care workers. A health professional is a specialist who provides a practical service needed by society. Health professions seek to maintain high standards of conduct and service by means of organization, education, and certification or licensure.

481.

E. The ADA of 1990 (American Disabilities Act) requires all public facilities to be accessible to persons with disabilities, including restrooms, entrances, and other facilities.

The medical office should provide efficiency, safety, and privacy for both the patients and staff. Physical hazards such as fire, falls, biohazards such as needle sticks and waste material, emergency phone numbers and prevention of crime must all be considered.

A medical assistant should have privacy so that telephone conversations with and about patients can be private—not in the reception room where outsiders may pick up on the conversation. A private area should be provided so patients may discuss bills, insurance, or appointments away from others. Any access to private patient information should be guarded. These sources, in addition to conversations regarding patients, include computer screens, fax machines, and private areas of the clinic. Computers and fax machines should have access codes known only to the clinic staff.

482.

D. Greeting patients by name makes them feel important. It is essential for the medical assistant to develop the ability to remember their names. Therapeutic communication begins with the patient's first introduction to the office. It includes both verbal and nonverbal clues. Good eye contact is a very important nonverbal clue.

A number of aspects influence the patient's opinion of the medical facility and its ability to provide quality medical care. They include (1) the caring attitude and professionalism of the staff and (2) the appearance of the physical plant including cleanliness, and high-tech equipment.

483.

C. The attitude of the medical assistant might be characterized best as empathetic—identifying with and understanding another's situation, feelings, and motives. The medical assistant should be sympathetic and kind. Empathy implies being objective without becoming emotionally involved in the patient's problems. Sick persons want to be taken seriously and to know that they have the full attention of the medical team. They are attuned to nonverbal clues as well as verbal ones and may choose to believe the nonverbal

clues if they conflict with the verbal ones. Therefore, the medical assistant should be aware that his or her mannerisms and moods, as well as speech, affect the patient whose anxiety is already heightened from the stress of illness.

484.

B. Closed questions typically begin with "do," "is," or "are" and can be answered with a simple "yes" or "no" or a brief explanation, i.e., "Is your throat still sore?" These questions are commonly used at the beginning of the interview to obtain basic information.

As the interview proceeds, open-ended questions are used to encourage the patient to elaborate more fully on the information. They typically begin with "how," "what," or "could" and invite the patient to be more open. The word "why" is often avoided because it requires the patient to justify or find a reason for his or her answers. A sick or puzzled patient may feel defensive or inadequate.

Open-ended questions may be worded so that they are indirect statements instead; i.e., "I'm anxious to hear about how you are responding to the medication." This reduces the monotony of questioning and still directs the conversation to answers the medical assistant is seeking.

Blocks to communication should be avoided. These include stereotype/cliche comments, imposing advice on a patient in a controlling manner, belittling the patient, defending the clinic, or changing the subject to avoid a discussion. All of these will tend to intimidate the patient.

An interview between a patient and a medical assistant may be divided into three parts. (1) It begins with the orientation, where the patient assumes the role of someone seeking answers and treatment and the medical assistant assumes the role of the agent of the physician who provides treatment and answers. (2) Identification of a problem proceeds as the patient provides clues and information to assist the physician in assessing objective and clinical findings. The medical assistant may draw out the needed information by asking the types of questions listed previously. (3) The final stage of the interview is the resolution of a problem. The patient may be directed to some area of the clinic for testing, to prepare for the physician's examination, or to receive patient education.

485.

E. Excellent articulation (the distinct pronunciation of words) is a verbal aspect of good communication, NOT nonverbal. Communication is a very complex process that succeeds in conveying a message from the sender to the receiver. The verbal message also has several other components, such as loudness, pitch, time between words, and speed of the speech. Names and numbers in particular should be enunciated more slowly and clearly in telephone messages.

The other four answer choices are aspects of non-verbal communication (sometimes referred to as body language). The type of clothing we wear, our posture, stance, eye contact, gestures, unconscious manner-isms, attitude, and accompanying facial expressions all convey nonverbal messages that accompany the spo-ken (verbal) message. The distance at which we stand to talk to the patient also sends a message; standing too close may be threatening, while standing too far away may be interpreted as avoidance.

Although nonverbal communication is more easily misinterpreted, people generally choose to believe the nonverbal message if it contradicts what we are saying. Therefore, medical workers should not allow body lan-guage to contradict the intended communication.

486.

D. Angry or aggressive clients should be treated in a way that will hopefully de-escalate their anger. First of all, do not take personal offense at the patient's remarks although they may be directed to you. Listen quietly and don't rush interactions. When appropriate, suggest to the patient ways to channel the anger into perhaps physical activity or to identify the causes such as writing down when it occurred and why. Always document the incident on the patient's chart for pro-tection in the event that it is referred to later or that it might be useful in building a patient profile for diag-nosis or treatment.

487.

A. The medical assistant is making it easier for the patient to pay for an office visit when she says, "The bill for today is $24." Most people are prepared to meet small cash bills on a cash basis. By communicating to the patient the need for immediate payment the med-ical assistant lowers billing, postage, and bookkeeping expenses and possibly makes it more convenient for the patient who does not have to mail a payment.

488.

B. The medical assistant is showing respect and also verifying the patient's identity when name and title are used to address the patient. The patient should be asked if another appointment is needed and if so, a choice given of two specific times. The appointment time is arranged before the patient leaves the office. This is more efficient than having patients telephone back later (if they remember). All patients should leave the office feeling that they received top quality care in a friendly and courteous manner.

489.

C. A medical assistant shows consideration for the waiting patients and enlists support and sympathy for the doctor from the patients when he or she expresses regret, explains the delay, and tells how long it will be. If possible, cancel appointments before the patients make the effort to come to the office only to find that the physician is not in.

490.

A. The medical assistant should check with the physi-cian when in doubt and call the patient back rather than attempting to assess how urgent the situation is and when the physician should see the patient. The doctor's policy about this type of call should be listed before-hand in the office procedure manual under standard procedures for telephone calls. Appointments are always necessarily assessed as to their urgency. (This is sometimes referred to as triaging although this term more accurately refers to ranking which emergency receives treatment first where resources are scarce.)

491.

C. First and most important the individual patient should be treated well. Existing satisfied patients will give referrals to their friends and co-workers. However, many other ways may help to maintain a competitive practice. The physician may keep a high profile by mailing newsletters and holiday remem-brances to patients, speaking at public meetings, and participating in community affairs. Office hours may be extended.

492.

B. The best way, generally, to control sexual harassment is to tell the harasser to stop the offensive behavior as soon as it starts. The next most effective way is to report the harassment to a supervisor or threaten the harasser with reporting it. Ignoring the offensive behavior is not effective. Employers should provide an atmosphere that makes reporting safe and easy. Sexual harassment on the job is unwanted sexual attention and may include patients as well as peers, supervisors, and subordinates. If harassment is reported for legal action, a record must be kept of the incidents to use as documentation and preferably witnesses will be available who will testify for the victim. The victim of on-job sexual harassment should realize that there is a risk of reprisal from the accused or others who side with the harasser.

If the harasser is a patient, the medical assistant should tell the patient that the behavior is inappropriate but she should retain her authority, dignity, and therapeutic approach. The patient may be under emotional stress from illness or suffering from mental disability.

493.

E. Medical assistants should be aware of a variety of special patient problems for sight-impaired persons and be prepared to manage them. With partially or totally blind patients, it is important for the medical assistant to inform the patient what is to be done beforehand, to speak directly to the patient, to walk a half-step ahead of the patient, and generally prevent the patient from possible injury. On return visits, these patients might appreciate having the same seating and examination areas so they can anticipate their moves. If a friend or family member does not accompany the patient, transportation may also need to be arranged to and from the office. All patients should be treated with dignity and their capabilities respected.

494.

E. All of these changes occur in some elderly patients but not uniformly nor at any given age. Some patients in their seventies and eighties appear more vigorous than others much younger do. The medical assistant must first assess the patient as to the help he or she will need with physical disabilities and communication problems. This requires knowledge of the aging process and the changes it brings, physically, emotionally, and mentally. In general, aging changes can be divided into several categories. Physical problems such as failing senses of sight, hearing, taste, smell, and touch result in lack of communication ability and of the ability to move easily or avoid obstacles. A failing memory may require written instructions about medication. Financial problems may create anxieties.

495.

E. The medical assistant should prepare carefully for a collection telephone call. Be certain that the unpaid bill is discussed only with the person responsible, and be particularly courteous, calm, and unemotional. Without pleading or threatening, the assistant should presume that the patient will pay the bill and try to establish a date when payment will be made and the exact amount that will be paid. The medical assistant must not call the patient who owes a bill at work if there is a likelihood that this will be considered harassment.

496.

C. Codependency, defined as the chronic stress of living in close association with a dependent person, can become a problem for medical assistants. The day in and day out giving during work may eventually drain their energy and create a hostile attitude toward patients. To counteract the effects of codependency, medical assistants must develop empathy that permits them to remain objective while maintaining the positive characteristics of sensitivity, a firm gentleness, and a pleasant disposition. They must also learn what their limitations are of energy and time and not go beyond these to the point of chronic fatigue.

In addition to clinical and administrative skills learned during training, medical assistants must be dependable and have good judgment. They must have good communication skills, be flexible, and genuinely like people. They should inspire confidence, which precludes negative grooming, irritating mannerisms, and nonverbal clues that conflict with their oral conversation.

497.

C. When children who are patients ask questions they should receive short, truthful, and honest answers. They should not be treated in such a way that they feel unimportant or too young to participate in their health care. To be successful as a care giver, medical assistants who work with children, or any other age group for that matter, should enjoy the age group and the type of work they do. If they do not, they should try to adjust their employment.

Some guidelines for working with children in a therapeutic manner are (1) establish a friendly relationship with the child, (2) try not to keep parents and children waiting, (3) listen to the parents' concerns, (4) help the children with their emotions—let them express their feelings, (5) keep an interesting environment with bright colors and toys, (6) give rewards, (7) do not give children a choice if they may make the wrong one (i.e., they should not be given a choice about having injections and tests), (8) hold infants lovingly (if they are receptive) for a few moments after stressful events and during every office visit. This will create positive associations with the office. Remember that children, especially younger ones, have an even harder time than adults understanding their illnesses and treatments. They, like everyone else, fear most what they do not understand.

498.

A. Maslow arranges human needs into a hierarchy (ranking) of five (some authorities list seven) levels, with necessities such as food, water, shelter, and clothing as the most basic. Next is safety and security followed by the next level of belonging to a group, finding a mate, and so on. Above this level are the prestige and esteem needs followed by self-actualization (where the individual achieves the highest level of potential). Some authorities consider knowledge acquisition and the need for balance and artistic quality as two additional levels above level five. Others consider the last two as part of self-actualization.

As a person's more basic needs are met, a person desires the next higher level of the hierarchy. This model helps to explain the behavior and motivation of patients. Medical assistants find it useful to remember these levels of desire or motivation as they work with patients under stress or with other employees whose actions may be puzzling.

499.

A. Denial is the first stage of accepting the certainty of one's impending death according to the Elizabeth Kubler-Ross theory of grief and loss, which divides the process into five stages. After denial and disbelief that the diagnosis could be true, the second stage, anger with hostility, is often expressed at themselves or medical care personnel. Stage 3 is bargaining or seeking drastic changes that may alter the course of events. Stage 4 is depression, loss, and grief, as the outcome seems more inevitable. Stage 5, the final stage, is acceptance and a realistic acknowledgment of the loss. Not all persons go through all the stages. For instance, some astute persons will not deny that death is imminent while others may never move from the denial stage.

The therapeutic response by medical assistants for persons facing a life-threatening illness and potential death has some general guidelines. Acknowledge the patient's beliefs and values. Do not give false assurances or seek to avoid discussing a problem. However, if a person is in denial, do not remove hope but help the patient remain as close to reality as possible. Promote dignity and self-esteem—do not "pity." Enable the sick person to remain independent as long as possible. Help the sick person conserve his or her energy. The words "I'm sorry" or "What can I do to help you?" may be the only appropriate words in certain grieving situations.

A medical professional must not internalize the death of a patient as a failure. Death is part of the life cycle.

Administrative Procedures

CHAPTER

4 Oral and Written Communications

chapter objectives

Major areas of knowledge/content included in this chapter are:

I. Applying professional oral communication standards to administrative medical office tasks

➤ types of communication devices and telephone setups

➤ office procedural manual as a guide to effective procedures

➤ telephone techniques used in triaging/handling emergencies/ problem calls/bill collection

➤ scheduling and appointment guidelines

II. Applying professional written communication standards to administrative office tasks

➤ incoming mail guidelines, including annotation and distribution, and receipt of bill payments

➤ outgoing mail guidelines including types of postage, classes of mail, and mail economy

➤ guidelines for letters and interoffice memos, addresses, and envelopes

➤ preparing reports and scientific papers, arranging meetings, and planning travel itineraries

➤ patient education

DIRECTIONS (Questions 1 through 122): Each of the numbered items or incomplete statements in this section is followed by answers or by completions of the statement. Select the ONE lettered answer or completion that is BEST in each case.

1. A matrix in a schedule is the
   A. available facilities
   B. time not available
   C. hospital rounds
   D. available schedule time
   E. pattern of cancellations
   (Fordney and Follis, pp 96–101; Kinn and Woods, p 121)

2. Which of the following is NOT a good means of time management except for emergencies?
   A. double booking
   B. modified wave scheduling
   C. advanced booking
   D. appointment time pattern
   E. same-day service
   (Fordney and Follis, p 84; Humphrey, p 128)

3. Scheduling patients with the same medical problem on the same day is
   A. modified wave scheduling
   B. advanced booking
   C. appointment time pattern
   D. wave scheduling
   E. grouping or categorization scheduling
   (Fordney and Follis, p 104; Kinn and Woods, p 127)

4. The medical assistant has opened and sorted the physician's daily mail. When the assistant places it on the physician's desk, what piece should be placed on top?
   A. an envelope marked "personal"
   B. a special delivery letter
   C. first class mail
   D. most important mail
   E. referrals from another physician
   (Frew et al, p 140; Humphrey, p 169; Fordney and Follis, pp 226–227)

5. A medical assistant whose responsibilities include opening the daily mail should do all of the following EXCEPT
   A. sort the letters to be opened
   B. open all the envelopes first
   C. read each letter as the contents are removed
   D. date stamp each letter or write the date in pencil at the top
   E. check to be sure enclosures are included
   (Frew et al, p 139; Humphrey, pp 167–169; Fordney and Follis, pp 226–227)

6. If a medical assistant accidentally opens a piece of personal mail to his or her employer, he or she should
   A. put it back in the envelope and tape the opened edge
   B. reseal the envelope with tape and put it with the outgoing mail
   C. put it in a new envelope and seal it
   D. give it to the physician immediately and explain what happened
   E. fold it and put it back in the envelope and write across the outside "opened in error"
   (Fordney and Follis, p 226; Frew et al, p 139; Humphrey, p 167)

7. Anything that the post office will accept for mailing can be sent by
   A. special handling
   B. second class mail
   C. third class mail
   D. air mail
   E. priority mail
   (Fordney and Follis, pp 226–228; Frew et al, p 137; Humphrey, p 164)

8. The least expensive proof of mailing is to
   A. obtain a certificate of mailing
   B. use a mailgram
   C. use certified mail
   D. use registered mail
   E. use insured mail
   (Fordney and Follis, pp 178–179; Frew et al, p 137; Humphrey, p 164)

9. Special handling applies to
   A. first class mail
   B. second class mail
   C. third class mail
   D. fourth class mail
   E. standard mail including insured and COD
   (Frew et al, p 137; Humphrey, p 164; Fordney and Follis, p 229)

10. You can purchase money orders at one time in amounts up to
    A. $100
    B. $500
    C. $700
    D. $1000
    E. limited only by local restrictions
    (Postal Consumer's Guide, pp 35–36)

11. The safest way to mail valuables is
    A. priority mail
    B. certified mail
    C. express mail
    D. registered mail
    E. Intelpost Service
    (Fordney and Follis, p 229; Humphrey, p 164; Kinn and Woods, pp 157–158)

12. If a medical assistant is mailing a package with an accompanying letter, he or she should send the items by
    A. parcel post
    B. certified mail
    C. a combination mailing
    D. second class mail

E. mail at a special rate for educational materials
   (Fordney and Follis, p 228; Frew et al, p 137; Kinn and Woods, p 157)

13. The fastest type of delivery by the United Postal Service is
    A. express mail
    B. priority mail
    C. first class mail
    D. standard mail A. and B.
    E. international mail
    (Postal Consumer's Guide, p 10)

14. Fees for special handling of mail are determined according to
    A. size of parcel
    B. distance of travel
    C. weight of parcel
    D. size of post office
    E. class of mail
    (Frew et al, p 137; Humphrey, p 164; Ratefold, p 10)

15. A medical assistant has mailed a letter and wants it back. He or she should
    A. ask the mail collector to return it
    B. attempt to retrieve it
    C. contact the local police department for assistance in retrieving it
    D. make application at the post office
    E. call the local postmaster
    (Frew et al, p 142; Humphrey, p 166; Kinn and Woods, p 159)

16. Which of the following statements about postage meters is NOT true?
    A. a postage meter prints its own postage
    B. some postage meters seal envelopes
    C. the mailer leases the machine and purchases the meter mechanism
    D. the meter locks when the postage is used up
    E. to use a postage meter, the mailer applies to the post office for a license
    (Fordney and Follis, p 224; Frew et al, p 124)

17. Since the cost of sending mail is a sizable expense in the medical office, the medical assistant should
    A. buy a postage meter
    B. avoid sending certified mail
    C. avoid mailings if at all possible
    D. keep current information about postal rates and categories
    E. send letters second class

    (Fordney and Follis, p 224; Keir et al, pp 134–135)

18. Responsibility for incoming mail requires judgment in handling cash payments. What procedure should be followed?
    A. open this mail separately
    B. post the payment immediately
    C. record payments immediately in the day's receipts
    D. both B and C
    E. none of the above

    (Frew et al, p 139; Keir et al, p 110)

19. Which of the following statements is NOT true about postal services?
    A. postcards are considered first class mail
    B. special handling is available for standard mail only
    C. a refund is made if registered mail is lost
    D. standard as well as express, priority, and registered mail may be insured against theft, damage, or loss
    E. printed books should be mailed as first class items

    (Consumer's Guide, pp 10, 20–30)

20. Items, such as contracts, deeds, collection letters, etc., which are not valuable intrinsically but for which proof of delivery is needed, would best be sent by
    A. express mail
    B. certificates of mailing
    C. certified mail

    D. registered mail
    E. special handling

    (Humphrey, pp 163–164; Kinn et al, p 178)

21. To speed up mail processing with automated envelope readers (optical character recognition, or OCR), the postal service issued guidelines for addressing envelopes. Which is INCORRECT as a postal service guideline?
    A. use only capital letters throughout the address
    B. use only recognized abbreviations
    C. use the standard two-letter state code
    D. on standard-size No. 6 3/4 envelopes, begin the address 12 lines down from the top and 2 1/2 inches from the left edge
    E. place only the state and ZIP code on the last line

    (Fordney and Follis, pp 185, 187–188; Frew et al, p 138)

22. Which is not true of postage meters?
    A. the meter can be used for all classes of mail
    B. metered mail can be deposited at a designated post office
    C. metered mail is canceled at the post office
    D. daily postage use can be monitored
    E. a postage refund can be requested if the meter makes an error

    (Fordney and Follis, p 174)

23. How much postage is required for a first class letter that weighs 2 ounces if the first ounce costs 33 cents and the rate for additional ounces is 22 cents?
    A. 50 cents
    B. 55 cents
    C. 64 cents
    D. $1.00
    E. 32 cents

    (US Postal Ratefold, p 1; Fordney and Follis, p 177)

24. Lost mail is traced by
    A. notifying the post office that a trace is requested
    B. writing the postmaster general
    C. checking telephone books and other sources for possible leads
    D. none of the above
    E. all of the above
    (Frew et al, p 142)

25. The fastest delivery of messages is by
    A. major airlines
    B. special delivery trains
    C. express mail
    D. telecommunications
    E. ZIP mail
    (Frew et al, pp 135–136; Humphrey, pp 160–162)

26. The two-letter abbreviation for Alaska, which can be found in US Postal Publication 65, is
    A. AL
    B. AK
    C. AS
    D. AA
    E. AI
    (Fordney and Follis, p 187; Consumer's Guide, p 26)

27. When the word "Personal" or "Confidential" is to appear on the envelope, it should be typed
    A. in the lower left corner
    B. in the lower right corner
    C. below the return address
    D. below the zip code
    E. both A and C are correct
    (Fordney and Follis, p 187)

28. Which of the following letter styles requires that the complimentary close and typed signature be placed in line with the left margin of the body of the letter?
    A. indented style
    B. semi-indented style
    C. block style
    D. semi-block style
    E. full block style
    (Frew et al, pp 125–132)

29. Which of the following represents an incorrect use of figures in expressing time?
    A. she made an appointment for ten-thirty
    B. he made an appointment for one o'clock
    C. she made an appointment for 8:45 A.M.
    D. dateline in letter "September first, '96"
    E. the office opened at five minutes after nine
    (Frew et al, p 128)

30. Which combination of the following forms of titles and names would be inappropriate for an inside address for a letter?
    A. Dr. William A. Andrews
    B. William A. Andrews, M.D.
    C. Dr. William A. Andrews, M.D.
    D. Representative James Blackburn
    E. General Lee Pickens
    (Frew et al, p 128)

31. A notation involving special services requested (i.e., special delivery) should be placed on the envelope
    A. in the lower left corner
    B. two lines below the return address
    C. two lines above the addressee's name
    D. below the stamp
    E. in the lower right corner
    (Fordney and Follis, p 179)

32. A small envelope is sometimes referred to as
    A. No. 5 1/4
    B. No. 6 3/4
    C. No. 8 1/2
    D. No. 9
    E. No. 10
    (Fordney and Follis, p 187; Frew et al, p 124)

33. A letter printed on 8 1/2″ × 11″ stationery may be folded twice to fit into a large envelope, sometimes called a No.
    A. 6 1/4
    B. 6 3/4
    C. 7 3/4
    D. 8
    E. 10
    (Frew et al, p 124)

34. Which of the following is NOT included on a memorandum?
    A. subject
    B. date
    C. complimentary close
    D. reference initials
    E. writer's name
    (Fordney and Follis, p 166; Humphrey, pp 209–210)

35. The salutation and complimentary close are omitted on written communications of
    A. full block letters
    B. interoffice memos
    C. semi-block letters
    D. indented letters
    E. none of the above
    (Frew et al, p 166)

36. Of the following, the most formal complimentary closing is
    A. Sincerely
    B. Warm wishes
    C. Sincerely yours
    D. Cordially yours
    E. Very truly yours
    (Fordney and Follis, p 170)

37. A patient calls and asks, "Is the doctor in?" He is not and the medical assistant answers
    A. "Who's calling?"
    B. "He's still seeing patients at the hospital."
    C. "I don't have any idea." (end of conversation)

D. "No, he's out at the country club playing golf."
    E. by providing medical advice
    (Kinn and Woods, p 105; Fordney and Follis, p 82)

38. Which office appointment system have physicians preferred in the past?
    A. open office hours system
    B. wave system
    C. time-specified (blocking) system
    D. modified wave system
    E. double-booking system
    (Fordney and Follis, p 83; Frew et al, p 185)

39. If a patient calls and cancels an appointment, the medical assistant should
    A. note the cancellation in the appointment book
    B. ask the patient to reschedule
    C. immediately offer a new appointment
    D. note the cancellation in the patient's record
    E. all of the above
    (Frew et al, pp 201, 204)

40. When the appointment schedule does not run smoothly, a medical assistant should
    A. make fewer appointments
    B. set aside a free interval at different times in the morning and afternoon
    C. make no lengthy appointments
    D. request the physician to speed up the schedule
    E. request that the physician employ an additional medical assistant
    (Frew et al, p 198)

41. Which of the following words is spelled INCORRECTLY?
    A. capillary
    B. chromosome
    C. cirrhosis
    D. curettage
    E. calcanius

42. Which of the following words is spelled INCORRECTLY?

    A. hemorrhage
    B. hemorrhoids
    C. homostasis
    D. humorous
    E. grain

    (Kinn and Woods, p 144)

43. Which of the following plural words is spelled INCORRECTLY?

    A. gulfs
    B. halfs
    C. thieves
    D. beliefs
    E. loaves

    (Keir et al, pp 93–94)

44. A list of the specific items under each division of the order of business is the

    A. minutes
    B. amendment
    C. question
    D. endorsement
    E. agenda

    (Fordney and Follis, p 133)

45. In preparing the minutes of a meeting, motions should be

    A. summarized with both pro and con points of view
    B. reported verbatim
    C. summarized with the name of the party seconding the motion
    D. reported as to number in favor and number against
    E. included only if they are passed by a quorum

46. The first paragraph of the minutes (proceedings) of a meeting should record

    A. kind of meeting (regular or special)
    B. name of organization
    C. date, time, and place
    D. presence or absence of presiding officers
    E. all of the above

    (Kinn and Woods, pp 350–351; Fordney and Follis, pp 187–188)

47. If there is only one minor surgery facility available, how many patients can be scheduled at a time for surgery?

    A. one
    B. two
    C. three
    D. four
    E. all of the above

    (Kinn and Woods, p 125)

48. The minutes of a formal business meeting should contain all of the following EXCEPT

    A. list of those present
    B. place of the meeting
    C. date of the meeting
    D. time of the meeting
    E. all main motions, points of order, and appeals

    (Fordney and Follis, pp 133–134)

49. When a patient is referred to another physician for diagnosis or treatment, the following is sent

    A. a personal note from the referring physician
    B. a copy of the patient's entire health history
    C. a summary of the patient's financial history with the clinic
    D. the reason for referral along with pertinent medical information on the patient
    E. nothing is sent

    (Becklin and Sunnarborg, pp 127–128)

50. At a meeting, a quorum generally represents
    A. half of the membership
    B. more than half of the membership
    C. two-thirds or more of the membership
    D. all of the membership
    E. whatever number of the membership attend the meeting

    (Robert, pp 16, 17)

51. The proper words to use when a medical assistant is making a motion at a business meeting are
    A. I propose
    B. I suggest
    C. I make a motion
    D. I recommend
    E. I move

    (Robert, pp 26–32)

52. There is a usual order of business followed by most organizations during a regular business meeting. Which of the following would be handled first after the chair has called the meeting to order?
    A. reports of officers, board, and standing committees
    B. new business
    C. unfinished (old) business
    D. reading and approval of minutes
    E. reports of special committees (either select or ad hoc)

    (Robert, pp 300–308)

53. Which one of the following is INCORRECTLY capitalized?
    A. Minute Maid
    B. Bab-O
    C. Genesis
    D. the East Side
    E. the City of Pittsburgh

    (Kinn and Woods, p 176)

54. Which of the following is INCORRECTLY capitalized?
    A. Streptococci
    B. Algebra II
    C. Ivory soap
    D. hepatitis
    E. staph

    (Keir et al, p 125; Kinn and Woods, p 176)

55. What information is contained in the heading of the second page of a two-page letter?
    A. name of addressee and page number
    B. subject, page number, and date
    C. name of addressee and date
    D. name of addressee, page number, date, and subject
    E. name of addressee, name of writer, subject, and date

    (Fordney and Follis, p 213; Kinn and Woods, p 150)

56. If a medical assistant is typing his or her own name for the typewritten signature in a letter,
    A. it should be preceded by a title in parentheses (Miss, Ms., Mrs., or Mr.)
    B. it should be preceded by a title that is not in parentheses
    C. it should be followed by a title in parentheses
    D. his or her first and last name should be typed on one line and his or her title on the next line
    E. he or she should type only his or her name but include a title in the hand-written signature

    (Fordney and Follis, p 211; Kinn and Woods, p 149)

57. A subject line in a letter
    A. is placed on the second line below the salutation
    B. must be typed in capital letters
    C. must be centered

D. is placed on the second line below the inside address

E. indicates the name that will be used in the salutation

(Fordney and Follis, p 211; Frew et al, p 129; Kinn and Woods, pp 149–150)

58. More than one-half of the calls received in the doctor's office are for appointments and can be handled by the medical assistant. Which of the following items is/are needed in making an appointment?

A. patient's name

B. availability

C. patient's telephone number

D. type of insurance payment

E. all of the above

(Kinn and Woods, p 128)

59. The medical assistant can establish an important impression with the patient by the way he or she greets the patients. Which of the following is a poor greeting technique?

A. greet the patient immediately when he or she arrives

B. introduce yourself to any new patient

C. ask prying personal questions

D. greet a regular patient by name

E. be sure to pronounce the patient's name correctly

(Fordney and Follis, pp 62–63; Frew et al, pp 53–54; Kinn and Woods, p 82)

60. When you are typing footnotes in a manuscript, which of the following entries would NOT be included?

A. author(s) names

B. title of the work

C. place where research was conducted

D. facts about the publication

E. pages cited

(Fordney and Follis, pp 250–251; Kinn et al, p 347)

61. An appropriate salutation for a female representative, Mrs. Jane Black, would be all of the following EXCEPT

A. Madam

B. My Dear Mrs. Black

C. Dear Madam

D. Dear Representative Black

E. Dear Madam Representative

(Kinn and Woods, p 149; Fordney and Follis, p 211)

62. Professional degrees should

A. not be used in the inside address

B. always be abbreviated in the inside address

C. precede the name in the inside address

D. appear on the line following the name in the inside address

E. be used only in correspondence between professionals with the same degrees

(Fordney and Follis, p 210; Frew et al, p 128)

63. A proofreader's mark that means "move to left" is

A. #

B. /

C. [

D.]

E. lc

(Fordney and Follis, p 216; Frew et al, p 135; Kinn and Woods, p 179)

64. A proofreader who has circled an abbreviation wants the printer to

A. underline the abbreviation

B. omit the abbreviation

C. italicize the abbreviation

D. capitalize the abbreviation

E. spell out the abbreviation

(Humphrey, p 199; Kinn et al, p 179)

65. A medical assistant is typing a manuscript for his or her physician-employer and sees a word with a line drawn through it and dots underneath. This means
   A. insert a hyphen
   B. insert a dash
   C. insert spaced periods
   D. let the word stand
   E. underline the word
   (Kinn and Woods, p 179; Fordney and Follis, p 246)

66. The approximate time required to read out loud a page of copy on which there are about 200 to 250 words is
   A. 1 minute
   B. 2 minutes
   C. 3 minutes
   D. 4 minutes
   E. 5 minutes
   (Fordney and Follis, p 253; Frew et al, p 149)

67. The first copy of a written article to be sent to a publisher is called the
   A. preliminary copy
   B. manuscript
   C. article
   D. rough draft
   E. none of the above
   (Becklin and Sunnarborg, p 229; Kinn and Woods, p 346)

68. The medical assistant should keep a calendar of all meetings that the physician plans to attend. Which of the following would NOT be included?
   A. name of meeting
   B. name of speaker
   C. date
   D. place
   E. time
   (Frew et al, pp 149–150; Kinn and Woods, p 350)

69. If your physician-employer wants to send copies (reprints) of an article he/she has written to colleagues, which of the following references would furnish their addresses?
   A. Abridged Index Medicus
   B. American Medical Association
   C. Cumulative Index Medicus
   D. Excerpta Medica Index
   E. American Medical Directory
   (Kinn et al, pp 347–348)

70. Which of the following letters would be signed by the medical assistant?
   A. medical reports to an insurance company
   B. an order of office supplies
   C. consultation and referral reports
   D. the physician's personal letters
   E. letter to the medical society officers
   (Kinn and Woods, p 151)

71. In a letter with a special mailing notation, a carbon copy notation, an enclosure, and reference initials, the proper sequence of these items at the end of the letter is
   A. reference initials, mailing notation, enclosure, carbon copy notation
   B. reference initials, enclosure, mailing notation, carbon copy notation
   C. enclosure, mailing notation, reference initials, carbon copy notation
   D. enclosure, mailing notation, carbon copy notation, reference initials
   E. carbon copy notation, enclosure, mailing notation, reference initials
   (Fordney and Follis, p 212; Frew et al, p 129; Kinn and Woods, p 150)

72. Written statements delivered by the sheriff's department serving notice that a lawsuit has been filed against a defendant are
   A. affidavits
   B. legal summons and complaint
   C. affirmative statements
   D. confidential statements
   E. truth statements
   (Humphrey, pp 69–70)

73. A telephone setup where each telephone receives, initiates, and holds calls, as well as makes an intercom possible is
    A. a key telephone setup
    B. a PBX
    C. a WATS
    D. a telex
    E. all of the above
    (Fordney and Follis, pp 77–78; Frew et al, p 173)

74. A mobile device attached to a belt or kept in a pocket to alert the wearer to a waiting telephone message is a
    A. fax
    B. pager
    C. touch-tone
    D. touch-a-matic
    E. telex
    (Fordney and Follis, p 76; Frew et al, p 175; Becklin and Sunnarborg, p 87)

75. Telephone calls that may be handled by the medical assistant include all of the following EXCEPT
    A. office administration matters
    B. routine reports from hospitals and other sources
    C. patients who will not reveal symptoms
    D. receiving x-ray and laboratory reports
    E. return appointments
    (Kinn and Woods, pp 107–110)

76. In answering the telephone, all of the following would be acceptable on the part of the medical assistant EXCEPT
    A. answer on the second ring
    B. identify the office first, then ask, "May I help you?"
    C. if there are two doctors in the office, answer "Doctors Jones and Smith"
    D. say "good morning" or "good afternoon" first, then identify the office, then self

E. answer by repeating the telephone number and then asking, "May I help you?"
(Frew et al, p 164; Becklin and Sunnarborg, pp 62–72)

77. The minimum information required when taking a telephone message includes
    A. the caller's name
    B. his or her telephone number
    C. the reason for the call
    D. actions needed
    E. all of the above
    (Frew et al, pp 164–165; Fordney and Follis, p 83)

78. Telephone calls that may be handled by a medical assistant include all of the following EXCEPT those regarding
    A. appointments
    B. requests for insurance assistance
    C. satisfactory progress reports from patients
    D. inquiries about bills
    E. calls from other physicians
    (Fordney and Follis, p 87; Frew et al, p 168; Kinn and Woods, pp 110–111)

79. If an angry telephone caller who complains that the fees are too high cannot be appeased, then the next step should be to
    A. tell the patient the fees are standard
    B. tell the caller to call back at the end of the day
    C. take the telephone number and promise that his or her call will be returned as soon as possible
    D. suggest that the caller write a letter to the doctor
    E. suggest that he or she call the doctor at home in the evening
    (Fordney and Follis, p 82; Frew et al, p 167; Kinn and Woods, p 111)

80. Habitual latecomers and patients who make a habit of canceling their appointments should be scheduled
    A. first thing in the morning
    B. just before lunch
    C. in the middle of the afternoon
    D. at the end of the day
    E. immediately after lunch
    (Fordney and Follis, p 102; Kinn and Woods, p 131)

81. A type of telephone caller who is least likely to be transferred to the physician is
    A. another physician
    B. a patient who you know has unfavorable test results
    C. a patient with an unsatisfactory progress report
    D. a patient complaining about the medical care or fees
    E. an unidentified caller
    (Frew et al, pp 168–171; Becklin and Sunnarborg, p 67)

82. A system used within the clinic to call into the different rooms to give messages to the staff is
    A. an intercom
    B. call pickup
    C. voice mail
    D. automatic hold recall
    E. automatic call distribution
    (Becklin and Sunnarborg, p 67)

83. When a medical assistant is talking with one patient on the telephone and another call comes in, he or she should
    A. answer the other call but immediately put the caller on hold
    B. answer the other call, identify the office, and tell the caller to hold
    C. answer the other call, identify the office, get the patient's name, and ask the caller to hold
    D. answer the other call, identify the office, quickly identify the caller and

reason for calling, and ask the caller to please wait a moment
    E. ignore the other call—the caller will undoubtedly call back
    (Frew et al, p 164; Fordney and Follis, p 81)

84. To search and access pages of printed data from the Center for Disease or other distant health center in a matter of minutes the medical assistant would use the
    A. World Wide Web
    B. pager
    C. cellular telephone
    D. telegraph
    E. all of the above
    (Keir et al, p 139)

85. When a patient does not understand English but speaks Spanish, Italian, French, or German, a reference available that could help with the doctor's office visit is a
    A. medical journal
    B. medical speller
    C. medical dictionary
    D. medical terminology text
    E. medical transcription guide
    (Becklin and Sunnarborg, pp 30–31)

86. What is the best procedure for communicating with the profoundly deaf patient?
    A. sign language
    B. use a written form and answers
    C. use a deaf sign manual
    D. shout at them
    E. all of the above
    (Becklin and Sunnarborg, pp 30–31; Fordney and Follis, p 63)

87. If a medical assistant is requested to plan the travel itinerary for a long trip, including the purchase of tickets, where does he or she find information?
    A. a recommended travel agency
    B. American Medical Association
    C. hotels

D. airlines

E. travel magazines

(Fordney and Follis, p 253; Frew et al, pp 150–151; Kinn and Woods, p 349)

88. If the medical assistant's employer prefers that he or she plan the travel itinerary rather than a travel agency, where does he or she obtain information?

A. ask employer for his or her preferences

B. the airlines' toll-free numbers

C. the hotel chains' toll-free numbers

D. travel guidebooks

E. all of the above

(Fordney and Follis, pp 256–259; Frew et al, p 150; Kinn and Woods, pp 348–350)

89. A good way to organize the details concerning trips by an employer is to

A. prepare an itinerary

B. consult a travel directory

C. call the airlines and hotels

D. keep a travel file for current and past trips

E. prepare a flight schedule

(Frew et al, p 150; Kinn and Woods, p 349)

90. Which of the following should the person arranging a meeting attend to first?

A. calendar notations

B. preparing a mailing list

C. composing the notice

D. reserving the meeting room

E. posting location and time of meeting

(Frew et al, p 150; Kinn and Woods, pp 350–351)

91. Which of the following statements about the typing of footnotes in a manuscript is NOT true?

A. the footnotes are placed at the bottom of the page on which reference is made

B. footnotes are double spaced

C. each footnote is preceded by the number used to refer to the footnote

D. footnotes are separated from the text by an underscored line

E. superior numbers are used in the manuscript to refer to footnotes

(Fordney and Follis, pp 250–257)

92. The proofreader's mark that indicates a hyphen should be inserted is

A. -

B. = or - /

C. =/

D. -]

E. -)

(Fordney and Follis, p 245; Frew et al, p 135; Kinn and Woods, p 179)

93. On a No. 10 envelope, the address should be typed beginning on line

A. 10

B. 12

C. 14

D. 16

E. 18

(Fordney and Follis, p 236; Frew et al, p 138)

94. A detailed outline of a trip is called a/an

A. itinerary

B. schedule

C. guide

D. agenda

E. journal

(Sunnarborg and Becklin, p 244; Frew et al, pp 150–151)

95. A proofreader's mark indicating that a word should be fully capitalized is

A. uc

B. cap

C. three lines drawn below the first letter of a word

D. three lines drawn below the word to be capitalized

E. a circle around the first letter of the word to be capitalized

(Fordney and Follis, p 241; Frew et al, p 135; Kinn and Woods, p 179)

96. A proofreader's symbol that means "insert space" is
    A. ^
    B. /
    C. -/
    D. x
    E. #
    (Fordney and Follis, p 246; Frew et al, p 135; Kinn and Woods, p 179)

97. The proofreader's mark] means
    A. insert parenthesis
    B. move to the left
    C. move to the right
    D. extend the left margin
    E. extend the right margin
    (Fordney and Follis, p 216; Frew et al, p 135; Kinn and Woods, p 179)

98. An appropriate complimentary close in a letter where the salutation is "Dear John" is
    A. Very sincerely yours
    B. Cordially
    C. Yours truly
    D. Yours very truly
    E. Respectfully yours
    (Fordney and Follis, p 211; Kinn and Woods, p 150)

99. An appropriate complimentary close in a letter where the salutation is "Dear Mr. Smith" is
    A. Respectfully yours
    B. Very truly yours
    C. Cordially yours
    D. Sincerely yours
    E. Cordially
    (Fordney and Follis, p 211; Frew et al, p 129)

100. Which of the following is a proper way to express a street number and name in an inside address?
    A. 439 North 13th Street

B. 4309–19th Street
    C. 8 Maple Avenue
    D. 4 Vermont Avenue, Southeast
    E. 305 Sixty-Sixth Street
    (Fordney and Follis, p 210)

101. When there is no colon after the salutation and no comma after the complimentary close, the style is referred to as
    A. closed
    B. open
    C. formal
    D. informal
    E. personal
    (Fordney and Follis, p 211; Frew et al, p 125)

102. Which of the following statements about a small, desktop switchboard (call director) for small to medium offices is FALSE?
    A. the operator takes all incoming calls
    B. outgoing calls can be dialed directly from each extension
    C. a headphone can be used
    D. a maximum of 110 extensions can be accommodated
    E. the call director is a desktop model
    (Frew et al, p 173)

103. OCR is an abbreviation that is associated with
    A. operating room procedures
    B. orthopedic surgery
    C. computers and the U.S. Postal Service
    D. telephones
    E. optometric examinations
    (Fordney and Follis, p 236; Frew et al, p 138)

104. A mailing notation on an envelope, such as "special delivery," should be
    A. typed in all capital letters
    B. printed on a sticker that is affixed to the envelope
    C. typed with initial capital letters

D. printed in red ink and underlined

E. placed on the envelope by a postal worker

(Fordney and Follis, p 239; Kinn and Woods, pp 153–154)

105. Which is the best scheduling (appointment) system for any one practice?

A. the one which meets the specific goals of the physicians and staff

B. time-allotted slots

C. category scheduling

D. modified wave

E. open hours

(Keir et al, p 110)

106. If you are typing a letter for your doctor and the letter requires more than one page, which of the following would NOT appear on the second and subsequent pages?

A. name of addressee

B. date

C. page number

D. subject of the letter

E. all of the above

(Fordney and Follis, p 213; Frew et al, p 130; Kinn and Woods, p 150)

107. The final draft of a manuscript is printed on 8 1/2″ × 11″ good quality, white paper. It also

A. is double spaced

B. is neat with no obvious corrections

C. is prepared in duplicate or triplicate

D. has generous margins

E. has all of the above

(Frew et al, p 149: Kinn and Woods, pp 346–347)

108. Open slots in the appointment schedule of a medical practice may be used to

A. allow time for emergency patients

B. allow time for other unscheduled patients

C. catch up on delays in the schedule

D. catch up on other work in the office

E. all of the above

(Sunnarborg and Becklin, p 96)

109. Express mail

A. guarantees next-day delivery

B. supplies a special address label

C. accepts up to 70 pounds

D. includes insurance (up to $500) in the fee

E. all of the above

(Frew et al, p 137; Kinn and Woods, p 157)

110. The complimentary close for a formal letter should be

A. Warm regards

B. Sincerely

C. Best wishes

D. Very truly yours

E. none of the above

(Fordney and Follis, p 211; Frew et al, p 129; Kinn and Woods, p 150)

111. When the medical assistant who is transcribing medical notes cannot hear or understand a certain phrase or it appears wrong, he or she should

A. flag, tag, or mark the passage or leave it blank

B. use the dictionary

C. rely on past experience with the person dictating the message

D. change it to a suitable terminology

E. none of the above

(Fordney and Follis, p 219; Frew et al, p 146; Kinn and Woods, p 178)

112. Errors made on electronic typewriters with correcting tape capability are corrected by

A. depressing the correction key

B. applying correction fluid

C. using separate correction paper

D. none of the above

E. B or C

(Kinn and Woods, p 143)

113. Which of the following are essential skills of the medical assistant who transcribes medical dictation?
   A. English grammar
   B. spelling
   C. typing
   D. medical terminology
   E. all of the above
   (Fordney and Follis, p 215; Frew et al, p 146; Kinn and Woods, p 166)

114. Which of the following is a disadvantage of the open office hours schedule used in rural areas and 24-hour emergency centers?
   A. patient interviews are at a steady pace
   B. this method results in poor collections
   C. both doctor and staff may be overburdened
   D. patients will take more of the doctor's time
   E. none of the above
   (Fordney and Follis, p 104; Kinn and Woods, p 122)

115. Efficient scheduling is dependent on an understanding of
   A. the practice
   B. the physician's habits and personality
   C. time needed for each patient
   D. available facilities
   E. all of the above
   (Fordney and Follis, pp 80, 81; Frew et al, p 201; Kinn and Woods, p 121)

116. To obtain the name of a telephone caller, the medical assistant might ask
   A. "What's your name?"
   B. "Who is this?"
   C. "May I tell Dr. ____ who is calling?"
   D. "Who are you?"
   E. none of the above
   (Frew et al, p 169; Kinn and Woods, pp 104–105)

117. When working with an elderly patient, you may find that they require a little more time than with other patients. Which of the following rules should be followed?
   A. talk in a normal tone unless they are hearing impaired
   B. talk slowly and have the elderly patient repeat directions
   C. give each elderly patient an individual assessment
   D. talk distinctly
   E. all of the above
   (Fordney and Follis, p 219; Frew et al, p 61; Kinn and Woods, pp 781–783)

118. When working with a hearing-impaired patient who lip reads, which of the following suggestions will help you communicate?
   A. stand or sit directly in front of the patient
   B. speak slowly
   C. speak distinctly
   D. shout
   E. A, B, and C
   (Frew et al, p 60)

119. After-hours telephone messages to the physician's office may be handled by
   A. personal answering services
   B. answering machine
   C. pager
   D. all of the above
   E. none of the above
   (Fordney and Follis, pp 80–81; Kinn and Woods, pp 114–115)

120. When a patient cancels an appointment, the medical assistant should
   A. draw a line through the appointment
   B. erase the patient's name
   C. make a note on the financial ledger
   D. write a letter to the patient
   E. none of the above
   (Fordney and Follis, p 102; Frew et al, pp 197–198; Kinn and Woods, p 133)

121. In addition to recording house calls in a regular appointment book, a notebook should be used to record the following information for each call so that the doctor can take the notebook with him or her.
    A. directions for reaching the home
    B. patient's name and address
    C. name of person making the request
    D. patient's telephone number
    E. all of the above

    (Fordney and Follis, p 106; Kinn and Woods, p 134)

122. A criterion statement with terms such as acute onset, or recently discovered—symptoms not present at previous examination—might be used when making what type of appointment?
    A. referral to a specialist
    B. an appointment with a gatekeeper
    C. HMO
    D. hospital
    E. none of the above

    (Fordney and Follis, p 151)

STUDY HINTS

1. Obtain a copy of the United States Postal Service RATEFOLD, Notice 123 (or the most current one), from your local post office. This folder lists the different classes of postage and services offered, the fees charged per weight or piece, and the methods used to calculate charges for different mailings. It is very useful for reviewing postal requirements for this test and is also a practical reference for the office or home.

    The Consumer's Guide to Postal Services and Products explains the many services available and also gives helpful tips on packaging, addressing, etc.

2. Learn the following proofreader's marks:
    New paragraph
    No paragraph
    Insert the word, letter, or punctuation that is listed in the margin where the caret is placed in the text
    Insert comma
    Insert apostrophe
    Insert quotation marks
    Insert period
    Insert colon
    Insert semicolon
    Insert question mark
    Insert hyphen
    Insert space
    Transpose
    Delete space
    Delete material that is crossed out
    Move to left
    Move to right
    Move up
    Move down
    Align
    Spell out
    Transpose words or letter
    Transpose space
    Small capitals
    Capitals
    Set in lowercase
    Subscript
    Superscript
    Wrong font
    One-em dash
    Two-em dash
    En dash
    Ellipsis
    Lowercase

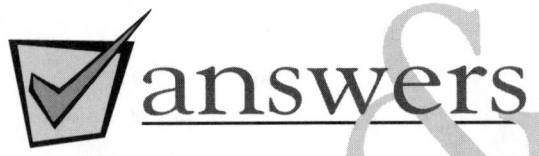

answers & rationales

1.

B. The matrix of a schedule is the time already allotted to other events and, therefore, not available for scheduling patients. The schedule must be built around these nonavailable blocks. Therefore, the first step in preparing an appointment book is to block off these times and "establish a matrix." The following guidelines are used for patient scheduling: (1) patient's needs, (2) physician's preferences, (3) available facilities, and (4) patients' preferences.

2.

A. Double booking, when two patients are scheduled at exactly the same time for the same doctor, is poor practice and makes for poor public relations. Patients may discover from talking to each other that they were scheduled at the same time and become angry if they have to wait a long time. Long waits for patients should be avoided since the office staff may, as a result, appear uncaring. Scheduling that serves both the physician and the patient should be used. Wave scheduling, a modification of time-allotted (stream) scheduling, is often used to average out the actual appointment time deviations. These deviations creep into the schedule in different ways. Walk-ins or work-ins who are sick must be triaged (screened) according to the urgency of their illnesses.

3.

E. The scheduling of patients together by category is often more efficient. For example, one morning a week might be devoted to expectant mothers in a general practice, or an internist might reserve the mornings for physical examinations. These particular blocks of patients might be highlighted with a light color in the appointment book for better recognition. Advance booking is the scheduling of appointments weeks or months ahead.

4.

D. The most important mail is placed on top of the stack of mail, with the least important on the bottom. Probably a special delivery letter would be the most important. The medical assistant should know the office policy concerning mail before opening it; for example, mail he or she should routinely handle and that which the physician wants to inspect. Do not open mail that may be personal or off limits. If the mail contains cash payments for medical bills, follow the office policy dictated in the office procedure manual. If it is office policy, have a co-worker cosign for cash received. Follow an efficient plan that will save time. Collect the needed supplies before beginning the task.

5.

C. A medical assistant should not read each letter as it is removed, since it is more time efficient to group tasks, such as opening the letters, date stamping the letters, and checking for other details, such as enclosures. If annotating the mail, proceed with reading the mail after it has been opened, noting the action that is needed. The most important words or phrases should be underlined or highlighted sparingly as the medical assistant looks for the answers to what, why, where, who, and when. All checks are stamped immediately for deposit only. Cash and checks are forwarded to the bookkeeper according to office policy.

6.

E. Personal mail belonging to others should not be opened, of course. If mail that was sent either to the physician personally or to another office is accidentally opened, put it back in the envelope and write across the envelope "opened in error." If the mail belongs to another office, seal it with tape and return it to the carrier.

7.

E. Anything up to and including 70 pounds (the maximum weight accepted) and 108 combined length and girth can be sent by Priority Mail, but the expense is greater. The post office uses the fastest means of transportation to deliver Priority Mail (2-day delivery guaranteed). Use green diamond-bordered envelopes to assure first class handling.

8.

A. A certificate of mailing is the least expensive proof of mailing if the sender does not need to prove receipt of an item and is not concerned with valuables being lost. The certificate may be purchased at the post office when mailing tax reports, collection letters, or other items requiring proof of mailing by a certain date.

9.

E. Special handling applies to standard mail parcels including insured and COD mail. It is not required by parcels sent first class, express or by priority mail class. It provides preferential handling as far as is practical in transportation but does not include special delivery. A special handling fee must be paid on all parcels that require special care.

10.

E. The total amount that can be purchased in postal money orders at one time is limited by temporary restrictions that the post office might impose. However, at this time, the maximum amount of one postal money order is $700. Additional amounts must be purchased with additional money orders of $700 or less. There is a $10,000 daily limit.

11.

D. Registered mail buys security because this mail is accounted for by number throughout the mailing process and is transported separately under a special lock. Restricted delivery and a return receipt may be requested for an additional fee. Insurance also may be purchased to a maximum of $25,000 based on declared value.

12.

C. If a package with an accompanying letter is being mailed, the letter should be attached to the outside of the package or placed in the package and "letter enclosed" should be marked on the outside of the package just below the space for the postage. First class postage is paid for the letter, and postage for the parcel is based on the class in which it falls. The combination travels in the class designated for the parcel.

13.

A. The fastest mail service available is express mail. Delivery is guaranteed for a specific time period 365 days a year including weekends and holidays. There is automatic insurance of $500 for contents. On demand pickup and information about services is available by calling 1-800-222-1811. The other answer choices are types of mail services that are available. For specific information refer to U.S. Postal Service literature including Consumer's Guide and United States Postal Service Ratefold.

14.

C. Fees for special handling are in addition to the regular postage and are determined according to the weight of the parcel. Currently two classes are charged for—(1) 10 pounds or less and (2) over 10 pounds. Special handling is available only for standard mail, which includes packages.

15.

D. Written application for the return of the letter should be made at the post office, together with an identically addressed envelope. If the mail has already left the post office, the receiving post office may be telephoned at the sender's expense. Under no circumstances should an individual attempt to retrieve mail that has already been deposited in a post office mailbox, since this is a federal offense.

16.

C. The mailer purchases the machine and then leases the meter mechanism. The user must apply to the post office for a license where a certain amount of postage is purchased and recorded on the dials of the meter.

17.

D. Postage and freight fees are a sizable expense for the medical office. The medical assistant in charge of mail should keep information current about postal rates, regulations, and categories. This should include information on private delivery companies as well. To reduce postage (1) encourage patients to pay fees at the time of their office visit; (2) avoid surcharges by using standard-size envelopes and cards; (3) use current addresses; (4) avoid mail damage by automated equipment due to the use of staples and paper clips, which may tear envelopes (use taping closures if needed, and write "Please Hand Stamp" on mailings not compatible with automated equipment); (5) weigh nonmetered mail on a postage scale so that correct postage for the weight is used; and (6) indicate correct class of mail for cheaper non-first class mail.

Surcharges are placed on large envelopes (more than 6 1/8″ wide × 11″ long × 1/8″ thick) of first class mail weighing less than 1 ounce and Standard Mail (B). single mail weighing less than 16 ounces.

18.

C. Payments should be recorded immediately in the day's receipts to prevent mix-ups due to procrastination. Realistically, the policy concerning mail-ins, including payments, is decided by either the physicians/directors or the clinic office manager and should be written in the office policy manual for reference by the employees.

19.

E. Standard Mail (B) should be used to send printed books without advertising because it is cheaper. Principal classes of mail service are as *express mail—the fastest type of traditional postal service; generally items that are deposited or picked up by 5 P.M. the previous day are delivered by noon, the next day to the receiving post office or, if designated by, 3 P.M. to the addressee. *Priority mail—preferential handling and delivery on all packages with a maximum 70 pounds and size limit size of 108 inches of combined length and girth. It is cheaper than express mail. *First-class mail—letters and so on weighing up to 11 ounces; envelopes must be at least 3″ × 5″. *Periodicals—often used to mail magazines and periodicals by retailers and advertisers. Medical offices seldom use this class for mailing items. **Standard Mail (A)**—used to mail newsletters to patients.

Standard Mail (B) includes parcel post. Standard Mail (B) and priority mail are charged by the zone and weight. **Registered mail**—is guaranteed against loss or damage; fees are based on value. Priority or first class postage is required. **Insured mail**—standard mail, first class, express and priority mail that is valued up to $5,000 can be insured by the post office. **Certified mail**—the postal service will provide proof of mailing and, for an additional fee, proof of delivery. **COD (collect on delivery)** is an additional service provided for express mail, priority mail, first class mail, and standard mail. International mail includes several classes of mail offered in the U.S. and also some additional classes. Metered mail has postage affixed by a postage meter machine at the medical office, reducing handling time at the post office. Metered mail must be bundled separately with the coding labels provided by the postal service. Letters and packages, if not first class, should be labeled with the type of service desired such as "Registered," written beneath the stamp area. Some of these classes of mail, such as registered mail, will require personal service at the post office.

Private services, such as the United Parcel Service (UPS) and Federal Express, also offer services and should be surveyed for cost efficiency, convenience, and delivery speed. The post office will furnish a United States Postal Service Ratefold, Notice 123, upon request. This folder includes a large amount of information in a quick, easy-to-read chart form. The U.S. Postal Service can be accessed on its website, www.usps.com for needed information.

20.

C. Certified mail is the best way to send documents, contracts, mortgages, or bank books that are not valuable intrinsically but for which proof of mailing and/or delivery is needed. It does not offer insurance protection. Domestic mail on which postage has been paid at the first class or priority mail rate will be accepted as certified mail. This method provides the sender with a receipt of delivery if requested.

21.

E. The postal service guidelines for addressing an envelope for an automated envelope reader require that the last line of the address contain the city, two-letter state abbreviation, and ZIP code. The total number of spaces on the last line should not exceed 26, including blanks between words. The ZIP (zone improvement plan) code consists of either five or nine digits and can be found for cities and streets by looking in ZIP code directories.

Other guidelines for optical scanning are that the first line of the three- or four-line address must be typed at least 2 inches from the top of the envelope and the bottom 5/8 of an inch of the envelope should be blank. Left and right margins should be at least 1/2 of an inch. All words in the address should be capitalized. Where both a street address and post office box are provided, the site to which the mail is to be delivered should be directly above the line with the city, state, and zip code.

22.

C. Metered mail does not have to be canceled at the post office since the meter imprints the amount of postage, postmark, and cancellation mark. All classes of mail can be mailed via metered mail by affixing adhesive strips with metered postage onto the packages. The mail should be deposited at a designated post office on the date shown. If the meter makes errors, a refund can be requested. (Do not use the meter afterward until the problem is corrected.) A refund can also be requested for spoiled and unused postage tapes and envelopes. The post office can direct the office to a list of meter suppliers and take an application for a license. The meter is set for the amount of postage and sealed by a postal employee.

23.

B. The cost is 55 cents—a 33-cent stamp for the first ounce and a 22-cent stamp for each additional ounce. If the letter had weighed 3 ounces, the cost would have been 77 cents—33 cents for the first ounce, 22 cents for the second ounce, and 22 cents for the third ounce. The fee for first class mail is charged by weight (but not distance), with the first ounce having a higher charge. Therefore, you would add the cost of the first ounce at the higher rate to the cost of all additional ounces at the lower rate. This rate structure applies to packages weighing 11 ounces or less. Postcards cost less to send than letters and envelopes.

Cost of parcel post (Standard Mail B) is charged according to both the package weight and the distance to its destination. The post office will weigh the package and assign postage, or the office can figure its own postage from the Ratefold. All mail should be weighed

with a postal scale (if not available with a postage meter) so that the exact postage needed can be calculated to avoid paying excess amounts.

24.

A. The post office is notified that a trace is requested of a particular piece of mail. The customer may have to fill out a special written form from the post office to trace mail. If a receipt of delivery was requested when the article was mailed the tracing will be easier. An attempt to trace ordinary first class mail can be made but it may not be successful.

Mail can also be recalled before it reaches the addressee. A written form must be filled out at the local post office. The post office master will call the postmaster at the letter's destination who will attempt to recover it. This will be at the expense of the sender. An envelope with an address identical to the letter being recalled must be furnished to the post office. In no event should anyone try to recover a letter from a postal mailbox since it is illegal to do so.

An address correction can be requested under the return address. When the post office forwards first class mail to the new address it will send a card with a postage due stamp and the new address to the sender.

25.

D. Telecommunications such as the fax machine and electronic computer-to-computer transmissions (e-mail) are the fastest methods of sending written messages, offering immediate communication. Cellular phones also are used widely because of their convenience. The staff and physician may wish to create a code that protects confidentiality since others in the vicinity with cellular phones can listen in on the messages.

26.

B. The two-letter abbreviation for Alaska is AK. All states have a two-letter abbreviation that must be adhered to when addressing mail. Abbreviations should be memorized or a list referred to since some abbreviations use the second letter of the state while others use a letter from elsewhere in the name. This is necessary to avoid confusion since some states such as Alabama and Alaska, Arkansas and Arizona, and Missouri, Michigan, and Mississippi, have the same first and second letters in their names.

27.

E. Personal notations (personal, please hold, confidential, and address correction requested) should be typed three lines below the return address (or line 9 from top) and aligned with the return address on the left margin. They may also be stamped or typed well to the left of the address in the lower left-hand corner. Each main word should begin with a capital letter.

28.

E. The full block style requires that the complimentary close and the typed signature appear on the left side in line with the left margin of the body. The paragraphs are not indented on either block or full block styles. The complimentary close and typed signature of the block style begin at the center point of the page. (Terminology describing letter styles may vary from author to author.) Other letter styles and formats are variations of the block where paragraphs are indented, such as the modified semi-block style or modified block style with indented paragraphs; the hanging indentation style in which the first line of the paragraph is extended to the left five or so spaces, the opposite of indented paragraphs; and the simplified style where the complimentary closing is eliminated and the salutation may be replaced by the subject line.

The physician will choose the style that he or she believes best projects a professional image, while also being easy to read.

29.

D. Dates should be expressed in figures when the day follows the month. Datelines in letters are not abbreviated. It would be correct to write "September 1, 2000" in a date line. Ordinals (numbers that give rank: first, second, third, etc.) are never spelled out after the month.

30.

C. "Dr. William A. Andrews, M.D." is an example of using incorrectly both a courtesy title (Dr.) and an academic title (M.D.). One or the other, preferably the academic title, should be used—never both. "Dr. William A. Andrews" is an acceptable form, as is "William A. Andrews, M.D."

31.

D. A notation requesting special services, such as special handling or airmail, should be placed on the envelope below the stamp. Such a notice should be entirely in capital letters. If there is an attention line, it should appear on the second line of the address.

32.

B. A small envelope is sometimes referred to as No. 6 3/4, referring to its length in inches. When an address is typed on a No. 6 3/4 envelope, it should begin 12 lines from the top and 2 1/2 inches from the left edge. These envelopes are often used for mailing statements. Other envelope sizes are the No. 10 (large) for mailing 8 1/2″ × 11″ stationery, and the No. 7 (monarch), for mailing smaller 7″ × 10″ stationery. All envelopes should be light enough in color to be able to be read by the postal service's optical scanners.

33.

E. A letter typed on 8 1/2″ × 11″ stationery may be folded twice to fit into a large, or No. 10, envelope. This fold is sometimes called a trifold because the letter has three sections after folding.

34.

C. An interoffice memorandum omits a salutation and complimentary close. A memorandum, less formal than a letter, is addressed to members within an organization. A standard memorandum format is used, containing a to, from, date, and subject line before the body of the memo. Its purpose is to convey routine information quickly and economically when background formalities are not necessary.

35.

B. The form for writing an interoffice memo does not include a salutation, or complimentary close, as in a letter. Besides the message, it contains the to, from, date, and subject lines at the top of the memo. It is quicker to write and, therefore, less expensive than the traditional and more formal letter.

36.

E. Complimentary closings that are formal in tone include Yours very truly, Yours truly, Very truly yours,

Very sincerely yours, and Respectfully yours. The following closings are informal in tone: Warm wishes, Cordially, and Cordially yours. The extent of formality in a closing is determined by the tone of the letter. Strangers are generally treated with more formality than acquaintances and friends.

37.

B. An appropriate response by a medical assistant to a patient who calls and wishes to speak to the physician is, "He's still seeing patients at the hospital." You also might say, "No, I'm sorry, Dr. Smith is not in. May I take a message?" However, do not under any circumstances offer a medical judgment over the phone even if symptoms are recited to you. Even a physician is careful about giving advice over the phone.

38.

C. The time-specified (blocking) system of appointments, the most structured and controlled system, is most efficient if it is respected and if it provides time for unplanned events. The amount of time allowed depends on the service to be provided during the visit. However, many things can create time lapses.

The wave system adjusts more to the variances of patients who arrive late, who take more time than anticipated, or who must be worked in without an appointment. In the wave system, several patients are scheduled simultaneously (probably on the hour) and rotated among the different facilities. While one has vital signs taken, another may complete paperwork, another may meet with the office manager, or have laboratory work done. A modified wave system combines the features of both the time-specified (blocking) system and the wave system. Patients may be scheduled 10 minutes apart for the first half-hour, leaving the second half of the hour open for catching up.

Categorizing, or grouping procedures, may be efficient, scheduling patients with common needs together. For example, all maternity cases could be scheduled one morning per week.

Offices that use a time-specified or wave system, often schedule a buffer time with no appointments in the morning and afternoon to catch up on a schedule that has been disrupted with unexpected emergencies.

The least structured scheduling system is open office hours, which is equivalent to a drop-in situation. Open office hours can be stressful and are usually the most inefficient of all schedules. The staff's and doctor's schedules are at the mercy of the unplanned flow of patients.

The physician determines the type of scheduling according to his or her preferences and needs.

39.

E. If a patient calls and cancels an appointment, the medical assistant should immediately offer a new appointment, inquiring tactfully as to the reason for the cancellation. No-show patients should be called on the telephone and offered another appointment. The cancellation should be documented in both the appointment book and the patient's medical record. Both are legal documents that can verify the facts in case of a legal suit later. If a patient repeatedly cancels, it is important to learn why by gently inquiring and perhaps reminding the patient that the visit is important healthwise. The exact policy, of course, is determined by each medical office and should be noted in the office policy manual.

40.

B. If a medical assistant finds that the appointment schedule does not run smoothly, he or she should experiment and set aside free intervals (buffer time) of perhaps 15 or 20 minutes at different times of the day. This may be in midmorning and midafternoon or at the end of the morning or afternoon. Open scheduling time frames at different times of the day may be especially important if the physician is in a family medical practice or other unpredictable specialty. Up to 25% of the schedule may be reserved for these buffer time slots. Some days such as Mondays and Fridays are more hectic and may require more buffer time.

41.

E. Calcaneus is the correct spelling, not calcanius. Obviously, there are thousands of medical terms that can be misspelled, but a doctor's specialty has a smaller group of more frequently used words. A small, loose leaf, indexed notebook in which all troublesome words are recorded as they occur is useful for overcoming spelling and word usage problems. Because word processors and electronic typewriters are being used more extensively, medical terminology spelling checkers can be utilized to aid in spelling. An understanding of the more common medical prefixes and suffixes also simplifies the spelling of medical terms.

42.

C. The word homeostasis is misspelled. A knowledge of medical prefixes and suffixes is useful in spelling medical terms. The word root "homeo-" is combined with the suffix "-stasis" to spell the word, homeostasis, which means a state of equilibrium (health) in the internal environment of the body.

43.

B. The plural of the word "half" is "halves." The plural of some nouns with an "f" ending is formed by adding "s," while others change the "f" to "v" and add "es." These variances in spelling are best coped with by consulting a dictionary or spelling checker.

44.

E. A list of specific items under each division of the order of business is called an agenda, which is presented at a meeting by the officers or the board. The agenda should include topics to be discussed, and should be typed and duplicated so everyone at the meeting has a copy.

45.

B. In preparing minutes of a meeting, motions should be reported verbatim. Other significant happenings and action are not reported verbatim in most meetings. The minutes should tell what the motion vote was and the name of the mover.

46.

E. All of the listed items should be reported in the first paragraph of the minutes, as should information concerning whether the previous meeting's minutes were approved. The body (not the first paragraph) of the minutes should contain a separate paragraph for each subject considered. The last paragraph states the hour of adjournment.

47.

A. Only one patient can be scheduled for the length of time required for the particular surgery. Available facil-ities affect the number of patients that can be scheduled as do the availability of the physicians and the length of time required for different procedures. This also applies to examination rooms, x-ray facilities, and special equipment. The easiest way to make these appointments is in addition to the main appointment schedule, to keep a separate list for the item that is limited. Practice will help to master this skill.

48.

A. The minutes of a formal business meeting do not contain a list of those present, but they do contain the type of meeting, the place, the date, the time, the purpose, and any action taken. The number of members and guests attending may be noted.

49.

D. The reason for referring the patient along with any pertinent medical information is sent to the referring physician so that the patient's visit will not be a surprise and the physician will have the information he or she needs. This information may be transmitted by either letter or by a telephone call from the referring physician. The patient must sign a release letter before his records are released to the new doctor.

50.

B. A quorum generally represents more than half the membership at a meeting. However, organizations may set the quorum at any number. The requirement of a quorum is a protection against an unduly small number of persons taking action in the name of the organization.

51.

E. The proper words to use when a medical assistant is making a motion at a business meeting is "I move." You make a motion, but you do not say, "I make a motion." The motion requires a second, and after discussion, it is voted on. A procedure for disposing of a motion without voting on it is to lay it on the table (or table it). Another procedure for accomplishing the same objective is to call for an adjournment. Robert's

Rules of Order has long been the accepted manual of parliamentary procedure for most organizations and should be referred to whenever questions of parliamentary procedure arise.

52.

D. In the standard order of a business meeting, the minutes are read and approved right after the meeting is called to order by the chair. It is possible to take up business out of its proper order, but it requires a two-thirds vote or unanimous consent. The standard order of a business meeting is reading and approving minutes; reports of officers, boards, and standing committees; and reports of special committees, special orders, unfinished business, and new business.

53.

E. A descriptive word that precedes the proper name of a geographic term is not capitalized. It would be proper to write "the city of Pittsburgh."

54.

A. The plural of a genus name is not capitalized, although the singular form is capitalized. Ex: Streptococcus, the singular form, is capitalized, the plural form, streptococci, is not. A medical office reference should be kept on hand, since there are specialized rules of capitalization for medical terms.

55.

D. The second page of a two-page letter contains the following information in the heading: name of addressee, page number, date, and subject (if needed). The data may be typed in either block or horizontal form. This provides identification if the page becomes separated from the cover (first) page. Be aware, however, that these rules vary with individual offices and their particular needs, experiences, and preferences. Textbooks can give only general guidelines.

56.

B. If a medical assistant is typing his or her own name for the typewritten signature in a letter, it should be preceded by a title without parentheses. When handwriting the signature, the courtesy titles of Miss, Ms., Mrs., or Mr. are not necessary.

57.

A. The subject line is typed on the second line below the salutation because it is considered part of the body of the letter. The letter often concerns a patient. Sometimes the word "subject" is used and sometimes it is omitted before the name. However, the attention line directing the letter addressed to a group or corporation, or to a particular person is placed on the second line below the inside address and above the salutation.

58.

E. All of the listed information and any other relevant information should be collected at the time of the appointment. Since a great percentage of patients have insurance, this is also valuable information. This information is obtained when the patient arrives at the office for the appointment. The reason for the visit is needed so that the medical assistant can decide the urgency of an appointment and whether more time will be needed, for example, as with a complete physical examination. Other essential information is who the person is, why the appointment was requested, time of the office visit, duration of the office visit, and the patient's home and work telephone numbers in case of a cancellation, in case of a schedule change, or if the patient is new.

59.

C. You should never appear overcurious about the patient's personal life. You should also avoid controversial subjects, such as religion and politics. It is important to have a personal touch when greeting and receiving patients regardless of their economic or social status, while also allowing them to maintain privacy.

60.

C. When you are typing footnotes in a manuscript, the place where the research was conducted would not be included. It would be necessary to look at the material cited to obtain this type of information. The footnotes appear at the bottom of the page, one line below the last line of the text.

61.

E. The titles of Madam and Representative are redundant. The courtesy titles of Madam, Mrs., Mr., and Dr. are dropped if another title is used. Any of the following salutations are acceptable in addressing a female member of the House of Representatives: Madam, My Dear Mrs. Black, Dear Madam, Dear Representative Black, and Dear Mrs. Black.

62.

B. Degree designations should always follow the name, and they are always abbreviated (e.g., Joe Brown, M.D.). When a professional degree is used, no title should appear before the name.

63.

C. A proofreader's mark that means "move to left" is [. "Move to the right" is indicated by the symbol].

64.

E. A proofreader who has circled an abbreviation wants the printer to spell it out.

65.

D. A word with a line drawn through it and dots underneath should be left in the copy. The term "stet," written in the margin, is also used to mean "let it stand."

66.

B. The approximate time required to read out loud a page of copy with about 200 to 250 words is two minutes. If slides or other illustrations are to be used in conjunction with a talk, more time must be allowed.

67.

D. The first copy of an article to be submitted to a journal for publication is called a rough draft, the first complete, consecutive typing of the article. Other drafts follow according to the style of doctor until the article meets the journal's guidelines for publication. To keep each draft separate, different colors of paper may be used. The style of articles for publication is generally more formal, omitting slang, and personal allusions although these may add a personal tone to oral presentations.

Speeches are also typed for presentation. Speeches should always be at least double spaced. In some offices, a jumbo or magnatype machine is used so the speech will be easier to read. Most word-processing programs and printers now allow control over varying print sizes in the same document. It takes about two minutes to read a page of about 250 words. The two or three words beginning the next page should be typed at the end of the preceding page in order to allow the speaker to move without a pause to the next page.

68.

B. The name of the speaker, unless of special interest, need not be included in the information that the medical assistant places on the physician's meeting calendar. However, the time, place, date, and name of meeting must be included for clarity. The medical assistant and the physician should both keep a copy. All changes must be made on both copies to avoid confusion.

69.

E. The American Medical Directory supplies addresses of colleagues to whom the physician wishes to mail reprints. The medical assistant should keep a record of reprint mailings and also keep a list of acknowledgments. If a person does not acknowledge receipt after two or three different reprints have been mailed, he or she should be removed from the mailing list.

70.

B. The medical assistant would usually sign a letter ordering office supplies. All of the other choices would be signed by the physician. Things that are strictly routine or business matters of the office usually are signed by the medical assistant.

71.

B. The proper sequence is reference initials, enclosure, mailing notation, and carbon copy notation.

72.

B. A legal summons and complaint is hand delivered by a member of the local sheriff's department to the physicians' office if the physician(s) is sued. If the physician(s) is unavailable the papers may be left with the medical assistant who is an agent of the physician(s). These papers are extremely important and the physician(s) must be notified of their delivery as soon as possible. The physicians will notify their liability insurance carriers and attorneys at once. If the professional liability insurance carriers decide not to settle out of court or cannot reach an agreement with the plaintiffs, the case will go to trial. Expert witnesses will be presented by the liability carrier to defend the position of their clients (the physicians). Eventually a judge or jury will decide if the physicians were innocent or at fault. If a guilty verdict is given, the judge or jury will set monetary damages. The court may also dismiss the case if a cause of action is not established against the physicians or the argument against the physicians is not strong enough.

73.

A. A key telephone setup makes an intercom possible by linking a group of phones together. Each telephone may use an outside line or an intercom line and can receive, initiate, or hold a call. Other features are available such as multi-line conferences, automatic dialing, and privacy. These setups are customized for the practice by the phone company. The telephone equipment needed depends on the medical clinic. Setups may include (1) the 6- or 10-button key system with several lines devoted to either incoming or interoffice calls; (2) desktop switchboards (call director) for larger facilities, which accommodate from 12 to 30 or more lines; (3) touch-a-matic phones that store frequently called numbers; and (4) speaker phones that free an individual from holding a receiver.

74.

B. A pager, sometimes called a beeper, may be carried by a physician for use as a signal to go to the telephone and dial the office or telephone answering service. The medical assistant or answering service dials a predetermined telephone number to reach the pager. This permits the physician to keep in touch with the office while having freedom of movement.

75.

C. When patients will not reveal symptoms, the medical assistant should put the calls through to the doctor or ask them to call back. Some patients prefer the additional confidentiality. The best responses to various kinds of telephone calls should be specified beforehand in the office manual. These include referrals, fee inquiries, confidential information requests, and test result reports.

76.

E. The phone should be answered by identifying the medical practice and offering to assist with a statement, such as "May I help you?" There should be a standard policy for answering the telephone that is efficient but avoids the appearance of being impersonal. The telephone should not be answered with the telephone number or a non-identifying "Hello."

77.

E. The minimum information required in taking a telephone message includes the caller's name, telephone number, reason for the call, and the action needed. A standard method (perhaps a standard form) for recording the telephone messages should be used to avoid a sloppy blizzard of memo slips, which may be lost.

78.

E. It is a professional courtesy to put through to the physician immediately any calls from other physicians. If the physician is not available, offer to call back as soon as possible. The office procedure manual may contain policy regarding these telephone calls.

79.

C. An angry telephone caller can be told that you will have to have time to pull his or her chart and that the call will be returned. The doctor may prefer to talk directly to an angry patient. The medical assistant must avoid getting angry. He or she must identify the actual problem and provide the best answer. Be sure to really listen, express interest, and take careful notes.

80.

D. Habitual latecomers and patients who make a habit of canceling their appointments should be scheduled at the end of the day. This will not create a vacancy or schedule problem during the day and will enable the physician to leave earlier if the patients do not appear.

81.

E. A type of telephone call that would usually not be transferred to the doctor is one from a person who refuses to give his or her name or business. These callers frequently are salespersons who know that if they identify themselves the call will not be transferred to the doctor. If they will not give you a message, one alternative is to suggest that they write a letter to the doctor. All of the other choices will sometimes, if not always, be transferred to physicians. However, in the final analysis, whether the calls are accepted or not depends on the office policy established by the physician(s). The policy for handling different types of calls should be recorded in the SOP (standard operating procedures) manual of the office.

82.

A. The intercom system is used by the staff to send messages to other rooms by pushing the appropriate intercom button. Other devices used in telephone communication are (1) voice mail which records messages so that they can be answered later; (2) call pickup which allows calls to be answered from an extension other than that which they were directed to; (3) automatic hold recall which reminds you at short intervals that another caller is waiting on the line; and (4) automatic call distribution which allows calls to be taken in the order received.

83.

D. When a medical assistant is talking with one patient on the telephone and another call comes in, he or she should triage the call; that is, identify the office, identify the caller and reason for the call, and ask the caller to please wait a moment if the call is not an emergency. Always give the person on the line the opportunity to say who is calling and if it is an emergency. If it is an emergency, the established procedure for an emergency is then followed. The term, triage, describes the categorizing of patients according to their need for medical care and the allocation of medical resources so that all may be treated most effectively.

If the caller cannot wait for some reason but it is not an emergency, the medical assistant should take the number and return the call as soon as possible. Callers should be treated impartially and under ordinary circumstances it is fair that the first caller receive the attention of the medical assistant first.

84.

A. The Internet/World Wide Web permits a person with a computer, modem, software, and Internet connection to use search engines such as Yahoo or Alta Vista to search for desired topics, access the information posted on the Internet and then to print off what is needed. Other electronic means such as e-mail and faxing are also being used increasingly to send and receive messages and gather information quickly and inexpensively. However, the problem of security both in medical facilities and on the Internet limits the use of these electronic messages at the current time.

85.

C. Some medical dictionaries, such as Taber's, have an interpreter section. This section provides the medical assistant with the basic questions for medical history, examinations, treatment, and medications. *Taber's Cyclopedic Medical Dictionary* includes an interpreter section for Spanish, Italian, French, and German. Newer advances in computer devices also are providing electronic multi-language dictionaries. However, it is still more efficient to ask if a relative or community volunteer can act as an interpreter.

86.

B. The best procedure for communicating with the deaf patient is probably to use a preprinted form with general questions so the patient can write answers. This avoids the problem of inept sign language or distorted speech patterns. If the local community has interpreters for the deaf, they may assist.

87.

A. Travel agencies that have been recommended by a trusted business associate and have a proven record of service are good places to start when planning a trip. They specialize in travel arrangements and can access information quickly about constantly changing fares and flight schedules, hotels, car rentals, and so on. Their service usually is free and generally includes free delivery of the tickets and itinerary to the traveler. Their income is from commissions paid by airlines and hotels.

88.

E. The employee planning a travel itinerary begins with the traveler's preferences. Then, there are many sources of information, such as the toll-free telephone services operated by airlines, hotel chains, and so on. Extensive guidebooks, such as *Crampton's International Airport Transit Guide*, are helpful in planning transit between airports and city centers when timing is crucial.

89.

D. A travel file should be kept for trips. A travel worksheet, a form with spaces for the trip's details, such as dates, modes of travel, travel time, reservations, travel funds, and appointments, is prepared. Keep a list of all required trip details such as packing a briefcase; personal items, such as eyeglasses; detailed and thumbnail itineraries; and a calendar of meetings.

90.

D. The first detail to attend to in arranging a meeting is reserving the meeting room (if it is away from the clinic); otherwise, it may not be available. After this, take care of other details such as a calendar notation, mailing list, and posting the time and place. The mailout should be made in time for the participants to make plans but not so far ahead that the meeting is forgotten.

91.

B. Footnotes are single-spaced. However, a double space separates each footnote. The manuscript narrative is also double-spaced. Details of how to write footnotes (and other technical tasks) are hard to remember if you seldom type manuscripts. The *Gregg Reference Manual* or other reference resources should be referred to when beginning a manuscript, if the task is not a familiar one. The use of reference material is always a good idea in such cases.

92.

B. The proofreader's mark that indicates a hyphen should be inserted is =. The correction should be made in the margin next to the error. Proofreading galley proofs is easier with two persons working together, one with the galley proof and one with the original manuscript. Some corrections may be indicated by the use of other symbols depending on the authority relied upon.

93.

B. The address on a large envelope (No. 10) should be started on about line 12 (2 inches) from the top edge. The address should be started just below the center of the envelope and just to the left of center. The address should be single spaced, and in all capital letters. The same rules apply to smaller envelopes (No. 6).

94.

A. An itinerary is a detailed, written outline of a trip and should contain the following information: the time of departure and arrival for each stop and terminal changes, accommodations and reservations, time changes, confirmations, interviews, or appointments. In other words, details that are needed during the trip should not be left to the traveler's memory. Medical assistants arranging travel details will consult the traveler for preferences in airlines, hotels, and so on. The traveler will probably use a travel agency and charge the expenses of travel to a credit card number. Factors considered when making travel arrangements are type of travel—e.g., coach or first class airline travel; cost range of tickets and hotels; type of hotel room (size, access to meetings, restaurants etc.); handling of baggage (weight requirements, etc.); waiting periods between flights; potential weather problems; and time between arrival and attending a conference.

Steps in arranging travel are as follows: (1) learn travel preferences; (2) obtain and confirm transportation and hotel; (3) prepare itinerary; (4) record itinerary in schedule book and reschedule patients that will be affected; (5) arrange travel funds; (6) prepare a travel folder for the traveler with maps, tickets, information about confirmations of hotel, packet on meeting, or conference materials; (7) arrange for funds for traveler; (8) confirm the arrangements for practice coverage during the physician's absence; and (9) notify the answering service of the dates of travel and provide the names of the covering physicians.

95.

D. Drawing three lines under a word indicates that it should be capitalized.

96.

E. The number symbol (#) is a proofreader's mark meaning "insert space." Proofreading corrections should be entered in a different color pencil in the margin of the proof next to the line with the error to be corrected.

97.

C. The proofreader's mark] means "move to the right." The opposite symbol [means "move to the left."

98.

B. An appropriate complimentary close in a letter where the salutation is "Dear John" is Cordially, Cordially yours, or Yours cordially. The complimentary close of a letter is determined by the formality of the salutation. "Cordially" is considered an informal closing and, therefore, belongs with "Dear John."

99.

B. An appropriate complimentary close in a letter to a business associate where the salutation is "Dear Mr. Smith" is "Very truly yours." The degree of formality in the closing should match that in the salutation.

100.

A. The correct street address is 439 North 13th Street. (The names of streets and street numbers are always written as figures except for street numbers when they are one through ten.) Ordinals (e.g., first, second, third) are not written out in street numbers above 10.

101.

B. In open punctuation, there is no colon after the salutation and no comma after the complimentary close. This pattern is always used with simplified letter styles and sometimes with the full block style.

102.

D. A call director, a small desktop switchboard most often installed in larger offices, can accommodate from as few as 12 extensions to up to 30 or more. Even the smallest switchboard has more labor and hardware expenses. Therefore, a typical smaller medical office will instead use a multiline 6- or 10-button telephone system, which allows for phones in various rooms and optional features such as conference calls, memory dial, and holding. Telephone service is an important part of a medical practice and much of the medical practice's connection to patients is over the phone.

The physicians set the policy, which should be outlined in a list of specific phone scenarios and the recommended responses. The medical assistant should project a positive image as well as manage the phone service efficiently. In addition to office phones, medical assistants must coordinate cellular and beeper service, answering services, and patient education regarding phones. Legal concerns for the physician and his or her staff include protecting the confidentiality of patients, especially over cellular and pager phones, not diagnosing over the phone, responding to emergencies, not abandoning patients by not being available when on call, not making specific promises, and not harassing patients by calling at inopportune times.

Mobile communications include cellular phone and the beeper or pager service for the physician on call. Answering services may be as simple as a taped recording identifying the office with its hours and inviting the caller to leave a message. A more professional answering service has an operator answer the call, screen the message, and call the physician, if indicated. The medical assistant is responsible for informing the answering service of the physician's whereabouts and seeing that the physician receives important phone messages left for him or her.

Patient education about the phone may use a tactfully worded brochure listing the clinic's phone policies with the phone hours and the most advantageous time to call. Patients may be instructed to keep a pen and pad handy for taking the doctor's messages and to perform home tests such as urine tests or the taking of temperatures before calling the medical office.

103.

C. Optical character recognition (OCR) is used by the peripheral devices of computers (scanners) to recognize optical characters, such as numbers on bank checks, bar codes on merchandise, and handwritten characters on tests. The post office is introducing an automated mail system requiring that envelopes' addresses conform to optical character recognition requirements. Everything in the address should be written in ALL CAPITAL LETTERS. Do not use script or italic type. Black print on white envelopes is preferred, as is use of the two-letter code for the state. Type the envelope in a block format in the area the scanner is programmed to read.

104.

A. Mailing notations (special delivery, certified, hand cancel, etc.) should be typed in ALL CAPITAL LETTERS in the right upper corner of the envelope 9 lines from the top of the envelope or 3 lines below the stamp. It should end about one-half of an inch from the right edge of the envelope.

105.

A. Whatever system works best for that individual practice is the best one. The personalities of the physicians, the community customs, and the types of patients all affect scheduling. On the one hand, some family practices in rural communities without phones find that open hours (unstructured blocks of time) with few appointments work best. Referral practices, on the other hand, may rely wholly on time-allotted appointments. An effective patient schedule meets three sets of goals—those of the physician, the patients, and the medical assistants. The physician desires time for all demands (e.g., emergencies, sufficient, uninterrupted time with patients, cost effectiveness). The patient desires a minimum waiting period for the appointment date, a minimum wait in the office, and maximum time with the physician. The medical assistant wants a smooth running office that closes on time, provides a lunch hour, and meets the approval of both the patients and the physicians.

Improper scheduling may cause patients to wait a long time and become angry. However, time must be set aside for urgent cases and for returning phone calls. An experienced medical assistant studies the practice's scheduling from past appointment books. Over the period of weeks, months, and seasons, distinct patterns of scheduling emerge. The medical assistant experiments until the most workable schedule evolves.

Computers are useful for coordinating appointments when the clinic has several practitioners. They eliminate the need for a separate appointment book for each physician, as well as for specialized equipment procedures such as electrocardiograms. A list should be kept beside the appointment book of the times required for different presenting complaints (e.g., routine office call—15 min.; minor office surgery, gynecological exam/pap smear, or annual physical exam—30 min.; new patient exam—60 min.).

Procedures for appointment scheduling should be kept in the office manual. The appointment record, because it is part of the office's legal documentation, is maintained as neatly as possible and kept for three years. Brochures for patient education concerning the general details of the medical office may be mailed after the initial appointment is made or given to the patient at the first visit.

106.

D. When you are typing a letter of one or more pages for your physician-employer, the name of the addressee, the page number, and the date should appear in this order on all subsequent pages. This information identifies each page in the event they become separated. Most authorities do not believe it is necessary to list the subject on subsequent pages (and not having to list this additional line of information would eventually save time). However, each individual office has its own rules regarding such procedural details and these rules will be followed as a matter of conformity.

107.

E. The final draft of a manuscript is double spaced, is neat with no obvious corrections (preferably prepared on a word processor), has margins of 1 inch or more on all sides, is provided in the number of copies requested, and is printed on good quality paper with the pages numbered consecutively. Each new section should begin on a new page. Paragraphs should be indented by five spaces. Grammar should be meticulous, with no slang, and the style should be straightforward and simple. The manuscript should not be folded or stapled for mailing but instead stiffened with a piece of cardboard and inserted into a large, page-size envelope. Several copies should be retained for the medical office records. During preparation, use the publisher's style guidelines, if available, for capitalization and other requirements. Otherwise, consult a reference book for complete details on how to prepare a manuscript.

108.

E. All of the choices are valid reasons for leaving open slots in a schedule. Experience will indicate what works best for an individual practice. Some specialties, such as family practice, require more free time than others. Leaving a 15- or 20-minute open slot in the morning and afternoon is a common practice in many offices.

109.

E. Express mail guarantees next-day delivery for mail received before 5 P.M. The service is available between larger cities, and confirmation of delivery can be supplied. A special address label is supplied, parcels up to 70 pounds are accepted, and letters may be included at no extra fee. Private services such as Federal Express also offer similar services.

110.

D. The complimentary close for a formal letter should be "Very truly yours." Complimentary closures for informal letters may be "Sincerely," "Warm regards," or "Best wishes." More formal closings are generally used when addressing strangers and strictly business or legal situations. Informal closures are generally reserved for friends and acquaintances. The complimentary close should be placed two lines below the last line of the body of the letter in the position that is appropriate to the style being used.

111.

A. An indistinct or wrong sounding phrase in the medical transcription should be flagged or marked so that it can be easily found again. It should also be left blank in the transcription until it can be accurately transcribed. The medical assistant then should refer it to the dictator or make certain that the phrase was what was intended. The notes must not be altered in any manner without permission from the dictator.

112.

A. The correction key is used to correct errors on electronic typewriters that have correcting tape capability. Different models operate slightly differently; therefore, the operating manual or an experienced user should be consulted for exact methods. It is very difficult to eliminate the use of typewriters even in offices with full word-processing and database capabilities because the typewriter is useful for one-of-a-kind, quick, odd jobs. Corrections even on typewriters with correcting abilities may be made in several ways depending on whether the paper has been removed from the typewriter and on the purpose of the finished typewritten material.

Each correcting method has its drawbacks. The neatest and the easiest is the correction made with a correction ribbon while the typed material is still aligned in the typewriter. However, typed material taken from the typewriter can be re-inserted and aligned, a paper inserted above the message, retyped with the message, and then removed to trick the electronic typewriter into correcting the message. Correction fluid is messy but quick. Small correction slips that act the same as correction ribbons can be purchased but the typing must be realigned with the original spacing.

Whenever possible, the word processor should be used for any sort of typing since corrections are more easily made.

113.

E. All of the listed skills are essential. The transcriber must be able to type correct English grammar, spell difficult medical terms from their pronunciation, type at an acceptable speed, and have a mastery of medical terminology. These skills are developed by practice, referencing, and taking courses.

114.

C. Without appointments, the staff sometimes finds itself working long hours some days to see everyone, and the patients must be hurried through. Other days there may be a scarcity of patients. However, the open-hours policy may result in good collections, since few patients are turned away. Some types of medical offices, such as family practices, are difficult even with appointments to schedule efficiently since they treat emergencies and unanticipated illnesses. The physician decides what the most efficient scheduling policy is. Whatever type of scheduling is decided on, the details should be written in the standard operating procedure (SOP) manual with a mutual understanding of the rules.

115.

E. Efficient scheduling is individualized to the practice with consideration to the many factors affecting appointments. The goal is to make the best use of both the physician's and the patient's time and the office resources. Different types of practices vary greatly in their scheduling needs. The patient's needs and the physician's habits must be considered. For example, emergencies such as suspected heart attacks cannot be neatly scheduled or postponed but must be attended to.

Medical assistants may be required to triage their patient load (allocate treatment to patients according to need) and adjust the schedule accordingly. Some other complaints, while not emergencies, should receive a same-day evaluation. Although the medical assistant schedules blocks of buffer time, the best plans may be defeated. The accessibility or delays of the physician must be considered. For example, the physician who attends noontime meetings of civic clubs will have a different schedule. The lack of facilities, such as extra surgical areas or examining rooms, limits the number of patients that can be scheduled together. Different complaints and treatments require varying lengths of time. A list with the times allotted to different types of exams and standard procedures should be kept by the appointment book for use when scheduling. Certain patients such as the elderly or disabled require extra appointment time.

Several other factors are also considered. From a legal standpoint, the patient with an emergency cannot be turned away because the schedule is full. The patient who needs a laboratory test requiring fasting should obviously not be scheduled in the afternoon. Referrals from other physicians are given scheduling priority, if possible within 24 hours. Patients seeking second opinions before surgery are also given priority. In certain practices, patients may be scheduled in groups according to their category (e.g., prenatal exams are scheduled on one day of the week).

116.

C. Callers should be asked to identify themselves and the purpose of their calls. If the caller does not identify him- or herself, the medical assistant should ask "May I ask who is calling, please?" or "May I tell Dr. ____ who is calling?" It is always important to use good telephone etiquette at all times and to sound polite when talking to a patient on the phone. If the caller persists in not identifying him- or herself or his or her purpose, then the medical assistant might instruct the caller to write a letter to the physician if that is in accordance with office policy. The medical assistant's goal in telephone screening is to avoid interrupting the physician and to handle independently calls that should not require the physician's attention. However, some calls will require the judgment of the physician. An established written office policy should guide the medical assistant in responding to such situations.

117.

E. When working with an elderly patient, it is important to talk slowly and speak distinctly while looking directly at the patient. It is also a good idea to have an elderly patient paraphrase important instructions so that you can make sure that the patient understands. One should not assume that all elderly people are deaf or impaired in movement. Each elderly patient should receive an assessment as an individual because of the great variation among persons who are advanced in age. Some are relatively unimpaired, although many do suffer loss of memory or sensory ability in the area of hearing, sight, taste, and smell.

118.

E. When dealing with a hearing-impaired patient, it is important to stand or sit directly in front of him or her and speak slowly and distinctly. Many hearing-impaired patients can lip read. Therefore, it is important that they see your mouth. Shouting or talking loudly will not help. It is also helpful to have access to community resources to help communicate with hearing-impaired and non-English-speaking patients.

119.

D. Most physicians use a personal answering service where a person listens to the caller and interprets the message. A less frequently used method is the answering machine, which records the message for a future time. The pager is used when the doctor wants to respond immediately. A cellular or mobile phone may also be used. The medical assistant's role as the office resource person is to be sure that the answering service is advised of the physician's whereabouts (if the physician assigns the task) and that the physician receives all the messages on time from the answering service. The confidentiality of messages that may be overheard by others through mobile communications must be respected.

120.

A. In addition to drawing a line through the appointment, the medical assistant should write "canceled" across it. In recording the cancellation in the patient's record, the date, hour, and reason should be noted. These become part of the progress notes section of the patient's record. Both the appointment book and the patient's record are legal documents that may be used later to document medical care.

121.

E. In addition to recording the information in a notebook for the physician to take with him or her on the house call, the medical assistant should make a copy of each page for follow-up and billing purposes. The same procedure should be used if the physician regularly sees patients in convalescent homes. A special block of time should be allotted on the appointment schedule for the trip. You should note the reason for the visit in the doctor's notebook.

122.

D. Hospitals require a **criterion** statement with specific terminology describing the symptoms in order to admit the patient on the level required for treatment. Many government and insurance programs require this pre-admission evaluation of the need for hospitalization in order to decide whether to pay the claim. The hospital needs the criterion (pre-admission evaluation) in order to place the patient in the appropriate facility. For example, the patient may be treated in an outpatient facility if appropriate, thus saving expense. Regarding the other choices, a gatekeeper is a primary care physician in some managed health care plans who is required to make a referral to a specialist before the plan will accept the expense. An HMO is a health management organization, a type of health care plan.

5 Bookkeeping, Credits, and Collections

chapter objectives

Major areas of knowledge/content included in this chapter are:

I. Bookkeeping and accounting types and procedures

➤ basic methods

➤ tools

II. Accounts receivable and other practice analyses

➤ aging accounts

➤ collection ratio

III. Debt collection and collection of demographic information

➤ billing cycle

➤ efficient office collection/collection calls/and letters/ tracing skips

➤ collection agencies

➤ state statutes of limitations; consumer protection against harassment; Truth in Lending Act

IV. Banking guidelines and procedures:

➤ check writing/patient check acceptance or rejection/ deposits/reconciling checking account/banking security policies, etc.

DIRECTIONS (Questions 123 through 200): Each of the numbered items or incomplete statements in this section is followed by answers or by completions of the statement. Select the ONE lettered answer or completion that is BEST in each case.

123. Information about a patient, such as date of birth, sex, address, telephone number, current primary diagnosis, current medications, and date last seen, is known as
    A. data processing
    B. the tickler file
    C. hard copy
    D. ROM
    E. demographic information
    (Fordney and Follis, pp 66–68; Kinn and Woods, pp 95–96)

124. Which of the following statements about double-entry bookkeeping is NOT true?
    A. it has checks and balances
    B. it is expensive
    C. it requires skill
    D. it is accurate
    E. it requires more time
    (Fordney and Follis, p 366; Kinn and Woods, pp 248–250)

125. A bookkeeping term synonymous with "debit" is
    A. charge
    B. discount
    C. adjustment
    D. balance
    E. receipt
    (Fordney and Follis, p 366; Kinn and Woods, p 204)

126. The one-write system of check writing is a feature of
    A. single-entry bookkeeping
    B. double-entry bookkeeping
    C. pegboard bookkeeping
    D. savings and loan accounts
    E. checking accounts
    (Frew et al, pp 249–254; Kinn and Woods, p 271)

127. If the blank checks from the medical office are stolen, the medical assistant might
    A. close the current account
    B. notify the bank
    C. notify the police
    D. ascertain the number of the first and last check in the batch
    E. all of the above
    (Fordney and Follis, pp 367–368; Kinn and Woods, p 270)

128. Which of the following statements about safe deposit boxes is NOT true?
    A. the box itself is a metal container
    B. the box is locked with a key
    C. the box is obtainable in various sizes
    D. the cost of a safe deposit box is deductible
    E. copies of the accounts receivable ledgers may be protected there
    (Hurlburt, p 196)

129. The individual record of the amounts owed and paid by each patient is found in the
    A. combined journal
    B. general ledger
    C. day book (daily journal)
    D. patient's ledger
    E. worksheet
    (Fordney and Follis, p 371; Kinn and Woods, p 243)

130. Posting to the patients' ledger and to the combined journal is made from the
    A. day book (daily journal)
    B. general ledger
    C. special journal
    D. trial balance
    E. worksheet
    (Fordney and Follis, pp 369–371; Frew et al, pp 267–268)

131. The process of transferring an amount from one record, such as a journal, to another record, such as a ledger, is called
    A. debiting
    B. crediting
    C. posting
    D. extension
    E. verification

    (Fordney and Follis, p 364; Kinn and Woods, p 241)

132. The word "debit" means
    A. add
    B. subtract
    C. debt
    D. right
    E. total

    (Fordney and Follis, p 364; Frew et al, p 266)

133. Medical equipment, professional services income, and rent expenses are all examples of accounts found in the
    A. patients' ledger
    B. general ledger
    C. blue book
    D. daily earnings record
    E. income statement

    (Frew et al, p 268; Kinn and Woods, p 240)

134. The pegboard bookkeeping system is sometimes called
    A. "write-it-once"
    B. "single entry"
    C. "double entry"
    D. "checks and balances"
    E. "hunt and peck"

    (Fordney and Follis, p 367; Frew et al, p 249)

135. The procedure for proving the correctness of the general ledger is called taking a
    A. posting
    B. balance

C. subtotal
D. total
E. trial balance

(Frew et al, p 269; Kinn and Woods, p 365)

136. Owners' equity is a term used interchangeably with
    A. proprietorship
    B. liability
    C. professional income
    D. an asset
    E. income statement

    (Fordney and Follis, p 366; Frew et al, p 267; Kinn and Woods, p 250)

137. A daily journal is where
    A. source documents are recorded
    B. items from the general ledger are transferred
    C. financial statements originate
    D. the trial balance is derived
    E. the petty cash account is credited

    (Kinn and Woods, p 243)

138. A liability is
    A. an expense
    B. opposite of credit
    C. recorded in the left column
    D. a debit
    E. all of these

    (Fordney and Follis, p 364; Frew et al, p 267)

139. The credit column in an accounting system is always
    A. the accounting base
    B. recorded in the left column
    C. recorded in the right column
    D. payments from the practice for expenses
    E. the patient's account due

    (Fordney and Follis, p 366; Kinn and Woods, p 243)

140. The balance column of an accounting system is
    A. the accounting base
    B. recorded in the left column
    C. recorded in the right column
    D. the difference between debit and credit columns
    E. payments for professional services

    (Fordney and Follis, p 364; Kinn and Woods, p 242)

141. In accounting terminology, "posting" means to
    A. transfer amounts from one record to another
    B. record in the left column
    C. record in the right column
    D. make a bank deposit
    E. pay expenses

    (Fordney and Follis, p 365; Kinn and Woods, p 242)

142. Transaction is a bookkeeping and accounting term that means
    A. transferral of amounts from one account to another
    B. an amount or event that must be recorded
    C. payment from practice for expenses
    D. payments by the patients
    E. discount

    (Frew et al, p 266; Kinn and Woods, p 241)

143. Receipts are
    A. amounts transferred from one account to another
    B. records of patients' financial accounts
    C. the difference between the debit and credit columns
    D. payment for professional services
    E. daily bank deposits from practice

    (Frew et al, p 266; Kinn and Woods, p 241)

144. Disbursements are another term for
    A. payments by the patient
    B. expenses owed

    C. discounts to patients
    D. cash amounts paid out
    E. payables

    (Frew et al, p 266; Kinn and Woods, p 259)

145. An accounts receivable ledger consists of
    A. a book of original entry
    B. a payment for professional services
    C. records of patients' current financial status
    D. a journal of disbursements
    E. expenses owed by the practice

    (Fordney and Follis, pp 371–373; Frew et al, p 268; Kinn and Woods, p 240)

146. The cash basis accounting system
    A. is the same as the accrual basis
    B. uses the formula, income = payment received
    C. is used by merchants
    D. is recorded in the left column
    E. is the difference between debit and credit columns

    (Fordney, p 366)

147. To replenish the petty cash fund
    A. cash is added
    B. a check is written
    C. money is transferred from daily collections
    D. the physician contributes currency each day
    E. the physician contributes currency when the fund falls below $5

    (Fordney and Follis, p 328; Frew et al, p 272–273; Kinn and Woods, p 247)

148. To stop payment on a check, it is necessary to
    A. go in person to the bank on which the check is written
    B. write to the nearest federal reserve bank
    C. call the payee's bank

D. call the bank on which the check is written and then confirm in writing

E. complete a form available at any bank

(Fordney and Follis, p 359; Kinn and Woods, p 276)

149. A patients' ledger is actually a/an
   A. accounts payable ledger
   B. accounts receivable ledger
   C. general ledger
   D. daily earnings record
   E. income account

   (Fordney and Follis, p 364)

150. A depositor's own check that is guaranteed by the bank is called a
   A. bank draft
   B. certified check
   C. counter check
   D. limited check
   E. cashier's check

   (Fordney and Follis, p 352)

151. The accounts receivable trial balance is a/an
   A. annual summary
   B. daily summary
   C. monthly accounting
   D. weekly statement
   E. income tax preliminary

   (Fordney and Follis, pp 369–370)

152. Which of the following are financial summaries?
   A. trial balance
   B. aging analysis of accounts receivable
   C. cash flow statement
   D. statement of income and expense
   E. all of these

   (Fordney and Follis, pp 381, 385–386)

153. A negotiable instrument is
   A. a warrant
   B. a check or draft

C. purchased only at U.S. post offices

D. MICR

E. a receipt

(Fordney and Follis, p 352)

154. A type of check that requires the signature of the purchaser at both the time of purchase and the time of use is the
   A. bank draft
   B. warrant
   C. voucher check
   D. traveler's check
   E. limited check

   (Fordney and Follis, p 352)

155. The legal term for the person who signs his or her name on the back of a check for the purpose of transferring title to the check to another person is
   A. agent
   B. restrictive
   C. endorser
   D. qualified
   E. unqualified

   (Fordney and Follis, p 353; Kinn and Woods, p 273)

156. "For deposit only to the account of Dr. F. Makewell" is an example of what kind of endorsement on a check?
   A. blank
   B. restrictive
   C. special
   D. qualified
   E. unqualified

   (Fordney and Follis, p 353; Kinn and Woods, p 274)

157. The most active financial record in the medical office is the
   A. general journal
   B. worksheet
   C. cash payment journal
   D. accounts receivable ledger
   E. trial balance

   (Fordney and Follis, pp 364–365; Frew et al, pp 268–269; Kinn and Woods, p 253)

158. The general journal, which is a record of the physician's practice, includes records of services rendered, charges made, and monies received. The general journal may be known by several other names. Which of the following is NOT another name for the general journal?
    A. daily log
    B. day book
    C. day sheet
    D. charge journal
    E. accrual accounting system
    (Fordney and Follis, p 240)

159. The word "credit" means
    A. add
    B. subtract
    C. far right
    D. paid
    E. total
    (Fordney and Follis, p 364; Kinn and Woods, p 240)

160. Cash amounts that are paid out are
    A. payables
    B. disbursements
    C. receivables
    D. receipts
    E. discounts
    (Fordney and Follis, p 364; Kinn and Woods, p 240)

161. The cash and checks taken as payment for professional services rendered are called
    A. payables
    B. disbursements
    C. receivables
    D. receipts
    E. discounts
    (Fordney and Follis, p 364; Kinn and Woods, p 240)

162. Payments made by patients are regarded as the physician's
    A. earnings
    B. gross income

C. drawing
    D. proprietorship
    E. equity
    (Frew et al, p 270)

163. The home position for the fingers on the 10-key calculator keyboard on computers and calculators is
    A. the full keyboard
    B. 1, 2, 3 keys
    C. 7, 8, 9 keys
    D. 4, 5, 6 keys
    E. 2, 5, 8 keys
    (Frew et al, p 213)

164. Complete information regarding the filing of reports and taxes from the employee's earnings and employer's tax contributions can be found in
    A. *Physician's Desk Reference*
    B. *Medical Office Handbook*
    C. *IRS Income Tax Guide*
    D. *IRS Employer's Tax Guide*
    E. *Federal Tax Deposits*
    (Fordney and Follis, p 396; Frew et al, pp 276–277)

165. When you are attempting to collect over-due accounts, there are several options available. Which of the following is considered the LEAST desirable method?
    A. personal interview
    B. telephone
    C. personal notes
    D. preprinted form letters
    E. collection agencies
    (Fordney and Follis, p 286; Frew et al, p 257)

166. Which one of the following procedures is the most time consuming when attempting to collect an overdue account?
    A. personal interview
    B. telephone
    C. personal notes

D. preprinted form letters

E. collection agencies

(Fordney and Follis, p 276; Frew et al, p 256; Kinn and Woods, p 393)

167. Collection agencies may retain up to ___% of the account collected on an overdue medical bill

A. 70 to 80

B. 40 to 60

C. 20 to 30

D. 10 to 25

E. 5 to 15

(Fordney and Follis, p 287; Frew et al, p 257; Kinn and Woods, p 299)

168. Which of the following statements is most appropriate for a collection letter?

A. "Unless we receive your check within 10 days . . ."

B. "I am disappointed that you have not paid your account."

C. "I feel sure you must have overlooked the last statement."

D. "In order for us to meet our bills, it is necessary for you to pay your account."

E. "Please send us your check or an explanation within 10 days."

(Fordney and Follis, pp 285–286)

169. Which of the following is NOT typical of an effective collection letter?

A. the letter is brief

B. the language is simple

C. the sentences are short

D. the amount you expect the patient to pay is stated

E. four or five appeals to such values as pride or cooperation are made

(Fordney and Follis, p 285; Frew et al, p 256)

170. A formula that is used for measuring how quickly outstanding accounts are being paid is known as the

A. accounts receivable ledger

B. accounting equation

C. accounts receivable ratio

D. accounts owed

E. accounts payable

(Fordney and Follis, p 385; Frew et al, p 267; Kinn and Woods, p 290)

171. Which of the following should NOT be used as a guide in selecting a collection agency?

A. the owner is a well-established businessman

B. the owner is a member of civic and business clubs

C. the owner is a member of an organization, such as the American Collectors Association

D. magazine advertisement of low monthly fees

E. a visit to the collection agency to observe procedures used

(Fordney and Follis, p 286; Frew et al, p 256; Kinn and Woods, p 299)

172. Most collection agencies work on a principle described as

A. accrual basis

B. contingency fee basis

C. capitation

D. professional fee basis

E. percentage basis

(Fordney and Follis, p 287; Frew et al, p 257; Kinn and Woods, p 299)

173. Patients who owe money and who have moved, failing to leave forwarding addresses, are called

A. freeloaders

B. beats

C. gilders

D. fliers

E. skips

(Fordney and Follis, p 290; Frew et al, p 258; Kinn and Woods, p 295)

174. It is recommended that only impersonal reminder notices be attached to patient bills, starting with the third billing, for at least the first
    A. 60 days
    B. 90 days
    C. 120 days
    D. 150 days
    E. 180 days
    (Kinn and Woods, p 293)

175. If a patient calls the office after his or her account has been turned over to a collection agency and wants to make payment arrangements, the medical assistant should
    A. suggest that the patient come to the office to discuss the matter
    B. schedule a series of dates for payments up to a period of 2 months
    C. tell the patient that only the total amount due can be accepted
    D. tell the patient all discussion must be with the agency
    E. tell the patient that only the total amount due plus the agency fee can be accepted
    (Frew et al, p 206; Kinn and Woods, p 299)

176. Billing statements to the patients and the patients' insurance company are made from the
    A. general journal
    B. worksheet
    C. cash payment journal
    D. accounts receivable ledger
    E. trial balance
    (Kinn and Woods, p 287; Zakus et al, p 168)

177. The most common method of payment by patients is
    A. cash
    B. money orders
    C. personal checks
    D. drafts
    E. warrants
    (Kinn and Woods, p 264)

178. The agreement by a third party to pay for a patient's medical services must be
    A. oral
    B. made after treatment
    C. written out prior to treatment
    D. notarized
    E. a special type of contract
    (Fordney and Follis, p 296; Frew et al, pp 248–262; Kinn and Woods, p 288)

179. Medical-Dental-Hospital Bureaus of America is concerned with
    A. health insurance
    B. collection services
    C. accounting practices
    D. appointment systems
    E. professional fees
    (Kinn and Woods, p 237)

180. Regulation Z of the Truth in Lending Act applies to physicians who accept payment from patients
    A. in cash
    B. in two installments
    C. in more than four installments
    D. in six or more installments
    E. with credit cards
    (Fordney and Follis, p 277; Frew et al, p 259; Kinn and Woods, p 236)

181. Statutes of limitations vary from one state to another and may range from
    A. 2 to 8 years
    B. 3 to 8 years
    C. 4 to 7 years
    D. 5 to 7 years
    E. 6 to 9 years
    (Fordney and Follis, p 56; Frew et al, p 37; Kinn and Woods, p 297)

182. Another term meaning "payroll register" is
    A. payroll journal
    B. payroll check
    C. employee's earnings record
    D. patient ledger
    E. financial record
    (Fordney and Follis, pp 403–404; Frew et al, p 273)

183. The collection percentage is obtained for a given period of time by dividing
    A. accounts receivable by amount collected
    B. amount collected by accounts receivable
    C. accounts receivable by total charges for all services
    D. total charges for all services by accounts receivable
    E. number of accounts receivable by total number of patients
    (Fordney and Follis, pp 266–270; Frew et al, pp 255–256; Kinn and Woods, p 290)

184. An age analysis is done to determine
    A. when patients should be scheduled for recall appointments
    B. complaints of various age groups of patients
    C. how much patients owe on their accounts and for how long
    D. which records may be destroyed or placed in inactive files
    E. insurance rates for different age groups of patients
    (Fordney and Follis, p 280; Frew et al, p 256; Kinn and Woods, p 292)

185. A legal device that permits a person to allow someone else to act for him or her in legal matters is a
    A. notary public
    B. power of attorney
    C. trust

    D. res ipsa loquitur
    E. non compos mentis
    (Fordney and Follis, p 52; Kinn and Woods, p 783)

186. Financial summaries are compiled on monthly and yearly bases. One of the common financial summary reports is a statement of income and expenses, which is also known as
    A. cash flow statement
    B. trial balance
    C. balance sheet
    D. statement of financial condition
    E. profit and loss statement
    (Frew et al, p 266; Kinn and Woods, p 261)

187. When a check is returned because of lack of funds, the medical assistant should
    A. determine from an accountant the action to take
    B. immediately redeposit the check
    C. immediately call the person who wrote the check
    D. deduct the amount of the check from the day sheet totals
    E. send the check to a collection agency
    (Fordney and Follis, p 267; Frew et al, p 241; Kinn and Woods, p 254)

188. A list of accounts showing the title and balance of each account is called a/an
    A. income statement
    B. balance sheet
    C. trial balance
    D. ledger
    E. chart of accounts
    (Frew et al, p 269; Kinn and Woods, p 240)

189. In completing a bank statement reconciliation, the medical assistant should
    A. add service charges to the checkbook balance
    B. deduct outstanding checks from the checkbook balance
    C. deduct deposits from the checkbook balance that are not included on the statement
    D. deduct service charges from the checkbook balance
    E. none of the above

    (Frew et al, p 240; Kinn and Woods, p 280)

190. Entries that include the patient's name, service rendered, charges, and receipts are made in the
    A. day sheet
    B. cash payments journal
    C. combined cash journal
    D. general ledger
    E. worksheet

    (Fordney and Follis, p 276; Frew et al, pp 240–241; Kinn and Woods, pp 240–241)

191. Which of the following equations is correct?
    A. assets plus liabilities equals proprietorship
    B. assets plus proprietorship equals liabilities
    C. assets equals liabilities plus proprietorship
    D. assets equals liabilities minus proprietorship
    E. assets equals proprietorship minus liabilities

    (Fordney and Follis, p 276; Frew et al, p 267; Kinn and Woods, p 248)

192. Which of the following represents the proper sequence of activity in the accounting cycle?
    A. adjusting, issuing financial statements, closing, and posting
    B. posting, adjusting, issuing financial statements, and closing
    C. posting, closing, adjusting, and issuing financial statements
    D. adjusting, posting, issuing financial statements, and closing
    E. posting, adjusting, closing, and issuing financial statements

    (Kinn and Woods, pp 160–161)

193. The simplest manual way to prepare payroll checks and create the necessary bookkeeping entries is to
    A. post them to individual accounts
    B. use a write-it-once check writing system
    C. set up a separate journal
    D. keep an individual file for taxes
    E. none of the above

    (Frew et al, pp 249–250)

194. A record of checks issued in a medical practice that shows the date of the checks, the number of each check, the account being paid, and the amount of the check is called a
    A. check register
    B. ledger
    C. journal
    D. source document
    E. accounts receivable document

    (Humphrey, p 270)

195. An employee who fails to complete the following form will have his or her income tax figured on the basis of being single with no exemptions.
    A. form 941
    B. form W-4
    C. form W-2
    D. form W-3
    E. form 940

    (Humphrey, p 270; Kinn and Woods, p 382)

196. Another term meaning employees' earnings record is
  A. payroll journal
  B. payroll check
  C. payroll register
  D. patient ledger
  E. financial record
  (Frew et al, pp 275–276; Kinn and Woods, p 261)

197. Fee reductions or cancellations should follow established policy guidelines of the physician. Which of the following might serve as a guideline to determine if fee reduction or cancellation is warranted?
  A. inquire through an open and honest discussion with the patient about his or her financial problem
  B. verify and recheck the initial information and the patient's credit rating to see if there have been any major changes
  C. check into the possibility of the patient's qualifying for any type of public assistance program
  D. investigate the possibility of the patient being covered by or entitled to an insurance settlement
  E. all of the above
  (Fordney and Follis, p 270; Kinn and Woods, pp 231–232)

198. Action(s) to avoid in making telephone collection calls to patients with delinquent accounts is/are
  A. calling between 9 P.M. and 8 A.M.
  B. calling the person again and again
  C. showing contempt
  D. leaving a message about the overdue bill at the patient's workplace
  E. all of the above
  (Humphrey, p 283)

199. The superbill often is used in medical practice and may be personalized for the practice. It is a combination
  A. statement
  B. insurance filing report
  C. charge slip
  D. patient receipt
  E. all of the above
  (Humphrey, pp 264–265; Kinn and Woods, p 242)

200. Which of the following is/are cardinal rule(s) of bookkeeping?
  A. enter all transactions immediately into the daily record (journal)
  B. stamp all checks with a restricted endorsement when received and deposit as soon as possible
  C. pay all sizable expenses by check
  D. using same color of ink each time, write legibly and keep columns straight
  E. all of the above
  (Fordney and Follis, pp 364–368)

STUDY HINTS

Review the basic vocabulary and principles of financial record keeping. If any area is hazy, look up the subject in your administrative office textbook.

Principles of Bookkeeping

➤ Physicians use cash basis method of accounting as opposed to accrual basis. In the cash basis method

  Income = receipt of payment

  Expense = payment for payroll, supplies, utilities, etc.

➤ **Computerized financial record keeping** is an extension of the principles of traditional manual bookkeeping.

➤ Manual bookkeeping systems vary with the simplicity or sophistication needed.

  Two basic types are (1) **single entry bookkeeping** which includes "**write it once**" (**pegboard**) systems and (2) **double-entry bookkeeping** which has more checks and balances to prevent **errors and is used by accountants**.

DOUBLE-ENTRY BOOKKEEPING IS BASED ON THE ACCOUNTING EQUATION

Assets = liabilities + proprietorship (capital).

The two sides must balance.

Accounting cycle in both single- and double-entry bookkeeping = sequence of activity for transactions. Steps in cycle include:

1. Record source document (transaction) into journal (diary) also called daily log or day-book which will serve as a reference in case of errors or disputes.
2. Transfer (post) journal entries into individual ledger accounts (on computer or by hand). Two broad categories of individual accounts are the **accounts receivable** (money owed to practice) and **accounts payable** (debts owed by practice).
3. Prepare trial balances on daily and monthly basis to test accuracy.
4. **Bill patients and third party payers** (example: insurance, Workers' Compensation, patient's relatives)
5. **Pay practice debts** such as utilities, payrolls, medical supplies, etc.6. Prepare **financial reports**
6. Prepare **financial reports**

Periodic summaries and analyses easily generated on the computer include:

Cash flow statement = cash on hand at beginning and end of month (or other period)

Collection ratio = total collections divided by net charges = percent collected

Accounts receivable ratio = current accounts receivable balance divided by average gross monthly charge

Age analysis = computer-generated age labeling of individual patient accounts so that lagging schedules of payments can be immediately recognized

Banking Services

Review the following:

➤ **Types of accounts**
➤ **Types of checks**
➤ **Types of endorsements**
➤ **Lost or stolen checks—how to handle**
➤ **Stop payment on checks**
➤ **Insufficient funds or no existing account for checks**
➤ **Types of checks to reject**
➤ **ABA (American Banker's Association) number**
➤ **Magnetic Imaging Character Recognition**
➤ **Returned checks—how to post**
➤ **Reconciling bank statements**
➤ **Security policies regarding bank accounts, and making deposits**

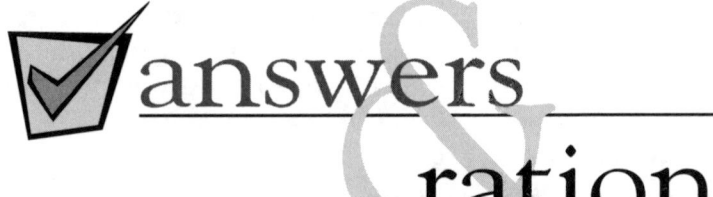
answers & rationales

This system is well suited to smaller medical practices because it saves time, requires less training than more complex systems and reduces the possibility of error. It does not have the checks and balances of double-entry bookkeeping. However, an accountant can take the financial transactions recorded by a medical assistant and transfer them to the accounts of a double-entry accounting system. From these, the accountant obtains the various reports that physicians use to evaluate the medical practice's financial state. The accountant also prepares tax summaries.

123.

E. Demographic information includes date of birth, sex, address, telephone number, and whatever else the physician considers important in the patient profile. (Demography is the study of the characteristics of human populations, such as vital statistics, distribution, growth, etc.) The information may be essential to the medical records and for collection of delinquent bills.

124.

B. The materials required for a double-entry bookkeeping system are inexpensive. However, it is time consuming, and requires more skill and knowledge of accounting procedures. Accounting, particularly in the area of tax law, is a complex field that requires a professional accountant. Many small practices hire an outside accounting service to supplement the bookkeeping of the medical assistant.

125.

A. A term synonymous with "debit" is "charge." This is opposed to "credit," which means payment or income. The debit (charge) is recorded in the left column, whereas the credit (income) is recorded in the right column.

126.

C. The one-write check system is a feature of the pegboard system of bookkeeping. (Bookkeeping is defined as recording the financial data on selected forms according to established procedure.) The pegboard system uses a one-write check system to write the check and record the transaction on the record of checks drawn. If it is an employee paycheck, it can be recorded on the payroll record. When used for patient accounts the pegboard system records the entry through pressure sensitive paper to four different source documents: a daily earnings summary, a deposit slip, a ledger card, and a charge/receipt slip (superbill) for the patient.

127.

E. All of these steps might be taken. The police should be notified in the town where the theft occurred, and the bank where the account is located should be notified of the police report and the check numbers that are unaccounted for. The account will be placed under surveillance, and possibly a new account will be opened. The account will not suffer after the loss is reported.

128.

B. The safe deposit box is locked into a compartment in the bank's vault using two keys (one belonging to the medical office employee and one that remains at the bank servicing the safe deposit box). A bank employee will only unlock the compartment after the approved medical office employee has provided identification, signed a ledger, and provided one of the safe deposit box keys. This system is designed to prevent theft of the contents of the safe deposit box. The bank vault is an excellent place to keep important papers, such as copies of the accounts receivable ledger. The accounts receivable ledger is especially important because in the case of an office fire, the practice still has a list of its debtors and the amounts owed. Space, however, will be limited.

129.

D. The patient's ledger (day sheet) contains the individual records of the amounts owed and paid by each patient. Because all transactions for professional services are posted daily, the ledger can be used to answer inquiries from patients about their accounts. The balance (summary) of the patient's ledger (day sheet) is transferred to the general ledger's accounts receivable category.

130.

A. The first record of services rendered to patients is the physician's daybook, also known as the daily journal, from which postings are made to the patients' ledger and to the combined journal. It is a chronological record (diary) of services rendered, charges, and receipts that can be referred to as needed to locate information or correct errors. Vocabulary and procedures for bookkeeping will differ from office to office—for instance, larger medical offices usually use a computerized system of bookkeeping, while smaller medical offices may still use a pegboard system and depend on an outside accounting firm for other accounting work. However, the general principles of bookkeeping are the same for both small and large offices and are needed in both the computerized and pegboard systems.

131.

C. "Posting" is the term used to describe the process of transferring an amount from one record to another, such as from a journal to a ledger. Debiting and crediting are the posting of debits (charges) and credits (payments).

132.

C. The word "debit" is derived from the Latin word for debt. It also has come to mean "to the left" in accounting procedures, since an item of debt is always recorded in the left (charge) column of an accounting ledger. Credit is a payment and is always entered on the right side of the ledger. The balance is the difference between the debits (debt) and the credits (payments).

133.

B. General accounts, such as medical equipment, professional services income, and rent expense, are found in the general ledger.

134.

A. The pegboard bookkeeping system is sometimes called a "write-it-once" system. The name "pegboard" comes from the board with pegs that hold multiple forms in place. With one writing (and the help of carbons or copy paper), an entry can be made in the journal day sheet, a deposit slip, the patient ledger, and the patient charge slip/receipt or superbill. Since the forms must align exactly for the system to work, they are obtained from a medical supply house that carries pegboard supplies. This system, requiring the least writing time, is a single-entry bookkeeping system. Single-entry bookkeeping is the oldest and simplest system, whereas double-entry bookkeeping is the most sophisticated and requires the most training.

135.

E. Proving the correctness of the general ledger is called taking a trial balance and includes listing all of the account balances to determine if the debit balances equal the credit balances. This is a check and balance in double-entry bookkeeping.

136.

A. Owner's equity, proprietorship, net worth, and capital all describe what remains of value (what a practice is worth) after the liabilities (expenses and debts) are subtracted. This includes anything of value, such as accounts receivable, buildings, equipment, and furniture. Assets = liabilities (debts and expenses) + proprietorship (capital, owner's equity, net worth). This is referred to as the accounting equation. Reports based on this equation are very important because they show the profitability of the medical practice.

The accounting cycle follows the medical practice's financial data from start to finish as the accountants process it. The accounting cycle can be summarized as follows: transactions, journal, general ledger, accounts, financial statements. Transaction information comes from source documents (e.g., utility bills, patient payment for services, patient charges, check stubs, invoices for supplies).

137.

A. Source documents are the original documents, such as patient payments for services, utility bills, rent notices, and insurance copayments, that provide information to post transactions. They are first posted to the daily chronological (general) journal and then to the appropriate accounts in the general ledger.

138.

E. A liability, an expense, or a debt can be a debit, which is recorded on the left column of the account. The credit is recorded on the right side of the account ledger. The trial balance compares the right (credit) and left (debit) sides of the general ledger accounts and is a very important control used to locate errors in accounting.

139.

C. The credit column is always to the right, whereas the debit column of an account is always to the left. The credit column is the payment-received column, and the debit column is the expense column. The far right column is reserved for the balance column. In double-entry bookkeeping, each transaction is recorded twice—in a debit column and in a credit column of the account—hence the name, double-entry bookkeeping, and the built-in check-and-balance system.

140.

D. The balance column of an accounting system is at the far right of the page and records the difference between debit (left) and credit (right) columns. It shows the financial condition of the practice at the time it is prepared.

141.

A. "Posting" is the transferring of amounts from one account to another. The daily receipts from the patients are posted from the daily (general) journal to the accounts receivable ledger to keep the patients' accounts up to date. In the write-it-once system (pegboard system), these postings are simultaneous.

142.

B. A business transaction is an amount or event that must be recorded in the accounting or bookkeeping accounts. This may be an expense, income received, a major purchase of capital equipment, or the monthly rent. Transactions are the elementary units of the financial records of businesses. They occur when something of value is exchanged for something else of equal value (e.g., the patient exchanges cash for a medical consultation with a physician).

143.

D. Receipts are the cash and check payments received for professional services. These and all other payments are entered daily into the general ledger, sometimes called the daily journal, which is a chronological record from which other accounts receive their data. This record may be referred to if there is a question involving other bookkeeping accounts.

144.

D. Cash amounts paid out are disbursements. Payables are owed amounts and have not yet been paid. Expenses are the cost of running a business whether or not they have been paid.

145.

C. The records of the patients' current financial status comprises the accounts receivable ledger and is kept current by daily postings. It is a reliable source for reference when patients inquire about their accounts. A "ledger" in accounting terminology is a book into which transactions are posted from another source.

146.

B. The cash basis method of accounting is used by physicians. Charges for services are considered income when payment is received, and expenses are entered when they have been paid. This system of accounting contrasts with the accrual basis used by merchants, where goods sold are considered income even though payment has not been received and expenses are recorded when incurred and before they are actually paid.

147.

B. To replenish the petty cash fund, a check would be written for the amount spent and posted to the various accounts in the general ledger for which the expense occurred. However, policies regarding petty cash may be outlined in the office policy manual and may vary from office to office. The physician or office director determines the amount of cash placed in the petty cash fund and the types of expenses that are paid from it.

148.

D. If it is necessary to stop payment on a check, one must call the bank on which the check is written and then confirm the stop payment order in writing. There generally will be a charge for a stop payment order.

149.

B. A patient's ledger is actually an accounts receivable ledger. The major source of income (and, therefore, accounts receivable) in a medical practice is from service to patients. The term ledger means an accounting book to which figures are posted. Therefore, the accounts receivable or patients' ledger describes the accounting book holding these accounts.

150.

B. A certified check is a depositor's own check that is guaranteed by the bank. The amount of the check is immediately deducted from the depositor's account.

151.

C. The accounts receivable trial balance is totaled before sending out the monthly patient statements. The previous month's total is recorded, and the current month's payments and charges are recorded.

152.

E. All of these answer selections are some type of financial summary report. Some, such as trial balance, cash flow statements, and aging analysis of accounts receivable, are monthly reports. Some are yearly reports, such as the statement of income and expense (profit and loss statement). All are important tools with which the physicians can judge the financial state of the practice.

153.

B. A check or draft is a negotiable instrument, since it meets the following criteria: it must be written and signed by its originator, must promise to pay a sum of money, and must be payable to the bearer either on demand or at a future date.

There are several types of checks designed to meet different needs (e.g., traveler's checks for security and acceptance, cashier's checks purchased from a bank, personal checks for convenience, a certified check on the payer's account guaranteed by the bank). The most common check is the personal check. It may be personalized, with the payer's name, address, and account number printed on it. A counter check is less secure with no printed personalization or account number, and therefore, no proof that the person has gone through the time and procedure to have personalized checks printed.

A bank draft is a check written by a bank on its funds in another bank. It is one of several types of checks that the cashier in a medical clinic should be acquainted with.

154.

D. The traveler's check requires the user to sign at time of purchase and time of cashing (use). This type of check is used where the use of cash is inadvisable because of security reasons or where personal checks are not accepted. They are purchased from banks and other sources.

155.

C. The endorser is the person who signs his or her name on the back of a check for the purpose of transferring title to the check to another person or a bank. The endorsement should be made as soon as it is received with ink or a rubber stamp on the back of the check on the left end (end nearest the name of payee). Endorsement may be of three types: the open endorsement where a person signs but adds no restrictions; the limited endorsement where the person signs and also indicates to whom the check should be paid; and the restricted endorsement, generally used by medical offices, with the wording "For deposit only to the account of, at Bank." This endorsement restricts the check funds to a particular account, thus preventing transfer to another account or person in case of theft. The policy concerning endorsement of checks will be dictated by office policy.

156.

B. A restrictive endorsement specifies the purpose of the endorsement, and "For deposit only" is such an endorsement. The endorsement for fullest protection should also contain the name of the account and the bank where the deposit will be made. In case the checks were lost, this prevents another person from cashing or depositing the checks.

157.

D. The most active financial record is the accounts receivable (accounts payable) ledger. It is the record of all charges and payments for professional services to the patient. It is the best source of information for patients inquiring about their accounts.

158.

E. The general journal is also known by the names daily log, daybook, day sheet, daily journal, or charge journal. This journal is called the book of original entry because it is where all transactions are first recorded. A journal is a chronological record, whereas a ledger is a book where numbers are posted.

159.

D. The word "credit" is sometimes called "paid." The credit column, located to the right, is used to enter payments received. The left column is for debits (debts). The far right column is the balance column.

The abbreviation for the word "credit" on an account card system is Cr. The abbreviation for the word debit is Dr, from the word debtor. It is the column to the left, sometimes called the charge column.

160.

B. Cash amounts that are paid out are disbursements. Receipts are payments in cash and check for professional services. Payables refer to the amounts owed to others that have not been paid.

161.

D. The cash and checks taken as payment for professional services rendered are called receipts. Receivables are charges for which the payment has not been received.

162.

B. Payments made by patients are regarded as the physician's gross income. The net income is the gross income minus the expenses. The individual cash and checks payments are *receipts* for professional services rendered. Receivables are charges for which the payment has not been received.

163.

D. The keys numbered 4, 5, and 6 are the home keys for the index, middle, and ring fingers on the 10-key calculator boards. The thumb activates the zero key. Practice will develop the skill of rapid touch operation that is similar to touch typing so that the operator will not need to look at the keyboard.

Adding machines and calculators come in a wide variety from hand-held calculators to computers; however, they all include the basic 10-key keyboard.

164.

D. The *IRS Employer's Tax Guide* gives complete tax information about filing the needed forms and deposits. The payment for federal income taxes, employee FICA taxes, employer FICA taxes, and unemployment taxes must be made periodically by depositing the proper amount in a federal depository institution, probably a nearby bank.

165.

E. When you are attempting to collect overdue accounts, the least desirable method available is the collection agency. It is important for the physician to determine if the ill will that could result from this method of collection is worth it in the long run. The physician must know what technique the agency uses because he or she can be held liable for illegal collection practices.

166.

C. The personal note technique is the most time consuming and costly for collecting overdue accounts. This method should be used only if a very few accounts are involved or if it involves only a few accounts where very large amounts are due. It also may be used if telephone contact is impossible.

167.

B. In the past it was common for collection agencies to retain 40% to 60% of the amount collected. Some collection agencies have now reduced their percentage because this encourages physicians to turn over accounts earlier, which increases the possibility for collecting the amount owed.

168.

E. An appropriate statement for a collection letter is, "Please send us your check or an explanation within 10 days." It is neither trite nor threatening. It tells the patient in a very clear manner what you expect of him or her.

169.

E. In an effective collection letter, only one appeal to the patient's sense of pride or spirit of cooperation would typically be made. A patient with good paying habits would never be sent the same type of collection letter that would be sent to a person who is known to neglect his or her doctor bill.

170.

C. Accounts receivable ratio refers to a formula used to measure how fast outstanding accounts are being paid. It is calculated by dividing the average gross monthly charges into the current accounts receivable balance.

171.

D. Rather than using a written contract of monthly fees, most agencies work on a contingency fee basis. This means that the agencies are paid a percentage on the claims that they collect.

172.

B. Most collection agencies work on a contingency fee basis (contingent on the collection of the outstanding debt). They keep a percentage of the amount collected. The percentage rate typically varies from 40% to 60% for the agency, which is why physicians choose the collection agency method as the final resort. Some agencies are reducing their fee to encourage physicians to turn over their overdue accounts earlier. The older an overdue account is, the greater the chance it will never be paid.

173.

E. Patients who owe money and who have moved, failing to give the physician their forwarding address, are called skips. They show the need for complete patient information (demographic data) at the time of the initial appointment. Telephoning personal references, friends, or relatives, checking the telephone company for new listings, with other physicians who treated the patient, or with the place of employment may help in locating skips. The first check of each new patient may be photocopied and retained for use of a driver's license number in tracing. If the skip cannot be located, the account should be turned over to a collection agency.

174.

B. It is recommended that only impersonal reminder notices that the bill is owed, such as printed stickers or rubber stamps, be attached to patient bills, starting with the third billing, for at least the first 90 days. However, the patient's past financial payment record and other factors, such as the type of practice, are taken into account when the physician decides on collection procedures.

175.

D. Once an account has been turned over to a collection agency, all further dealings should be between the patient and the agency. If patients call the office afterward about their bills, they should be referred to the collection agency.

176.

D. The most active financial record is the accounts receivable ledger, since it contains all the patients' account balances. This ledger is posted daily so that it is always up to date when patients inquire about their balance.

177.

C. Most patients pay with personal checks to be drawn on their bank accounts. A check policy should be decided on in advance, since occasionally third-party checks (which are risky) and checks larger than the account balance are offered. Postdated checks also may be offered.

178.

C. An agreement by a third party to pay for another's medical services must be in writing to be enforceable and must be made prior to treatment. The agreement may be typewritten or written in longhand.

179.

B. The Medical-Dental-Hospital Bureaus of America (MDHBA) is a national organization of agencies that is committed to following the collection methods most acceptable to physicians. The headquarters of MDHBA is in Chicago, Illinois.

180.

C. Regulation Z of the Truth in Lending Act, enforced by the Federal Trade Commission, requires the doctor to provide disclosure of information regarding finance charges when there is an agreement between the physician and patient to accept payment in more than four installments.

181.

B. Statutes of limitations vary from state to state and may range from 3 to 8 years. The time limit in Texas is 3 years, and in Wyoming it is 8 years. The other states fall between these two with regard to the time limit.

182.

C. The payroll register is used to prepare the entries in the payroll journal. The payroll register is an itemized list of all employees' total earnings and all deductions. The entries into the payroll journal consist of the pay period's total salary expenses for the federal income tax, social security tax (FICA), and any other deductibles, such as life insurance.

183.

B. The collection percentage, which can be an indication of the soundness of a physician's collection procedures, is obtained by dividing the amount collected by accounts receivable. This may be done monthly by taking the amount collected during the month and dividing it by the amount outstanding on the first of the same month.

184.

C. An age analysis (sometimes called "aging accounts") is done to determine how long and how much patients have owed on their accounts and may also list actions taken for collection on various accounts, and so on. It will show which patient accounts should be followed up, trends in time required for bill collection, and insurance claims that are outstanding. The collection percentage for a time period can also be determined. It is a valuable tool for analyzing the amount collected compared to amount of medical services rendered and the effectiveness of collection procedures.

185.

B. A power of attorney is a legal device that permits a person to allow someone else to act for him or her in legal matters. Sometimes a physician will grant a power of attorney limited in amount and time to an employee who is charged with writing checks.

186.

E. The statement of income and expense is also referred to as the profit and loss statement. It covers a specific period, with total income called gross income or earnings and income after deductions of all expenses called net income. The financial picture of the practice on a specific date is shown on a statement of financial condition or the balance sheet.

187.

C. The medical assistant should immediately call the person who wrote the check. Then the assistant should post the amount of the check that is returned for lack of funds as a new charge on the patient's ledger card.

188.

C. A trial balance is a list of accounts showing the title and balance of each account. The total of accounts with debit balances should equal the total of accounts with credit balances (in double-entry bookkeeping).

189.

D. In completing a bank statement reconciliation, the medical assistant should deduct any bank service charges from the checkbook balance to bring it into line with the bank balance. Other factors that may cause the bank balance to differ from the medical practice's checkbook balance are outstanding checks that make the bank statement higher than the checkbook, deposits after the date of the bank statement that will make the checkbook balance higher, errors by either the medical office bookkeeper or the bank, and dishonored checks (insufficient or nonexistent funds) that make the bank statement lower than the checkbook.

190.

A. Entries made in the day sheet include the patient's name, service rendered, charges, and receipts. This record is known as the book of original entry because it is where every transaction is first recorded. Other names for it include general journal, financial diary, daily journal, and the chronological record.

191.

C. The correct accounting equation is Assets equals Liabilities plus Proprietorship (A = L + P). A similar wording with the same meaning is Assets = Liabilities + Owner's equity. This equation means that all things of value in a business or medical practice are equal to the liabilities owed to creditors plus the owner's claims. The left side of the equation must always equal the right.

192.

E. The proper sequence of activity in the accounting cycle, of those steps included in the question, is posting, adjusting, closing, and issuing financial statements. A similar wording of the accounting cycle in double-entry bookkeeping is as follows: transactions (original service and payment analyzed) recorded on source document—record source document information into journal—transfer journal information into general ledger accounts (posting)—prepare trial balances to prove accuracy—prepare financial statements from trial balances.

193.

B. A write-it-once combination check writing system is the simplest manual way to prepare payroll checks and generate the required accounting records. An employee's compensation record is automatically prepared, and an entry is made on the records of checks drawn. The check is addressed to the employee and can be mailed. Summaries are made at the end of the month from the records of checks drawn.

194.

A. A check register is a record of checks written on the medical office account that provides essential information such as date, number and amount of check, payee receiving the check and the reason, a

place for bank deposits, and any other information that is valuable. The write-it-once pegboard system allows the check to be placed over the register so that information from the check is automatically transferred to the check register. The check register is used to show the current checking balance, to reconcile the bank statements, and to answer any questions that arise about the checks issued.

195.

B. Before the end of the first period, the employee must complete a form W-4 (Employee's Withholding Exemption Certificate) or be charged at the rate of a single taxpayer with no exemptions. Some employees elect to take no exemptions and have more tax withheld, which is refunded later when their income tax reports are filed.

The W-2 form (wage and tax statement) is distributed by the employer to the employees no later than January 31 of the next year. It must list total wages for the year; all FICA, state, and local income taxes; and all voluntary deductions withheld.

196.

C. The payroll register, an itemized list of all employees' total earnings and all deductions, is used to prepare the entries in the payroll journal in single-entry and double-entry bookkeeping. The pegboard, write-it-once system can prepare the payroll register at the same time the entries are made.

197.

E. All of the statements made should be used as guidelines to determine if fee reduction or cancellation of fees is warranted. If these are established and the information is obtained at the time, it will help to eliminate the need for recording a fee on the books and then reducing it.

198.

E. All of these actions should be avoided. The clinic and medical assistant may be accused of harassment if repeated phone calls are made or if calls are made between 9 P.M. and 8 A.M. Leaving a message at the patient's workplace about the overdue bill is an invasion of privacy and might also be considered harassment. Showing contempt or losing one's temper does not accomplish the desired goal, since an angry or insulted patient may not make an effort to pay.

Do not apologize for calling but assume a dignified and respectful tone. Be sure the person is the correct party, avoid threats, keep promises to call back, and assume the positive attitude that the person is going to pay as soon as suitable arrangements are worked out. The call should be made in private, and the called party should be asked if now is a convenient time to talk.

199.

E. The superbill is all of the listed answer selections. It may be personalized for a specific practice. Often used with a pegboard, it is a combination charge slip, statement, receipt, and insurance reporting form, which includes the diagnosis and physician's signature. The amount of the fee is written by the doctor or the medical assistant on the superbill. The superbill is filled out with demographic data at the beginning of the patient's office visit and follows the patient from registration until after the exam is completed; then the charges are calculated. A copy is given to the patient to serve as a receipt or statement after financial arrangements have been made. Another copy may document medical service for an HMO or be attached to a partially completed insurance claim saving time in completing the form.

CPT-4 codes to identify each procedure are printed on the superbill and marked or circled by the physician to identify the procedure performed. The CPT-4 codes are standard to the industry, recognized by most insurance companies and individualized for each medical specialty (e.g., urology, a medical specialty, has its own listing, which is different than family practice). ICD-9 codes are also printed on superbills in some offices since Medicare may require these codes.

200.

E. All charges and receipts concerning patients should be posted daily to keep the patients' accounts current. Otherwise, there will be confusion, a loss of income, and probably a loss of confidence in the medical assistant. All transactions should be recorded immediately to prevent errors. Checks are protected from loss by a restrictive endorsement and deposited in the bank daily.

6 Medical Records and Office Management

chapter objectives

Major areas of knowledge/content included in this chapter are:

I. Types and purpose of medical records

- ➤ Weed system/ POMR/traditional/computer-generated medical records

- ➤ legal and medical uses of medical records

II. Filing systems for patient records and other documents

- ➤ commonly used filing systems for patients—alphabetic, numerical, and electronic

- ➤ application of special filing system aids such as tickler files, color, and master indexes

III. Filing guidelines—storage, protection, transfer, retention, and purging

IV. Documentation and error correction

V. Office administration

- ➤ overseeing and replenishing inventory of drugs and supplies

- ➤ equipment servicing and repair/supervising janitorial service

- ➤ work schedules

- ➤ personal attributes of successful administrators

DIRECTIONS (Questions 201 through 261): Each of the numbered items or incomplete statements in this section is followed by answers or by completions of the statement. Select the ONE lettered answer or completion that is BEST in each case.

201. MEDLARS (Medical Literature Analysis and Retrieval System) is a bibliographic retrieval system based at the
    A. Library of Congress
    B. National Library of Medicine
    C. American Hospital Association
    D. American Medical Association
    E. American College of Surgeons
    (Fordney and Follis, p 241; Frew et al, p 220; Kinn and Woods, p 345)

202. The problem-oriented medical record (POMR) is also called the
    A. SOAP system
    B. source-oriented system
    C. traditional method
    D. Weed system
    E. none of these
    (Kinn and Woods, p 213)

203. SOAP is an acronym (formed from beginning letters of a compound term) that pertains to
    A. sterilization techniques
    B. telephone equipment
    C. dictation equipment
    D. patient records
    E. malpractice
    (Fordney and Follis, p 127; Kinn and Woods, pp 216–217)

204. The "S" and "O" of the acronym SOAP, which is a format for progress notes, mean "subjective" and "objective," respectively. Which of the following is classified as objective information?
    A. examination and diagnostic tests
    B. routine personal data about the patient
    C. the patient's personal and medical history
    D. the patient's family history
    E. the chief complaint and date of onset
    (Fordney and Follis, p 147; Kinn and Woods, p 217)

205. An example of subjective information included in the patient record is the
    A. patient's complaint
    B. physical examination
    C. laboratory reports
    D. diagnosis
    E. progress notes
    (Fordney and Follis, p 133; Kinn et al, p 217)

206. A system of patient records developed by Lawrence L. Weed, MD, is called
    A. POMR
    B. MICR
    C. ADP
    D. OCR
    E. IDP
    (Fordney and Follis, p 146; Kinn and Woods, p 213)

207. A number such as 616.9 is used in a classification system known as the
    A. Barnard classification
    B. Cunningham classification
    C. Boston Medical Library classification
    D. Library of Congress
    E. Dewey decimal system
    (Fordney and Follis, p 242; Kinn and Woods, p 343)

208. A type of monthly reader's guide to medical literature, published by the National Library of Medicine, is the
    A. *American Medical Directory*
    B. *Cumulative Index to Hospital Literature*
    C. *Cunningham Classification*
    D. *Cumulative Index Medicus*
    E. *Practical Medicine*
    (Fordney and Follis, p 241; Frew et al, pp 220–221; Kinn and Woods, p 344)

209. Hard disks, floppy disks, or compact discs (CD-ROM) are used to store medical office files in the following type of filing system:
    A. electronic
    B. Moran
    C. numerical
    D. color coding
    E. alphabetical
    (Becklin and Sonnarborg, p 106)

210. The most common method of filing is
    A. alphabetical
    B. geographic
    C. numerical
    D. by subject
    E. by sound
    (Fordney and Follis, p 167; Kinn and Woods, p 202)

211. If the same material is filed in more than one place, the medical assistant should fill out a form called a/an
    A. index
    B. intrafile
    C. integral record
    D. cross-reference
    E. multiple reference
    (Fordney and Follis, p 167; Frew et al, p 110)

212. To indicate that a folder has been removed from a file, a medical assistant should substitute in its place
    A. an "in guide"
    B. an "out guide"
    C. a tab
    D. a flag
    E. a retrieval card
    (Kinn and Woods, p 197)

213. Pieces of stiff cardboard that separate file folders and bear captions such as "A-Al" or "Am-Az" are called
    A. tabs
    B. guides

C. references
D. cards
E. dividers
(Fordney and Follis, pp 171–172; Frew et al, pp 104–106; Kinn and Woods, p 197)

214. Probably the best practical method of filing reports, clippings, excerpts, and pamphlets relating to medical and scientific topics is
    A. alphabetically
    B. numerically
    C. by subject
    D. chronologically
    E. alphabetically with numerical cross-reference
    (Kinn and Woods, p 204; Zakus et al, p 137; Fordney and Follis, p 177)

215. A space-saving card filing system is the
    A. rotary
    B. vertical
    C. horizontal
    D. visible
    E. phonetic
    (Becklin and Sunnarborg, p 104)

216. Which of the following is NOT an advantage of the open-shelf filing system?
    A. creation of a quiet working environment
    B. lower equipment costs
    C. fast retrieval of records
    D. maximum record security
    E. easy access to files
    (Kinn and Woods, pp 195–196; Fordney and Follis, p 171)

217. When you have misplaced a file and after you have made a complete and methodical search through the proper folder, there are several places you may look for a misplaced paper. Which of the following sites may prove to be beneficial?
    A. in the folder in front of the correct folder
    B. on the bottom of the file under all of the folders

C. in the folder behind the correct folder

D. between the folders

E. all of the above

(Fordney and Follis, p 178)

218. A type of file setup to remind patients to come in for regular checkups is commonly called a

A. reminder file

B. recall file

C. tickler file

D. follow-up file

E. checkup file

(Fordney and Follis, p 178; Kinn and Woods, p 206)

219. In the individual folder of a patient, correspondence is filed

A. randomly

B. chronologically, with the most recent paper in the front of the folder

C. chronologically, with the most recent paper in the back of the folder

D. by subject

E. with larger papers in the back of the folder and smaller papers in the front

(Fordney and Follis, p 173; Kinn and Woods, p 206)

220. Indexing is a step in alphabetical filing that

A. places a mark indicating the paper is ready to file

B. cross-references a paper

C. arranges paper in filing sequence

D. labels

E. decides where to file papers

(Fordney and Follis, pp 176–177; Frew et al, p 105; Kinn and Woods, p 199)

221. Which of the following titles is considered an indexing unit?

A. Dr.

B. Mrs.

C. Capt.

D. Sir

E. Sister

(Fordney and Follis, pp 168–169; Kinn and Woods, p 202)

222. When the names of two or more individuals are exactly the same, the first consideration after the name is the

A. street number

B. street name

C. county

D. state

E. ZIP code

(Fordney and Follis, p 169)

223. Indicate the third indexing unit in the following name: Mr. Evans Thomas Boyatsis, Jr.

A. Mr.

B. Evans

C. Thomas

D. Boyatsis

E. Jr.

(Fordney and Follis, p 168; Kinn and Woods, p 201)

224. A medical assistant must file correspondence of the following two individuals: Mr. Bruce Turner, 148 Spring Boulevard, Chattanooga, TN 37404, and Mr. Bruce Turner, 239 First Avenue, Chattanooga, TN 37420. Which of the following is the last indexing unit?

A. Bruce

B. Turner

C. 148

D. TN

E. ZIP code

(Becklin and Sunnarborg, pp 110–113)

225. Which indexing unit determines the order in which the two names in the previous question are filed?

A. second

B. third

C. fourth

D. fifth

E. sixth

(Becklin and Sunnarborg, pp 110–113)

226. Referring to Question 224, what is the third indexing unit?

A. Bruce

B. Turner

C. Chattanooga

D. TN

E. ZIP code

(Becklin and Sunnarborg, pp 110–113; Fordney and Follis, p 169)

227. If each indexing unit is identical up to and including the city, the next unit to be considered is the

A. ZIP code

B. street number

C. street name

D. state

E. personal title

(Becklin and Sunnarborg, pp 110–113; Fordney and Follis, p 169)

228. The procedure for filing reports and letters requires several steps. Which is the last or final step in the filing process?

A. index the material

B. inspect each record or piece of correspondence to determine if it has been released for filing

C. code the material by marking the index caption on the papers to be filed

D. locate the file drawer or shelf, place the papers with heading to the left, with the most current on top

E. sort the material by placing in a desk sorter

(Fordney and Follis, p 176; Kinn and Woods, p 199)

229. The procedure for filing reports and letters requires several steps. Which one of the following steps is the first step in the filing process?

A. index the material

B. inspect each record or piece of correspondence to determine if it has been released for filing

C. code the material by marking the index caption on the papers to be filed

D. locate the file drawer or shelf, place the papers with heading to the left, with the most current on top

E. sort the material by placing in a desk sorter

(Fordney and Follis, p 167; Kinn and Woods, p 199)

230. Which of the following names would come first when indexing a set of files?

A. Brown, J.

B. Brown, James

C. Brown, Sarah (Mrs. Brian L.)

D. Brown, William

E. Brown, Robert

(Fordney and Follis, p 168; Frew et al, p 108)

231. The order in which progress notes, laboratory reports, x-ray reports, and so on are added to the patient's medical record is

A. objective

B. subjective

C. chronologic

D. problem oriented

E. diagnosis related

(Fordney and Follis, pp 138–139; Kinn and Woods, p 218)

232. When the doctor visits patients outside the office in hospitals or nursing homes

A. an outfolder is placed in the file

B. the patient record is carried in a wearproof folder

C. duplicate patient records are maintained

D. the record does not leave the office

E. the patient record is sent beforehand

(Fordney and Follis, p 106)

233. Removing pins, mending damaged records, and stapling like papers together in preparation for filing is called

A. conditioning

B. releasing

C. indexing

D. coding

E. assembling

(Fordney and Follis, p 176; Kinn and Woods, p 199)

234. When a system of color coding is used in filing business records, the code should be known by
    A. only the medical assistant
    B. only the physician and the medical assistant
    C. everyone who uses the files
    D. the physician, staff, and patients
    E. the local chapter of the medical society

    (Frew et al, pp 103–104; Kinn and Woods, pp 204–205; Fordney and Follis, pp 174–175)

235. The system of filing that would be used in a medical office where a great degree of privacy is desired is
    A. alphabetical
    B. geographic
    C. chronologic
    D. by subject
    E. numerical

    (Fordney and Follis, p 170; Frew et al, pp 107–108)

236. Generally, medical records of a practice are classified into three groups: active files, inactive files, and closed files. After what period of inactivity is a file placed in the inactive group of files?
    A. 1 year
    B. 5 years
    C. 6 months
    D. 3 months
    E. at end of treatment

    (Fordney and Follis, p 179; Kinn and Woods, p 223)

237. The type of filing system that is very expensive initially and also requires more maintenance is the
    A. drawer type

B. shelf files with doors

C. rotary-circular files

D. lateral files

E. automated files

(Kinn and Woods, p 196; Fordney and Follis, p 171)

238. Which type of filing equipment will use more wall space and not extend out into the room as far?
    A. drawer files
    B. shelf files
    C. rotary-circular files
    D. lateral files
    E. automated files

    (Kinn and Woods, pp 195–196; Fordney and Follis, p 171)

239. When errors about information are noted in the chart, they must be corrected using a legally acceptable technique. Which is correct?
    A. mark through the mistake at least ten times
    B. only initial the strikeout
    C. if there are incorrect data, enter the correct information on a new page
    D. date and sign only explanations, not strikeouts
    E. if the entry has been made in the wrong chart, draw a single line through the data and note, "Recorded in this chart by error. This information has been transferred to the chart of Tom Dowell."

    (Fordney and Follis, p 143; Frew et al, p 88; Kinn and Woods, p 219)

240. Of the following records, which should be kept in a desk file or file cabinet for 3 years?
    A. real estate deeds
    B. bank deposit slips
    C. powers of attorney
    D. passports
    E. promissory notes

    (Fordney and Follis, p 179; Kinn and Woods, p 223)

241. All of the following are true regarding microfilming records for storage EXCEPT
    A. less space is required for storage
    B. less time is required in searching
    C. it requires special equipment
    D. they are considered paperless files
    E. it is easier to produce a microfilm in court than traditional records

    (Fordney and Follis, p 181)

242. Of the following records, which is kept permanently?
    A. correspondence
    B. receipts for business equipment
    C. professional liability policies
    D. announcements of meetings
    E. letters of transmittal

    (Fordney and Follis, p 179; Kinn and Woods, p 223)

243. Which of the following statements is INCORRECT?
    A. folders to be filed should be arranged in indexing order before going to the file cabinet
    B. only one file drawer should be opened at a time
    C. the top edge of items in the folders should be to the right
    D. in making a search for a misfiled paper, the medical assistant might look in the folder in front of and behind the correct folder
    E. before material is dropped into a folder in a drawer, the folder should be lifted an inch or two

    (Fordney and Follis, p 174; Frew et al, pp 104–105; Kinn and Woods, p 200)

244. Filing should be done
    A. daily
    B. twice daily
    C. when the file basket is full
    D. every other day
    E. weekly

    (Fordney, p 173; Kinn and Woods, p 219)

245. Which of the following statements about the firing of an employee is NOT accepted protocol?
    A. the employee is warned verbally of unacceptable performance
    B. the employee is warned in writing if behavior continues
    C. the employee is given notice
    D. termination both verbally and in writing if behavior continues
    E. the person who hired does not fire the person

    (Kinn and Woods, p 373; Fordney and Follis, p 424)

246. A medical assistant should be certain that the cleaning firm contracted to perform major cleaning of the office on a regular basis is performing according to the agreement. Which of the following is NOT considered to be a daily or weekly housekeeping operation?
    A. dust
    B. empty trash baskets
    C. cleaning of delicate equipment
    D. clean mirrors and pictures
    E. wash sinks, basins, and toilets

    (Fordney and Follis, pp 191–192)

247. Supplies absolutely necessary to the medical practice are classified as
    A. critical supplies
    B. periodic supplies
    C. incidental supplies
    D. basic supplies
    E. temporary supplies

    (Fordney and Follis, pp 194–195; Frew et al, pp 101–102)

248. Drug samples should be organized into categories in a sample cupboard or drawer. A good way to categorize free drug samples would be by
    A. tablets, pills, liquids, and creams
    B. injectables, oral medication, suppositories

C. drug action

D. alphabetically

E. medications by age groups

(Fordney and Follis, p 200; Kinn and Woods, p 360)

249. Salesmen and pharmaceutical representatives generally should see the physician

A. by appointment

B. between patient appointments

C. only if the medical assistant deems it necessary

D. only if they are showing new products

E. only if they are new to their jobs

(Fordney and Follis, p 101)

250. Which federal act oversees the safety of health facilities including protection against occupational exposure to Hepatitis B virus and human immunodeficiency virus?

A. OSHA

B. CLIA '88

C. DEA

D. CDC

E. COLA

(Fordney and Follis, p 201; Kinn and Woods, pp 73, 420)

251. The filing system that offers the most even distribution of folders throughout the file is

A. geographic

B. alphabetical

C. by subject

D. terminal-digit

E. color

(Fordney and Follis, p 170; Frew et al, pp 107–108; Kinn and Woods, p 205)

252. Maintaining medical records accomplishes which of the following objectives?

A. serves as a defense against malpractice suits

B. affords continuity of medical care

C. justifies payment for services rendered

D. documents that high-quality care has been provided

E. all of the above

(Frew et al, pp 109–112; Kinn and Woods, pp 209–211; Fordney and Follis, p 127)

253. A tickler file is useful for the following purposes

A. ordering of supplies

B. follow-up items

C. paying dues and subscriptions

D. housekeeping tasks

E. all of the above

(Fordney and Follis, p 178; Kinn and Woods, p 206)

254. A file should be maintained for information concerning servicing of equipment. Information in the service file should include which of the following?

A. warranty dates

B. frequency of service

C. cost of service

D. who last serviced the equipment and when

E. all of the above

(Fordney and Follis, p 199; Kinn and Woods, p 357)

255. Which of the following are functions of the office procedure manual?

A. it lists the tasks required of the personnel

B. it serves to standardize procedures

C. it lists titles and responsibilities for the office staff

D. it instructs temporary personnel in office procedures

E. all of the above

(Frew et al, pp 97–99; Kinn and Woods, pp 366–368; Fordney and Follis, pp 188–189)

256. A master list of equipment items would include
    A. cost of service and maintenance
    B. operating manuals, including instructions
    C. purchase date, cost, and description and estimated life of equipment
    D. repair and maintenance instructions
    E. the SOP manual

    (Frew et al, p 100; Kinn and Woods, pp 256–258; Fordney and Follis, pp 199–200)

257. Two aids to maintaining an adequate supply of critical supplies are
    A. *Standard Suppliers Dictionary*
    B. a critical supply items list and supply inventory cards
    C. equipment maintenance list
    D. maintenance manual
    E. all of the above

    (Fordney and Follis, pp 194–195)

258. The forms necessary for the physician's registration with the Drug Enforcement Agency (DEA) can be obtained from
    A. the local police
    B. State Attorney General's office
    C. any regional DEA office or DEA Section, P.O. Box 28083, Central Station, Washington, DC 20005
    D. the local health unit
    E. all of the above

    (Kinn and Woods, p 1002; Fordney and Follis, p 158)

259. To make the workday proceed more efficiently and ensure that everything essential gets done, the medical assistant should
    A. enlist the help of a coworker to remind him or her of tasks
    B. make a work schedule and follow it as closely as possible
    C. try to hurry
    D. not allow interruptions
    E. make a tickler file

    (Frew et al, p 21; Fordney and Follis, pp 186–187)

260. If you have questions or a complaint about medical supplies that have been received, which of the following information should be on hand before contacting the supplier?
    A. invoice number
    B. date ordered
    C. person who placed order
    D. catalog, if used for order
    E. all of the above

    (Frew et al, pp 219–220; Kinn and Woods, p 359; Fordney and Follis, p 195)

261. Which of the following is NOT typical of assertive individuals who have the capacity for professional growth and management?
    A. assuming a modest attitude that lets others have credit for your ideas
    B. saying no to unrealistic or unreasonable demands
    C. speaking up for what they deserve such as a promotion
    D. asking employers for necessary supplies to perform their jobs well
    E. identifying and acquiring desirable skills for job performance and advancement

    (Frew et al, p 25; Fordney, p 424)

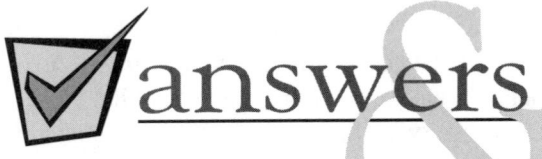

201.

B. MEDLARS is a computer-based system operating at the National Library of Medicine. It has computer access also to MEDLINE (biomedical referencing system) and TOXLINE (toxicology information), CHEMLINE (dictionary of chemical substances), and Cancerlit (cancer literature).

202.

D. The POMR is also called the Weed system after its originator, Lawrence Weed, MD. It imposes logic on the medical record by dividing a medical action into four bases: (1) the database that includes the chief complaint (CC = chief complaint), present illness, and patient profile; (2) a list of patient problems that require workup; (3) treatment plan; and (4) progress notes that are numbered to match problem numbers in the problem list.

203.

D. SOAP is an acronym that pertains to patient records, more particularly to the POMR. The POMR originated as a way to organize medical records in an orderly and easy-to-understand fashion. Each patient problem is given a number as it is identified, which is used for reference in treatment. As new problems occur, new numbers are assigned. They are placed before the doctor's notes about the patient visit. The POMR method is most useful where several people are involved with one person's medical record. An alternative method of organizing material is the source-oriented medical record, which groups information according to its source. For instance, all laboratory reports are grouped and shingled together in one place

in the chart, all nurse's or doctor's notes together in another part of the chart, and so on.

The doctor's notes in a POMR medical record are organized according to the plan SOAP. The letters represent the words *subjective* data (patient-generated information), *objective* findings, *assessment* of the patient's status, and *plan* for treatment.

204.

A. The examination and diagnostic tests supplied by the doctor are classified as objective information and are based on clinical evidence. The "A" in SOAP stands for assessment or diagnosis. The "P" in SOAP refers to plans for further studies, treatment, or management of the patient's problem.

205.

A. An example of subjective information included in the patient record is the patient's complaint. In addition, other subjective information includes routine personal data about the patient, the patient's personal and medical history, and the patient's family history. The subjective information is provided by the patient, and the objective information is supplied by the doctor.

206.

A. A system of patient records developed by Lawrence L. Weed, MD, is called POMR, or the problem-oriented medical record. This type of record, with a database, problem list, treatment plan for each problem, and progress notes correlated with the problems, is a departure from the traditional source-oriented medical record.

207.

E. A number such as 616.9 is used to label books in the Dewey decimal system, a classification system that has very wide usage in both medical and other libraries. Whereas the Dewey decimal system uses numbers and decimals to categorize the books according to subjects, the Library of Congress uses a combination of letters and numerals (e.g., Library of Congress classification RC 321-431 is diseases of the nervous system). A glance at the library card catalog and some assistance from the librarian will acquaint you with the system used.

208.

D. A type of monthly reader's guide to medical literature, published by the National Library of Medicine, is the *Cumulative Index Medicus*. It includes author and subject indexes for more than 3000 periodicals published both in the United States and abroad. MEDLINE is the computer equivalent of *Cumulative Index Medicus*.

209.

A. Electronic files are stored in a system connected to a personal computer or word processor. These may consist of hard disks, floppy disks, compact discs (CD-ROMs), or tapes. A *password* protects the confidentiality of the patients' records. Care must be taken in naming the files (labeling), using passwords, and deleting nonessential files. The usual precautions used with other electronic data must be used with patient files. Many medical offices have retained the printed medical patient charts. However, the widespread use of computers and the exchange of medical information will undoubtedly increase the prevalence of electronic files.

Another process of storing records in a manner other than the conventional printed page is micrographics in which the paper records are miniaturized to very small images on film and stored in a card file or a book-type binder. *Microfiche* (90 frames on a sheet of film) and *ultrafice* (up to 1000 frames on a sheet) can obviously store immense amounts of information in a small space. However, machines are necessary for enlarging the frames. This type of media is popular for storage of records that would otherwise require immense and costly space.

210.

A. The most common method of filing is alphabetical, especially in small offices. It is straightforward and easy to understand but does not conceal the identity of the patients. Unfortunately, some people have difficulty alphabetizing and wreak havoc with the files. Indexing rules standardize the alphabetizing procedure (i.e., the surname (last name) is always considered first, numbers are filed as though spelled out, etc.).

Numerical is the second most common method of filing. It assigns each patient a number as they are registered the first time. An alphabetical cross-reference index is always maintained to find the number of the file. Other various refinements may be used (e.g., the two terminal digits of the number may correspond to the shelf or drawer that should hold the record). The number system also provides more privacy than a record labeled with the patient's name.

Color coding, commonly used in the medical office, has many different applications. However, every employee using the records should know the color system. Color coding used with both alphabetical and numerical filing systems makes both filing and retrieving quicker. Out-of-place files are obvious when they are a different color. Among the applications of color are (1) alphabetical filing—dividing the letters of the alphabet into different colors so that there is an almost equal distribution of files between the colors; (2) numerical filing—assigning a color to a segment of numbers; and (3) each digit from 0 to 9 may be assigned a color. Colors are then used with either the beginning or terminal digits. In the two terminal digit system, the last two digits are each assigned a color. Two colors representing the last two digits of the medical records number are placed on the file. They become color bands that are obvious when looking at files stored on shelves.

Other ways of making color work are to assign different colors to Medicaid and Champus files or to use dividers in different colors (e.g., each doctor's patients may have a different color). Health conditions such as allergies also can be indicated by color.

General correspondence is often filed by subject matter. Generally, there is a cross-index to help locate subjects that might be filed under different headings.

Files may also be separated geographically—that is, by the area where the patient lives or works. For example, all workers from a company might be housed in a separate area or files could be arranged by street addresses.

211.

D. A cross-reference should be filled out if the same material is filed in more than one place. A cross-reference is a good idea with names that are unusual and possibly may have the given name filed as the surname. For example, a cross-reference would be filed for the name James Mark under the heading Mark James, "see James Mark."

The purpose of cross-referencing is to make the document trail easy to find in case one clue such as a number or name is misunderstood or lost. Numerical and alphabetized files are cross-referenced to avoid losing a file due to misunderstanding. Subject files may be either cross-referenced to a number or to another subject that the file is related to.

212.

B. An out guide with the borrower's name is substituted for a folder that has been removed from a file. This serves as a reminder that it has not been returned. Because patients' files are legal documents, they must not be allowed to disappear and must be traced if necessary.

213.

B. Guides are pieces of stiff cardboard that separate file folders and bear captions such as "A-Al" or "Am-Az." It is a good idea to purchase good quality guides, since they receive much wear. Guides are one of several types of equipment that make filing more efficient.

Other equipment needed for files is as follows: (1) shelves, file cabinets, etc., to hold the total number of files used; (2) guides of heavy cardboard or plastic with the section indicated that will subdivide the shelf or file drawer into smaller sections for ease in referencing files; (3) file folders (manila folders) hold the document of one patient, personnel documents for each employee, or other unit that is filed; (4) labels to identify the individual files, the guide units, and the file drawers or shelves according to the file system used, usually alphabetical or numerical; and (5) a smaller tickler file that cross-indexes all the other files.

214.

C. Probably the best practical method of filing reports, clippings, and excerpts and pamphlets relating to medical and scientific topics is by subject using numerous cross-references. A miscellaneous file is used until the volume requires a larger system of filing and then the file is subdivided into topics.

215.

A. A rotary system, whereby cards are cut to fit a curved rod and hooked onto a circular axle, is the most space-saving card filing system. Any system of filing storage has its advantages and disadvantages. Some are more expensive, occupy more space, provide more security, are more easily adapted to changing needs, and/or are easily referenced.

Some of the more common types of file holders are storage for **card files** in a smaller box or cabinet; **vertical file** units, which are housed in the usual file cabinet with drawers; **lateral files** in cabinets, which open to the side to allow easy access to the files; **open shelf files**, which make good use of space and **mobile aisle files**, which are **open shelf files** that move together or apart in order to save space. There are also **electronic files**, which are stored on compact disks or other electronic storage.

216.

D. Open-shelf filing does have the advantage of creating a quiet working environment, reducing equipment costs, conserving space, and speeding up the retrieval of records, as well as conserving effort, since there is no opening or closing of drawers. However, open-shelf units without doors offer little protection or confidentiality of records and are susceptible to water and flame damage in the event of fire.

217.

E. When you have completed a methodical search for a misplaced file, you may find it beneficial to look in both the folders in front of and behind the correct folder. The file may have slipped to the bottom, and files may have been placed over it. It may be in a patient's folder with a similar name, or it may still be in the sorter waiting to be filed.

218.

C. A tickler file is used to remind patients to schedule an office visit and also to bring other events to the medical assistant's attention. The tickler file always has a chronologic order, often in the format of a calendar. It should be referred to each morning. Tickler files (checklists of office tasks that need to be performed on a time schedule) are often found in the front section of the office procedure manual and include a wide array of topics, from the date for renewing licenses to reminding patients to come in.

219.

B. In an individual folder (one folder for one individual person or firm), correspondence is filed chronologically with the most recent paper in the front. The papers are categorized into different subjects, such as laboratory, but the chronologic order of each category is maintained. A method called "shingling" is used to save space with laboratory reports. Each report almost overlaps the one before it with only the dates at the bottom line of the older reports showing. In this manner, the dates of each report can be seen, as well as the full report of the most recent test. The reports can be lifted like pages of a book to see the test reports of previous dates. The progress notes are placed one on top of another with the most recent one always on top.

220.

E. Indexing is deciding where to file the paper according to its position in the alphabet. In the filing system based on alphabetical order (most commonly used in doctors' offices), there are 12 standard indexing (alphabetizing) rules. (Some texts give as many as 19 rules that may vary according to the clinic or authority. They may also be changed for convenience by a particular filing department.) These rules standardize the filing process so that different people's judgment or a lapse in one's own memory will not cause the filing system to vary. For instance, one rule to prevent confusion is to always file a surname with a foreign prefix as though it were one word (e.g., De Labretonne is filed as one word, DeLabretonne, disregarding the capitalization). Keep a written list of the rules until you have memorized them through practice in filing.

An abbreviated list of rules follows. (Consult a textbook, if possible, explaining the indexing rules.) (1) Order of indexing units (parts of a name) is surname first; first name or initial, second unit; and middle name or initial is third unit. (2) Names of businesses are indexed in the order the name is written. (3) Symbols and coordinating words such as "the," "a," and "an" are separate units or are disregarded. (4) Initials precede a name beginning with the same letter (the librarian's "nothing comes before something" rule). (5) The apostrophe is disregarded in filing. (6) Hyphenated words are considered one unit. (7) "Mac" and "Mc" are filed in their regular places in the alphabet. (8) The name of a married woman is indexed by her legal name (husband's surname, her given name, and middle name or maiden surname). (9) Titles followed by a full name are disregarded in indexing. Titles without complete names (e.g., Sister Mary) are considered the first indexing unit. (10) Addresses (state, city, street, street number) are used to distinguish between identical names. (11) When numbers are part of the business name such as 9th St. Computer Shop, the numbers are spelled out and then indexed. (12) Names of businesses are indexed as written. National (first unit) Association (second unit) of (third unit) Pathologists (fourth unit).

221.

E. "Sister" is considered an indexing unit, and it is the first unit when followed by a given name only.

222.

D. When the names of two or more individuals are exactly the same, the first consideration after the name is the address, indexing the city first, the state second, the street third, and the ZIP code last. References differ on whether the city or state is the part of the address considered first. Office policy would be followed in these cases.

223.

C. The indexing units in order would be as follows: Boyatsis, Evans, Thomas because "Jr." is considered an identifying element and not an indexing unit. Last name is the first indexing unit, first name is second, and middle initial or name is third.

224.

E. The ZIP code is the last indexing unit used. The components of the address (state, city, street, and ZIP code) are used to differentiate in case of identical names.

225.

D. The indexing order for these two individuals is as follows: surname, given name, city, state, street name, and street number. It is necessary to consider the street name because all of the preceding units are identical. Office policy regarding indexing of names will vary somewhat from office to office as will other aspects of office procedure such as filing. The important principle to understand is that all co-workers must follow the same rules. Otherwise confusion will result in lost files, lost time, and wasted effort.

226.

C. The third indexing unit is the city, Chattanooga. (The first unit was the surname, the second the given name, the third the city, the fourth the state, and the fifth the street.)

227.

D. The next unit to be considered after the city is the state, then the street name, and then the street number. (The units of city and state may be reversed in order.)

228.

D. The last step in the filing procedure is to locate the proper file drawer or shelf with the appropriate caption and place the papers with the heading to the left. The most recent material should be placed on top. This last step would be preceded by conditioning or inspecting (taking out paper clips, stapling related papers together, mending damaged records, etc.); releasing (indicating the paper is ready for filing by initialing or stamping FILE, etc.); indexing (deciding where the paper goes in the file, writing the decision somewhere on the paper [coding] and preparing a cross-reference sheet if needed for a second location). Also, make sure all papers in the file have the patient's name on them, usually in upper right corner; and sorting (arranging the papers in filing sequence) before going to the file cabinet. A desk sorter on a tray may be used for larger numbers of papers. The final step is storing and filing, face up, top edge to the left, with most recent date to the front of the folder.

229.

B. The first step in the filing procedure is to inspect each record or piece of correspondence and determine if it has been released for filing. Physicians usually place a checkmark or initials in the upper right-hand corner.

230.

A. Brown, J., would precede Brown, James, because of the rule that initials come before a name beginning with the same letter ("nothing comes before something" in indexing). Brown, Robert, comes before Brown, Sarah (Mrs. Brian L.), because Robert comes before Sarah, the given name of the woman used for indexing (not her husband's name). Brown, William, comes last because it is last in alphabetical order.

231.

C. All information collected about the patient is added to the file in chronologic order with the latest always on top. Information, such as laboratory reports, may be separated according to category, but the newest will be on the top and the oldest on the bottom. All progress reports, notations, laboratory reports, and so on must be dated.

232.

D. The patient's record should not leave the office, since it is a valuable legal document. A Physician's Pocket Call Record, a printed form with a space for the necessary information, may be used instead. Another alternative is to photocopy the record.

233.

A. Removing pins, mending damaged records, and stapling like papers together in preparation for filing are called conditioning or inspecting. Other steps in the filing process include releasing, indexing and cross-referencing, coding, sorting, and storing.

234.

C. When a system of color coding is used in filing, the code should be known by everyone in the office who uses the files. The key should be written in the agency's procedure manual. The uses of this system of filing are limited only by the imagination.

235.

E. The numerical system of filing would be used in a medical office where a great degree of privacy is desired. Generally, most patient records are filed alphabetically. Alphabetical filing is most common in small practices.

236.

C. At the end of 6 months of inactivity, a file is generally placed in the inactive status. It will remain there until the patient receives treatment, again placing the file in active status, or ends his or her relationship with the physician by moving away, dying, or otherwise terminating the relationship. This is the perpetual transfer method.

237.

E. The type of filing system that is very expensive initially and also will require more maintenance is the automated file. This file system brings the record to the operator instead of the operator going to the record. This filing system usually is found only in large clinics or hospitals.

238.

D. Lateral files use more wall space than vertical files and do not extend into the room so far. This type of filing equipment is especially attractive for the physician's private office.

239.

E. When errors about information are noted in the chart, including an entry into the wrong chart, a proper correction technique is as follows: draw a single line through the error so that the information recorded can still be read and always date and initial the strikeout. If the error is incorrect data, strike it out (single line), enter the correct information directly below the strikeout, and date and initial the entry. If you have recorded in the wrong chart, strike out with a single line and write that the information was charted by error and explain where the information has been transferred. Then date and sign the strikeout and the explanation.

240.

B. Among the records that should be kept for 3 years before being transferred to dead storage are current bank statements, bank deposit slips, and receipts for paid bills if needed for tax purposes. Real estate deeds, promissory notes, and powers of attorney should be kept in a safer place, such as a safe deposit box.

241.

E. It is difficult to produce microfilm in court. Other disadvantages of microfilming records are that the cost is high, microfilm is difficult to read for prolonged periods of time, and the microfilm is too small for refiling if a patient returns. However, microfilm storage is sometimes chosen when storage space is very costly.

242.

C. Professional liability policies (which ensure against malpractice suits) should be kept permanently. Some authorities also believe that all previous patient records should be kept (in auxiliary storage) permanently as protection against malpractice suits.

243.

C. When papers are filed in folders, the top edge of items should be to the left (not the right) for easier reading, with the most recent date to the front of the folder. File drawers left open, even just a little, can cause injury to a passerby or tilt, spilling the contents. Office safety mandates that they be either secured to the floor or wall or that other precautions be observed to prevent accidents.

244.

A. Filing should be orderly and systematic to keep records accessible and prevent confusion. It is best to return records to the filing cabinet at the end of the day for security purposes. This also protects them from the cleaning crew in the evening and possibly against fire. The complete filing procedure including examination, indexing, coding, sorting, and storing should be carefully developed and outlined in the office procedure manual.

245.

E. Usually the same person who hired the individual also fires the individual. The employee is given a warning at least twice that his or her performance is jeopardizing the job unless the offense is a gross breach of ethics or a legal issue. He or she should be given notice of termination according to written office policy.

246.

C. Cleaning of expensive and delicate equipment is not a task that is delegated to the cleaning service. The maintenance service should have written instructions concerning the disposal of contaminated waste, what areas are off-limits, and what supplies will be furnished. It is important that the medical office be attractive, pleasant, and clean.

247.

A. Critical supplies are those necessary for the medical practice that require special orders and perhaps long delays. Other items that are easily and quickly acquired are incidental supplies, and items required only at the beginning of each year are periodic supplies.

248.

C. Drug samples received from drug representatives and in the mail should be categorized according to drug action. For example, all sedative samples should be stored together, all stimulant samples together, and so on. The new samples should be at the back, with the oldest samples in front to be used first. Periodically, the samples' expiration dates should be checked, and expired samples should be destroyed.

249.

A. Salespersons and pharmaceutical representatives should see the physician by appointment. They will be screened by the medical assistant according to office policy. Some physicians want to see the salesperson for a very brief period between patients; others will prefer seeing the persons after the last patient at the noon break or at the end of the day. Most company representatives understand the time factor and want to cooperate so that they may be welcomed again at a later date.

250.

A. OSHA, a synonym for Occupational Safety and Health Act, sets standards of safety for all health facilities. It mandates information and training of employees about AIDS and hepatitis. Employers must identify, in writing, tasks and procedures as well as job positions where occupational exposure to blood occurs. It mandates universal precautions, which include engineering and work practice controls. Handwashing is emphasized. Procedures are defined that minimize splashing and spraying of blood. Employers must offer employees at no cost the Hepatitis B vaccination within 10 days of beginning occupational exposure. Postexposure evaluation and follow-up must be provided to any employee who has had an exposure incident. OSHA also provides guidelines for labeling and handling chemicals.

251.

D. Terminal-digit is regarded as being the most effective numerical filing system, and there is usually a nearly perfect distribution of folders throughout the file. This system of filing is a simple and accurate method that increases the productivity of file clerks.

252.

E. Adequate medical records will meet all of the objectives stated. Accurate and complete medical records are essential for continuing excellent medical care. They will also save the physician's and patient's time.

253.

E. A tickler file is useful as a reminder for a variety of purposes, including all of those mentioned. Tasks can be better organized by using such a file, and it is easy to set up with 3″ × 5″ cards and guides to represent the months and days.

254.

E. It is important to keep a special file or folder that keeps up with servicing of office equipment. This file should contain the following: warranty dates, frequency of service recommended, the cost of the service, and when and by whom the equipment was last serviced.

255.

E. All of the listed items are functions of the office procedure manual, which every practice needs to organize the large number of activities and to standardize the work of the different staff members. If a manual does not exist, the medical assistant should approach the physician about its design before starting one.

256.

C. The equipment master list would include date of purchase, the cost, a description of the equipment, and its estimated life. A separate record is maintained for each piece of equipment with such particulars as receipts, operating manuals, instructions, guarantees, repair and maintenance information, dates repaired, and service personnel with their phone numbers.

257.

B. A critical supply items list should be kept with quantities needed, reorder levels, and where to reorder. An inventory card is used to keep up with groups of similar items. It is updated whenever an order is placed.

258.

C. The forms necessary for the physician's registration with the Drug Enforcement Agency (DEA) can be obtained from either any DEA regional office or from DEA Section, P.O. Box 28083, Central Station, Washington, DC 20005

259.

B. To work efficiently and not overlook essential tasks, the medical assistant should create a written sample work schedule and daily reminder list. A medical assistant should not depend on memory to assure that the needed tasks are performed. Emergencies and disruptions often distract from the usual tasks creating forgetfulness and inefficiency.

The daily reminder list should include every necessary task and may consist of some or all of the following: upon arriving at the office, call the physician's answering service for overnight messages; check all the rooms for appearance; prepare tray and set-ups for daily work; sort and open the mail; place list of appointments on physician's desk; pull and prepare the needed files for today's appointments; type office dictation; work on bookkeeping; check supplies; prepare bank deposit; file today's patient charts at end of day; and lock up office and check security. If several employees work together in the office, they should each have access to the work schedule and understand the work assignments.

Time management skills must be used to organize and prioritize the work. The job list should be reviewed during the day, completed tasks marked off, and the remaining tasks prioritized with perhaps an asterisk or numbers. Whenever possible, the inefficiency of double work should be avoided by following through with the task at hand. However, emergencies may prevent this.

260.

E. All the necessary information, such as invoice number, date ordered, person who placed order, catalog information, etc., should be collected together before making a call about an order. These facts are more easily gathered if good housekeeping practices are used. Packages when received should be stored in a storeroom and opened when time permits. The contents should be checked, with comparisons made to the order list of number of items ordered, price listed, and so on.

261.

A. Assertive individuals do not assume a false (dishonest) modesty and allow others to falsely take credit for work that belongs to them. They can express themselves constructively in the face of disagreement. Medical assistants who wish to achieve personal growth and management skills will (1) take credit for their own ideas, (2) say no to unrealistic demands, (3) make reasonable but firm requests, and (4) speak up for what they need or deserve such as a timely promotion or needed supplies for jobs they are expected to perform.

The assertive person endeavors to (1) be knowledgeable and competent on the job; (2) study and master the job skills necessary for promotion; (3) take the necessary courses, do research, and practice to acquire these skills; (4) ask the employer for necessary items for performing the job efficiently; and (5) assume an assertive but pleasant demeanor.

The medical assistant should distinguish between assertiveness, which is constructive, and aggressiveness, which is destructive. The goal of assertiveness is to keep relationships with co-workers smooth and productive. Assertiveness may call for letter writing or cooperation with supervisors rather than face-to-face confrontation.

7 Insurance and Coding

chapter objectives

Major areas of knowledge/content included in this chapter are:

I. Vocabulary of insurance and coding

II. Types of third party payers:

- insurance • health maintenance organizations • government programs

➤ Traditional indemnity plans and managed care plans

III. Translating medical problems and solutions into numerical data for computer processing required by third party payers

➤ types of codes used to process claims

IV. Insurance specialists' tasks

V. Processing claims

➤ advantages of manual versus electronic preparation and submission of claims; use of universal claim forms

➤ preventing errors, tracing claims; insurance claims log

➤ coordination of benefits/payment by primary versus secondary carriers

➤ researching rejections • making inquiries to insurance companies • appeals

DIRECTIONS (Questions 262 through 333): Each of the numbered items or incomplete statements in this section is followed by answers or by completions of the statement. Select the ONE lettered answer or completion that is BEST in each case.

262. A physician's usual fee is
    A. the charge he or she makes to private patients
    B. the range of charges made by the majority of physicians in a given area
    C. the average charge made by the majority of physicians in a given area
    D. the charge specified by an insurance council
    E. the charge set by a government agency
    (Kinn and Woods, pp 228–229)

263. When patients become members of a health maintenance organization (HMO), they have several rights. Which of the following is NOT one of these rights?
    A. the right to accept or reject treatment
    B. the right to choose any physician as their doctor
    C. the right to know if the treatment prescribed has side effects
    D. the right to know what effect the treatment will have on the body
    E. the right to know if there are alternatives to treatment
    (Humphrey, pp 286–287; Kinn and Woods, p 313; Rowell, p 25)

264. The fiscal agents for Medicare and other government-sponsored insurance programs keep a continuous list of the usual and customary charges by individual doctors for specific procedures. This is used to determine the
    A. insurance allowance
    B. customary fee
    C. prevailing rate
    D. reasonable fee
    E. fee profile
    (Frew et al, pp 287–288; Kinn and Woods, p 229)

265. Dr. Schuyler charges his patients $38 for the first office visit. Other doctors with similar training and experience in the same community charge from $34 to $42 for the same service. An insurance company that pays a U&C (usual and customary) fee would pay Dr. Schuyler
    A. $34
    B. $35
    C. $38
    D. $42
    E. an amount that cannot be determined from the facts presented
    (Fordney and Follis, pp 295, 297; Kinn and Woods, p 229)

266. If the range of U&C fees in the community is from $30 to $36 and Dr. Schuyler charges $38, the insurance company would pay
    A. $30
    B. $32
    C. $34
    D. $36
    E. $38
    (Fordney and Follis, pp 295–297; Kinn and Woods, p 229)

267. Medicare forms must be signed by the
    A. physician only
    B. medical assistant only
    C. patient only
    D. patient and the medical assistant
    E. patient and the physician
    (Fordney and Follis, pp 340–341; Frew et al, pp 288–294; Rowell, pp 318–327)

268. The proportion of a patient's charge billed to Medicare Part B that will be paid is
    A. varied
    B. total amount of bill

C. 80%

D. 80% of the reasonable charge minus a deductible

E. 70% of reasonable charge

(*Fordney and Follis, p 304; Kinn and Woods, p 380; Rowell, p 299*)

269. A reason for the return of insurance claim forms to the physician's office might be

A. a missing or incorrect procedure code number

B. a missing or incorrect diagnostic code number

C. provider number not imprinted on forms

D. beneficiary's name missing or incorrect

E. all of the above

(*Fordney and Follis, pp 335–345; Kinn and Woods, p 330; Rowell, pp 60–61*)

270. Copies of Medicare forms may be obtained from the

A. office supply firm

B. fiscal agent

C. patient

D. Social Security Administration

E. Internal Revenue Service

(*Fordney and Follis, p 335*)

271. Which of the following is NOT a duty of a medical assistant acting as the medical insurance specialist in a medical office?

A. inform patients of the amount their insurance payment will pay on their clinic bill

B. gather information and signatures for insurance claims

C. submit the insurance claim form

D. review insurance payments

E. help clients

(*Collins et al, pp 19–20*)

272. If a medical insurance policy has a deductible of $50

A. the patient has to pay this amount

B. the patient may deduct this amount from the physician's bill

C. the patient does not have to pay the first $50 of service

D. the physician is reimbursed for $50 only

E. the patient is reimbursed for $50 only

(*Becklin and Sonnarborg, pp 177, 187; Fordney and Follis, pp 293, 304; Rowell, pp 25, 61*)

273. In a Worker's Compensation case, the medical assistant should

A. bill the patient for the deductible

B. file a bill with the insurance carrier every 2 weeks

C. send no bill to the patient

D. bill the patient for the unpaid portion

E. bill carrier in one lump sum

(*Frew et al, p 297; Kinn and Woods, p 332; Rowell, pp 399–400*)

274. To collect payment for a doctor's fee under Medicare, the medical assistant should send the claim form to the

A. head office of the fiscal agent

B. patient

C. Social Security Administration (SSA)

D. Internal Revenue Service (IRS)

E. State Welfare Agency

(*Fordney and Follis, p 311; Frew et al, pp 288–289; Kinn and Woods, pp 322, 336*)

275. The CPT-4 method of procedural coding became the procedural coding of choice when

A. the AMA promoted it

B. the Medicare program used it as the first level

C. the states adopted it

D. Blue Shield adopted it

E. the Food and Drug Administration adopted it

(*Frew et al, p 306; Rowell, p 26*)

276. Assuming a doctor actually charged for a given service in a year's time $28, $30, $32, $32, and $35, the usual fee would be
    A. $28
    B. $30
    C. $32
    D. $35
    E. an average
    (Becklin and Sonnarborg, p 177; Frew et al, p 311)

277. Insurance that provides weekly or monthly cash benefits to employed policyholders who become unable to work because of accident or illness is called
    A. special risk insurance
    B. loss of income protection or disability insurance
    C. personal accident insurance
    D. surgical insurance
    E. medical insurance
    (Becklin and Sonnarborg, p 158; Rowell, p 22)

278. Catastrophic coverage is referred to as
    A. major medical insurance
    B. hospital insurance
    C. medical insurance
    D. surgical insurance
    E. special risk insurance
    (Becklin and Sonnarborg, p 175; Kinn and Woods, p 305)

279. Blue Shield makes direct payment to
    A. physician members
    B. all physicians
    C. all policyholders
    D. whomever the patient specifies
    E. the hospital
    (Frew et al, p 301; Kinn and Woods, p 331; Rowell, pp 264–265)

280. Hospital insurance is included under Medicare
    A. in Part A
    B. in Part B
    C. only for those who are older than 70 years of age
    D. only for those who pay an additional premium
    E. for those who do not receive monthly Social Security benefits
    (Becklin and Sonnarborg, pp 186–187; Kinn and Woods, p 307; Rowell, p 294)

281. The insurance program authorizing treatment by civilian physicians at the expense of the government for dependents of military personnel is
    A. Foundation of Medical Care
    B. American Association of Foundations and Medical Care
    C. Medicaid
    D. CHAMPUS
    E. Medicare
    (Kinn and Woods, pp 309–310)

282. Part B of Medicare is
    A. voluntary
    B. compulsory
    C. automatically included with Part A
    D. free to the policyholder
    E. required for hospital benefits
    (Fordney and Follis, p 303; Frew et al, pp 288–289; Rowell, p 295)

283. When a new patient comes into an office and says he or she is covered by Medicare, the medical assistant should ask for an identification card. The card includes all the following information except
    A. name
    B. identification number
    C. whether hospital coverage is included
    D. whether medical coverage is included and effective date
    E. annual premium to be paid
    (Frew et al, p 289)

284. Patients may qualify for Medicaid depending on
    A. amount of Social Security being collected
    B. other insurance carried
    C. their income
    D. nature of illness or surgery
    E. whether they are covered by Medicare
    (Collins et al, pp 139–140; Frew et al, pp 291–294; Rowell, p 341)

285. Within the time limit set by the state after a physician has seen a Worker's Compensation patient for the first time, a report, Doctor's First Report of Occupational Injury or Illness, is typed. It should have
    A. two copies
    B. three copies
    C. at least four copies signed by the doctor
    D. two copies signed by the doctor
    E. four copies signed by the patient
    (Frew et al, p 297; Kinn and Woods, p 332; Rowell, pp 400–402)

286. A bill is never sent to the patient in which type of case?
    A. Medicare
    B. Worker's Compensation
    C. Blue Cross
    D. Blue Shield
    E. indemnity insurance plan
    (Frew et al, pp 297–300; Kinn and Woods, p 332; Rowell, pp 399–400)

287. In a severe or prolonged case involving Worker's Compensation, reports should be sent to the insurance carrier at least
    A. once a week
    B. once a month
    C. once a year
    D. quarterly
    E. twice a year
    (Kinn and Woods, p 332)

288. An insurance term used to describe the payment by an insurance company of a certain percentage of the actual expense (perhaps 75% to 80%), with the patient paying the remaining amount, is
    A. assignment of insurance benefits
    B. deductible
    C. insuring clause
    D. coinsurance
    E. income limit
    (Collins et al, pp 4–5; Kinn and Woods, p 303; Rowell, pp 25, 53)

289. Which one of the following helps insured persons when illness or accident results in wage loss?
    A. regular medical expense protection
    B. major medical expense protection
    C. disability income protection
    D. surgical expense protection
    E. hospital expense protection
    (Collins et al, p 176; Kinn and Woods, p 305; Rowell, pp 265–266)

290. The amount charged for a medical insurance policy is called a
    A. beneficiary
    B. claim
    C. fee schedule
    D. premium
    E. usual and customary (U&C) fee
    (Kinn and Woods, p 303; Rowell, pp 21–22)

291. Coordination of benefits is also known as
    A. preexisting conditions
    B. exclusions
    C. assignment of insurance benefits
    D. coinsurance
    E. nonduplication of benefits
    (Frew et al, p 290; Kinn and Woods, pp 303–304)

292. A standard form for both group and individual insurance claims, acceptable to almost all insurance companies, is referred to as
   A. 1490 form
   B. DA 1863-2 form
   C. Title XVIII form
   D. HCFA form 1500
   E. fee schedule
   (Frew et al, p 294; Kinn and Woods, p 327; Rowell, pp 26–27)

293. Provider-sponsored health insurance refers to plans developed by
   A. patients
   B. hospitals and physicians
   C. insurance companies
   D. government agencies
   E. religious organizations
   (Frew et al, p 301; Kinn and Woods, pp 306–307; Rowell, p 35)

294. Blue Cross offers which method of reimbursement?
   A. fee for service
   B. capitation
   C. closed panel
   D. salary
   E. indemnity method
   (Frew et al, pp 301–302; Kinn and Woods, p 331; Rowell, p 265)

295. Retrospective reimbursement whereby charges are made by the medical professional for each professional service rendered is also known as
   A. fee for service
   B. capitation
   C. closed panel
   D. salary
   E. indemnity method
   (Kinn and Woods, p 43; Rowell, p 29)

296. Reimbursement (payment) for medical services from the insurance carrier (company) is known as
   A. coordination of benefits
   B. indemnity
   C. assignment of benefits
   D. adjustment
   E. salary
   (Frew et al, p 892; Kinn and Woods, p 306)

297. Private patients are not accepted for treatment in the type of plan referred to as
   A. prepaid group practice
   B. Blue Cross
   C. Blue Shield
   D. indemnity plans
   E. fee for service
   (Frew et al, p 301; Kinn and Woods, p 304; Rowell, pp 33–34)

298. The Kaiser Foundation Health Plan is an example of
   A. a closed panel contract
   B. fee for service
   C. capitation
   D. Worker's Compensation
   E. an indirect type of service plan
   (Kinn and Woods, p 313)

299. Part A of Medicare does NOT pay for
   A. a bed in a semiprivate room
   B. private duty nurses
   C. physical, occupational, and speech therapy
   D. medical supplies, such as splints and casts
   E. medical social services
   (Rowell, pp 296–298)

300. Under the provisions of Part A of Medicare, there is a lifetime limit for care in a psychiatric hospital of
   A. 85 hospital benefit days
   B. 190 hospital benefit days
   C. 240 hospital benefit days
   D. 3 years
   E. 5 years
   (Rowell, p 296)

301. The number of benefit periods under Part A of Medicare is
    A. limited to 120 days
    B. limited to one per 6-month period
    C. limited to one per year
    D. limited to three per year
    E. unlimited
    (Rowell, p 296)

302. Part B of Medicare does NOT pay for
    A. medical and surgical services by a doctor of medicine
    B. medical and surgical services by a doctor of osteopathy
    C. drugs that cannot be self-administered
    D. hearing examinations for prescribing hearing aids
    E. limited services by chiropractors
    (Rowell, pp 298–299)

303. Under Part B of Medicare, reasonable charges are determined by the
    A. Social Security Administration
    B. insurance commissioner in each state
    C. Medicare carriers
    D. Health Insurance Council
    E. Public Health Service
    (Rowell, pp 303–304)

304. Overall responsibility for administration of the Medicare program rests with the
    A. Commissioner of Public Health
    B. Social Security Administration
    C. Director of Internal Revenue
    D. Health Care Financing Administration (HCFA)
    E. health commissioner in each state
    (Frew et al, p 88; Rowell, p 294)

305. Medicaid is financed by
    A. federal, state, and local taxes
    B. employer-contributed funds
    C. employee-contributed funds
    D. premiums paid by policyholders
    E. closed-panel contracts
    (Frew et al, pp 290–294; Kinn and Woods, p 304; Rowell, pp 341–342)

306. Which of the following statements about Worker's Compensation is FALSE?
    A. the Worker's Compensation law is the same in each state
    B. an employee may lose his or her rights to benefits if he or she does not accept medical attention offered in a Worker's Compensation case
    C. under the Worker's Compensation law, medical bills are paid if the injury suffered by the employee was caused by both accident and carelessness
    D. a physician's office should always have a supply of blank Worker's Compensation insurance forms
    E. bills for patients under the Worker's Compensation law are sent to the insurance carrier
    (Frew et al, p 297; Kinn and Woods, p 310)

307. The payment to the physician of a fixed sum per patient per month, regardless of the services rendered, is an application of
    A. fee for service
    B. closed-panel contract
    C. capitation
    D. salary method of payment
    E. provider-sponsored plan
    (Rowell, p 29)

308. Under many Blue Shield plans, patients entitled to "paid-in-full benefits," meaning there will be no additional charges, must go to
    A. participating physicians
    B. nonparticipating physicians
    C. specialists
    D. physicians listed by the Social Security Administration
    E. doctors associated with clinics
    (Rowell, pp 264–265, 306–307)

309. When a patient has insurance coverage under both CHAMPUS and a private or group health insurance policy, which is the primary carrier who pays first?
    A. CHAMPUS
    B. the private or group insurance carrier
    C. Medicare
    D. primary carrier is determined by birthdate
    E. none of these

    (Collins et al, p 191)

310. The medical program for needy persons is called
    A. Medicaid
    B. Medicare
    C. CHAMPUS
    D. Worker's Compensation
    E. indemnity insurance

    (Frew et al, p 291; Kinn and Woods, p 304; Rowell, pp 341, 346)

311. Which is the FIRST step in analyzing diagnoses and using the correct ICD code to file an insurance claim?
    A. find the diagnosis in the patient's chart
    B. locate the diagnosis in the ICD's alphabetical index
    C. find the code in the alphabetical index of the tabular list
    D. comb the subclassifications for the code that describes the patient's precise disease or condition
    E. type the ICD diagnostic code on the claim form and proofread for errors

    (Collins et al, p 50)

312. To compensate for dishonesty on the part of employees, physicians may purchase
    A. term insurance
    B. umbrella coverage
    C. fidelity insurance
    D. office overhead insurance
    E. Worker's Compensation insurance

    (Fordney, pp 39–40)

313. An assignment of benefits from the patient means that the insurance company will
    A. pay the patient directly
    B. pay the physician directly
    C. reimburse the patient for coinsurance requirements
    D. not pay for medical services
    E. not pay for hospital services

    (Frew et al, p 892; Rowell, p 496)

314. An individual or corporation that makes payment on an obligation or debt but is not a party to the contract that created the obligation or debt is known as a
    A. first-party payer
    B. second-party payer
    C. third-party payer
    D. fourth-party payer
    E. none of the above

    (Fordney and Follis, pp 295–296; Frew et al, p 248)

315. A federally funded third-party payer program that pays the medical bills of spouses and dependents of persons on active duty in the uniformed services is called
    A. Medicare
    B. Worker's Compensation
    C. CHAMPUS
    D. Medicaid
    E. CHAMPVA

    (Fordney and Follis, p 311; Frew et al, pp 294–295)

316. A third-party payer program jointly funded by the states and federal government to provide medical care to citizens on public assistance/welfare, Aid to Dependent Children programs is
    A. CHAMPVA
    B. CHAMPUS
    C. Worker's Compensation
    D. Medicare
    E. Medicaid

    (Frew et al, p 291; Fordney and Follis, p 302)

317. How often is the Physician's Current Procedural Terminology (CPT-4) published by the American Medical Association?
   A. every 3 months
   B. every 6 months
   C. once every year
   D. once every 2 years
   E. when deemed necessary
   (Collins et al, p 62)

318. The CPT-4 code book is divided into how many coding sections?
   A. three
   B. four
   C. five
   D. six
   E. seven
   (Collins et al, p 62)

319. In the *CPT 2000* manual, descriptors for the level of evaluation and management services include which of the following?
   A. history
   B. examination
   C. medical decision making
   D. nature of the presenting problem
   E. all of the above
   (CPT 2000, p 2)

320. In the *CPT 2000* manual, what modifiers are available in E/M (evaluation and management)?
   A. prolonged E/M services
   B. unrelated E/M services by the same physician during a postoperative period
   C. significant separately identifiable E/M services by the same physician on the same day of a procedure or other service
   D. reduced services
   E. all of the above
   (CPT 2000, p 3)

321. In the *CPT 2000* manual, the services listed at the time of wound repair should include
   A. the size of the wound in centimeters
   B. the shape of the wound (i.e., curved, angular, or stellate)
   C. if the wound was debrided because of gross contamination
   D. if nerves, blood vessels, or tendons were involved
   E. all of the above
   (CPT 2000, pp 57–58)

322. What are the primary classes of main terms in the *CPT 2000* index?
   A. procedure or service
   B. organ or other anatomic site
   C. condition (i.e., abscess, entropion)
   D. synonyms, eponyms, and abbreviations
   E. all of the above
   (CPT 2000, p 459)

323. A summary of additions, deletions, and revisions of CPT codes can be found in
   A. Appendix A
   B. Appendix B
   C. Appendix C
   D. index
   E. Introduction
   (CPT 2000, p 409, Appendix B)

324. The CPT-4 coding system uses a main number to describe particular services. This main number uses a base of
   A. three digits
   B. four digits
   C. five digits
   D. six digits
   E. seven digits
   (Rowell, p 115)

325. How many levels are used in the Health Care Financing Administration, Common Procedure Coding System (HCPCS)?
    A. one
    B. two
    C. three
    D. four
    E. five
    (Rowell, p 112)

326. What coding classification is used to identify diseases and code diagnoses on medical insurance claims?
    A. CPT-4
    B. ICD-9-CM
    C. HCPCS
    D. HCFA
    E. NCHS
    (Frew et al, p 306; Rowell, pp 68–69)

327. Which of the following incidents, if performed by a medical assistant, may be considered fraud or insurance abuse?
    A. putting different diagnoses on the insurance claim and patient's chart
    B. adding additional treatments to the insurance claim not listed on the patient's chart or ledger
    C. raising the fee for insurance coverage only
    D. altering the date of patient treatment on patient's insurance claim and account
    E. all of the above
    (Frew et al, pp 314–315; Rowell, pp 16–17)

328. Prior authorization by the insurance company that must be obtained before admitting a patient into the hospital is called
    A. precertification
    B. patient status
    C. a deductible
    D. preexisting condition
    E. none of the above
    (Keir et al, p 114)

329. The diagnostic-related groups (DRGs) are divided by body systems into 470 groups. What purposes does the DRG system serve?
    A. a revised Health Care Financing Administration code
    B. a substitute for CPT coding
    C. a substitute for ICD-9 classification
    D. strict guidelines for hospital admissions and stays
    E. none of the above
    (Keir et al, p 336)

330. A claims inquiry (tracer) is made for what reason?
    A. payment is not received within the time limit
    B. carrier may still be investigating the claim
    C. amount of payment was incorrect
    D. payment was made for the wrong person
    E. all of the above
    (Fordney, p 187)

331. If an insurance claim has been denied by a private insurance company and the physician believes it is unfair, what recourse does he or she have?

    A. report it to the AMA
    B. contact the Medicare program
    C. contact the CHAMPUS program
    D. begin a review and appeal process
    E. begin a lawsuit

    (Fordney, pp 187–188)

332. A Relative Value Scale (RVS) adapted for the Health Care Financing Administration (HCFA) that is the basis for the Medicare fee schedule is known as

    A. current procedural terminology
    B. resource-based RVS
    C. the insurance claims registry
    D. all of the above
    E. none of the above

    (Fordney, pp 300–306; Fordney and Follis, pp 304–305)

333. An insurance specialist coded a patient's diagnosis of acute appendicitis with the number 540.9. What system of coding was she using?

    A. CPT-4
    B. HCPCS
    C. CHAMP
    D. Medicaid
    E. ICD-9

    (Keir et al, pp 181–182)

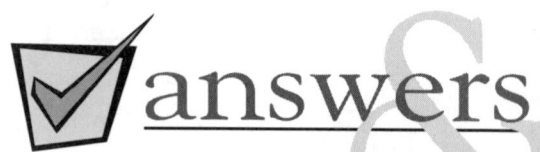

answers & rationales

262.

A. A physician's usual fee is the charge he or she makes to private patients. The customary fee is the range of charges made by the majority of physicians practicing in the same geographic and socioeconomic area who have similar training and experience.

263.

B. Patients who become members of an HMO (Health Maintenance Organization) do not have the freedom to choose their physician and still receive the benefits of the HMO. They are restricted to physicians who are members of the chosen HMO. All the other answer selections are the rights of all patients.

Health organizations that provide protection against illness and loss of related income manage cost containment and receive compensation in different ways. Among the *managed-care* types are HMOs, preferred provider organizations (PPOs), and independent practice associations (IPAs).

The increasingly common HMOs place their priority on maintaining health with preventive medicine and thereby containing costs. Their physicians are often salaried or receive fixed sums. Patients pay a set periodic amount. The HMO's compensation for health care is limited to physicians inside the HMO.

The PPOs contract with physicians, hospitals, and other providers to accept lowered fees in exchange for membership in the network. Blue Cross/Blue Shield is an example of a PPO.

The IPA is an HMO where the physicians are self-employed in their own offices and receive fees from the program on a per-patient basis. The amount of money received depends on the number of patients seen.

The traditional *indemnity plans* include medical insurance companies that paid most of a medical bill and compensated physicians on a fee-for-service basis. Their cost-containment practices include second opinions before surgery, precertification for hospital admission for nonemergency services, shorter hospital stays, and outpatient surgeries where possible.

264.

E. The fee profile of an individual doctor for Medicare and other insurance programs is established by the continuous list that he or she submits of the usual (most frequent) charge for a specific service. The customary fee is the range of usual fees charged by doctors in the same locality.

265.

C. An insurance company that pays a U&C fee would pay Dr. Schuyler $38 because his fee falls within the range established by other doctors with the same specialty and in the same locality.

266.

D. The insurance company in this situation would pay Dr. Schuyler $36, the upper limit of the range of fees charged by other physicians with similar training and experience in the same community.

267.

E. Medicare forms must be signed by both the patient and the physician. Forms that are not signed by both parties will not be processed. It is not legal for the medical assistant to sign the physician's name.

268.

D. Medicare pays 80% of the reasonable physician's charge after subtracting a deductible. The patient must pay the remaining 20% as well as the deductible amount to the physician.

269.

E. Common reasons for the return of insurance claim forms to the physician's office are missing procedure codes or missing diagnostic code numbers. Any number of typographical or incorrect errors may also cause the return of a claim. The name of the patient may be incorrect or incomplete (no nicknames allowed), or the policy identification number may be incorrect. The following will also cause a delay in processing: the current diagnosis is missing because of failure to change the default diagnosis in the computer program, missing fourth or fifth digits of the ICD code, missing treatment dates, missing hospital admission or discharge dates, missing required prior authorization numbers, staples in the bar code area, failure to print on proper lines of the form, and attachments that do not have the patient and policy identification on each page.

An insurance claims register (diary) should be maintained so that the status of insurance claims submissions is known and inquiries can be made to the appropriate parties when questions arise. Thirty days is the usual time to wait until inquiries are made into why the insurance company has not responded. After the 30-day period, there is a choice of billing again, calling the field representative of the company, or sending a tracer (a memo containing the basic billing information).

There are a number of reasons to inquire about an insurance claim form: a denial of payment that is not understood, the payment amount is incorrect, you do not recognize the payee (he or she may be the policy-holder for a patient), or you do not receive a breakdown showing for how much the patient is still responsible.

There are also a number of reasons to rebill an insurance claim.

270.

B. Copies of Medicare forms may be obtained from the fiscal agents for Medicare, which are listed in the Medicare Fiscal Agents or Carrier Directory. The claims form, known as HCFA-1500 (1-84) in the Medicare program and Champus-501 in the CHAMPUS program, is a universal claims form accepted by most insurance companies on the majority of claims.

271.

A. The office medical insurance specialist will not attempt to predict how much an insurance company will pay on a patient's policy because there is no way to review the insurance policy and the many variables connected, such as cancellations, restrictive clauses, previous billing, and so on. Although the individual clinic managers and physicians determine the job description of each insurance specialist, the same basic tasks are generally performed. The medical assistant who has the position of a medical insurance specialist performs the following tasks: (1) gathers information and signatures, (2) submits the insurance claims to the insurance companies, (3) reviews insurance payments when they arrive, and (4) assists clients.

Information gathering includes the following: (1) obtaining personal and insurance information on the patient information form in the patient's chart; (2) obtaining and using the right forms to file the insurance; (3) gathering the appropriate signatures for release of information and assignment of benefits; and (4) collecting the diagnosis, treatment, and charges from the patient service slip.

Submitting the insurance claims form to the insurance company includes (1) finding and recording the correct diagnosis (ICD-CM codes) and procedure (CPT codes); (2) filling out the insurance claim form and photocopying and filing a copy in the patient's chart; and (3) logging a diary of the form into the insurance logbook for future reference. The completed insurance claim then is submitted to the correct insurance company and address by mail or by electronic claims transmission through the modem of a computer.

Reviewing insurance payments includes the duties of (1) reviewing the EOB (explanation of benefits) and making sure the insurance company has considered all charges and has not made an error, (2) requesting reviews by the insurance company when errors appear to have been made, (3) recording the check amount or rejection of the claim in the insurance log next to the submission entry, and (4) making sure the payment is credited to the patient's account. If additional forms should be submitted with more information or physician reports, work with the physician or office staff to accomplish this.

Helping clients with insurance claims includes answering clients' questions about insurance reimbursement and assisting clients with insurance problems.

272.

A. If a medical insurance policy has a deductible of $50, the patient has to pay this amount. Once the deductible has been paid in a calendar year, the insurance company will begin to pay either all or, in many cases, 80% of the charges from that point on. The insurance company will keep a running total of the patient's charges until the deductible is met. The medical assistant who files the insurance will not know whether the patient has met his or her deductible until the explanation of benefits (EOB) is received (along with a check if the deductible has been met).

273.

C. The patient is not billed for any unpaid portion of the account. There is no deductible; the physician agrees to accept the compensation carrier's approved fees for services as payment in full. Carefully itemized and coded bills should be filed with the compensation carrier every 30 days until the bill is paid.

Worker's Compensation insurance programs that compensate medical costs, lost wages, and disability benefits for work-related injury or illness are different for individual states. In addition, the federal government has a separate program for its civilian employees. Some general types of information needed for filing these forms are as follows: become familiar with the regulations in your state and with which forms and records are needed; learn which agencies (with addresses) receive the claim forms; review reimbursement and billing regulations; become familiar with filing deadlines; and find out whether the employee can choose his or her physician.

Medical reports for injured employees generally contain the following: dates of exam and treatment, patient's history as given to physician, physician's account of his or her findings, x-ray and diagnostic test results, diagnosis, clinical treatment, and physician's explanation of relationship between injury or illness and work environment.

274.

A. To collect payment for a doctor's fee under Medicare—a federal program for people who are 65 or older and some disabled persons—the medical assistant should send the claim form to the head office of the fiscal agent, which is an intermediary for the federal government. These are listed in the Medicare fiscal agents and carrier directory, which is available from the local Social Security Administration.

275.

B. The CPT-4 coding system came to the forefront when the federal government designated the Health Care Financing Administration Common Procedure Coding System (HCPCS), with three levels of codes as the official Medicare code. The CPT codes and modifiers previously developed by the AMA comprised the first level. The HCFA-designated codes were the second level, and the third level contains codes of individual insurance companies.

276.

C. The usual fee would be $32 because a usual fee is the fee that is most frequently charged by a particular doctor for a service. The customary fee is the range of fees charged by physicians in the same area with similar training and experience. The term reasonable fee applies to difficult procedures that require extra time and effort by the physician.

277.

B. Loss of income protection is insurance that provides weekly or monthly cash benefits to employed policyholders who become unable to work because of accident or illness. This type of insurance is not intended for payment of specific medical bills.

278.

A. Major medical insurance is sometimes referred to as "catastrophic" coverage. It provides protection against very expensive medical bills for prolonged catastrophic illnesses. It may be separate or combined with a basic medical protection plan.

279.

A. Blue Shield makes direct payment to physician members, but payment is made to the subscriber (patient) if the physician is a nonmember. Blue Cross/Blue Shield plans are nonprofit PPOs, widely available to individuals and small groups, who contract with health care providers. They determine physician payments by using three fee categories: (1) usual, customary, and reasonable fees; (2) customary maximums based on charges by most physicians in a community; and (3) fixed fee schedules (a list of maximum fees for specific services). Individual members carry an identification card from which the medical assistant should gather this information for filing a claim: subscriber's name, certificate number, group name and number, and name of the area Blue Cross/Blue Shield that handles contract.

280.

A. Hospital insurance is included under Part A of Medicare as well as care in a skilled nursing facility, home health care, and hospice care. Part A of Medicare automatically enrolls any person receiving monthly Social Security or railroad retirement. There is no charge for this insurance.

Medicare also has a Part B, which is optional and has a deductible. It must be paid for through premiums. Part B helps pay physician services, outpatient hospital services, durable medical equipment, and other services and supplies. The patient's Medicare card should show if the patient is enrolled in Part B.

Medigap policies are written by private insurance companies to fill in the "gaps" in Medicare coverage. These generally pay the Medicare deductible and coinsurance, and some cover services that Medicare does not cover. If a patient has *Medigap*, the primary payer is *Medicare*. The claim is filed with Medicare first.

281.

D. CHAMPUS is the insurance program authorizing treatment of military personnel's dependents by civilian physicians at the expense of the government. CHAMPVA shares health costs for dependents and survivors of veterans with 100% service-connected disabilities. CHAMPUS stands for Civilian Health and Medical Program of the Uniformed Services.

282.

A. Part B of Medicare is voluntary, and the insured person must apply for coverage within a specified period and pay a monthly premium.

283.

E. The identification card for Medicare patients includes the name of the beneficiary, claim number, sex, whether hospital or medical insurance (or both), effective date of coverage, and signature of the insured. The cost of the annual premium is not included.

284.

C. Medicaid is a medical care program for people of all ages who cannot pay their medical bills and who meet certain low-income requirements. Medicaid is paid by both the state and federal government and regulations vary from state to state. A physician chooses whether to participate in the total Medicaid program and accepts their fees as total payment if he or she participates. However, he or she also bills for services not covered under the program. Four areas the medical assistant should pay special attention to when filing Medicaid claims are (1) eligibility, which can vary with income; (2) preauthorization for specific services; (3) filing deadlines; and (4) third-party liability (Medicare is the secondary carrier when other insurance or coverage is available).

285.

C. Within the time limit set by the state, after a physician has seen a Worker's Compensation patient for the first time, a report, Doctor's First Report of Occupational Injury or Illness, is typed with at least four copies. (First, however, the patient must report the injury to the employer before seeking medical care. The medical assistant should check to see that this was done.) One copy of the doctor's report is forwarded to the insurance carrier, one to the patient's employer, one to the state Worker's Compensation Board, and one is retained in the physician's file. The Worker's Compensation file on the patient is kept separate from any other information on the patient that the clinic may have on treatment unrelated to the Worker's Compensation injury.

286.

B. A bill is never sent to the patient in a Worker's Compensation case. When treatment is terminated, a final report and bill are sent to the insurance carrier. The physician accepting Worker's Compensation cases agrees that the insurance company's approved fees are payment in full.

287.

B. In a severe or prolonged case involving Worker's Compensation, reports should be sent to the insurance carrier at least once a month.

288.

D. Coinsurance is a term used to describe the payment by an insurance company of a certain percentage of the actual expense (75% to 80%), with the patient paying the remaining amount. A deductible is the amount the patient must pay *before* the insurance payment begins. This and other terms often appear in the EOB (explanation of benefits) statement sent with the insurance payment.

Other terms needed to understand the EOB are as follows: *allowable charge* (maximum amount insurer allows); *deductible* (amount patient must pay first); and *disallowed, nonallowed,* or *"not eligible for payment"* (the difference between payment and what the physician charged for the service). Allowable charges are often based on the usual, customary, and reasonable (UCR) payment, which is an amount the insurance company determines.

289.

C. Disability income protection does not help insured persons to pay hospital and physician bills, but it does provide workers with regular weekly or monthly cash payments in the event that wages are cut off as a result of accident or illness.

290.

D. The amount charged for a medical insurance policy is called a premium. The insurer agrees to provide certain benefits in return for the premium. The real cost of medical care to an individual is the insurance premium plus deductibles, co-payments, and medical expenses not covered.

291.

E. Coordination of benefits is also known as nonduplication of benefits. The provision in many group plans prevents the available benefits from exceeding the covered medical expenses. In the case in which a child is covered by both parents' insurance policies, a primary carrier is designated (generally the father's insurance or the one whose birthday is first in the year) to pay the full benefits.

292.

D. HCFA Form 1500 is accepted by most insurance companies, states, and the federal government. The Health Care Financing Administration (HCFA) administers Medicare.

293.

B. Provider-sponsored health insurance, such as Blue Cross/Blue Shield, is developed by hospitals and physicians. The "providers" in this case are the providers of health care. There are also private insurance company plans and health maintenance organizations (HMOs). HMOs employ both physicians on a salary and independent physicians' associations.

294.

A. Blue Cross (and Blue Shield) is referred to as a fee-for-service type of plan. The plan pays the care providers for each service rendered to the member patient. Blue Cross/Blue Shield also is a provider-sponsored insurance plan.

295.

A. Retrospective reimbursement, or fee for service, is the billing method of physicians in private practice. This includes Blue Shield insurance plans, as well as many other private insurance plans.

296.

B. Indemnity is the payment or reimbursement from the insurance carrier for medical services provided the insured patient. Assignment of benefits by the patient permits payment of the indemnity directly to the doctor.

Coordination of benefits is the sharing of costs between the *primary carrier,* who pays benefits according to its contract, and the *secondary carrier,* who pays the rest of the covered charges. This prevents overpayment of benefits beyond the cost of the medical service.

297.

A. Specified health services are rendered to an enrolled group of persons by the physician. The structure of prepaid group practices varies. In some, the physicians form an independent group, whereas in others, the physicians are paid a salary by the health plan. They are also known as health maintenance organizations (HMOs).

298.

A. The Kaiser Foundation Health Plan is an example of the closed-panel or salary contract, a type of prepaid group practice model (or HMO). Kaiser Foundation was a pioneer of prepaid group practice beginning in California in 1933.

299.

B. Part A of Medicare, which pays hospital costs, does not pay for some additional expenses such as private duty nurses, personal comfort or convenience items, extra charges for use of a private room unless needed for medical reasons, noncovered levels of care, and doctors' services.

300.

B. Under the provisions of Part A of Medicare, there is a lifetime limit for care in a psychiatric hospital of 190 hospital benefit days. Other hospitalizations under Part A of Medicare are covered by benefit periods, and the patient pays a deductible for each period.

301.

E. The number of benefit periods under Part A of Medicare is unlimited. However, hospice care for terminally ill patients has special limited benefit periods.

302.

D. Part B of Medicare does not pay for hearing examinations for prescribing hearing aids or for fitting or changing hearing aids. There also are other exclusions.

303.

C. "Reasonable charges" is the approved charge determined by Medicare insurance carriers under Part B of Medicare. The Medicare "reasonable charge" that the insurance carrier approves will be the lowest of the three: the customary charge (the amount the physician most frequently charges), the prevailing charge (based on all customary charges in a locality), or the actual charge. The customary charge is the charge most frequently made for the service in the previous calendar year by the physician; the prevailing charge is determined by the carrier.

304.

D. The Health Care Financing Administration (HCFA) of the federal government administers the Medicare program. Application for benefits must be made by eligible persons. The local Social Security Administration offices will take applications and provide information about Medicare.

305.

A. Medicaid is financed by federal, state, and local taxes. Benefits and coverage vary from state to state. It provides medical care for those on public assistance and certain other low-income people.

306.

A. Each state has its own individual regulations concerning Worker's Compensation insurance, which insures workers against the cost of on-the-job injury. Federal law requires that states meet minimum standards regarding Worker's Compensation insurance. The employer pays the premium.

307.

C. Capitation is a payment plan used by some HMOs whereby a fixed sum is paid for each patient or participant regardless of the amount of service rendered. This contrasts with the salary some physicians receive as HMO employees and the fee-for-service payment of Blue Cross/Blue Shield.

308.

A. Under many Blue Shield plans, the participating physicians agree to accept Blue Shield's payment as payment in full for services. However, if the patient goes to a nonparticipating physician, this may not be true, since the physician is not obligated to accept these terms.

309.

B. The other health insurance carrier pays before CHAMPUS if it is a private health insurance carrier. However, CHAMPUS pays first if the other insurance is Medicaid or insurance designed to supplement CHAMPUS. CHAMPUS provides hospital and medical services for dependents of service persons, retired service persons and their dependents, and dependents of service persons who died in active duty.

310.

A. Medicaid is the medical assistance program for the medically indigent. (The term indigent means needy or lacking.) A Medicaid identification card is issued to the beneficiary showing the dates of coverage and should always be checked if the patient indicates he or she is covered. Benefits and restrictions vary from state to state.

311.

A. The first step to filling in the diagnostic (ICD-9-CM) code of an insurance claim form is to locate the diagnosis (or diagnoses if more than one) in the patient's chart. The diagnostic code is the number assigned to a diagnosis in the International Classification of Diseases book(s). The other steps are looking up the diagnosis and corresponding code in the alphabetic index in the ICD, finding the number code in the tabular list in the ICD for the diagnosis you located in the alphabetic index, combing the subclassifications of number codes in the tabular list to get the exact code numbers for the precise disease or condition, and filling in the ICD numbers of the diagnostic code on the correct line of the claims form. Then proofread the insurance claim form for accuracy.

312.

C. To compensate for employee dishonesty, a physician might purchase, as insurance, either individual fidelity bonds or a blanket fidelity bond for all employees in the event of embezzlement. (Fidelity is a word for loyalty.) The insurance company selling the fidelity or honesty bonds will prosecute any guilty employees. Bonding also means that the physician will be paid a fixed sum of money if a financial loss is due to an employee embezzling funds or certain other contingencies. A medical assistant who files insurance claims should always initial the bottom of the claims so that the work can be identified. It is also wise to insist on precise bookkeeping and record keeping with numbered encounter forms, transaction slips, and cash receipts. It is imperative that forms be numbered if a physician's signature stamp is used so that the claims can be traced.

313.

B. An assignment of benefits form usually attached to the insurance claims form states that the payment is to be made to the physician. It is dated and signed by the patient.

314.

C. An individual or corporation that makes payment on an obligation or debt but is not a party to the contract that created the obligation or debt is known as a third-party payer. A medical insurance company that pays a policy holder's medical bills is a third-party payer. Most medical bills paid in medical offices today are paid by third-party payers. There are also other types of third-party payers such as relatives that agree to the original contract.

315.

C. CHAMPUS is a federally funded third-party payer medical insurance for spouses and dependents of persons on active duty in the uniformed services. This includes the Armed Forces, Public Health Service, Oceanic and Atmosphere Administration, and the North Atlantic Treaty Organization (NATO). Retired personnel from these services as well as their spouses and dependents are covered by CHAMPUS. CHAMPVA is a federally funded third-party payer for spouses and dependents of veterans with total service-connected disabilities or who died as a result of service-connected disabilities.

316.

E. Medicaid is a program that provides medical care to individuals who are on public assistance (welfare), Aid to Dependent Children program, and to certain other medically needy individuals who meet the states' special requirements. Medicaid is funded jointly by the state and the federal government. Medicare is a federally funded program for persons older than the age of 65 who are retired on Social Security, Federal Civil Service, or Railroad Retirement. The program also covers their spouses older than the age of 62, persons who qualify for the federal disability program, the End-Stage Renal Disease program, and persons older than the age of 65 on Medicaid.

317.

C. The CPT-4 coding book is published yearly and released every December. Each new volume contains many changes in the narrative description of existing codes as well as the addition of new codes to the system. Medical offices should not use outdated CPT-4 volumes. Outdated volumes may result in rejected insurance claims and, therefore, be more costly than a new CPT-4 volume. Source documents and computer code files should be updated.

318.

D. The CPT coding book is divided into six coding sections. Each section has its own set of guidelines at the beginning of the section. The six main sections in the CPT book appear in the following order: (1) evaluation and management, (2) anesthesia, (3) surgery, (4) radiology, (5) nuclear medicine and diagnostic ultrasound, and (6) pathology and laboratory medicine.

319.

E. The *CPT 2000* manual lists and explains the seven descriptors used to determine the levels of evaluation and management services. The key components are history, examination, and medical decision making. The next three components, counseling, coordination of care, and the nature of the presenting problem, are contributory factors. Time is the final component.

320.

E. All of the listed answer choices are modifiers that are available in E/M (Evaluation and Management). The modifiers can be reported by adding a hyphen and the two-digit number identifier, or they can be listed by a separate five-digit code in addition to the procedure number.

321.

E. Detailed instructions are given in *CPT 2000* for reporting the services listed at the time of wound repair. They include the size of the wound—length and shape; the length of multiple wounds and which to report as the primary or secondary procedure with a modifier; decontamination or debridement and how to report the procedure; involvement of nerves, blood vessels, and tendons; and systems to report under and modifiers to use.

322.

E. All of the above listed answer choices are main terms in the CPT index: procedure or service (e.g., endoscopy, anastomosis, splint); organ or other anatomic site (e.g., tibia, color, salivary gland); condition (e.g., abscess, entropion, tetralogy of Fallot); synonyms, eponyms, and abbreviations (e.g., Brickler operation, Clagett procedure). Page 459 of the *CPT 2000* provides instructions for the use of the CPT index.

323.

B. A summary of additions, deletions, and revisions of CPT codes are found in Appendix B, page 409, of *CPT 2000*. For instance, the code 00520 has had its terminology revised since the previous publication.

324.

C. The CPT-4 coding system is based on a five-digit main number. A two-digit modifier may be added after the five-digit main number. This additional number is used when it is necessary to indicate that the service performed deviated from the average service for that specific code number. Each modifier is used to describe a specific variation from the normal service.

325.

C. The HCPCS (Health Care Financing Administration Common Procedural Coding System), with three levels, is a national system of uniform coding for reporting health care services to the Medicare program. HCPCS is a trilevel system. Level one codes represent existing CPT-4 codes. Level two codes are new nationwide codes that augment CPT-4. Level two codes allow for more definitive reporting of physician services, such as the injections of specific medication. The level three codes are generally used by each regional Medicare fiscal intermediary. A fiscal intermediary is a large private insurance company that has been awarded a federal contract for processing the claims for programs, such as Medicare, that are administered by the federal government.

326.

B. ICD-9-CM (*International Classification of Diseases*, 9th edition, Clinical Modification) has been used since 1979 for all coding of diagnoses in the United States. This system (ICD-9-CM) distinguishes the coding of diagnoses from the coding of the physician's services (CPT-4). However, the diagnosis (ICD-9-CM) must agree with the physician's services (CPT-4), which was rendered to treat the disease. Otherwise, the insurance company will reject the claim because the two sets of codes are inconsistent.

327.

E. The medical assistant would become a party to fraud or insurance abuse if he or she participated in any of these incidents listed. Fraud is defined by the Medicare and Medicaid Anti-Fraud and Abuse Act of 1977 as an intentional misrepresentation or concealment of facts. This same act defines insurance abuse as incidents or misrepresentations that do not fall into the fraud classification but are considered to be inconsistent with acceptable practice of medicine. These lead to improper reimbursement, treatments that are not medically necessary for the disorder, or procedures that are considered to be harmful or of poor quality.

The medical assistant, as well as the physician, can be prosecuted for insurance fraud or abuse.

328.

A. Precertification is the process of notifying insurance companies of pending hospitalization and receiving their approval before the actual hospitalization. Without prior review and approval by the insurance company, the claim will be denied for nonemergency hospitalization. This practice began in an effort to hold down costs by preventing unnecessary hospitalizations.

329.

D. DRGs (diagnosis-related groups) used by Medicare provide guidelines for physicians regarding hospital admission and the length of the hospital stay. The system attempts to standardize payment for medical care by making a lump sum payment for individuals within the same DRG regardless of the actual cost to the health care facility.

The DRG worksheet supplied by the hospital is often used in clinics to assist in completing medical records for patients.

330.

E. All of the reasons listed—no payment, incorrect payment, payment to the wrong person, or insufficient explanation of benefits—may be cause for the medical assistant to make a claims inquiry. The insurance carrier may be contacted by writing (include all necessary forms) or by telephone. If you phone, document the name of the insurance representative contacted and details of the conversation.

331.

D. If an appeal for payment has been made and no satisfactory agreement was reached, then the physician may proceed with a peer review of the claim. The explanation of benefits furnished by the insurance company will give the time limits for appealing. A peer review by unbiased physicians will evaluate the claim and decide on the payment. When the review is in progress, the insurance specialist should keep a record of the claim's progress.

If the appeal is for CHAMPUS, Medicaid, Medicare, or Worker's Compensation claims, the insurance carriers for those programs should be contacted for the necessary forms and procedures to follow.

332.

B. Medicare's Resource-Based Relative Value Scale (RBRVS) became the basis for the Medicare fee schedule for nonsurgeons for evaluation and management of patients. It is based on several factors such as the total work required for a service and cost of the physician's practice and liability insurance. The RBRVS was based on earlier RVS (relative value studies) charges made by physicians.

333.

E. The insurance specialist is using the ICD-9 (International Classification of Diseases) coding system, which is used to report diagnoses. ICD-9 uses a base of three to five digits, depending on the level of specification (third, fourth or fifth, with five being the highest). Any diagnosis that affects the care, is a reason for treatment, or influences the health status of the patient should be coded.

8 Computers and Office Machines

chapter objectives

Major areas of knowledge/content included in this chapter are:

I. Understanding computer components
➤   input devices
➤   central processing unit
➤   output devices
➤   storage capacity and backup of records
➤   transmission devices
➤   software programs and basic commands to control computer

II. Maintenance
➤   care of computers
➤   maintenance agreements

III. Security precautions to safeguard medical information
➤   passwords, identification devices, and work with barriers

IV. Computer applications and medical management software
➤   menus
➤   new patient entries
➤   practice information
➤   insurance billing

V. Other office machines

DIRECTIONS (Questions 334 through 382): Each of the numbered items or incomplete statements in this section is followed by answers or by completions of the statement. Select the ONE lettered answer or completion that is BEST in each case.

334. The most difficult part of learning a computer applications program is
   A. learning the commands
   B. number alignment
   C. information retrieval
   D. corrections
   E. editing

   (Kinn and Woods, p 186)

335. The "roadmap" and most important component of a computer system is the
   A. mainframe
   B. on-line system
   C. peripheral accessories
   D. software
   E. central processing unit (CPU)

   (Baptist et al, p 25; Kinn and Woods, p 183)

336. Which of the following functions is performed with computer software in the physician's office?
   A. processing insurance claims
   B. accounting processes
   C. checking spelling of documents
   D. typing form letters
   E. all of the above

   (Gylys, p 2)

337. Before purchasing a computer or other office machine, which of the following should be analyzed?
   A. training needed
   B. ease and speed of operation
   C. cost
   D. office procedures modified by the machine
   E. all of the above

   (Keir et al, p 73)

338. The detailed instructions that tell the computer what to do are called the
   A. mainframe
   B. on-line system
   C. peripheral accessories
   D. software
   E. central processing unit (CPU)

   (Baptist et al, p 25)

339. To protect against loss of information processed on a computer, the medical assistant should
   A. make back-up copies
   B. format a disk
   C. learn the program commands
   D. debug the program
   E. use electronic mail

   (Baptist et al, pp 37–38)

340. When insurance claim information is transferred directly from the medical practice's computer over a telephone line to an insurance carrier, it is known as
   A. electronic claims submission
   B. information retrieval
   C. kilobytes
   D. read-only memory
   E. data processing

   (Bonewit-West #2, pp 255–256)

341. To prepare a floppy disk to receive information from the computer's operating system, it must be
   A. booted
   B. debugged
   C. cataloged
   D. initialized (formatted)
   E. saved

   (Bonewit-West #2, pp 74–76; Gylys, p 8)

342. In the word processor program, the typed material is corrected with the
    A. daisy wheel
    B. cursor, back space, and delete buttons
    C. monitor
    D. wraparound function
    E. clear button
    (Bonewit-West #2, p 88)

343. Moving through the information in a document, either horizontally or vertically, is known as
    A. scrolling
    B. editing
    C. booting
    D. filing
    E. processing
    (Bonewit-West #2, pp 88–89)

344. The patient's bill whether prepared by the computer or manually is always mailed to the
    A. patient
    B. employer
    C. guarantor
    D. caregiver
    E. none of the above
    (Bonewit-West #2, p 240)

345. A list of computer program functions that provides a way to move from one part of the program to another is a
    A. computer application
    B. menu
    C. transaction
    D. file maintenance
    E. report
    (Bonewit-West #2, p 120)

346. Software programs that are designed especially for the front office in medical clinics are known as
    A. medical office management software programs
    B. patient registration systems
    C. appointment systems
    D. multi-user computer systems
    E. database management
    (Bonewit-West #2, p 120)

347. A computer system that allows people in different offices to work on different tasks at the same time is known as a/an
    A. data field
    B. menu-driven program
    C. networked system
    D. numeric field
    E. all of the above
    (Baptist et al, pp 9–10; Bonewit-West #2, p 106)

348. What distinguishes a numeric field in a computer program?
    A. it accepts only numbers
    B. it is a date-only field
    C. it performs calculations
    D. it is the sum of other numbers
    E. it is performed with the numeric keyboard
    (Bonewit-West #2, p 124)

349. How is the numeric keypad activated on the IBM PC?
    A. press the number lock key
    B. press enter
    C. go to arithmetic-logic unit
    D. activate the function keys
    E. none of the above
    (Gylys #2, p 4)

350. The computer application most used in medical front office accounting is
    A. word processing
    B. a spreadsheet
    C. communications
    D. database management
    E. none of the above
    (Bonewit-West #2, p 112)

351. The computer program application that contains fields, records, and files is known as
    A. word processing
    B. a spreadsheet
    C. a database
    D. communications
    E. electronic claims submission
    (Bonewit-West #2, pp 113–117)

352. The computer application used to enter and edit text, and type letters and medical histories is
    A. word processing
    B. electronic mail
    C. a database
    D. a spreadsheet
    E. a modem
    (Baptist et al, p 6; Bonewit-West #2, pp 85–91, 112)

353. A multi-user/multitask computer system would always have these components
    A. electronic claims submission
    B. claim summary report
    C. multiple terminals
    D. line feed control
    E. tractor feed
    (Bonewit-West #2, p 106)

354. The various reports generated by the computer for the medical office are accessed from the
    A. word-processing program
    B. medical practice database
    C. file maintenance system
    D. patient registration system
    E. none of the above
    (Bonewit-West #2, p 106)

355. To prevent unauthorized computer access to confidential patient and financial records the staff must
    A. keep the computer terminal locations secret
    B. lock the computer at night
    C. assign each user a password
    D. limit computer use to one person
    E. none of the above
    (Bonewit-West #2, pp 151, 153)

356. Documentation for a computer medical management program does NOT include
    A. program user manuals
    B. on-line help screen
    C. reference cards
    D. manufacturer's support
    E. file names
    (Bonewit-West #2, pp 97, 103, 105)

357. The source document placed on the patient's chart by the receptionist and used to post charges for payment at time of service is known as a/an
    A. route slip
    B. encounter form
    C. charge slip
    D. superbill
    E. all of the above
    (Bonewit-West #2, p 218; Gylys, pp 151–152)

358. The computer patient registration system should allow access to
    A. demographic information
    B. insurance information
    C. financial records
    D. appointments
    E. all of the above
    (Bonewit-West #2, p 105)

359. A set of commands organized into a step-by-step sequence to guide the computer in performing a task is a
    A. database
    B. program
    C. processor
    D. keyboard
    E. numeric field
    (Bonewit-West #2, pp 5, 8)

360. The main menu of a medical office management program would list
    A. specific tasks
    B. the alphanumeric field
    C. a source document
    D. text formatting
    E. the program's systems
    (Bonewit-West #2, p 121)

361. Which of the following start-up tasks in the file maintenance system are required when a medical computer program is installed?
    A. medical practice identification
    B. user passwords
    C. physician's ID number
    D. insurance carriers
    E. all of these
    (Bonewit-West #2, pp 138–139)

362. Which of the following is NOT a term used for patient bill statements?
    A. insert statements
    B. mailer statements
    C. speed mailers
    D. data mailers
    E. accounting reports
    (Bonewit-West #2, p 241)

363. Diagnostic and procedural code entry refers to the
    A. insurance carrier identification
    B. patient scheduling
    C. physician's practice category
    D. CPT-4
    E. accounting codes
    (Bonewit-West #2, p 171; Gylys #2, p 22)

364. After the computer prepares the insurance claim, it must be submitted by mail or electronically. Which of the following is NOT a step in submitting electronic claims?

    A. computer displays message that claims are ready for transmission
    B. cooperating insurance carriers are notified
    C. message is displayed on screen during transmission
    D. final message indicates that process has been completed
    E. the amount is deducted from patient's account
    (Bonewit-West #2, pp 254–256)

365. Which of the following is NOT included in pieces of hardware for a medical office computer system?
    A. keyboard
    B. video screen (monitor)
    C. central processing unit (CPU)
    D. printer
    E. DOS
    (Bonewit-West #2, p 13)

366. Which of the following is an input device for computers?
    A. monitor
    B. keyboard
    C. CPU
    D. printer
    E. modem
    (Bonewit-West #2, pp 8, 9)

367. The primary cause of malfunctioning of computers and keyboards is
    A. environmental contaminants
    B. poor programming
    C. insufficient wiring
    D. electrical surges
    E. none of the above
    (Bonewit-West #2, pp 16, 26)

368. How are the function keys on the IBM computer keyboard used?

    A. to write programs
    B. expedite accounting
    C. set up original computer tasks
    D. software program commands
    E. none of the above

    (Bonewit-West #2, pp 27–28)

369. What is a computer "prompt"?

    A. a hurry-up command
    B. a date reminder
    C. a request for input
    D. a transition to another program
    E. a timer

    (Bonewit-West #2, p 125)

370. What is a default value?

    A. error message
    B. help screen
    C. failure of program
    D. the usual response of the program
    E. none of the above

    (Bonewit-West #2, p 126)

371. If you forget commands in a program, what is the quickest way to refresh your memory?

    A. look in the program manual
    B. ask a co-worker
    C. consult the HELP screen
    D. call the technical representative
    E. consult another program

    (Bonewit-West #2, p 126)

372. The information displayed at any one time on the computer monitor is known as a

    A. screen
    B. menu
    C. prompt
    D. record
    E. program

    (Bonewit-West #2, p 122)

373. Which term does NOT refer to a type of printer?

    A. laser
    B. ink jet
    C. dot matrix
    D. thermal
    E. tractor feed

    (Bonewit-West #2, pp 31–34; Keir et al, p 69)

374. Which of the following are printer controls?

    A. on/off
    B. on-line
    C. line feed
    D. form feed
    E. all of the above

    (Bonewit-West #2, p 36)

375. Which of the following is NOT a part of copy machine operation?

    A. number of copies control
    B. regular/light/dark adjustment
    C. line feed
    D. paper supply level
    E. legal or letter-size control

    (Keir et al, pp 63–64)

376. What office machine uses the terms fast forward, backup, and rewind?

    A. typewriter
    B. microfilm machine
    C. computer
    D. transcriber
    E. postage meter

    (Keir et al, p 65)

377. The machine that sends and receives copies of printed documents over the telephone is the

    A. computer
    B. transcriber
    C. photocopier
    D. fax machine
    E. scanner

    (Keir et al, p 136)

378. Which of the following should be considered when purchasing a computer system for the office?
    A. kinds of software available
    B. how long supplier has been in business
    C. support offered after installation
    D. all of the above
    E. none of the above
    (Keir et al, p 73)

379. Which of the following may be important when negotiating a maintenance agreement for office equipment?
    A. renewal time frame
    B. contract terms for labor and parts
    C. exclusions and restrictions
    D. temporary equipment loans
    E. all of the above
    (Keir et al, p 73)

380. Which key signals the computer to accept your response to an on-screen prompt?
    A. alternate key
    B. control key
    C. exit key
    D. enter key
    E. shift key
    (Baptist et al, p 49)

381. Which command is used when turning off a computer?
    A. cancel
    B. exit or quit
    C. list
    D. leave text
    E. delete
    (Baptist et al, p 47)

382. The hard disk on an office computer system is
    A. the power unit of the computer
    B. the primary storage site for electronic file storage
    C. a 3″ rigid plastic disk
    D. a portable detachable memory device
    E. none of the above
    (Baptist et al, pp 23, 24)

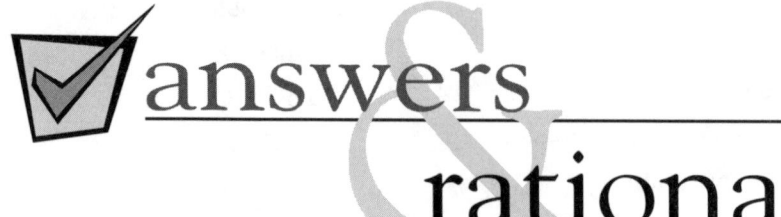
334.

A. The most difficult part of learning a computer applications program such as word processing is mastering the commands that take the operator from one part of the program to another and that execute the desired tasks. The easiest way to master a new program is to receive personalized instructions from a knowledgeable person while spending time with the computer working through the program. Either a formal class or assistance from a co-worker can provide the needed guidance. When this personal assistance is not available, time spent with tutorial manuals and working with the program's built-in HELP screen will suffice. Manuals and HELP screens should also be used later when questions arise regarding program use.

335.

D. The software is the roadmap that tells the computer what to do with the data it receives. Without instruction, the computer cannot function. Therefore, the roadmap of instructions (computer application program) for the tasks expected of the computer is the first consideration when buying a computer system.

336.

E. All of these functions are performed with specially designed software. Specialized medical office management programs permit computerizing of most front office tasks. In addition, useful reports on financial areas and other areas of the medical practice are possible that would be too time-consuming to do by hand. Almost all physicians' offices are now computerized to some extent.

337.

E. Many factors must be analyzed when making a major purchase such as a computer. Some factors include cost, training needed, the ease and speed of operation, and the affected office procedures. The physician, as director of the clinic, decides when to computerize or buy other major equipment. However, he or she will probably consult key assistants from the beginning. The transition period of training and "breaking in" must be carefully planned. Technical back-up by professionals is advisable during this period. Office tasks must be completed using both manual and computer methods until the computer methods are judged to be trouble free. However, after the transition, increased productivity, accuracy, and easier analysis should result.

338.

D. The software (or programs) of the computer gives the computer instructions about what to do with the data it receives. Without instructions (software), the computer hardware cannot function. Therefore, computer application programs are the first aspect to be considered when buying a computer system. The hardware (computer, monitor, printer) is bought to be compatible with the software. Specialized medical office management software that is customized to an individual medical practice can be purchased. However, off-the-shelf programs that are less expensive initially can also be purchased for many medical office tasks.

339.

A. Back-ups (additional copies) of all data files, documents, and other important work should be made daily in addition to storage on the hard disk within the computer. Floppy disks or tapes may be used. These duplicate back-up records should be stored in a separate location for security reasons. (Files may be erased by operator error, computer malfunction, or electrical failure.) Other devices protecting the medical records are antistatic devices and voltage regulators. The files are protected from outside human intervention by passwords given only to trusted employees.

340.

A. Electronic claims submissions forward insurance claims by computer or fax to a cooperating insurance carrier. Such submissions require either a modem or a fax machine at both the origin and the destination. Insurance claims are processed faster in this manner, which in turn means quicker payment. Electronic mail by either computer or fax consists of electronic messages sent from one place to another.

341.

D. A blank floppy disk (5 1/4- or 3 1/2-inch size) must be initialized (formatted) to accept information generated by the particular program in use such as DOS. Certain application programs have a menu choice that may be used to format new blank disks or erase and reuse those with old, unwanted information. In other programs, another systems disk supplied by the software vendor is used. Formatting erases old information so that a disk may store newer, pertinent information. A disk is easily protected against accidental formatting and loss of information by following instructions for the type of disk.

Preformatted disks are now commonly used. The disk must be of the right type for the computer and disk drive being used.

342.

B. The cursor (a blinking symbol on the monitor screen) may be toggled back and forth between either the insert mode or replace (type-over) mode. The arrow keys move the cursor to the page position where text is inserted or typed over. The insert mode allows additional text to be inserted. The replace mode allows you to type over the character at the cursor point. The cursor can be moved around the display screen one space at a time in any direction without changing the text by using the arrow keys (cursor movement keys)

or "mouse." (The mouse is an efficient hand-held device that permits quicker access to different parts of the text and program commands.) Keyboard commands allow quick scrolling to different pages of the document.

343.

A. Scrolling moves the cursor and the monitor screen up and down through the text, thus permitting rapid access to different parts of the document. Scrolling upward moves the cursor and screen nearer to the beginning of the document, while scrolling downward moves toward the end. Pressing the directional keys moves the cursor, and keyboard commands can also change the location of the cursor. Movement may be by the line, page, and paragraph, or to the beginning or end of the document.

344.

C. The statement of the amount owed by the patient is always sent to the guarantor who has taken responsibility for paying the bill. The guarantor is usually the patient. However, it may be a third party such as a parent, guardian, or insurance company. The statement is always itemized.

345.

B. A menu provides a list (selection) of functions needed for the user to go from one task to another within a program. The main menu provides the primary functions such as accessing and saving the files, removing files from the screen, and exiting. A submenu allows an item on the main menu to be divided again into several more specific tasks. For example, a submenu about printing formats may give information about spacing, margins, page numbers, indenting, and letter styles and sizes. The first menu viewed after turning on a computer is generally a choice of the application programs stored on the computer.

The menus are either controlled by keyboard commands or accessed by a mouse or trackball.

346.

A. Medical office management software programs automate the front office tasks of appointments, patient registration, recording chart notes, accounting, billing, and analysis reports. For insurance purposes, the software program should also include the CPT-4 medical services code list with fees and the ICD-9-CM diagnostic codes list. This software will include the database of patients with their demographic information.

347.

C. A network (multi-user/multitask) system has several terminals for operator access connected to the same central processing unit (CPU). Several people can work at different tasks while accessing the same program and database. Thus, an appointment for a new patient, a bill payment, insurance claim submissions, and medical transcription of patient records can all be underway in different offices of the health organization using the same CPU and database. Larger systems provide convenience and efficiency.

The network generally requires its users to have passwords to gain access to the information stored in the system. This policy protects the privacy of patient records and other sensitive material.

348.

A. A numeric field accepts numbers only. Some screens in medical software such as those that accept CPT codes will accept only numbers and are called numeric fields. If attempts are made to enter letters into these fields, an error message appears on the screen. Some fields are alphanumeric, which means they accept both letters and numbers. A date-only field requires the entry of a date in a standard format.

349.

A. Pressing the number lock key on the IBM PC activates the numeric keypad numbers located separately to the right of the alphanumeric keyboard. Some operators prefer the efficiency of the keypad to the numbers across the top of the regular keyboard. On the computer 10-key calculator keypads, the middle keys numbered 4, 5, and 6 are the home keys for the index, middle, and ring fingers. The thumb activates the zero key. Practicing with the fingers in this position will develop a rapid touch skill similar to touch typing. The operator will not need to look at the keypad.

350.

B. The spreadsheet is an electronic bookkeeping ledger that does repetitive calculations quickly. It permits quick generation of financial reports, such as the daily accounts receivable, the aged accounts receivable, and practice analyses. The spreadsheet, the database, and the word processor are the three main divisions of basic computer office programs. However, the terminology referring to these basic divisions may vary with different software.

351.

C. The database computer application contains the field (a single item of information), the record (a set of related items), and the file (a collection of related records). Databases allow large amounts of data to be easily retrieved, compared, and manipulated. Databases can rearrange files by the processes of alphabetizing, number selection, and other programmed criteria. The ability to sort and rearrange information makes database applications valuable office tools. Information can be sorted and quickly reported in a variety of ways.

352.

A. Word processing is similar to typing except that it has many functions that are not possible with typewriters. These functions include editing (deleting, copying, and moving), filing, and formatting of text. The difference between computer and typewriter keyboards are the additional special keys and key combinations for the computer. All computer keyboards have the enter (return) key and the arrow keys. Other special keys and their functions vary according to the brand of computer and software program.

353.

C. A network (multi-user/multitask) system has two or more terminals. Each terminal has a keyboard and monitor that connects directly by cables with a central processing unit. This enables several persons to use the same program simultaneously from different locations. These computer systems are always larger than the microcomputers designed for use with only one terminal and one person at a time. To protect confidential information, the network system generally requires that its users have a password to access the system.

354.

B. The bulk of information contained in the reports comes from the medical practice databases. The databases allow the physician to analyze many aspects of the practice. These reports may include any data that can be organized by number or alphabet into lists and compared. These reports allow the physician to control his or her practice more accurately.

355.

C. Passwords protect the computer information system from unauthorized entry. Each employee is assigned a password with which he or she gains entry into the system. The password also attaches the operator's identification to each transaction, which enables the questionable transactions to be traced. Common-sense precautions should also be followed. Outsiders should not be allowed to watch the password being keyed in. Monitors displaying confidential information should not be left unattended.

Hard copy (paper records) generated by the computer should be treated confidentially. This includes using a paper shredder or some similar means to protect confidentiality when disposing of discarded papers.

356.

E. Documentation does not include file names. Documentation is for the purpose of assisting the operator in mastering the software program and must include a written set of program instructions. A HELP screen on the computer monitor, reference cards for quick review, student tutorial manuals, and a more complex program manual are included in documentation.

357.

E. All of these terms—route slip, encounter form, charge slip, and superbill—refer to the slip also called a source document, which is attached to the patient's chart at the beginning of the visit. The physician checks off the appropriate diagnoses and procedures. The medical assistant posts the charges during the patient's departure or by later batching the route slips together.

358.

E. All of these items—demographic data, insurance information, financial records, and appointments—should be available through the computer's patient registration system. For convenience, any type of patient information should be accessible by name or with social security information. Demographic information includes sex, date of birth, social security numbers, addresses, telephone numbers, and insurance policy and group numbers. Demographic information is essential for a number of tasks such as filing insurance claims and contacting patients.

359.

B. A program is a set of instructions organized into a logical step-by-step sequence to guide the computer in performing a specific task. An example is Word Perfect, an IBM word-processing program. Programs can be designed for many different types of tasks. In addition to word processing, accounting, and databases, programs exist for drafting, art, games, spelling correction, and so on. Programs may be either stored within the computer on a hard disk or on a floppy disk.

360.

E. The main menu of a medical office management program lists the different systems that comprise the program. These include patient registration, appointment scheduling, posting transactions, patient billing, insurance billing, reports, and file maintenance. Each of these systems in turn is further classified into a submenu, which lists specific tasks. For example, the patient registration system on the main menu has a submenu that will allow new patient entry, editing of existing patient record, deleting of patient record, and reviewing of patient record. The submenu also has a means of exiting back to the main menu.

361.

E. All of these are part of the file maintenance system. They must be inserted before front office procedures can be entered into the computer system. In addition to the listed items, procedure and diagnostic codes and referring physicians' information are also entered. During the transition period after the installation of a front office computer both manual and computer methods are used for the office work. This allows the office staff time to note any deficiencies in the computer program.

362.

E. Accounting reports summarize different accounting aspects such as daily transactions, aged accounts receivable, and outstanding insurance claims. The other terms listed do refer to patient bill statements. Computerized patient statements processed on the computer may be printed in a variety of formats. One format is the insert statement with the guarantor's (payer's) name, address, and amount owed. This is inserted into a window envelope or an addressed envelope. The other type known as a mailer statement, speed mailer, or data mailer comes off the printer already inserted into a mailing envelope.

363.

D. CPT-4 is a coding system that provides a uniform language for physicians to report their medical, surgical, and diagnostic services. Most government and private insurance companies require the claim forms to use numerical CPT codes to identify patient procedures instead of writing out the information. The CPT consists of five digits for each procedure plus a two-digit code modifier for further identification.

364.

E. The amount requested from the insurance company is not deducted from the patient's account until payment is actually received. The insurance company might refuse to pay the claim for some reason. The first four steps listed in the question are necessary for submitting the insurance claim.

365.

E. DOS, classified as software, is an operating system program stored on a floppy disk. There are four different operating systems, and the one you have depends on the kind of computer you use. The four main pieces of equipment included in the hardware of the computer are (1) the keyboard where data is entered; (2) the video screen, which displays information (soft copy); (3) the central processing unit (CPU), which performs the functions of the program; and (4) the printer, which produces hardcopy.

366.

B. The keyboard is the most commonly used device for entering data into the computer in medical clinics. Less common methods are scanners, which enter printed digits, words, and graphics, and the mouse. Input is information that is entered into the computer. Output is processed data from computers that is either printed (hard copy) or displayed on the monitor screen (soft copy).

367.

A. Environmental contaminants are most often responsible for computer malfunctioning although lightning strikes and electrical surges also cause damage. Smoke, dust, dirt, and spilled beverages can penetrate the electronic connections. Soft drinks and coffee should not be placed where they may be spilled into the keyboard or computer hardware. Smoking should be banned from the computer room (if not already from the entire medical clinic). Computers should be protected from electrical surges and lightning by surge protectors at the plug-in. Keyboards and other computer surfaces may be cleaned with a damp cloth but never cleaning fluids. Aerosol sprays, solvents, and abrasives should never be used.

368.

D. The function keys on the IBM keyboards are used in software programs to issue commands such as accessing menus, printing, HELP screen, and so on. Because the commands vary, the operator must know the individual program's commands. Special keys that make the computer keyboard different than a typewriter also include the enter (return) key and the arrow keys.

369.

C. A prompt is a message on the computer screen that requests the operator to enter information. The cursor should be moved to the right of the command to enter information. Sometimes the prompt is indicated by a question mark. Prompts make the program easier and more "user friendly."

370.

D. A default value is the usual response of the program to a certain task. The computer will use this value unless the operator overrides it by entering another value. For instance, page margins and spacing have default values that are automatically used in printing documents unless they are changed by the operator. Default values that appear on the monitor screen within a prompt can be accepted by simply pushing the enter (return) key. Drive A is the default disk drive because when the computer looks for disk information it automatically goes to this drive first.

371.

C. Consulting the HELP screen included in most computer programs is the quickest way to refresh your memory. The program user manual will indicate how the HELP screen can be accessed on screen. Usually, the HELP screen lists all the program commands alphabetically or by function. If more information and instruction is still needed after seeing the HELP screen, consult the program manual. If this also fails then consult a knowledgeable co-worker or a technical representative.

372.

A. A "screen" is the information shown on the monitor screen at any one time. Any particular part of the program can be identified by its "screen." Data-entry screens may be "fill-in-the-blank" with little difference from printed forms except that they are completed on the computer, not on paper. They may be printed if a hard copy is needed, changed when needed or deleted altogether. The screen also has identifying information as to the type of function being utilized, and the position of the cursor in the program.

373.

E. Tractor feed refers to a method of feeding continuous sheets of paper into the printer. The other methods are automatic and single-sheet feeding. The other answer choices were types of printers. The laser printer provides high-quality printing. Impact printers such as the dot matrix may give a choice of near letter-quality printing or of draft mode, which is faster but of poorer quality. The ink jet printers give excellent quality printing and also allow for color printing.

What is new technology today in printers and computers may be outdated in a few years because of the rapid changes in technology.

374.

E. All of these are printer controls. Most printers have these basic controls. If a printer is on-line, it can accept data from the computer for printing. The line-feed control can be activated only when the computer is off-line. It advances the paper one line at a time. The form-feed control advances the paper one page at a time. Many printers also have menus that use the listed controls to select print styles and control other advanced printer features. The printer manual should be consulted for maintenance tasks.

375.

C. The line feed is a line-by-line adjustment on the computer printer, not a photocopier. The other choices are all adjustments for the photocopier. The paper supply level is checked to prevent paper from running low and/or jamming in some models. The size of the copy, legal or letter size, can be selected, as can the number of copies. Some machines also can be adjusted for darkness of the copy. Models of photocopiers vary with some having automatic feeders; the ability to enlarge or decrease size of copy; the ability to collate, staple, or print two-sided copies; as well as other features. A maintenance agreement should be negotiated because the copier requires routine maintenance.

376.

D. The transcriber enables the medical assistant to listen to notes the physician has recorded on audiotape and transcribe them into written records. It has earphones, a foot pedal, start, stop, and back-up controls. It also has fast forward and rewind controls. The transcriber frees the hands to type the notes into a computer or typewriter. Taping medical notes into a recorder is convenient because it enables the doctor to make notes as the patients are examined and when he or she is away from the office.

377.

D. The fax (facsimile) machine scans a document and converts the image to electronic pulses, which are sent over telephone lines. The receiving fax machine converts the electronic pulses back to an identical copy of the original document. The first page of the fax transmission is the cover page. It lists the vital information of date, recipient's name and address, fax number and number of pages sent, sender's name, and fax number, along with any other routing instructions.

When sending confidential patient records to another fax station, ask that they acknowledge receipt. Otherwise it may be necessary to call them. A note may be included stating that the material is confidential and if missent or received by unintended persons that its confidentiality should be protected. The office should formulate a policy covering faxed information. One possibility is to arrange for the material to be identified by number instead of by the patient's name.

378.

D. Adequate support by the vendor and the right kind of software for a medical office and hardware to process the software are essential in the purchase of a computer. The vendor should be knowledgeable and experienced in the field of health care as well as in general computer software. The vendor should be willing to listen to the office's needs and ideas for improvements. Although not essential, automatic upgrades and subscription service may be desirable.

When starting up a computer system to replace a manual office routine, both methods must be maintained in duplicate. When it is apparent that the computer system is working satisfactorily, the manual system may be discontinued. This duplication of effort is stressful to the office staff but a necessary step.

379.

E. All of these considerations, renewal timeframe, effectiveness, contract terms for labor and parts, exclusions and restrictions, and temporary equipment loans, are important when deciding on maintenance agreements for office equipment. Upgrade provisions and depreciation rates also should be considered. Decisions and information regarding warranties and maintenance agreements should be summarized in an office equipment manual for reference when needed.

380.

D. The enter key accepts data you have entered into a field and moves on to the next item. It also accepts default data or your choice of an item on a menu. In word processing, the enter key also acts as a carriage return when a new line is desired immediately instead of using the automatic return. Entering information on the screen does not save it into permanent memory such as the hard disk. This requires a "save" command. Other keys used on the keyboard are the shift key used (as on the typewriter) to capitalize letters and access uppercase symbols and keys used for special computer functions (e.g., the alternate and control keys used with the special function keys to give commands).

381.

B. The exit command (or quit command on some computers) would be used. This command initiates a sequence of orderly events that prompts the user to save or delete the file currently in use and then return to the main menu. Manufacturers recommend that the user follow these steps rather than "crashing" the computer by simply turning off the power switch.

The list command in some programs allows viewing and retrieval of files. The cancel command allows the user to cancel the last command and return to a previous situation. The save command copies the file on the monitor and "desktop" of the computer to storage on a permanent memory device such as a hard disk, a so-called floppy disk, or a tape. One function usually available is the HELP command that helps the user to identify the commands. The escape key may have various functions with different programs. It may act as a cancel command.

Some keys such as the caps lock and shift key are "toggle" keys that toggle back and forth between two functions such as capital or lowercase letters. In the case of the insert key, it is toggled between the insert (letters) mode and the overstrike (letters) mode. The IBM-compatible keyboards have a row of function keys across the top that perform commands alone and in combination with other keystrokes from the keyboard.

Names of commands vary from program to program. However, they are similar enough that a person who masters one program will usually find other programs of the same type easier to master.

382.

B. The hard disk, usually concealed inside the cabinet of the computer, is the primary storage for information. Hard disks (C or D) store very large amounts of information conveniently in electronic files that can be retrieved and altered as needed. Because crucial information should never be trusted to only one storage site, back-up floppy disks in disk drives (A or B) are used for back-up storage and are stored in a separate location. Floppy disks can also be transferred from one computer to another but have much less storage capacity than hard disks.

Floppy disks (usually 3 1/2-inch) must be purchased preformatted in the type suitable for the particular disk drive or formatted or initialized in the office.

III

Clinical Procedures

9 Examination Room Techniques

chapter objectives

Major areas of knowledge/content included in this chapter are:

I. Principles of infection control and aseptic techniques including disposal of contaminated materials

➤ medical asepsis including hand washing, sanitation, and chemical disinfection

➤ surgical asepsis including scrubbing, gowning, gloving, surgical assisting and equipment preparation

II. Treatment area instruments, supplies, and equipment— preparation and operation including

➤ autoclave/sterilizer/electrocardiograph/examination table

➤ ophthalmoscope/otoscope/sphygmomanometers/ spirometer/thermometers

➤ physical therapy including fitting of crutches

III. Vital signs/equipment and procedures

IV. Assisting the physician with patient histories, examinations, and procedures

➤ visual testing

➤ body positions

V. Procedural explanations and instructions to patients

DIRECTIONS (Questions 1 through 129): Each of the numbered items or incomplete statements in this section is followed by answers or by completions of the statement. Select the ONE lettered answer or completion that is BEST in each case.

1. The normal axillary (armpit) reading, which is lower than either the oral or rectal temperature, is
   A. 97.6°F
   B. 96.6°F
   C. 35.4°C
   D. 37.5°C
   E. 99.6°F
   (Frew et al, p 346; Keir et al, p 478)

2. The normal oral temperature is
   A. 99.6°F
   B. 96.6°F
   C. 97.6°F
   D. 98.6°F
   E. 99.0°F
   (Frew et al, p 346; Keir et al, p 475)

3. The normal rectal temperature reading, which is higher than the normal oral or axillary temperature, is
   A. 97.6°F
   B. 99.6°F
   C. 30.0°C
   D. 35.0°C
   E. 36.8°C
   (Frew et al, p 346; Keir et al, pp 475–476)

4. A patient has a temperature reading of 102.0°F. The equivalent temperature reading on the Celsius (centigrade) scale is
   A. 35.5°C
   B. 38.9°C
   C. 53.6°C
   D. 56.7°C
   E. 184.5°C
   (Frew et al, p 349)

5. In taking an oral temperature, the standard oral thermometer should be left in place for
   A. 1 minute
   B. 3 minutes
   C. 8 minutes
   D. 10 minutes
   E. 12 minutes
   (Frew et al, p 346; Keir et al, p 475)

6. Which federal clinical laboratory regulation has specific guidelines for quality control, quality assurance, record keeping, and personnel qualifications?
   A. DEA
   B. OSHA
   C. CLIA '88
   D. CDC
   E. COLA
   (Palko and Palko, p 97; Wedding and Toenjes, pp 25–27)

7. In which position is a patient placed to take an axillary temperature?
   A. prone
   B. supine
   C. Trendelenburg
   D. knee-chest
   E. lithotomy
   (Zakus, p 25)

8. The normal pulse rate (pulsations per minute) for adults is
   A. 40–60
   B. 60–90
   C. 80–100
   D. 90–100
   E. more than 100
   (Bonewit-West #1, p 98)

9. The normal pulse rate for children from 1 to 7 years of age is
   A. 60–100
   B. 70–110
   C. 80–120
   D. 90–130
   E. 100–130
   (Frew et al, p 352; Kinn and Woods, p 664)

10. At birth, the normal pulse rate is at least
    A. 60
    B. 80
    C. 100
    D. 110
    E. 130
    (Kinn and Woods, p 664)

11. Normally, the pulse rate is the same as the
    A. number of heartbeats in 1 minute
    B. number of heartbeats in 30 seconds
    C. average length of beats in 1 minute
    D. difference between systolic and diastolic pressure
    E. difference between hypertension and hypotension
    (Keir et al, pp 483–484)

12. Bradycardia is a term meaning
    A. abnormally fast heartbeat
    B. abnormally slow heartbeat
    C. average heartbeat
    D. diseased heart
    E. throbbing pulse
    (Bonewit-West #1, pp 100, 103; Frew et al, p 353; Keir et al, p 312)

13. If the pulse is taken at the wrist, the artery used is the
    A. radial artery
    B. temporal artery
    C. carotid artery
    D. facial artery
    E. femoral artery
    (Bonewit-West #1, p 99; Keir et al, pp 483–485)

14. An increase in one's pulse rate may be caused by
    A. fever
    B. poisons
    C. mental depression
    D. rest
    E. chronic disease
    (Frew et al, pp 351, 359; Keir et al, pp 453–484)

15. The preferred method to take a pulse rate is to count for
    A. 30 seconds and double the number
    B. 1 full minute
    C. 2 full minutes and take one-half of the number
    D. 30 seconds and multiply by 0.5
    E. 3 minutes, with a 30-second break between each count
    (Kinn and Woods, pp 461–462)

16. The normal rate of respiration per minute for adults is
    A. 6–10
    B. 10–13
    C. 14–20
    D. 18–22
    E. 22–28
    (Bonewit-West #1, p 106; Frew et al, p 354)

17. The normal rate of respiration for infants is approximately
    A. 8–14
    B. 15–22
    C. 18–24
    D. 24–32
    E. 30–60
    (Bonewit-West #1, p 106; Frew et al, p 354)

18. A decrease in respiration may be caused by
    A. excitement
    B. hemorrhage
    C. sleep
    D. obstruction of air passages
    E. exercise
    (Bonewit-West #1, p 106)

19. Difficult or labored breathing that may require the patient to be placed in a orthopneic or Fowler's position for comfort is
    A. apnea
    B. eupnea
    C. orthopnea
    D. dyspnea
    E. tachypnea
    (Bonewit-West #1, p 106)

20. Cheyne-Stokes describes
    A. a type of respiration
    B. a type of pulse
    C. the name of a thermometer
    D. a type of stethoscope
    E. the surnames of two surgeons who designed the first blood pressure apparatus
    (Frew et al, p 353; Keir et al, pp 486–487)

21. Systolic pressure of 160 or above is referred to as
    A. bradycardia
    B. tachycardia
    C. hypertension
    D. hypotension
    E. pulse pressure
    (Bonewit-West #1, p 109; Kinn and Woods, p 466)

22. The position used for a patient in shock is
    A. supine
    B. prone
    C. lithotomy
    D. jackknife
    E. Trendelenburg
    (Zakus, pp 89–90)

23. A patient who is to be examined vaginally should be placed in the
    A. lithotomy position
    B. Trendelenburg position
    C. supine position
    D. anatomic position
    E. prone position
    (Bonewit-West #1, p 364; Zakus, pp 84–85)

24. A patient is to have a flexible sigmoidoscopic examination. The medical assistant should assist the patient to assume the
    A. supine position
    B. Sims position
    C. dorsal recumbent position
    D. semi-Fowler's position
    E. Trendelenburg position
    (Frew et al, p 389; Kinn and Woods, pp 607–608; Keir et al, pp 363, 547–542)

25. The physician requests that a patient be positioned flat on her back on the examination table with the soles of her feet flat on the table. The legs are sharply flexed at the knees. The patient will be placed in which of these positions?
    A. horizontal recumbent
    B. dorsal recumbent
    C. prone
    D. jackknife (knee-chest)
    E. supine
    (Bonewit-West #1, p 137)

26. Which of the following requires consideration in addition to positioning a patient for surgery?
    A. where the physician and you will stand or sit for the surgery
    B. the comfort of the patient
    C. where instruments and other equipment will be placed
    D. removal of the patient's clothing
    E. comfort of surgery team
    (Kinn and Woods, p 1115)

27. Listening to sounds produced when the body is struck in a definite manner is called
    A. auscultation
    B. inspection
    C. percussion
    D. palpation
    E. palpitation
    (Bonewit-West #1, p 122; Frew et al, p 401)

28. An abnormally slow pulse is
    A. extrasystole
    B. tachycardia
    C. thready pulse
    D. pulse volume
    E. bradycardia
    (Frew et al, p 353; Bonewit #1, p 103)

29. Which of the following factors has an inverse ratio to the pulse rate?
    A. physical exercise
    B. anger
    C. increased metabolism
    D. increasing age
    E. fever
    (Frew et al, p 351)

30. Which of the following may describe the action of a specific poison, medication, or excess body chemical on the pulse rate?
    A. an increase in pulse rate
    B. a decrease in pulse rate
    C. a bounding pulse
    D. none of the above
    E. any of the above
    (Zakus, p 29)

31. The apical pulse is taken
    A. on the wrist
    B. on the thigh
    C. on the neck
    D. with a stethoscope
    E. on the temple
    (Bonewit-West #1, p 99; Frew et al, p 354)

32. The selection of one of the three available blood pressure cuff sizes depends on the
    A. age of patient
    B. diameter of limb
    C. position of patient
    D. pulse rate of patient
    E. weight of patient
    (Bonewit-West #1, p 114; Zakus, p 40)

33. Anthropometric measurements that are taken routinely on maternity patients, infants and children, dieting patients, and others would include which of the following?
    A. hormonal tests
    B. respiration, pulse, and blood pressure
    C. body dimensions, including height, weight, and size
    D. metabolic tests
    E. stress tests
    (Frew et al, p 359)

34. A patient's general medical history is obtained preferably
    A. at the beginning of the first office visit
    B. whenever the need arises
    C. before admission to a hospital
    D. at the reception desk
    E. at a convenient time
    (Bonewit-West #1, pp 57–65; Zakus, p 53)

35. The term "asepsis" means
    A. heterotroph
    B. optimum growth temperature
    C. neutral pH
    D. free from infection or pathogens
    E. infection
    (Bonewit-West #1, p 4; Frew et al, p 596)

36. Which of the following is a poor aseptic technique to follow in the medical office?
    A. keeping the medical office clean from dirt and dust
    B. wearing ornate jewelry
    C. carefully disposing of wastes, such as feces, etc.
    D. using waterproof bags to dispose of soiled items
    E. cleaning spills with household bleach and similar disinfectants
    (Bonewit-West #1, pp 5–7)

37. An organism that is infected with a pathogen and is a source of infection to others is a/an
    A. anaerobe
    B. microorganism
    C. reservoir host
    D. nonpathogen
    E. fomes

    (Bonewit-West #1, p 4; Zakus, p 172)

38. Health care workers who may acquire HIV (the AIDS virus) from occupational exposure are at greatest danger from which of the following?
    A. unprotected personal care
    B. contaminated blood that touches severely chapped hands
    C. accidental splattering of blood in the mouth
    D. contaminated blood from an open wound
    E. accidental needle sticks

    (Palko and Palko, pp 5–6)

39. Heat is created within tissues by converting electric energy in
    A. thermotherapy
    B. light therapy
    C. hydrotherapy
    D. ultrasonic therapy
    E. diathermy

    (Bonewit-West #1, p 827; Frew et al, p 660)

40. Which of the following dry heat treatments will produce surface heat that penetrates the skin to a depth of 3 to 10 mm?
    A. paraffin bath
    B. heating pads
    C. infrared radiation lamp
    D. ultraviolet radiation lamp
    E. hot water bottles

    (Bonewit-West #1, pp 825–926; Frew et al, p 660)

41. Whirlpool baths are used in
    A. electrotherapy
    B. ultrasonic therapy
    C. hydrotherapy
    D. thermotherapy
    E. diathermy

    (Bonewit-West #1, p 824; Frew et al, p 661)

42. A medical assistant helping a patient who requires short-wave diathermy should
    A. increase the volume of energy (heat) above the initial comfortable tolerance of the patient
    B. position the machine so that the patient can turn up the energy
    C. administer the treatment for as long as the patient can comfortably tolerate it
    D. be certain the area to be treated is exposed and examined for skin breaks, inflamed areas, and any metals
    E. encourage the patient to ask for more heat during the treatment

    (Frew et al, p 660)

43. Casts that immobilize musculoskeletal injuries do NOT utilize which of the following?
    A. plaster
    B. flexion
    C. synthetic material
    D. fiberglass
    E. air cast

    (Bonewit-West #1, pp 345–349; Kinn and Woods, pp 725–730)

44. The formation of prothrombin is a major function of
    A. vitamin A
    B. vitamin C
    C. vitamin D
    D. vitamin E
    E. vitamin K

    (Kinn and Woods, pp 978–979; Zakus, p 417)

45. Exposure to sunlight is considered adequate for adults as a source of
    A. vitamin A
    B. vitamin C
    C. vitamin D
    D. vitamin E
    E. vitamin K
    (Frew et al, p 522; Kinn and Woods, pp 972–978)

46. Ascorbic acid is synonymous with
    A. vitamin A
    B. vitamin C
    C. vitamin D
    D. vitamin E
    E. vitamin K
    (Frew et al, p 522; Zakus, pp 648–649)

47. Dermatitis, dementia, and diarrhea are characteristic of
    A. cheilosis
    B. niacin deficiency (pellagra)
    C. rickets
    D. tetany
    E. beriberi
    (Frew et al, p 521; Zakus, pp 648–649)

48. The fetal period of the life cycle lasts from
    A. the union of the ovum and sperm to the end of the second month of pregnancy
    B. the third month to the ninth month of pregnancy
    C. birth to 1 year of age
    D. 1 to 6 years of age
    E. the union of the ovum and sperm to the ninth month of pregnancy
    (Keir et al, p 412; Taber's, p 719)

49. Sickle-cell anemia occurs primarily in
    A. Jewish people
    B. English people
    C. young people
    D. African Americans
    E. elderly people
    (Palko and Palko, p 256; Wedding and Toenjes, p 264)

50. A disease that runs its course in years is
    A. acute
    B. subacute
    C. chronic
    D. fulminating
    E. explosive
    (Bonewit-West #1, p 123; Taber's, p 383)

51. The art of distinguishing between two allied diseases by contrasting their symptoms is called
    A. laboratory diagnosis
    B. clinical diagnosis
    C. physical diagnosis
    D. roentgen diagnosis
    E. differential diagnosis
    (Bonewit-West #1, p 122; Zakus, pp 61–62)

52. The study of the causes of disease is
    A. etiology
    B. embryology
    C. diagnosis
    D. exacerbation
    E. histology
    (Taber's, p 679; Zakus, p 169)

53. Organisms that cause disease are called
    A. subacute
    B. chronic
    C. acute
    D. pathogens
    E. fulminate
    (Keir et al, p 796; Zakus, p 169)

54. A diagnosis based solely on the evaluation of the health history of the patient and the physical examination findings is called a
    A. clinical diagnosis
    B. physical diagnosis
    C. laboratory diagnosis
    D. differential diagnosis
    E. pathologic diagnosis
    (Bonewit-West #1, p 128)

55. The first pack that the circulating assistant in office surgery opens is
    A. the instrument pack
    B. the sponge packs
    C. the sterile base for the other sterile items
    D. drapes
    E. syringes
    (Bonewit-West #1, pp 225–226; Kinn and Woods, p 1119)

56. A condition of a disease where symptoms increase in severity after an initial improvement or a regular course is called
    A. intercurrent
    B. intermittent
    C. benign
    D. exacerbation
    E. subacute
    (Taber's, p 682)

57. Rash diseases are referred to as
    A. exanthemas
    B. exacerbation
    C. explosive
    D. palpation
    E. sequelae
    (Miller and Keane, pp 565, 566)

58. The process of measuring is called
    A. inspection
    B. palpation
    C. palpitation
    D. mensuration
    E. manipulation
    (Kinn and Woods, p 486)

59. The complete destruction of all forms of microbial life is
    A. disinfection
    B. cleaning
    C. sanitization
    D. sterilization
    E. protection
    (Keir et al, p 449; Taber's, p 1831)

60. Chemical germicides, boiling water, and flowing steam are used in
    A. cleaning
    B. disinfection
    C. sterilization
    D. lubrication
    E. autoclaving
    (Bonewit-West #1, p 428; Kinn and Woods, p 428)

61. Dry heat, moderately heated chemical-gas mixtures, and saturated steam under pressure (autoclaves) are used in
    A. cleaning
    B. disinfection
    C. sterilization
    D. lubrication
    E. sanitization
    (Bonewit-West #1, pp 430–436; Keir et al, pp 449–451)

62. Which is an unacceptable guideline for hand scrubbing when assisting with surgery?
    A. use surgical soap
    B. use sterile brush
    C. hold hands down to allow water to drain off the fingertips
    D. scrub hands and forearms for 5 to 10 minutes
    E. dry hands by patting with sterile towels
    (Kinn and Woods, pp 1087–1093)

63. To be prepared for sterilization, hinged instruments, such as hemostats, must always be
    A. opened
    B. closed
    C. taped
    D. oiled
    E. disinfected
    (Kinn and Woods, p 431; Zakus, p 188)

64. How are falls prevented when a patient is getting into and out of a wheelchair?
    A. lock the wheels
    B. back into the chair using the armrests as braces
    C. to leave the chair, fold back the footrests and lock the wheels
    D. place the unaffected foot on the floor first when leaving the chair
    E. all of the above
    (Bonewit-West #1, p 734; Kinn and Woods, p 743)

65. An examination tray setup includes single-use exam gloves, K-Y jelly, an anoscope, cotton applicators, and a fecal occult blood kit. What type of examination is indicated?
    A. visual acuity examination
    B. eye, ear, and nose examination
    C. rectal examination
    D. pelvic examination
    E. none of the above
    (Zakus, p 106)

66. A medical assistant with clean, dry hands may remove from an autoclave
    A. dry wrapped packs
    B. instruments sterilized on a tray without wrapping
    C. nothing, unless he or she uses sterile forceps
    D. nothing, unless he or she uses sterile gloves
    E. only those instruments that are going to be used immediately
    (Kinn and Woods, p 436)

67. When autoclaving, the exposure period is timed beginning when
    A. instruments are placed in the autoclave
    B. adequate pressure has built up
    C. an adequate temperature has been reached

D. the instruments have been cleaned
E. the medical assistant pours water into the reservoir
(Bonewit-West #1, p 187)

68. Items should be placed in an autoclave to allow for contact with steam on
    A. upper surfaces only
    B. lower surfaces only
    C. all surfaces
    D. all surfaces except the edges on which the materials are placed
    E. any two sides of the package
    (Bonewit-West #1, pp 187–188)

69. Which of the following may be safely disinfected with germicidal solutions?
    A. instruments used in contact with outer skin
    B. the appropriate type of clothing to wear to the appointment
    C. percussion hammers and stethoscopes
    D. all of the above
    E. none of the above
    (Bonewit-West #1, p 189)

70. Scheduling a preoperative (preop) appointment should include special advice to the patient. Which of the following would be included in this type of patient education?
    A. advise patient of the approximate length of time for the procedure
    B. the appropriate type of clothing to wear to the appointment
    C. advise the patient to arrange for someone to accompany him/her to the appointment
    D. advise the patient as to the anticipated time to take off from work or arrange for home care
    E. all of the above
    (Keir et al, pp 635–637)

71. As three methods of controlling microbial life, sanitization, disinfection, and sterilization are
    A. used separately as methods of decontamination
    B. often used jointly as methods of decontamination
    C. all equally effective in combating viruses, such as that of serum hepatitis
    D. of no concern if disposable products are used
    E. not easily implemented in a physician's office
    (Keir et al, pp 448–449)

72. Inasmuch as an article cannot be partially sterile, objects should be categorized as either sterile or
    A. clean
    B. antiseptic
    C. disinfected
    D. fumigated
    E. nonsterile
    (Frew et al, p 611)

73. Which of these principles apply to maintaining a sterile surgical environment?
    A. touch only the outside of a sterile wrapper
    B. when in doubt consider an object nonsterile
    C. avoid talking and sneezing over a sterile field
    D. hold gloved hands above waist level
    E. all of the above
    (Kinn and Woods, pp 1085–1086; Frew et al, pp 611–612; Zakus, pp 203–204)

74. Incomplete sterilization in an autoclave may be caused by
    A. placing instruments too close together in the autoclave
    B. opening door too wide during the drying cycle
    C. trapping air pockets in the autoclave

D. starting the time period before the correct sterilization temperature is reached
    E. all of the above
    (Bonewit-West #1, pp 174–181; Kinn and Woods, pp 430–432)

75. Which of the following meet acceptable criteria for use as wrapping materials for autoclaving?
    A. muslin fabric
    B. nonwoven disposable materials, such as Kim wrap
    C. clear plastic with permeable paper facing envelope
    D. permeable paper envelopes
    E. all of the above
    (Bonewit-West #1, pp 178–179; Kinn and Woods, p 430)

76. The most widely used medical disinfectant is
    A. phenol
    B. alcohol
    C. chlorohexaphene
    D. formaldehyde
    E. detergent
    (Bonewit-West #1, p 170; Kinn and Woods, p 428)

77. Before reusing a uterine biopsy punch, uterine tenaculum, or a cervical biopsy forceps, these instruments, which penetrate the body, should be
    A. disinfected
    B. cleaned
    C. sterilized with dry heat
    D. sterilized by autoclaving
    E. sanitized
    (Bonewit-West #1, p 174)

78. To clean the chamber of the autoclave, which of the following should be used?
    A. steel wool
    B. commercial autoclave cleaner
    C. hydrogen peroxide
    D. fine sandpaper
    E. alcohol
    (Bonewit-West #1, p 186)

79. Which of the following is a poor practice when assisting with physical examinations?
    A. wash hands before setting up
    B. prepare all needed instruments and supplies
    C. check examination room
    D. assist patient as required
    E. leave a male doctor alone with the female patient
    (Kinn and Woods, pp 489–490)

80. When given properly, the method of injection that is safest and that provides gradual and optimal absorption is the
    A. intramuscular
    B. intravenous
    C. intradermal
    D. subcutaneous
    E. epidural
    (Keir et al, p 676; Zakus, p 278)

81. Drugs in the amounts of 2 mL or more are given
    A. intramuscularly
    B. intravenously
    C. intradermally
    D. subcutaneously
    E. any of the four ways
    (Bonewit-West #1, p 280;Keir et al, p 676; Zakus, p 278)

82. Which of the following would NOT be included in the vital signs?
    A. weight
    B. respiration
    C. pulse
    D. temperature
    E. blood pressure
    (Keir et al, p 470; Kinn and Woods, p 442; Zakus, p 19)

83. Standard limb lead I records the voltage through the heart from
    A. right arm to left arm
    B. right arm to left leg
    C. left arm to left leg
    D. midpoint between left arm and left leg to right arm
    E. midpoint between right arm and left leg to left arm
    (Burdick, pp 10, 11)

84. The augmented lead AVF records the voltage through the heart from
    A. right arm to left leg
    B. left arm to left leg
    C. midpoint between left arm and left leg to right arm
    D. midpoint between right arm and left leg to left arm
    E. midpoint between right arm and left arm to left leg
    (Bonewit-West #1, p 448; Burdick, p 11)

85. When a medical assistant is instructed to do an electrocardiogram (ECG) on a patient who has had an entire arm amputated, the electrode or sensor is placed on the torso. The other arm limb electrode or sensor should be
    A. placed on the outside of the arm
    B. placed on the inside of the arm
    C. placed on the torso at the opposite position to the other electrode
    D. placed next to the other electrode
    E. placed on the patient's side opposite the first electrode
    (Burdick, p 26)

86. The code representing lead VI in taking of ECGs is
    A. — —
    B. — ••
    C. — •••
    D. — ••••
    E. — •
    (Burdick, p 13)

87. Leads I, II, and III in a routine ECG require the use of
   A. two arms and two legs
   B. two arms and one leg
   C. one arm and two legs
   D. one arm and one leg
   E. the chest and all the limbs
   (Burdick, p 10)

88. Which one of these patient activities should NOT interfere with the taking of a proper ECG?
   A. touching ungrounded metal objects
   B. continuing to talk during the test
   C. moving during the test
   D. wearing jewelry and a wristwatch
   E. emotional excitement and apprehension
   (Burdick, p 25)

89. Which of the following statements is NOT a purpose of cardiac stress testing or the treadmill?
   A. to observe and record the patient's cardiovascular response to exercise
   B. to cause cardiac arrest
   C. to determine an individual's energy performance capacity
   D. to prescribe a specially designed exercise program
   E. to diagnose cardiac disease
   (Kinn and Woods, p 524; Zakus, pp 543–544)

90. Which of the following will cause an alternating current artifact on the ECG tracing?
   A. electrodes too tight or too loose
   B. corroded or dirty electrodes
   C. electrolytes unequal in amount on each electrode
   D. lotions, body creams, or oils on skin in the area where the electrode is placed
   E. an electrocardiograph that is improperly grounded
   (Bonewit-West #1, pp 451–452; Burdick, p 33)

91. An electrocardiograph lead designated as AVR is a type of
   A. limb lead
   B. chest lead
   C. unipolar lead
   D. precordial lead
   E. bipolar lead
   (Burdick, p 11)

92. When the standardization button is pressed on an electrocardiograph
   A. upward deflection appears on the graph paper
   B. the paper ceases to move
   C. a buzzer sounds
   D. the paper moves more rapidly
   E. the machine adjusts the baseline
   (Bonewit-West #1, pp 445–446; Burdick, p 24)

93. Lead V3 in electrocardiography is
   A. the third limb lead
   B. the third precordial lead
   C. located on the left anterior axillary line
   D. located in the fourth intercostal space at the level of lead V4
   E. located in the fourth intercostal space to the left of the sternum
   (Bonewit-West #1, p 448; Burdick, p 12)

94. In taking an ECG, the electrode used for grounding is identified as
   A. LA
   B. RA
   C. LL
   D. RL
   E. C
   (Burdick, p 10)

95. The position of the first standard chest lead (V1) is the
   A. third intercostal space, left sternal margin
   B. third intercostal space, right sternal margin

C. fourth intercostal space, left
sternal margin

D. fourth intercostal space, right
sternal margin

E. fifth intercostal space,
midclavicular line

(Bonewit-West #1, p 449; Burdick, p 12)

96. The centering device on an
electrocardiograph

A. standardizes the ECG

B. controls the position of the baseline
of the ECG

C. aids in the placement of chest
extremity leads

D. causes the stylus to record on the
moving paper

E. aids in the placement of limb leads

(Burdick, p 21)

97. The first wave of the ECG is the

A. S wave

B. Q wave

C. P wave

D. T wave

E. R wave

(Burdick, p 6)

98. The accepted standard of deflection on an
electrocardiograph for each millivolt (mV)
of heart potential is

A. 5.0 mm

B. 10.0 mm

C. 20.0 mm

D. 100.0 mm

E. 200.0 mm

(Bonewit-West #1, p 445; Burdick, p 24)

99. In cleaning the electrodes on an electrocardiograph, a medical assistant should use

A. silver polish

B. steel wool

C. fine scouring powder

D. sandpaper

E. soap and water

(Burdick, p 38)

100. When the ECG instrument is running at
"normal" speed, the paper is passing the
stylus (or going through the machine) at
the rate of

A. 10 mm/sec

B. 20 mm/sec

C. 25 mm/sec

D. 35 mm/sec

E. 50 mm/sec

(Burdick, p 18)

101. Towel clamps have

A. sharp points

B. curved tips

C. sharp points and curved tips

D. blunt points and curved tips

E. sharp points and straight tips

(Bonewit-West #1, p 199)

102. Abbreviations, such as s/s, b/b, b/s, str, and
cvd, are used to describe

A. scissors

B. forceps

C. clamps

D. needle holders

E. scalpels

(Bonewit-West #1, p 197)

103. The parts of the hemostatic forceps located
near the ring of the handle that keep the
hemostat tightly shut are called the

A. box lock

B. serrated tips

C. ratchets

D. blade tips

E. tooth assembly

(Bonewit-West #1, pp 197–198)

104. A viewing instrument that usually is equipped with a light source is called a/an
    A. probe
    B. scope
    C. director
    D. applicator
    E. obturator
    (Frew et al, p 606; Kinn and Woods, pp 1106–1107)

105. An instrument that fits inside a scope and protrudes forward to guide the scope into the canal or body cavity is a/an
    A. applicator
    B. probe
    C. lumen
    D. director
    E. obturator
    (Frew et al, p 606)

106. Shroeder uterine tenaculum forceps have
    A. three intermeshing teeth
    B. single sharp teeth on each jaw
    C. serrations and blunt ends on jaws
    D. a curette at the end of one jaw
    E. two sharp teeth on each jaw
    (Kinn and Woods, p 1075)

107. Scissors that use a beak or hook to facilitate the removal of sutures are
    A. all-purpose scissors
    B. bandage scissors
    C. gauze scissors
    D. iris scissors
    E. stitch scissors
    (Frew et al, p 605; Kinn and Woods, p 1069)

108. The instrument used by the physician to measure the pelvis of an expectant mother to determine the probability of a normal birth is called a
    A. Martin pelvimeter
    B. Hegar uterine dilator
    C. Sims uterine curette

    D. vulsellum forceps
    E. Novak biopsy curette
    (Bonewit-West #1, p 383; Frew et al, p 609)

109. The purpose of a trocar is to
    A. dilate the cervix for examination purposes
    B. withdraw fluids from cavities
    C. remove matter from the ear canals
    D. remove sutures
    E. separate tissue from bone or cartilage
    (Frew et al, p 607; Kinn and Woods, pp 1073–1074)

110. Of the following instruments, the one that might NOT be illuminated is the
    A. ophthalmoscope
    B. anoscope
    C. sigmoidoscope
    D. proctoscope
    E. otoscope
    (Kinn and Woods, pp 607–609)

111. An instrument used for measuring intraocular tension is the
    A. tonometer
    B. ophthalmoscope
    C. Martin pelvimeter
    D. Larry probe
    E. Dix eye spud
    (Kinn and Woods, pp 563–565)

112. A medical assistant who has been asked by her physician-employer to give an eye examination using a Snellen eye chart should instruct the patient to
    A. keep one eye closed when reading the chart
    B. hold one eye closed with his or her fingers
    C. keep both eyes open during the test, covering one of them at a time
    D. keep both eyes open and uncovered during the test
    E. none of the above
    (Keir et al, pp 504–505; Zakus, p 124)

113. When administering a Snellen eye chart examination, the medical assistant
    A. stands beside the patient
    B. stands beside the chart
    C. sits beside the patient
    D. stands wherever he or she feels most comfortable
    E. sits at a desk and calls out the numbers of each line to be read by the patient

    (Keir et al, pp 567–569; Zakus, p 122)

114. The numerator (top number) of the fraction indicating the patient's results on an eye examination represents the
    A. distance of the patient from the chart
    B. lowest line read satisfactorily
    C. lowest line read with no mistakes
    D. age of the patient
    E. first line read with no more than two mistakes

    (Frew et al, p 423; Keir et al, p 504)

115. On a Snellen eye chart, the symbol on the top line can be read by persons with normal vision at
    A. 50 feet
    B. 100 feet
    C. 150 feet
    D. 200 feet
    E. 250 feet

    (Bonewit-West #1, pp 306–307; Zakus, p 121)

116. Which type of physical examination will reveal abnormalities of the female reproductive system?
    A. neurological
    B. oncological
    C. urological
    D. pelvic
    E. proctological

    (Bonewit-West #1, pp 364–369; Zakus, p 98)

117. Antibody, Rh factor, syphilis, and perhaps gonorrhea screening, cytologic smears of the cervix, glucose, and maternal-fetal alphafetoproteins are laboratory tests for what type of patient?
    A. juvenile
    B. elderly
    C. pregnant
    D. male
    E. leukemic

    (Kinn and Woods, p 642)

118. An instrument handed by the medical assistant to the surgeon must
    A. be unpacked at the moment
    B. be in the position to use without repositioning
    C. always be identified orally
    D. be flipped into his/her hand
    E. none of the above

    (Bonewit-West #1, p 228)

119. Which of the following may interfere with a mammogram?
    A. body lotions or powders
    B. a lead apron over abdomen
    C. earrings
    D. two-piece dress
    E. diet

    (Bonewit-West #1, pp 488–489)

120. The first screening in private during the patient's visit to assess needs and symptoms and to determine the next time to be seen is known as the
    A. assessment
    B. interview
    C. triage
    D. review of symptoms
    E. history

    (Keir et al, pp 468–469)

121. Which of these conditions may result from improper care of a spirometer?

    A. angina
    B. acute coronary insufficiency
    C. recent myocardial infarction
    D. coronary embolism
    E. cross-contamination and infection

    (Kinn and Woods, p 547)

122. An examination tray setup contains a wide variety of instruments and supplies such as a nasal speculum, an otoscope with oph-thalmoscope attachments, percussion hammer, tongue depressors, vaginal speculum, and tuning fork. What type of examination is anticipated?

    A. sigmoidoscopy
    B. pelvic exam and Pap smear
    C. complete physical examination
    D. rectal examination
    E. neurological examination

    (Keir, p 523; Bonewit-West #1, p 125)

123. The prefixes centi-, milli-, micro-, nano-, and pico- are all used in what system of measurements?

    A. English
    B. metric (SI)
    C. apothecary
    D. Kelvin
    E. absolute

    (Palko and Palko, p 74; Estridge et al, p 30)

124. When fitting a patient for axillary crutches, which of the following statements are correct?

    A. the patient must be in a standing position
    B. the shoulder rests should allow for two or three fingers' width between crutch top and armpit (approximately 2 inches)

C. the angle of elbow flexion should be measured with a goniometer
    D. the patient should wear shoes
    E. all of the above

    (Bonewit-West #1, pp 351–352; Kinn and Woods, pp 732–733)

125. Leads I, II, and III use two limbs for recording the electrical force of the heart. These leads are called

    A. unipolar leads
    B. standard limb leads
    C. precordial leads
    D. bipolar leads
    E. both standard limb and bipolar leads

    (Burdick, p 10)

126. Which of the following are types of artifacts that can make the interpretation of the recording difficult?

    A. wandering baseline
    B. somatic tremor
    C. alternating current
    D. baseline interruption
    E. all of the above

    (Burdick, pp 32, 33)

127. The current choice most used by medical clinics for disposing of regulated waste (disposable items containing infectious waste) is

    A. autoclaving
    B. incineration
    C. a dry heat oven
    D. gas sterilization
    E. a contract with a commercial waste service

    (Bonewit-West #1, p 21)

128. When assisting in the examination room, which of the following duties is very important in preventing the spread of disease?

    A. prepare the exam room beforehand
    B. assemble the instruments and supplies to be used
    C. wash hands between patients
    D. assist the doctor during the exam
    E. attend the patient during and after the exam

    (Bonewit-West #1, pp 5–7)

129. Which of the following examination instruments is used for holding open a body canal so that it can be examined more thoroughly?

    A. otoscope
    B. audioscope
    C. ophthalmoscope
    D. speculum
    E. sphygmomanometer

    (Bonewit-West, p 122; Taber's, p 1794)

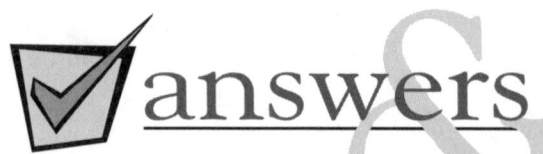

answers & rationales

1.

A. The normal axillary (armpit) temperature is 97.6°F, which is equal to 36.4°C on the Celsius scale. This is about 1°F less than the normal oral temperature. Body thermometers measure the heat produced by the body which in turn reflects the **metabolic rate** of the body. The **hypothalmic thermostat** in the brain regulates body temperature. Infections most commonly cause a rise in temperature (fever) but other causes include heat stroke, cancer, and CNS damage.

2.

D. The normal oral temperature with the thermometer placed under the tongue and with the lips held closed is 98.6°F. Temperature varies in health from 97.6°F to 99°F. It is usually lowest in early morning and highest in the evening.

Nondisposable thermometers can transmit infection if they are not properly disinfected between patients. A plastic sheath should always be used to cover a glass thermometer when taking a temperature to avoid this danger.

3.

B. The normal temperature when taken rectally is 99.6°F, or 37.5°C. The rectal temperature is the most accurate when you compare it with oral and axilla procedures; it is used in fevers when accurate temperature is of the utmost importance.

The traditional glass thermometers can be obtained with either slender tips for oral use; fat, stubby bulbs for rectal use; or a small bulb in the security thermometer. They may also be obtained with either Fahrenheit or Celsius (centigrade) scales. The oral thermometer should never be used rectally because of the danger of piercing the tissues or breaking.

4.

B. When converting a temperature reading on the Fahrenheit scale to a Celsius (centigrade) temperature, this formula is used:

$$C = (F - 32) \times 5/9$$

Conversely, to convert from a Celsius reading to Fahrenheit, the following formula would be used:

$$F = (C \times 9/5) + 32$$

In this particular example, the calculation would appear as follows:

$$C = (102.0°F - 32) \times 5/9$$
$$C = 38.9°C$$

5.

B. A standard oral thermometer should be kept in the mouth under the tongue, with the lips closed, for 3 minutes. A similar time period is required for a rectal temperature reading. The axillary (armpit) reading requires a much longer period (10 minutes). The reason for the time variations is that the rectum and mouth are enclosed cavities with a plentiful supply of surface blood vessels to warm the area quickly. The armpit, in contrast, is not enclosed and does not have surface blood vessels to warm the area. Because the axillary temperature is not as accurate as the oral or rectal temperatures, the axillary site is used only when the oral and rectal sites are contraindicated.

Thermometers should register 96°F or lower before they are used.

6.

C. CLIA '88 (Clinical Laboratory Improvement Amendments of 1988) apply to laboratories that test for disease prevention, diagnosis, or treatment of humans. All clinical laboratories are assigned to a test category according to their test complexity. The lowest level, waived tests, includes simple, stable tests that require little interpretation. The next level, moderate complexity, includes most clinical tests. The moderate complexity level requires proficiency testing, qualified personnel, and adequate record keeping to ensure documentation of adequate quality control and quality assurance. Proficiency testing requires testing of unknowns in the laboratory and submission to a designated agency that judges the tests' accuracy. The proficiency tests are performed three times per year.

7.

B. Lying in a supine position, the patient is able to enclose the thermometer by keeping an arm close to the side of the body and grasping the shoulder with the hand. The patient may also follow these directions while in a sitting position. To prepare the patient for an axillary temperature, the medical assistant should wipe the axilla with a soft, dry cloth or with absorbent cotton to remove moisture.

8.

B. The normal pulse rate for adults ranges from 60 to 90 pulsations per minute. The pulse rate is affected by the individual's activities and illnesses. The pulse is taken with the patient sitting or lying down, with the artery that is used for taking the pulse at the same level or lower than the heart.

9.

C. The normal pulse rate, or average number of pulsations per minute, for children between the ages of 1 and 7 years is 80 to 120. The faster pulse rate of children and infants helps to compensate for greater heat loss from their smaller bodies.

10.

E. At birth, an infant's pulse may range from 130 to 160 pulsations per minute, which is the fastest normal rate of a person's lifetime. It will decrease in rate until adulthood and then level off.

11.

A. The pulse rate is the average number of pulsations (expansion and relaxation of the arteries) that occur in 1 minute, and normally this is the same as the heartbeat (constriction and relaxation of the heart muscle). The pulse may vary according to age, sex, and condition of the patient.

12.

B. Bradycardia indicates an abnormally slow pulse. The pulse may be irregular in either its timing or its intensity. If the pulse rate is less than 60 pulsations per minute and regular, it is called a bradycardia; if it is greater than 100, it is called a tachycardia.

13.

A. The radial artery extends down the forearm through the wrist and may be pressed against the bones of the wrist and the arm. The pulse in the radial artery is the easiest location for most people to find and is, therefore, the most common site for taking the patient's pulse.

Another site for taking pulse is the carotid artery located in the neck. The temporal artery, in front of the ear on the side of the forehead, also is used frequently when the arms or hands are injured. The site where the pulse is taken should be noted if it is a site other than the radial artery.

14.

A. An elevated temperature will usually increase a patient's pulse rate. Other causes of increased pulse rate may include pain, shock, certain drugs, exercise, and hyperthyroidism. Pulse rates will decrease during sleep or rest, after brain injuries, as a result of hypothyroidism, and with certain drugs, such as digitalis.

15.

B. The preferred method for counting the pulsations is to count for 1 full minute rather than to count for 30 seconds and double the sum. The longer the pulse is taken, the better the chances of detecting pulse irregularities.

16.

C. The normal rate of respiration in adults is approximately 14 to 20 breaths per minute, lower than that of children (18 to 30 breaths per minute). One complete respiration includes inhalation, which is the taking of oxygen into the lungs, and exhalation, which is the release of carbon dioxide from the body. The respiration rate is usually in proportion to the pulse rate, one complete respiration with every four pulse beats (1:4).

17.

E. The normal rate of respiration for infants is approximately 30 to 60 breaths per minute. The respiration rate and pulse rate will rise as the body temperature rises. Note that similar to pulse, respiration slows as the individual ages, leveling off in adulthood. The respiration rate for children may range from about 18 to 30 breaths per minute. Important variations to observe when checking a person's respiration are rate (fast or slow), volume (deep or shallow), and rhythm (regular or irregular).

18.

C. Aside from sleep, several other factors may result in a decreased respiration rate (e.g., drugs, such as morphine or opium). The respiration rate may fall as low as 1 or 2 breaths per minute in cases of overdose. All of the other four answer choices would cause respiration to increase.

19.

C. A patient who suffers with orthopnea must either sit up or stand up to breathe. Patients who exhibit this type of condition often find it more comfortable to lean slightly forward. It also helps to rest their arms or shoulders on a support. Dyspnea is a word meaning difficult breathing. "Dys-" is a prefix meaning bad, difficult, or painful. The suffix "-pnea" means to breathe. The patient with dyspnea may become cyanotic from lack of oxygen.

20.

A. Cheyne-Stokes is a form of respiration usually found in patients with diseases of the kidneys and heart and in those with such conditions as brain injury, coma, and meningitis. In one type of Cheyne-Stokes respiration, the patient's breathing increases in rapidity and then decreases, followed by a pause before beginning again. In another type, the rate of breathing increases to a pausing point and then begins again.

21.

C. Hypertension usually is regarded as systolic pressure higher than 160 mm or diastolic pressure higher than 95 mm. These values were established by the World Health Organization. Hypertension for which no detectable cause can be diagnosed is called essential (or idiopathic) hypertension.

22.

E. The Trendelenburg position is used in cases of shock, in some abdominal surgery, and for patients with low blood pressure. The patient lies with legs or knees elevated and the head lower than the knees to increase circulation to the head.

23.

A. The lithotomy position is used for patients who are to be examined vaginally. This position is sometimes called the stirrups position, dorsosacral position, or dorsal recumbent position with knees flexed. This position is also used for cystoscope examinations.

24.

B. The Sims position is used for flexible sigmoidoscopic examinations because it is more comfortable. The alternative proctologic position requires the use of an examining table that can be elevated and tilted in the center and lowered at the head and legs. (The sigmoidoscope derives its name from the fact it is used to examine the colon, which is considered to have an "S" shape. (Sigmoid means shaped like the letter "s," actually the Greek letter sigma and scope = light.)

25.

B. In the dorsal (back) recumbent (reclining) position, the patient lies on the back with the legs sharply flexed at the knees. The soles of the feet are placed flat on the table. In the supine position, the legs are only slightly flexed at the knees.

26.

D. While important, the patient's clothing is a separate consideration. The possibility that clothing may interfere with the surgery requires thought. It may become stained, be in the way for the surgery team, be uncomfortable for the patient, act as a tourniquet on the body, or contaminate the site.

Positioning the patient for surgery also requires forethought. The comfort of the patient in one position for an extended time may be limited. Will he eventually become tired and have to move during surgery? Will the bandage fit properly when the patient returns to a normal position? Can you and the physician work comfortably with the patient's position? Are the instruments and supplies accessible?

27.

C. Percussion means the listening to sounds produced when the body is struck in a particular manner. The fingertips are used to tap the body lightly but sharply to determine the position, size, and consistency of an underlying structure. The presence of pus or fluid in a cavity can be diagnosed in this manner.

28.

E. The prefix "brady-" means slowness. A pulse rate below 60 pulsations/min usually is considered bradycardia. The word extrasystole means "extra contraction," but it causes the person to have the sensation of a skipped beat. The prefix "tachy-" means rapid, and the suffix "-cardia" refers to the heart. A pulse rate in excess of 90 pulsations/min is termed tachycardia. Pulse volume refers to strength of the heartbeat and the volume of blood pumped. A thready pulse, which is usually also rapid, is weak and hard to distinguish.

29.

D. Age has an inverse ratio to the pulse. Newborn infants have a pulse range of about 130 to 160, decreasing through adulthood with aging to a normal range of 60 to 90. Physical exercise, strong emotions, and increased metabolism, such as in pregnancy and fevers, increase the pulse beat.

30.

E. Some medications and chemicals depress the pulse rate, whereas others increase the pulse rate, and still others may cause a bounding pulse. Therefore, the specific chemical must be known to predict the reaction. Two drugs that affect the pulse rate are digitalis, which decreases the pulse rate and is used to treat arrhythmias, and atropine, which increases the pulse rate. A high blood calcium level increases the pulse rate.

31.

D. The apical pulse is taken with a stethoscope placed over the apex of the heart, which is below the left nipple. It is always taken on children younger than the age of 2 and on all patients with potential or known heart problems. It may also be taken when the pulse is difficult to obtain at the other usual sites.

32.

B. The diameter of the limb where the blood pressure is taken determines the size of cuff, since the cuff should be 20% greater than the diameter of the limb. The cuff comes in three sizes: pediatric, adult, and thigh. The thigh cuff is used for taking blood pressure from the thigh or from the arms of large adults, whereas pediatric cuffs are for children and very small adults. A too small cuff used on a large arm may cause a falsely elevated reading.

The blood pressure apparatus (sphygmomanometer) comes in 3 basic types: (1) the mercury column, (2) the anaeroid dial, and (3) the computerized models for home use. They must be recalibrated regularly to keep the reading accurate. The action of the blood pressure apparatus is to obliterate the arterial pressure of the arm in the same manner as a tourniquet. Then while the MA listens through a stethoscope the pressure is gradually released until sound is no longer heard. The beginning of the sound is the systolic pressure; the end is the diastolic pressure. The sounds in between are divided into five phases known as Korotkoff sounds. Blood pressure above normal produces hypertension; those below normal, hypotension.

33.

C. These measurements of body dimensions, an indication of general health, are monitored closely when they indicate important changes in the conditions of certain patients. A quick weight gain in a maternity patient may indicate fluid retention. In children, unusual growth patterns might indicate hormonal disturbances. A large increase in the head size of an infant would indicate hydrocephalus. The term, anthropometric, means reading from right to left, literally, measurement of man.

34.

A. The patient's general medical history, including allergies, demographic data, family history, past illnesses, lifestyle, and assessment of basic body systems, should be obtained at the first office visit so that it will be available thereafter for diagnosis and treatment. The patient interview should be conducted in a private area, probably an examination room, where patient confidentiality and privacy are protected.

35.

D. The term "asepsis" means that there are no pathogens (disease-causing microorganisms) on a surface or area, and it is free from infection. To maintain a surface free of pathogens, the nature of microorganisms and their life needs must be understood. Heterotrophs are organisms that use organic or living substances for food (e.g., bacteria that live in the body), whereas autotrophs use inorganic and nonliving substances (e.g., some soil bacteria). Optimum growth temperature at which a microorganism grows best is usually about 98.6°F (body temperature). Most microorganisms prefer a neutral pH (around 7.0 and similar to our bodies), neither too acid nor too basic.

36.

B. The wearing of ornate jewelry may transmit pathogens if they are harbored in the grooves and crevices of the jewelry. A medical assistant should always be alert to the possibility of disease transmission from one patient to another through fomites (objects that carry disease organisms).

37.

C. An organism that is infected with a pathogen (disease-carrying microorganism) and infects others is a reservoir host. Strep throat is sometimes transmitted by persons who do not show symptoms of an active streptococcal infection. Hepatitis, AIDS, and many other diseases are transmitted through reservoir hosts who may not show evidence of the illness. Other mammals, birds, insects, and lower life forms may also serve as reservoir hosts for microorganisms that cause disease in humans.

38.

E. Accidental needle sticks pose the greatest risk to health workers from occupational exposure. However, only 52 health care workers out of nearly 7 million have been documented as acquiring HIV through occupational exposure prior to 1997. Nevertheless, all health care personnel should follow Universal Precautions guidelines to protect themselves and others and prevent the spread of this virus and other disease. Because HIV lives within white blood cells (WBCs), any type of body fluid or tissue that might contain WBCs must be treated as contaminated. Every patient should be regarded as a potential HIV carrier rather than limiting the Universal Precautions to only known risks. Personal protective equipment, barrier devices, and an effective disinfection routine should be used. Needle sticks can be avoided. Do not recap or remove a used needle from a syringe but instead dispose of promptly into a sharps container. If removal is necessary, use clamps to keep the needle at a safe distance. Also give necessary working space to another employee who is drawing blood, disposing of needles or hazardous waste, or handling body tissue. By not crowding the worker, you will prevent being accidentally stuck or contaminated. Hepatitis B is also a blood-borne pathogen transmitted in much the same way as HIV. Every health worker should keep abreast of current developments in safety techniques and health education.

39.

E. Diathermy is a treatment that creates heat within tissues by converting short-wave, high-frequency electric energy into heat. It increases the blood circulation to the treated tissue, which, in turn, increases healing in many cases.

40.

C. Infrared radiation lamps will produce surface heat that penetrates the skin to a depth of 5 mm. Ultraviolet radiation treatments produce rays that penetrate to a depth of less than 0.1 mm. Heating pads and hot water bottles are examples of other dry heat treatments.

41.

C. Whirlpool baths are used in hydrotherapy. Also used are hot and cold showers, hot and cold wet compresses, contrast baths, or ice packs. The whirlpool provides heat to the immersed body parts along with a gentle massage action.

42.

D. A medical assistant aiding a patient who requires short-wave diathermy should be certain the area to be treated is exposed and examined for reactive areas, which would indicate that treatment should not be given there, such as inflamed areas or breaks, and any metal, including metal implants. (Metal becomes hot.) A towel should be placed over the patient between the skin and the electrode. This aids in preventing excessive perspiration, which would cause a steam blister.

43.

B. Flexion is the act of bending or being bent. The purpose of a cast is just the opposite—to immobilize the injured body part to allow it to heal. A fracture is the most common cause for a cast but it also may be used to correct deformities or to promote healing after surgery. Several types of casts are now in use but the two main categories are plaster and synthetic. Each type has its advantages. Plaster casts mold better to the body part so the injured body part is immobilized more securely. They are less expensive and smoother, less-ening the chance of hands or clothes being scratched.

Synthetic casts dry and set more quickly. They weigh less and are less bulky than plaster. Synthetic casts are also more moisture resistant.

The medical assistant assists the physician in applying casts and may educate the patient in the use and care of the cast.

44.

E. The formation of prothrombin, the clotting agent of the blood, is the primary function of vitamin K. The major source of vitamin K for the body is synthesized by the bacteria of the intestine. They supply about one-half to two-thirds of our vitamin K needs. The rest comes from food sources, such as green leafy vegetables and organ meats.

45.

C. Exposure to sunlight is considered an adequate source of vitamin D for most adults. (In some cases such as osteoporosis, additional Vitamin D may be prescribed.) Vitamin D is necessary for metabolism of calcium and phosphorus in normal nourishment and in the formation of bones and teeth. Rickets is a disease condition found especially in infants and children resulting from a deficiency of vitamin D.

46.

B. Ascorbic acid is another name for vitamin C. Vitamin C is necessary for proper wound healing, and it promotes resistance to bacterial infection. Prolonged lack of vitamin C in the diet will cause the disease scurvy, with irreversible skeletal malformations.

47.

B. The three Ds—dermatitis, dementia, diarrhea—are characteristic of pellagra. Pellagra is a disease that results from a deficiency of niacin. Niacin is one of the B vitamins and is formed from tryptophan, an essential amino acid that comes from meat and other complete sources of protein.

48.

B. The fetal period follows the embryonic period and extends from the third month to the end of the ninth month of pregnancy. During the first 8 weeks of pregnancy, the structure is called an embryo. Growth and development of the systems occur during the fetal period. (Authors may vary slightly on the period of time assigned to the embryonic stage.)

49.

D. Sickle-cell anemia is a hereditary chronic form of anemia caused by the formation of abnormal sickle or crescent-shaped erythrocytes or red blood cells (RBCs) in the bone marrow. The RBCs contain an abnormal type of hemoglobin known as "hemoglobin S." The frequency of the gene that causes sickle-cell disease is high in the African American population in the United States.

50.

C. Chronic diseases run their course over long periods of time (e.g., months, years). The word "chronic" is used to describe a disease that shows little change or a slow progression. Chronic means the opposite of acute. This term is used often in patient histories.

51.

E. A differential diagnosis is used when several diagnoses are possible. The most likely diagnosis is listed first, along with other alternatives. These various possible diagnoses are analyzed by comparing and contrasting all symptoms, signs, objective clinical findings, and laboratory test results to reach a primary or definitive diagnosis. A secondary diagnosis is a second health problem or condition that is less serious than the primary diagnosis.

52.

A. The etiologic agent is the pathogen that causes the disease and may be a virus, bacteria, protozoa, fungus, or larger microscopic parasite.

A study of the causes of disease is etiology. The suffix "-logy" means "the study of." The other two possible choices with the suffix "-logy" are the term embryology, which means the study of the embryo, and the term histology, which means the study of the microscopic structures of tissue.

53.

D. The word "pathogen" means something capable of producing a disease ("path-," disease; "-gen," creation). The other possible answers refer to conditions of a disease.

54.

A. Diagnosis based on the patient's history and the physical examination without the benefit of diagnostic tests, such as laboratory or radiology results, is known as a clinical diagnosis. The term 'diagnosis' alone often means the final diagnosis.

55.

C. A sterile surface must be provided for the remaining sterile items to be placed. The pack, which has a large wrapper whose inside surface will serve as a sterile base, is opened, inside sterile side up. The preparation for surgery must proceed in a step by step logical manner so that one is not "painted in a corner" so to speak. The first step in preparing a surgery set up is generally to read the indexed cards in the surgery file which describe the individual surgery set ups and procedures. Items, which are necessary but not sterile such as the anesthesia, are placed on an adjacent stand or table.

56.

D. When a disease increases in severity after displaying an improvement or a regular course, it has exacerbated. This is sometimes referred to as the aggravation of symptoms.

57.

A. Rash diseases, or exanthemas, involve illnesses, such as measles, chickenpox, or scarlet fever. Exanthemas refer to any eruptions of the skin that is accompanied by inflammation. (Exanthema is Greek for eruption.)

58.

D. Mensuration is a procedure of measuring as done in chest expansion as part of the physical examination of male patients. The procedure includes measuring the chest at the nipple line once with the chest cavity completely inflated and once completely deflated.

59.

D. Sterilization is the complete destruction of all forms of microbial life. There is no such thing as partial sterilization. Sanitization means to make something clean, not to destroy all microbes or bacteria. Disinfection is to free from the presence of disease-causing organisms (pathogens). Surgical instruments must be sterile because they penetrate into the body past the defenses of the skin. How the equipment will be used determines what method must be used.

60.

B. Disinfecting agents include chemical germicides, flowing steam, and boiling water.

61.

C. Methods of sterilization include dry heat, moderately heated chemical-gas mixtures, and saturated steam under pressure (autoclaves). Dry heat, moderately heated chemical-gas mixtures, and chemical agents are limited to certain applications and require longer exposure to achieve sterile conditions. Therefore, they are not usually the method of choice unless the article cannot withstand autoclaving.

62.

C. When hands are scrubbed for surgery, the hands are held **UP** to prevent water (and microbes) from the arms from running back onto the hands and contaminating them. Before scrubbing a file is used to clean the nails. The hands are scrubbed, with surgical soap and a sterile brush with attention given to the fingernails. After washing the hands are dried with a sterile towel with the hands still held above the waist. This surgical hand scrubbing contrasts with medical aseptic hand washing where the hands are held below the waist, not washed as long or thoroughly, and water is allowed to run off the arms. In the case of medical asepsis, the hands may be dried with a nonsterile paper towel.

63.

A. Hinged, handled instruments must always be opened when they are sterilized. It is important to have plenty of space between items being prepared for the autoclave so steam can circulate around all items.

64.

E. All of these wheelchair practices should be followed to avoid falls. The wheels must be locked when entering and leaving. The footrests must be folded out of the way when not being used to avoid tripping over them. The patient's body should be supported with the arms while getting in and out of the chair. The unaffected foot (if there is one) will help to support the body when leaving the chair. Most patients acquire wheelchair skills with practice.

65.

C. A rectal examination tray setup will include a rubber glove or finger cot, lubricant such as K-Y jelly, a rectal speculum or anoscope, cotton-tipped applicators, and probably a fecal occult blood kit. The rectal examination can give information such as the presence of polyps, early cancer, lesions, inflammatory conditions, and hemorrhoids. In addition, the exam can give information about the adjacent organs—the uterus in the female and the prostate gland in the male. Masses in the rectum or pelvic region and displacement of the uterus can be detected. In the male, the enlargement and texture of the prostate gland can be noted. The medical assistant may be expected to hand the physician the various instruments and supplies as needed and perhaps hold the light. If the anoscope is used, it will be lubricated. Other procedures such as cultures will be carried out if needed. After the exam, the patient is assisted as needed and given needed instructions. After the patient leaves, the medical assistant disposes of used equipment and supplies according to Universal Precautions guidelines, and takes care of all specimens and cultures according to policy. The exam table and room are cleaned and a fresh exam table cover and clean equipment furnished for the next patient.

66.

A. It is not necessary to use either forceps or gloves for dry wrapped items. Instruments that are sterilized without wrapping must be handled with sterile forceps or sterile gloves.

67.

C. The exposure period is timed beginning when an adequate temperature has been reached as opposed to a particular pressure. The proper operating temperature of the autoclave is 250°F (121°C).

68.

C. It is necessary for the medical assistant to properly position materials in the autoclave so that steam comes in contact with all surfaces. Materials and surrounding walls should be separated by 1 to 3 inches to allow for adequate steam penetration. During the sterilization process, all trapped air should flow out and be replaced by steam.

69.

D. Instruments and supplies may be safely disinfected with germicidal solution if they are used on the outer skin or if they are inserted into body orifices that do not bypass the body's natural defenses. However, there is a growing tendency to use disposable items for these procedures if they are available.

70.

E. When the medical assistant is scheduling a preop appointment, it is important that the patient understand the following facts about the procedure: (1) the approximate length of time required for the procedure; (2) the appropriate type of clothing to wear to the appointment; (3) the need to arrange for someone to accompany him or her; (4) the anticipated time to take off from work after surgery; and (5) the need for home care during the recovery period. In addition to these, it may be important to advise the patient about the amount of time that he/she must fast before the scheduled appointment.

71.

B. The three methods represent different levels of decontamination and often are used jointly. Sanitation is the process of cleaning items of all organic matter and dirt. Disinfection will destroy most infectious microorganisms but not all spore-forming bacteria or viruses such as those associated with infectious hepatitis. Sterilization results in complete destruction of all microbes.

72.

E. Because an article cannot be partially sterile, it is either sterile or contaminated (nonsterile). There is no in-between.

73.

E. All of the above principles help to maintain sterility in a surgical environment. You should also study other rules from a suitable textbook. In general, any object that has not been sterilized should not come near the sterile field or be passed over it. This includes air currents as well as ungloved hands, clothes, and so on. Sterile objects may not be taken out of the field and returned because they may be contaminated. Anything lower than the sterile field is considered nonsterile, so the hands or instruments must not drop below the waist. Moisture can conduct pathogens from one layer to another so wet objects must be considered contaminated and nonsterile. Sterile objects must remain dry. Five basic rules are (1) know what is sterile, (2) know what is not sterile, (3) keep sterile and nonsterile objects separated, (4) prevent contamination, and (5) remedy a contaminated situation immediately.

74.

E. All of the answers given will result in incomplete sterilization. It is also important that the correct sterilizing temperature of 250°F (121°C) be maintained throughout the entire cycle.

75.

E. All of the materials listed are used for autoclave wrappings. The wrapping material must permit steam to penetrate it while it keeps out contaminants during the period of storage. In addition to the four materials listed, there are rigid containers available for autoclaving use. These are expensive but are reusable. All materials should be approved specifically for autoclave use.

76.

B. The most widely used disinfectant is alcohol, usually a 70% solution. Isopropyl alcohol is replacing ethyl alcohol because it exhibits slightly greater germicidal action. Chlorohexaphene is replacing hexachlorophene in germicidal soap because hexachlorophene is completely soluble only in alcohol.

77.

D. These instruments must be sterilized because they penetrate the tissues of the patient. These instruments could be sterilized with dry heat, which does not rust the cutting edges, but it would greatly increase the time required for sterilization. Microorganisms and spores are more resistant to dry heat than to moist heat because it penetrates more slowly and unevenly.

78.

B. Strong abrasives, which would scratch the surface, should never be used in cleaning an autoclave. A commercial solution designed for autoclave cleaning should be used in cleaning the chamber, and then it should be rinsed thoroughly with clean, soft water. The chamber should be dried and the door left open.

79.

E. Most male doctors prefer that the medical assistant remain in the examination room to assist them and as a precaution against the possibility of charges that they acted improperly toward female patients. The other selections are guidelines. A general outline of medical assistant duties for a physical examination follows: Wash your hands before preparing the instruments and supplies to prevent the spread of pathogens. Next cover the examination table with clean covers. The patient is then assisted and positioned on the table. During the exam, the medical assistant observes the patient for various reactions such as pain or discomfort, and gives needed instructions and patient education afterwards. Specimens after collection are generally the responsibility of the medical assistant. The medical assistant may also be responsible for recording certain medical information. The used instruments and supplies should be placed in cleaning solution to be later sterilized or disposed of according to Universal Precaution guidelines. After the patient is assisted off the exam table and leaves, the exam room is cleaned and prepared for the next patient.

80.

A. The intramuscular injection is probably the easiest, safest, and best tolerated by patients. There is a better blood supply in muscular tissue than in subcutaneous tissue, and there is no danger of an unabsorbed accumulation of drugs. The intravenous injection is the most dangerous type of injection.

81.

A. Large doses of drugs, in amounts of 2 mL or more, are given intramuscularly. If the volume of dosage ordered is 3 to 5 mL, it should be divided and injected into two or more sites. Unabsorbed medicines can cause damage to the tissues.

82.

A. Weight and height are not included in the list known as vital signs. The vital signs (also called cardinal signs) include temperature, pulse, blood pressure, and respiration (abbreviated TPR for temperature, pulse, respiration and BP for blood pressure). Medical assistants must realize that accurately measured vital signs can tell much about the health or diseased condition of a patient.

83.

A. Standard limb lead I records the voltage through the heart from right arm to left arm. Lead II records voltage traveling down through the long axis of the heart from right arm to left leg. Lead III records voltage from left arm to left leg.

84.

E. The augmented lead AVF records the voltage through the heart from a midpoint between right arm and left arm to left leg. The AVR measures the midpoint between left arm and left leg to right arm. The AVL records an electrical current that is midpoint between right arm and left leg to left arm.

85.

C. When a medical assistant is doing an electrocardiogram (ECG) on a patient who has had an entire arm amputated, the electrode (sensor) is placed on the torso with tape or a Welsh self-retaining bulb. The other limb lead electrode (sensor) should be placed in the same manner on the torso opposite the first so that the triangle is retained. The electric vector will not be changed, and the results will not be affected.

86.

E. The code representing lead VI in the taking of ECGs is one dash and one dot. This is part of a code initiated by the Southern Association of Cardiology Technicians and has met with wide acceptance.

87.

B. Leads I, II, and III require the use of two arms and one leg. The left leg along with the right arm and left arm make up the triangle, which is called Einthoven's triangle.

88.

D. The wearing of jewelry or watches by patients who are having an ECG should have no bearing on the effectiveness of the recording. Jewelry will not affect an ECG unless it actually interferes with the placement of sensors or if the jewelry comes in contact with the electrolyte gel.

89.

B. The cardiac stress test is not performed for the purpose of causing cardiac arrest. (Cardiac arrest, where the heartbeat stops, causes immediate death if not reversed by cardiopulmonary resuscitation.) The cardiac stress test is performed to increase physical exertion to a point known as "target heart rate," where a deficiency of blood supply to the heart appears. All of the other choices are important aspects of the stress test.

90.

E. Improper grounding of the electrocardiograph will produce an alternating current artifact, not a wandering baseline. Corroded or dirty electrodes as well as electrodes that are too tight or too loose can cause the baseline to wander. Unequal amounts of electrolyte or lotions, body creams, or oils on the skin in the area of the electrode can cause the baseline to wander.

91.

C. An electrocardiograph lead designated as AVR is a type of unipolar lead. The other unipolar leads are AVL, AVF, and V. AVR, AVL, and AVF leads all visualize the heart from a frontal view, top to bottom. The V leads give us a third dimension, from front to rear, the horizontal plane.

92.

A. When the standardization button is pressed on an electrocardiograph, the 1-mV (one millivolt) signal is connected to the machine and causes a deflection upward on the graph paper. The ECG instrument must be standardized each time so that an ECG taken at one time on a patient can be compared to another made at a different time.

93.

B. Lead V3 in electrocardiography is the third precordial lead. The precordial, or chest, leads are identified as lead V1 through lead V6.

94.

D. RL is the lead wire connected to the right leg, and its purpose is to ground the patient. The RL lead is also called the "reference electrode," and it is necessary for proper operation of the instrument.

95.

D. The position of the first standard chest lead is the fourth intercostal space, right sternal margin. The position of the second standard chest lead is the fourth intercostal space at the left margin of the sternum.

96.

B. The centering device on an electrocardiograph controls the position of the baseline of the ECG. With most tracings, the centerline should be kept near the center of the page.

97.

C. The first wave of the ECG is the P wave. It is during this period that the auricles contract. This is also known as "atrial depolarization." The QRS complex represents ventricular depolarization. The T wave represents the repolarization of the ventricles.

98.

B. The accepted standard of deflection on an electrocardiograph for each millivolt of heart potential is 10.0 mm. This standard is accepted throughout the world.

99.

C. A medical assistant should be certain that the electrodes are not corroded. If cleaning is necessary, he or she should use a stiff brush and fine scouring powder. Silver polish or steel wool should not be used.

100.

C. The internationally accepted speed to run the ECG instrument is 25 mm/sec. This is known as "normal." The ECG is recorded at 50 mm/sec when the heart rate is too rapid or when certain segments of a complex are too close together to read clearly. This extends the recording to twice its normal width.

101.

C. Towel clamps have sharp points, which may be used to hold a sterile towel to the edge of an incision. The curved tips allow the clamps to hang freely without obstructing the physician's line of vision.

102.

A. The letters "str" means straight blades, and "cvd" refers to curved blades on scissors. The type of blade tip on scissors is indicated by s/s where both blades are sharp and b/b where both are blunt. The letters b/s mean one is blunt and one is sharp.

103.

C. The toothed clasps on the handle are known as ratchets. The ratchets keep the instrument tightly shut when it is closed. The hinge joint of the two parts of forceps or scissors is known as a box lock.

104.

B. The term "scope" indicates a viewing instrument that is equipped with a light source. Scopes are especially useful to physicians to see into dark cavities of the body. Examples of some of the scopes commonly used in physicians' offices are the sigmoidoscope, proctoscope, otoscope, ophthalmoscope, and microscope.

105.

E. The obturator is an instrument that fits inside a scope to close the lumen and guide the scope into the canal or body cavity. Obturators also may be used to puncture tissue for insertion. After the instrument is in place, the obturator (stylet) may be withdrawn to allow other instruments to pass through.

106.

B. Schroeder uterine tenaculum forceps contain single sharp teeth on each jaw. Schroeder uterine vulsellum forceps, which are also used for holding tissue, contain two sharp teeth on each jaw.

107.

E. Stitch scissors contain a hook or beak on one of the jaws to get under and to cut a suture when the wound is sufficiently healed.

108.

A. By using a Martin pelvimeter to measure the female pelvis, a physician can determine whether a baby can pass through the birth canal or whether a Caesarean section should be anticipated.

109.

B. A trocar, which is used to withdraw fluids from cavities, consists of a cannula (outer tube) and a sharp, pointed stylette (obturator). The stylette is withdrawn after the trocar is inserted.

110.

B. An anoscope may not be illuminated because of its shorter length as compared with a proctoscope or a sigmoidoscope. An anoscope may be approximately 3.5 inches (8.9 cm) in length. This length permits examination of the anal area and lower rectum.

111.

A. A tonometer is used to measure intraocular tension (pressure), and it is particularly helpful in identifying glaucoma. The instrument is expensive and very delicate and requires special care.

112.

C. Even though only one eye is tested at a time, both eyes should be kept open during a test. One eye would be covered with an eye occluder or a piece of cardboard. Do not have the patient use fingers to hold the eye closed for two reasons: (1) the fingers may not be clean; and (2) applied pressure will affect visual acuity of that eye when it is tested.

113.

B. A medical assistant should stand beside the chart so that he or she may point to the lines to be read by the patient. The chart should be illuminated with maximum light without glare on the chart. It should be at the patient's eye level.

114.

A. The numerator (top number) represents the distance of the patient from the eye chart, whereas the denominator (bottom number) represents the lowest line read satisfactorily by the patient. The initials OD means "right eye," OS means "left eye," and OU means "both eyes."

115.

D. Persons with normal vision can read the symbol on the top line of a Snellen eye chart (for distance vision) at a distance of 200 feet. The symbols on the second line can be read at 100 feet, and the bottom line can be read at 10 feet. Patients who are unable to read even the top letter of the Snellen chart are tested further to see how well, if at all, they distinguish light. If they can see well enough to count fingers (C.F.) or perceive light without seeing the fingers (L.P.) or see no light at all (N.L.P.), this is also recorded. Patients are blind when they cannot perceive light and are legally blind when their vision is less than 20/200 in both eyes when wearing correction glasses.

On the left side beside each set of letters is found a set of two numbers separated by a line to form a fraction. The top number indicates the distance the patient must stand from the chart. The bottom is the distance from the chart required by a normal person to read the chart.

Near vision, which often is a problem for the elderly (presbyopia), is tested by having the patient read a piece of paper with different sizes of print.

116.

D. A pelvic examination with a Papanicolaou (Pap) smear will reveal abnormalities of the female reproductive system. The Pap smear is used to detect precancerous conditions, unusual cell growths, and cancer of the cervix or uterus. The physician inspects the vulva, vagina, cervix, and palpates of the uterus, fallopian tubes, and ovaries. Condition of the organs is noted, including any masses, or other abnormality.

The medical assistant washes his or her hands first, as in any procedure, to prevent transfer of contagious disease, then assembles the needed instruments and supplies and prepares the room. The patient is given pre-exam instructions, which include emptying her bladder. Other pre-exam procedures include taking the patient's blood pressure and pulse, and providing a gown. Later she is positioned on the table in the manner specified, usually the lithotomy position.

The medical assistant assists the doctor with the instruments, supplies, and light, and observes the patient's reactions. Afterwards the medical assistant labels and processes the Pap smear and any other collections. The patient is assisted off the table and given instructions. The used instruments and supplies are cared for according to Universal Precaution guidelines. Last, the exam room is cleaned and prepared for the next patient.

117.

C. The pregnant patient may require in the first trimester of pregnancy these and other tests: antibody screening, Rh factor, syphilis and perhaps gonorrhea tests, cytologic smears of the cervix, glucose, and maternal-fetal alphafetoproteins. In addition, other care includes a pelvic examination with pelvimetry (measuring of the pelvis bone structure) to check for normal birth canal capacity. The estimated date of confinement (EDC) is calculated at this time. Consent forms regarding hospital confinement for the birth are signed. Appointments are scheduled regularly throughout the pregnancy. The patient is educated regarding suitable diet, exercise, rest, and bowel functions. She is cautioned against the harmful effects of alcohol, tobacco, and drugs. Teratogenicity is a term that describes a drug's potential to cause birth defects.

Symptoms such as nausea, vomiting, dizziness, swelling of limbs, and vaginal bleeding are monitored and brought to the doctor's attention. Care in the second trimester (15–28 weeks) will include abdominal palpation and fetal heart monitoring. During the third trimester (28th week to delivery), the patient and fetus are closely monitored. Childbirth preparation classes may be started. Labor, which ends the third trimester, has three stages (1) onset of labor to complete dilation of the cervix, (2) complete dilation of the cervix to birth of the fetus, and (3) from birth of fetus to expulsion of the placenta and membranes.

118.

B. Any instrument handed the physician should be in a functional position that is usable without having to reposition it. Whether it is identified orally is a matter of preference by the physician. The instrument will be already on a sterile field if its use is anticipated. It should be placed in his hand in a firm manner and not released until he has grasped it.

119.

A. The patient having a mammogram to detect breast tumors should NOT wear body lotions or powders. They tend to obscure details of the breast tissue on the x-ray. A two-piece dress is convenient for the patient since she will need to undress to the waist. A lead apron may be used to provide extra protection for the lower abdomen. The mammogram, a specialized type of x-ray, detects breast tumors much earlier than other methods. The medical assistant may offer the patient instructions regarding monthly self-examination of her breasts for lumps. Most breast tumors are discovered by the women, themselves.

120.

C. Triage is the term used to describe the initial screening in private of patients and the assessment of their needs. The term originated in wartime when injured soldiers were assessed as to the seriousness of their injuries and where to send them for treatment. Triage is the sorting out and classification of patients to determine priority of need and proper place of treatment. Phone triage refers to sorting patients' requests over the phone and scheduling them according to their need. The rules of prioritizing should follow the rules of first aid. The instructions concerning triaging should be written down as office policy, especially if the office handles emergencies.

121.

E. Because the danger of infection transferring from one patient to another exists, the spirometer must be disinfected after each patient. All parts must be cleaned according to instructions.

Spirometry measures vital capacity of the lungs (the greatest amount of air that can be expelled during a complete but unforced expiration following a maximum inspiration). Vital capacity aids in diagnosing functional and obstructive abnormalities that affect breathing (dyspnea). Patients should be advised not to eat a heavy meal or smoke for 6 hours before the test. Several conditions do not allow the extra stress of forced breathing. Among these are acute conditions affecting the heart.

122.

C. The wide variety of instruments indicates that a complete physical exam is anticipated. The nasal speculum will be used to examine the nose; the otoscope, the ears and throat; and with the ophthalmic attachments, the eyes. The percussion hammer and tuning fork will test neurological responses. The vaginal speculum indicates a pelvic exam with inspection of the female organs. In addition to these areas, the complete physical examination may include a rectal exam, visual acuity tests, and any other that the doctor believes is indicated.

123.

B. The metric system of measurement uses these prefixes. The medical laboratory uses these attached to the front of the basic units of length (the meter), weight (the gram) and volume (the liter) for convenient expression of a wide variety of measurements. All the given prefixes are divisions of the number 10, although others not commonly used in medical work are multiples of 10. The prefix centi = 1/10 or 0.1 (one tenth); milli = 1/1000 or 0.001 (one thousandth); micro = 1/1,000,000 or 0.000001 (one millionth); nano = 10^{-9} (one-billionth) and pico = 10^{-12} (one-trillionth). The measurements that use prefixes and units are generally expressed in metric or scientific notation. (See the terms nano and pico for the use of scientific notation in place of decimals or fractions). SI (System International) is a modern, updated version of the metric system, which added newer units of measurement and attempted to standardize the metric system's use among different countries. Be sure to review the metric system in a medical assistant textbook.

124.

E. The patient should be fitted for crutches while he or she is wearing shoes and in a standing position. The distance between the top of the crutch and the armpit should be about 2 inches, which is about two to three finger widths. The angle of the elbow flexion should be 30 degrees when holding the hand grip. This angle should be checked with a goniometer. (Goniometry is the measurement of joint motion.)

125.

E. Leads I, II, and III use two limbs for recording the electrical force of the heart. These leads are called standard limb leads or bipolar leads. The three limb leads that form the triangle are the right arm, left arm, and left leg. The right leg is the "ground" or "reference" electrode. The new trend is to refer to electrodes as sensors.

126.

E. Wandering baseline, somatic tremor, alternating current, and baseline interruption are all types of artifacts that can appear on the recording, making it difficult to interpret. Somatic tremor artifacts are very irregular, whereas alternating current interference is very regular. When AC interference is noted, the first thing to check is proper grounding of the instrument.

127.

E. The commercial services, which contract to dispose of medical waste, must be licensed by the Environmental Protection Agency. Records tracking the disposal of medical waste must be maintained for three years for the EPA. Federal regulations must be followed.

128.

C. Hands must be washed in between patients to break the chain of infection and prevent the transfer of microbes from one patient to another. All other duties in the examination room must also be performed in a manner that prevents disease. For example, biological waste material is disposed in the recommended way, reusable but contaminated instruments are immediately placed in a sanitizing solution or enclosed container, and work surfaces must be cleaned and sanitized.

The MA generally has the following assignments for physical exams: (1) prepare the examining room by seeing that it is clean with previously used supplies removed; (2) clean paper is rolled onto the exam table and clean drapes are made available if needed; (3) the patient is instructed about the procedure and readied for the exam; (4) the medical assistant remains near the patient and assists the physician as required; (5) after the exam, the medical assistant gives post-exam instructions to the patient; (6) after the patient is gone, the room is cleaned and supplies are disposed of according to good aseptic practice; and finally, (7) the medical assistant washes his or her hands.

129.

D. A speculum (often disposable) is used for examining and keeping open body canals such as a vagina or nasal passage. The speculum varies in size and shape according to its use (e.g., a nasal speculum for a small child is designed to fit a child's nostrils). Vaginal speculums are used to inspect the vagina and cervix and are usually lubricated for ease of insertion and removal. The speculum may be fitted with an obturator inside. The obturator may have a light when used in colon examinations.

10 | Laboratory Procedures

chapter objectives

Major areas of knowledge/content included in this chapter are:

I. Center for Disease Control and Prevention (CDC) guidelines and safety concerns

II. Clinical Laboratory Amendment (CLIA '88) guidelines

➤ quality control/quality assurance/documentation

➤ proficiency tests

III. Selected tests

➤ urinalysis, including methods of collection

➤ hematology, including methods of collection

➤ blood chemistry—glucose, blood urea nitrogen (BUN), cholesterol, and triglycerides

➤ immunology tests

➤ pregnancy testing

➤ microbiology including stains, culture and sensitivity

IV. Basic radiography

DIRECTIONS (Questions 130 through 267): Each of the numbered items or incomplete statements in this section is followed by answers or by completions of the statement. Select the ONE lettered answer or completion that is BEST in each case.

130. Pregnancy tests detect pregnancy by the presence in either urine or serum of
   A. human chorionic gonadotropin (hCG) hormone
   B. heterophile antibodies
   C. febrile agglutinations
   D. autoimmune antibodies
   E. none of the above
   (Palko and Palko, pp 459–460; Wedding and Toenjes, p 366)

131. Confirmatory (alternative) testing is performed on samples to increase the medical assistant's confidence that the result of a test is correct. Which of the following is NOT a correct statement about confirmatory tests?
   A. confirmatory testing is used to check validity of a test result
   B. confirmatory testing is a procedure for quality control
   C. confirmatory testing may involve repeating the test on the same specimen
   D. confirmatory testing may involve testing a new sample
   E. confirmatory testing would not be done when the sample results are normal
   (Palko and Palko, p 185; Wedding and Toenjes, p 166)

132. A test to determine the ability of the kidneys to concentrate or dilute the urine, according to the needs of the body, measures
   A. glucose
   B. ketone bodies
   C. occult blood
   D. protein
   E. specific gravity
   (Keir et al, p 580; Palko and Palko, pp 164–165, 197)

133. In routine urinalysis, all of the following are physical properties of the urine EXCEPT
   A. color
   B. appearance
   C. specific gravity
   D. odor
   E. sediment
   (Bonewit-West #1, pp 534–535; Palko and Palko, pp 162–166)

134. The range of the volume of urine voided by an adult during a 24-hour period is
   A. 30–60 mL
   B. 500–600 mL
   C. 750–2000 mL
   D. 250–2500 mL
   E. 1000–5000 mL
   (Palko and Palko, p 164)

135. Clinitest is a test to detect
   A. occult blood
   B. glucosuria
   C. hematuria
   D. acidity
   E. ketonuria
   (Keir et al, pp 583–584; Palko and Palko, p 186)

136. In performing a venipuncture, the medical assistant should not leave the tourniquet on the patient's arm, without releasing it, for longer than
   A. 30 seconds
   B. 60 seconds
   C. 2 minutes
   D. 3 minutes
   E. 5 minutes
   (Palko and Palko, p 234; Estridge et al, p 115)

137. Due to excess lipids in the blood, turbid (lipemic) serum appears
    A. light yellow straw color
    B. cloudy and milky
    C. dark yellow
    D. clear and transparent
    E. tinged with red

    (Palko and Palko, p 240)

138. If a blood sample is collected in a serum separator gel tube, the medical assistant generally should allow the clot to form for what period of minute(s) before centrifuging?
    A. 1
    B. 2
    C. 3
    D. 15
    E. 30

    (Palko and Palko, p 240)

139. In quantitative measurement of urobilinogen, the type of urine specimen required is a
    A. 24-hour specimen
    B. fresh specimen
    C. 2-hour postprandial specimen
    D. 12-hour specimen
    E. 2-hour volume specimen

    (Palko and Palko, pp 149, 183)

140. The organ in the body responsible for the production of insulin is the
    A. liver
    B. kidney
    C. stomach
    D. pancreas
    E. pituitary

    (Palko and Palko, pp 406–407; Estridge et al, p 212)

141. The storage form of glucose in the liver is
    A. amino acids
    B. fats

    C. glycogen
    D. proteins
    E. lipids

    (Palko and Palko, pp 406–407; Bonewit-West #1, p 643)

142. A glucose tolerance test (GTT) measures the response of the body to a sudden intake of glucose. The highest blood glucose reading for a normal person during the GTT will occur
    A. 15 minutes after the test starts
    B. 30–60 minutes after the test starts
    C. 60–90 minutes after the test starts
    D. 90–120 minutes after the test starts
    E. right before the test starts

    (Bonewit-West #1, p 560; Palko and Palko, p 409)

143. The blood urea nitrogen (BUN) test is a blood test used to assess function of the
    A. heart
    B. kidneys
    C. liver
    D. lungs
    E. intestine

    (Palko and Palko, pp 442–443; Estridge et al, pp 391–392)

144. High plasma cholesterol levels may be associated with which of the following?
    A. severe anemias
    B. hyperthyroidism
    C. atherosclerosis
    D. newborns
    E. cachexia

    (Bonewit-West #1, pp 642–643; Palko and Palko, p 439)

145. In structure and form, cocci bacteria are found in which of the following shapes?
    A. spherical
    B. spiral
    C. rod
    D. curved
    E. triangular

    (Bonewit-West #1, pp 441–442; Palko and Palko, p 486; Estridge et al, p 461)

146. Which procedure is inappropriate when performing venipunctures?
    A. instruct the patient to hold the arm straight and stiff
    B. apply the tourniquet just above the elbow
    C. swab the area of the puncture with an alcohol sponge
    D. insert the needle bevel up
    E. release the tourniquet after withdrawing the needle

    (Bonewit-West #1, pp 584–588; Palko and Palko, pp 234–238)

147. When doing a differential white cell count, the normal range of eosinophils is
    A. 1–3%
    B. 5–8%
    C. 10–12%
    D. 15–20%
    E. 20–25%

    (Palko and Palko, pp 310, 313; Wedding and Toenjes, p 254)

148. A term indicating that a disease has become widespread in a population and has increased in territory is
    A. endemic
    B. epidemic
    C. communicable
    D. pandemic
    E. contagious

    (Taber's, p 1397)

149. The invasion of the body by any pathogenic organism is called
    A. contagion
    B. infection
    C. endemic
    D. communicable
    E. pandemic

    (Bonewit-West #1, p 4; Taber's, pp 986–988)

150. Which of the following diseases is a fungus?
    A. German measles
    B. influenza
    C. hepatitis
    D. chickenpox
    E. dermatophytosis (e.g., athlete's foot)

    (Keir et al, pp 446–447; Palko and Palko, pp 486, 492)

151. The smallest of the microorganisms are the
    A. rickettsiae
    B. streptococci
    C. protozoa
    D. viruses
    E. fungi

    (Kinn and Woods, pp 946–947)

152. Cocci occurring in pairs are
    A. micrococci
    B. diplococci
    C. streptococci
    D. staphylococci
    E. sarcinae

    (Bonewit-West #1, p 664; Palko and Palko, p 486; Estridge et al, p 461)

153. Cocci occurring in chains are
    A. micrococci
    B. diplococci
    C. streptococci
    D. staphylococci
    E. sarcinae

    (Bonewit-West #1, p 664; Palko and Palko, p 486)

154. Which federal regulation for the clinical laboratory specifies guidelines for quality control, quality assurance, adequate record keeping, and qualified personnel?
    A. DEA
    B. OSHA
    C. CLIA '88
    D. CDC
    E. COLA

    (Bonewit-West #1, pp 517–518; Palko and Palko, pp 96–97; Walters, pp 5–6)

155. Viruses differ from bacteria in that they have
    A. both DNA and RNA
    B. only DNA
    C. only RNA
    D. either DNA or RNA
    E. neither DNA nor RNA
    (Palko and Palko, p 485; Estridge et al, p 464)

156. Which federal agency oversees the safety of health facilities including protection against occupational exposure to hepatitis B virus and human immunodeficiency virus?
    A. OSHA
    B. CLIA '88
    C. DEA
    D. CDC
    E. COLA
    (Bonewit-West #1, pp 1, 12–14; Estridge, pp 4–5)

157. The term used to indicate that two or more organisms are living together is
    A. symbiosis
    B. symphysis
    C. synapsis
    D. synergism
    E. syncope
    (Taber's, p 1877)

158. A term applied to bacteria that can adapt to an environment with or without oxygen is
    A. aerobic
    B. anaerobic
    C. facultative
    D. gram-positive
    E. gram-negative
    (Palko and Palko, p 489; Taber's, p 702)

159. Diseases that occur when the body apparently fails to recognize its own constituents and begins to produce antibodies to fight them are called
    A. anaphylaxis
    B. allergy
    C. latent infection
    D. autoimmune
    E. acquired immunodeficiency syndrome (AIDS)
    (Palko and Palko, pp 450–455; Taber's, p 178)

160. Direct contact, droplets, and fomites are ways in which viruses are transmitted to cause
    A. influenza
    B. malaria
    C. meningitis
    D. botulism
    E. Rocky Mountain spotted fever
    (Kinn and Woods, pp 417, 945)

161. Most rickettsial diseases are transmitted by
    A. coitus
    B. improperly prepared food
    C. fecal-food contamination
    D. direct contact
    E. insects and ticks
    (Kinn and Woods, p 945)

162. The disease of Coccidioidomycosis is commonly called
    A. San Joaquin fever
    B. athlete's foot
    C. malaria
    D. scarlet fever
    E. rabbit fever
    (Palko and Palko, p 492; Estridge et al, p 466)

163. An example of a pathogenic fungus that a medical assistant may see in a physician's office is
    A. tetanus
    B. *Trichomonas vaginalis*
    C. dysentery
    D. malaria
    E. ringworm
    (Kinn and Woods, p 946; Palko and Palko, pp 492–493)

164. Which temperature scale is used in the medical laboratory because it has smaller units and is easier to calculate?
    A. Fahrenheit
    B. Absolute
    C. centigrade or Celsius scale
    D. Kelvin
    E. none of the above
    (Palko and Palko, pp 54–55; Estridge et al, pp 404–405)

165. The test in microbiology or bacteriology that checks the susceptibility of an organism to specific antibiotics is the
    A. culture test
    B. isolation test
    C. sensitivity test
    D. screening test
    E. inoculation test
    (Bonewit-West #1, pp 678–680; Palko and Palko, pp 489–492)

166. The Mantoux test is used to screen for the pathogenic acid-fast organism, which causes
    A. gonorrhea and syphilis
    B. cholera and diphtheria
    C. measles and mumps
    D. tuberculosis and leprosy
    E. pneumonia and hepatitis
    (Bonewit-West #1, pp 287–289; Kinn and Woods, p 543)

167. A persistent viral infection in which the symptoms come and go is called a/an
    A. acute infection
    B. chronic infection
    C. fast infection
    D. latent infection
    E. slow infection
    (Kinn and Woods, p 418)

168. Which of the following is considered to be a CORRECT safety rule in the medical laboratory?
    A. hands should be washed frequently and thoroughly
    B. eating, drinking, and smoking are acceptable in the laboratory
    C. it is not necessary to ever wear rubber gloves in the laboratory
    D. it is all right to put pens, pencils, and fingers in your mouth while working in the laboratory
    E. it is not necessary to supervise inexperienced laboratory workers
    (Keir et al, pp 435–437; Palko and Palko, pp 7–8)

169. The stain most used to identify and study bacteria is the
    A. Gram stain
    B. acid-fast stain
    C. Wright's stain
    D. Giemsa stain
    E. none of the above
    (Palko and Palko, p 487; Estridge et al, p 461)

170. Glucose meters are used in the physician's office laboratory and the home to monitor blood glucose levels. Which of the following equipment would NOT be necessary to perform a blood glucose using a glucose meter?
    A. glucose reagent strips
    B. distilled water
    C. a manual or semiautomatic skin puncture device
    D. an electronic glucose meter
    E. a sample of blood
    (Kinn and Woods, pp 932–933; Palko and Palko, pp 411–412)

171. The normal range for a prothrombin time test is
    A. 5–10 seconds
    B. 11–13 seconds
    C. 18–20 seconds
    D. 25–30 seconds
    E. 30 seconds to 1 minute
    (Palko and Palko, p 378; Estridge et al, p 252)

172. Which of the following radiographs (x-ray exams) would produce numerous cross-sectional images of a body part?
    A. the CAT scan also known as computed tomography
    B. angiocardiogram
    C. bronchogram
    D. cystogram
    E. hysterosalpingogram
    (Bonewit-West #1, pp 495–496; Keir et al, p 279)

173. The procedure that provides an image of a developing fetus and thereby reveals its sex is
    A. magnetic reasonance imaging
    B. conventional x-ray
    C. CAT scan
    D. ultrasonography
    E. intravenous pyelography
    (Bonewit-West #1, pp 494–495)

174. A contrast media often used in radiographic diagnostic procedures of the gastric tract is
    A. fluoroscopy
    B. carbon dioxide
    C. air
    D. iodine
    E. barium sulfate
    (Bonewit-West #1, p 487; Keir et al, p 629)

175. The "chain of custody" referred to in drug testing in the workplace is
    A. a security system that protects the reliability and validity of the testing results
    B. another term for the drug-testing procedure
    C. a legal term used in the prosecution of drug addicts
    D. a description of a policy that discourages drug usage in the workplace
    E. a pre-employment drug screen program
    (Bonewit-West #1, p 540; Hurlbutt, p 276)

176. Which of the following diagnostic radiology machines does not use x-ray or ionizing radiation of any kind?
    A. fluoroscopy
    B. mammography
    C. xeroradiography
    D. computed tomography
    E. magnetic resonance imaging
    (Bonewit-West #1, p 515; Keir et al, p 279)

177. Which of the following statements about occult (hidden) blood in urine is FALSE?
    A. occult blood is not visible to the naked eye
    B. occult blood is the hemoglobin from disintegrated red blood cells
    C. hemoglobinuria is a term sometimes used to designate the presence of occult blood in urine
    D. a positive reaction on the reagent test strip occurs when sediment has more than the normal number of red cells
    E. if the urine sediment turns the reagent test strip block white, the test is positive for occult blood
    (Palko and Palko, p 181)

178. The presence of numerous leukocytes in the urine during microscopic examination is referred to as
    A. polyuria
    B. uremia
    C. albuminuria
    D. pyuria
    E. leukocytopenia
    (Bonewit-West #1, p 315; Palko and Palko, p 184)

179. On the N-Multistix 10 SG, most tests can be read
    A. in less than 2 minutes
    B. between 3 and 4 minutes
    C. between 5 and 10 minutes
    D. after 15 minutes
    E. after 1 hour
    (Bonewit-West #1, pp 330–331)

180. In a reagent dipstick test for ketone bodies in the urine, the largest amounts are represented by an intensified
    A. red color
    B. yellow color
    C. green color
    D. blue color
    E. maroon color
    (Kinn et al, p 864; Palko and Palko, p 180)

181. If a urine specimen is to be sent to a laboratory for a bacteriologic culture, a female patient should be instructed to
    A. collect the specimen in a sterile bottle
    B. collect a specimen midstream in a sterile bottle
    C. collect a specimen midstream in a clean bottle
    D. collect the entire specimen in a clean bottle
    E. forcibly void a small amount into a sterile bottle
    (Palko and Palko, pp 149–150)

182. The best urine sample to use for a pregnancy test is a
    A. random specimen
    B. first morning specimen
    C. second-voided specimen
    D. 2-hour postprandial
    E. 24-hour specimen
    (Palko and Palko, pp 459–460)

183. Ictotest is a tablet used to diagnose
    A. diabetes mellitus
    B. liver function
    C. kidney function
    D. pregnancy
    E. urinary output
    (Palko and Palko, pp 185–186)

184. Epithelial cells are reported as
    A. the number per high-power field
    B. the number per low-power field

C. 1+ to 2+
D. a particular color
E. a percentage
(Palko and Palko, p 199; Estridge et al, p 362)

185. An Addis count is done to determine
    A. whether a patient is pregnant
    B. a patient's urinary output of formed elements for 12 hours
    C. the number of red cells in urinary sediment
    D. the presence of occult blood
    E. the presence of ketone bodies
    (Palko and Palko, p 132)

186. A wound culture would be obtained to identify which of the following?
    A. strep bacteria
    B. staph bacteria
    C. Gram-negative organisms
    D. other pathogens
    E. any of the above
    (Kinn and Woods, pp 706–707)

187. X-rays may be potentially dangerous to employees in a physician's office where they are taken because
    A. most machines leak radiation
    B. walls cannot be protected
    C. the effect of radiation is cumulative
    D. the effect of radiation is difficult to determine symptomatically
    E. physicians do not explain the dangers
    (Kinn and Woods, p 816)

188. The most effective way of being certain that individuals employed in a physician's office are not receiving a dangerous amount of radiation is to
    A. subscribe to a film badge service
    B. attach a special paper clip to a film packet worn in a pocket

C. take x-rays while wearing a protective apron

D. wear protective gloves when using x-ray machines

E. turn your back to the patient

(Kinn and Woods, p 816; Zakus, p 486)

189. Specimens collected for drug or alcohol analysis should be accompanied by

A. purpose of test

B. collector's name

C. site of collection/date/time

D. pertinent comments about specimen

E. all of the above

(Bonewit-West #1, p 540; Palko and Palko, p 181)

190. The direct roentgen (x-ray) beam comes from the

A. cone

B. x-ray tube

C. film

D. lead screen

E. control panel

(Zakus, p 484)

191. Secondary radiation is

A. emitted by the patient being filmed

B. emitted by the direct roentgen beam

C. leakage from head of x-ray

D. emitted by the cone of the x-ray machine

E. emitted by the control panel of the x-ray machine

(Kinn and Woods, p 816; Zakus, p 485)

192. Which of the following is not used in collecting sputum for cultures?

A. expectoration

B. tracheal suctioning

C. bronchoscopy

D. nebulization

E. palpation

(Kinn and Woods, pp 552–553)

193. A radiograph is a/an

A. color photograph

B. permanent record of an x-ray image

C. black-and-white photograph

D. computer-coded card

E. opaque mass

(Bonewit-West #1, p 504)

194. A patient is scheduled for a retrograde pyelogram. The contrast medium will be administered

A. orally

B. intramuscularly

C. intravenously

D. directly

E. subcutaneously

(Bonewit-West #1, pp 512–513)

195. A patient has been scheduled for an intravenous pyelogram (IVP) on a Tuesday morning. The medical assistant's instructions to the patient about diet for the preceding evening should be to eat

A. a regular evening meal but no breakfast on Tuesday

B. a light meal with nothing after 9:00 P.M.

C. a regular evening meal and a light breakfast on Tuesday

D. nothing after midnight

E. nothing for 24 hours before the test on Tuesday

(Bonewit-West #1, p 493)

196. A patient has been scheduled for a cholecystogram. This is an examination of the

A. gallbladder

B. colon

C. small intestine

D. ureters

E. kidneys

(Bonewit-West #1, pp 492–493)

197. A patient who is having an upper gastrointestinal (GI) series will
    A. receive a dye by injection
    B. take dye tablets orally
    C. receive an enema of barium sulfate
    D. receive an injection of air in the colon
    E. drink a suspension of barium sulfate
    (Bonewit-West #1, p 491)

198. The system of scientific measurement used in medical laboratories is the
    A. metric system
    B. household system
    C. English
    D. apothecary
    E. none of the above
    (Palko and Palko, p 73; Estridge et al, pp 28–29)

199. Which of the following is not a component of blood?
    A. plasma
    B. erythrocytes (red blood cells)
    C. thrombocytes (platelets)
    D. leukocytes (white blood cells)
    E. epithelial cells
    (Bonewit-West #1, pp 618–622)

200. When a patient is placed in an AP (anteroposterior) position for radiography, the
    A. anterior (front of the body) is facing the tube
    B. anterior is facing the film
    C. posterior is facing the tube
    D. patient is on his or her side
    E. face and abdomen are down on the table
    (Bonewit-West #1, p 508; Zakus, p 484)

201. The fragments of blood cells that are counted on blood smears or in blood dilutions in order to predict the body's ability to clot blood are
    A. platelets

B. eosinophils
C. reticulocytes
D. basophils
E. neutrophils
(Kinn and Woods, p 904; Palko and Palko, pp 305–306)

202. Which of the following tests would not be performed on an automated hematology instrument?
    A. Ivy (template) bleeding time
    B. WBC count
    C. RBC count
    D. red blood cell indices
    E. platelet count
    (Palko and Palko, p 330)

203. A blood cell with a biconcave shape and no nucleus is a/an
    A. erythrocyte
    B. lymphocyte
    C. monocyte
    D. thrombocyte
    E. polymorphonuclear cell
    (Palko and Palko, p 305; Estridge et al, pp 185–186)

204. A blood cell that is very large with a nucleus that may be oval, indented, or horseshoe-shaped is a/an
    A. lymphocyte
    B. monocyte
    C. basophil
    D. eosinophil
    E. neutrophil
    (Palko and Palko, p 311; Estridge et al, p 186)

205. In a differential smear, platelets appear as very small azure-blue bodies when stained with
    A. Gram's stain
    B. Wright's stain
    C. iodine
    D. Ziehl-Neelsen stain
    E. merthiolate
    (Palko and Palko, pp 316–317)

206. RBC pipettes are made so that if blood is drawn to the 0.5 mark and diluted to the 101 mark, the dilution will be
    A. 1:50
    B. 1:100
    C. 1:150
    D. 1:200
    E. 1:500
    (Palko and Palko, p 285)

207. A hemocytometer is a counting chamber used to count cells microscopically. The total area on one side of the hemocytometer is
    A. 6 mm^2
    B. 4 mm^2
    C. 1 mm^1
    D. 9 mm^2
    E. 5 mm^2
    (Palko and Palko, p 281)

208. If you performed a white blood count using a hemocytometer and the average cell count was 120, the dilution was 1:20, and the area counted was 4 mm^2, what would be reported as the answer?
    A. 5000 WBC/mm^3
    B. 10,000 WBC/mm^3
    C. 8250 WBC/mm^3
    D. 6000 WBC/mm^3
    E. 12,500 WBC/mm^3
    (Palko and Palko, pp 282–283)

209. The normal WBCs per cubic millimeter for both men and women is
    A. 2500–5500
    B. 4500–6000
    C. 4500–12,000
    D. 6000–11,000
    E. 8000–12,000
    (Palko and Palko, p 278)

210. Automated blood cell counters are now commonly used not only in hospitals but also in physicians' offices. Which of the following statements about the automated instruments is FALSE?
    A. they count fewer numbers of cells
    B. they are more accurate than manual methods
    C. they have reduced the frequency of handling the blood samples
    D. they have reduced the risk of exposure to blood-borne pathogens
    E. they have increased the efficiency in the laboratory
    (Palko and Palko, pp 331–332)

211. A fibrometer is an automated analyzer that is used to perform
    A. glucose determinations
    B. coagulation determinations using clot formation
    C. platelet determinations
    D. hemoglobin determinations
    E. protein determinations
    (Palko and Palko, p 378)

212. The normal RBC count for men, reported as millions of cells per cubic millimeter, is
    A. 1.5–2.5
    B. 2.5–3.5
    C. 3.5–4.5
    D. 4.5–6.0
    E. 5.5–6.5
    (Palko and Palko, p 283; Estridge et al, p 142)

213. A complete blood cell (CBC) count consists of all of the following when capillary blood is used EXCEPT
    A. red blood cell (RBC) count
    B. white blood cell (WBC) count
    C. hemoglobin (Hgb) estimation
    D. differential count (diff)
    E. erythrocyte sedimentation rate (sed rate)
    (Palko and Palko, pp 255–256)

214. Which of the following is NOT an aspect of quality control in the medical laboratory?
    A. assurance of proper care and handling of specimens
    B. evaluation of the techniques and equipment used to perform the tests
    C. evaluation of the changes and/or errors that are commonly associated with routine clinical chemistry
    D. confidence that the variables that cause errors are in check or within an acceptable range
    E. quality control samples ensure that laboratory hazards have been eliminated
    (Palko and Palko, pp 6, 12, 14)

215. On long standing, urine becomes
    A. neutral
    B. acid
    C. alkaline (basic)
    D. clear
    E. balanced in acidity and alkalinity
    (Bonewit-West #1, p 325; Palko and Palko, p 151)

216. Usually the most concentrated urine (greatest specific gravity) is voided
    A. first thing in the morning
    B. 1 hour after breakfast
    C. 1 hour before meals
    D. early in the evening
    E. at bedtime
    (Palko and Palko, p 165)

217. A 2-hour postprandial urine specimen is commonly ordered by the physician when he or she is particularly interested in knowing the results for
    A. bilirubin
    B. protein
    C. specific gravity
    D. glucose
    E. nitrite
    (Palko and Palko, p 148)

218. If a urine specimen is not collected properly, blood might be found as a contaminant in the specimen of
    A. infants
    B. adolescents
    C. men older than 65 years of age
    D. women who are menstruating
    E. women older than 65 years of age
    (Palko and Palko, p 181)

219. Normal urine has a pH range of
    A. 1.5–3.5
    B. 2.5–4.0
    C. 4.5–8.0
    D. 0–9.0
    E. 10.0–14.0
    (Palko and Palko, p 178)

220. The normal specific gravity of urine usually ranges between
    A. 1.000 and 1.001
    B. 1.001 and 1.002
    C. 1.010 and 1.025
    D. 1.025 and 1.050
    E. 1.050 and 1.0075
    (Palko and Palko, pp 164–165)

221. The weight of a given volume of a substance divided by the weight of the same volume of water is the formula for
    A. specific gravity
    B. pH
    C. acidity
    D. alkalinity
    E. sedimentation
    (Palko and Palko, p 164)

222. For the highest possible magnification, the 100X oil immersion lens is used with an eyepiece (ocular) that gives a magnification of 10X. This allows the medical assistant to see an object
    A. 10 times its actual size
    B. 100 times its actual size
    C. 1,000 times its actual size
    D. 10,000 times its actual size
    E. 100,000 times its actual size
    (Palko and Palko, p 31)

223. Which of the following procedures represents proper handling or care of the microscope?
    A. store the microscope without a dust cover
    B. use only the coarse adjustment with the oil immersion objective
    C. carry the microscope with one hand
    D. store the microscope with the high power objective nearest the stage
    E. clean all excess oil from the oil immersion objective with lens paper
    (Palko and Palko, pp 34–35; Estridge et al, pp 87–88)

224. When a microscopic slide is to be examined, the field is found by
    A. lowering the low power objective using the coarse adjustment
    B. lowering the microscope head by using the micrometer head
    C. using the high power objective
    D. using the intermediate power objective
    E. using a 53 eyepiece
    (Palko and Palko, pp 33–34; Estridge et al, p 86)

225. For microscopic examination, slides are placed on the
    A. substage
    B. objective
    C. stage
    D. condenser
    E. diaphragm
    (Palko and Palko, p 33; Estridge et al, p 86)

226. The Centers for Disease Control and Prevention (CDC) issued recommendations known as Universal Precautions for the prevention of such diseases as
    A. AIDS and hepatitis
    B. smallpox
    C. influenza
    D. cancer
    E. scurvy
    (Palko and Palko, pp 6, 515)

227. From what area of the respiratory tract should sputum be collected?
    A. nose
    B. throat
    C. pharynx
    D. lungs
    E. mouth
    (Keir et al, p 297)

228. For examination of a stool specimen for occult blood, the specimen
    A. should be kept warm and examined immediately
    B. should be kept cold and examined immediately
    C. should be kept cold and examined within 2 hours
    D. need not be kept warm or examined immediately
    E. should be kept warm and examined within 2 hours
    (Keir et al, p 589; Estridge et al, p 539)

229. Papanicolaou smears are specimens of cells which are analyzed to detect
    A. cancer of the cervix
    B. endometriosis
    C. syphilis
    D. fibroid tumors
    E. vaginitis
    (Keir et al, pp 533–537)

230. Normal bleeding time using Duke's method is
    A. 1–3 minutes
    B. 5–10 minutes
    C. 10–15 minutes
    D. 15–30 minutes
    E. 30–60 minutes
    (Estridge et al, p 246)

231. In making a finger puncture, a medical assistant should be careful to avoid
    A. massaging the finger to promote circulation to the tip
    B. cleansing the puncture site with 70% alcohol
    C. squeezing the puncture to encourage bleeding
    D. wiping away the first drop or two of blood with a sterile sponge
    E. allowing a drop of blood to form that is large enough to carry out testing
    (Palko and Palko, p 233)

232. An example of a gram-negative organism is
    A. streptococcus
    B. pneumococcus
    C. tubercle bacillus
    D. diphtheria bacillus
    E. *Neisseria gonorrhoeae*
    (Palko and Palko, p 487)

233. An example of a gram-positive organism is
    A. gonococcus
    B. typhoid bacillus
    C. *Staphylococcus*
    D. dysentery bacillus
    E. *Meningococcus*
    (Palko and Palko, p 487)

234. A glucometer is designed to give readings of
    A. glucohemoglobin
    B. occult blood
    C. liver function
    D. granulation
    E. blood glucose values
    (Keir et al, pp 353, 555–557)

235. Expressed in terms of mm/hour, the normal range of Westergren erythrocyte sedimentation rates (ESR) for men older than 50 is
    A. 0–20
    B. 0–9
    C. 11–29
    D. 31–50
    E. 51–70
    (Palko and Palko, p 351; Estridge et al, p 218)

236. The average range of hemoglobin values for women, expressed as g/100 mL, is
    A. 6–10
    B. 12.5–15
    C. 18–22
    D. 24–28
    E. 30–34
    (Palko and Palko, p 261)

237. In a differential white blood cell count, basophils and eosinophils may average
    A. less than 5%
    B. 10–20%
    C. 25–33%
    D. 40–50%
    E. 50–70%
    (Palko and Palko, p 313; Estridge et al, p 187)

238. In differential white blood cell counts of adults, lymphocytes may average
    A. less than 5%
    B. 5–10%
    C. 10–20%
    D. 25–33%
    E. 60–80%
    (Palko and Palko, p 313)

239. In a normal differential WBC count, neutrophils average approximately
    A. 10–20%
    B. 20–40%
    C. 0–5%
    D. 50–70%
    E. 70–80%
    (Palko and Palko, p 313)

240. The normal hematocrit reading for men is approximately
    A. 30–40%
    B. 40–52%
    C. 50–60%
    D. 60–70%
    E. 70–80%
    (Palko and Palko, p 264)

241. Which of the following may result in accidental needle sticks to the medical assistant?
    A. carefully recap needles before disposal
    B. never push a needle into the red plastic needle disposal box with your hand
    C. never try to remove a needle or syringe from the red plastic needle box
    D. never put a needle down—dispose of it promptly
    E. never put needles or other sharp instruments in trash cans
    (Palko and Palko, p 11; Estridge et al, p 37)

242. One of the recommended AIDS-related precautions for the medical assistant is to disinfect work surfaces and equipment with
    A. soap and water
    B. 70% alcohol
    C. ether
    D. ammonia
    E. sodium hypochlorite (household bleach)
    (Palko and Palko, pp 8, 12)

243. The Center for Disease Control and Prevention (CDC) has developed guidelines recognizing the infectious potential of any patient specimen. Which of the following guidelines provides the single greatest protection against AIDS and other blood-borne pathogens?
    A. store personal items
    B. wear protective clothing
    C. isolate each biological specimen from the worker
    D. avoid spattering of biological specimens
    E. do not eat or drink in the laboratory
    (Palko and Palko, p 6)

244. A quality control program in a laboratory ensures the reliability of the tests and their results. Which of the following would cause errors in a quality control program?
    A. proper care and handling of specimens
    B. evaluation of the techniques and equipment used to perform the tests
    C. evaluation of the changes and/or errors commonly associated with routine clinical chemistry
    D. establishment of confidence that the variables that cause errors are within an acceptable range
    E. the quality control program should be posted weekly
    (Palko and Palko, p 103)

245. Levy-Jennings charts are used in the laboratory to make easy comparisons of test controls in order to have better
    A. quality control
    B. calibration of instruments
    C. statistical deviations
    D. a record of test values
    E. none of the above
    (Palko and Palko, p 98)

246. Blood serum
    A. may be separated from the blood cells by centrifugation
    B. is always collected in green-top tubes
    C. is obtained from clotted blood that has been mixed with an anticoagulant
    D. retains fibrinogen after centrifugation
    E. all of the above
    (Palko and Palko, p 240)

247. Plasma
    A. is always collected in red-top tubes
    B. is obtained from blood that has been mixed with an anticoagulant in the collection tube
    C. is obtained from clotted blood that has not been mixed with an anticoagulant
    D. does not contain fibrinogen
    E. none of the above
    (Palko and Palko, p 235)

248. When performing a venipuncture,
    A. if a vacuum tube is not filling properly, substitute another tube
    B. all tubes containing an anticoagulant or preservative should be allowed to fill to the exhaustion of the vacuum
    C. select a venipuncture site by the feel, not appearance, of the vein
    D. the patient's identification should be verified before the venipuncture
    E. all of the above
    (Palko and Palko, pp 236–238)

249. To inform and prepare a patient for a fasting glucose determination, the medical assistant should instruct the patient to
    A. drink fruit juice in the morning before the test
    B. fast for 8–12 hours
    C. eat a normal breakfast prior to the test
    D. drink only milk
    E. avoid exercise
    (Palko and Palko, p 409)

250. To perform a venipuncture, the medical assistant should
    A. swab the site with an alcohol sponge
    B. position herself in front or slightly to the side of the patient
    C. penetrate the skin about 1/4 inch below the point where the vein will be entered
    D. enter the skin and vein with the needle at a 15-degree angle to the skin surface
    E. all of the above
    (Bonewit-West #1, pp 584–588)

251. The medical assistant who prepares blood smears should
    A. keep the spreader slide at a 35- to 40-degree angle
    B. place one-half of a drop of blood about 1/2 to 3/4 inch from the end of the slide
    C. bring the spreader slide back into the drop to start the smear
    D. have a feathered edge at the thin end of the smear
    E. all of the above
    (Palko and Palko, pp 306–307)

252. Which of the following factors must be included when calculating a blood cell count that has been performed using the Unopette and the hemocytometer?
    A. number of cells counted
    B. the area counted
    C. dilution factor
    D. depth of the fluid on the hemacytometer
    E. all of the above
    (Palko and Palko, p 286; Estridge et al, p 140)

253. Which of the following blood parameters is performed with a colorimeter within an automatic blood cell counter?
    A. white blood cell determination
    B. red blood cell determination
    C. hematocrit determination
    D. hemoglobin determination
    E. white cell differential
    (Palko and Palko, p 333)

254. Physicians often order a clinical laboratory panel or profile on a patient when they are checking a particular body organ or system. Which of the following is NOT a common profile study ordered by the physician?
    A. cardiac profile
    B. liver profile
    C. thyroid profile
    D. skeletal profile
    E. diabetic screening
    (Palko and Palko, p 522)

255. Which venipuncture type is preferred to obtain blood from patients who are hard to stick?
    A. the butterfly method
    B. the vacuum tube method
    C. an arterial puncture
    D. none of the above
    E. all of the above
    (Keir et al, pp 588–594)

256. The reagent strip method for occult blood in urine is measuring amounts of
    A. bilirubin
    B. white blood cells
    C. intact red cells and free hemoglobin
    D. urobilinogen
    E. fibrinogen
    (Palko and Palko, p 181)

257. The part(s) of the microscope responsible for regulating the light that strikes the object are the
    A. ocular and objective
    B. condenser and iris diaphragm
    C. lens and barrel of the microscope
    D. stage
    E. eyepiece
    (Palko and Palko, pp 32–33)

258. Agglutination test kits used to detect the presence of heterophil antibodies that are found in the plasma or serum of patients with infectious mononucleosis (IM) contain the following
    A. slides
    B. reagents
    C. positive control
    D. negative control
    E. all of the above
    (Palko and Palko, pp 458–466; Estridge et al, pp 311–312)

259. Which of the following tests are used to diagnose the disease syphilis?
    A. latex slide agglutination test
    B. Epstein-Barr heterophile agglutinations
    C. RA test
    D. febrile agglutinations
    E. VDRL
    (Bonewit-West #2, p 652; Kinn et al, p 629)

260. To determine the specific gravity of a urine sample in a physician's office, a medical assistant might use which of the following?
    A. urinometer
    B. refractometer
    C. N-Multistix SG reagent strip
    D. falling drop method
    E. all of the above
    (Palko and Palko, pp 165–166)

261. A good blood cell differential smear includes which of the following?
    A. drop of blood is too large
    B. drop of blood is too small
    C. using a slide that is not entirely free of grease or dust
    D. using a spreader slide with a chipped end
    E. making a feathered edge
    (Palko and Palko, pp 306–307)

262. Which of the following written instructions will NOT be given to patients for 24-hour urine collections?
    A. urinate into a small container and transfer to a larger collection bottle
    B. do not collect the first sample of initial day on arising in the morning but write down the time
    C. follow directions given by the laboratory supplying the container for preserving the specimen
    D. void at exactly the same time the following morning and add the sample to the collection container
    E. add one-fourth of a cup of bleach to the container as a preservative
    (Frew et al, p 757; Palko and Palko, p 149)

263. Which instruction to a female patient for a clean-catch specimen is a poor practice?
    A. collect the first urine voided
    B. if menstruating, insert a fresh tampon or use cotton to stop the flow
    C. wash the urinary opening and its surroundings from back to front with a sterile antiseptic pad while separating the skin folds around the urinary opening
    D. begin urinating while keeping the skin folds apart with the fingers of one hand
    E. hold the container with the other hand, and collect only the midstream.
    (Bonewit-West #1, pp 318–319)

264. The following criteria must be met to obtain reliable pregnancy test results EXCEPT
    A. a first morning sample is preferred but a random sample can be used
    B. at least 60 days must have passed since the beginning of the patient's last menstrual period for a positive result
    C. the specimen should be collected in a dry glass or plastic container
    D. a clean-catch urine specimen is not essential
    E. the specimen should be tested immediately, refrigerated, or frozen for later testing
    (Palko and Palko, pp 459–460)

265. If a urine sample is permitted to stand for a period longer than 1 hour at room temperature without a preservative, which of the following will NOT occur?
    A. the sample will become alkaline (basic)
    B. glucose levels may increase
    C. bilirubin will undergo changes due to the effect of light
    D. bacteria will multiply rapidly, resulting in a cloudy specimen
    E. urea may be converted to ammonia
    (Palko and Palko, p 151)

266. The diagnostic ultrasound uses very high frequency inaudible sound waves that bounce off the body to record information on the structure of internal organs. The record produced is called a/an
    A. electrocardiogram
    B. diskogram
    C. sonogram or echogram
    D. urogram
    E. encephalogram

    (Zakus, pp 479–480)

267. Which of the following laboratory tests results indicates the need for immediate action (an action value)?
    A. a fasting blood sugar of 100 mg/ 100 mL
    B. a hematocrit of 50% in an adult male
    C. 1% eosinophils on a blood WBC differential slide
    D. 2–3 WBC in a urine specimen
    E. high protein level in a urine specimen

    (Palko and Palko, p 121)

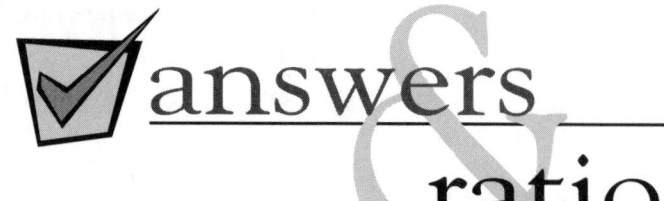
130.

A. The hormone, human chorionic gonadotropin (hCG), is produced by the placenta of the developing embryo and therefore provides evidence of pregnancy. The simplest and most modern test for pregnancy uses a test kit with enzymes that develop color to indicate pregnancy and the hCG hormone. Pregnancy can be detected as early as 10 days after conception using this test. The urine or serum provided for testing should be either tested immediately or refrigerated if testing is within the next 48 hours. If it is to be kept for a longer period of time, it should be frozen.

131.

E. Confirmatory testing using a different, more time-consuming or costly test might also be done on a sample that reads in the normal range. If the test result is normal but the medical assistant expected it to be abnormal because of the other factors known about the patient, the medical assistant would want to conduct a confirmatory test. Alternative testing is another term for this type of testing.

132.

E. Testing the specific gravity of urine indicates the ability of the kidneys to concentrate or dilute the urine. The average normal range of specific gravity is 1.010 to 1.025. Diabetes insipidus is a disease that causes loss of concentrating ability of the kidneys due to impaired function of the antidiuretic hormone (ADH).

133.

E. Physical characteristics of the urine include color, appearance, specific gravity, odor, and turbidity. The yellow color of normal urine is due to the presence of a yellow pigment, urochrome. The turbid appearance of a basic urine may be due to the presence of phosphates and carbonates.

134.

C. The average range of urine volume voided by a normal adult in a 24-hour period is 750–2000 mL. This is a little more than 1 1/2 quarts to four quarts. The amount can vary greatly depending on the individual's fluid intake, the temperature, and the climate, as well as the amount of perspiration.

Diseases affect the output of urine and may cause a lack of urine production (anuria in the disorders of renal obstruction and renal failure) or on the other hand an excessive amount (polyuria in diabetes and certain kidney disorders).

135.

B. Clinitest is a test for glucosuria using Clinitest tablets. It is a nonspecific test for glucose because in reality it will test positive for any reducing sugar. It is used along with the dip-and-read strip (enzymatic test), which is specific for glucose only. Clinitest is used to reveal lactose and galactose present in galactosemia, a metabolic disorder. The two sugars, lactose and galactose, present in this disorder will test negative with the enzymatic test but positive with the Clinitest.

136.

C. The medical assistant should never leave a tourniquet on the arm for more than 2 minutes without releasing it when performing a venipuncture. Not only will the patient suffer discomfort, but it may also alter the test results.

137.

B. Turbid serum appears cloudy and milky. This may be due to high lipid (fat) levels in the patient's blood.

138.

D. If a blood sample is collected in a **serum separator gel tube** (red-/black-stopper), the tube should be allowed to clot at room temperature for a period of 5–15 minutes. If the sample is collected in a plain red-stopper tube that does not contain serum separator gel the sample should be allowed to clot for 20–30 minutes at room temperature. This period is extended to 30–60 minutes if the sample is refrigerated.

When serum is required, the medical assistant generally should centrifuge the specimen for 15 minutes at the recommended speed of the manufacturer. Note that individual laboratories have their own guidelines that must be adhered to for uniform results. The over vigorous "ringing" of the clot or overlong exposure of the sample to higher temperatures may cause hemolysis to appear in the serum.

Several rules should be remembered regarding blood collection tubes: (1) blood collection tubes of the different types with different additives, etc., are distinguished by the different colors of their rubber stoppers; (2) a chart of the different tests, type of collection tube for that test, and correct processing steps should be posted at the blood draw station; (3) care should be taken to follow exact processing steps since hemolysis of the blood or the wrong additive may ruin the test results.

139.

E. In the quantitative measurement of urobilinogen, the type of urine specimen collected from the patient is a 2-hour volume specimen. Normal values for urobilinogen is 0.2–1.0 mg/dL. Increases above this value can be seen in urine of patients with both hemolytic and hepatic disease.

140.

D. The organ in the body that produces insulin is the pancreas. When blood glucose levels rise, this stimulates the pancreas to release insulin. Insulin enables glucose to leave the blood and enter muscle and liver (hepatic) cells. This causes the blood glucose level to fall.

141.

C. Glycogen in the liver cells is a storage form of glucose. Glycogen is a polysaccharide that is commonly called animal starch, which can be converted rapidly back to glucose when it is needed by the body for energy. This process is called glycogenolysis.

142.

B. A normal person without diabetes mellitus will have a peak concentration of glucose in his or her blood 30–60 minutes after drinking the glucose at the start of the GTT test. The blood glucose level will return to fasting levels (70–90 mg/dL) about 2.5–3 hours after the start of the test. Diabetes mellitus patients will not reach the peak concentration until 2–3 hours after the test starts, and they will have higher blood glucose levels (180 mg/dL or higher; dL = 100mL).

143.

B. The **BUN** test is a kidney function test. The physiologic role of the urea is to act as a carrier of waste nitrogen, which is the end product of protein metabolism. Remember that the element nitrogen is only present in protein molecules, not in sugars (saccharides) or fats (lipids). Adult normal BUN = 8–18 mg/dL (dL = 100 mL).

144.

C. An elevated plasma cholesterol level is often associated with **atherosclerosis** caused by cholesterol deposits in the blood vessels. An elevated cholesterol reading can also be considered a diagnostic tool in detecting liver malfunctions. Hypothyroidism also causes the cholesterol reading to elevate. The normal cholesterol range for males between the ages of 16 and 65 is 135–230 mg/dL (dL = 100 mL).

145.

A. In structure and in form, **cocci** are found in spherical shape. (The word form, cocci, means round.) Some common cocci pathogenic to humans are *Staphylococcus aureus*, which has the appearance of grape clusters and is associated with staph abscesses and a kind of food poisoning, and streptococci that grow in chains and cause strep throat and rheumatic fever. Other shapes of bacteria are bacilli (rod shaped) and spirilla (spiral). In reality, the bacterial shapes vary but these are the three general shapes.

146.

E. In performing venipunctures, the medical assistant must release the tourniquet *before* withdrawing the needle. A sterile gauze pad or dry sterile cotton is placed over the puncture site, the needle is removed, and pressure is applied to the site for several minutes. **Hematomas** (bruises) may be caused by incorrect technique, such as withdrawing the needle while the vein is still distended, before the tourniquet is released, or failing to keep pressure on the puncture site until clotting has occurred to prevent further bleeding.

147.

A. The normal range for eosinophils is 1–3%. The cytoplasm of eosinophils has light blue tinges and is covered with bright pink or red granules. The nucleus appears deep lavender to light blue on staining. Eosinophils will increase with a hypersensitive (allergic) reaction. The other types of white cells seen on a normal differential white count and recognized by their cellular structure are (1) the lymphocyte 25–33%, (2) mature neutrophils called polys 54–62%, (3) immature neutrophils called bands 3–5%, (4) basophils 0–1%, and (5) monocytes 3–7%.

148.

D. Pandemic (pan = all; dem = people; ic = adj.) is a term referring to an epidemic that has increased to cover a larger territory. A disease or condition that is epidemic at the same time in many parts of the world is known as pandemic. An epidemic refers to a rapidly spreading disease or a severe one that is only occasionally present, and endemic refers to a disease that is constantly present but only recognizable in a few people. AIDS is now a worldwide, pandemic disease.

149.

B. Infection is a term used to describe the invasion of the body by a pathogenic organism. If the conditions are favorable, the organisms will multiply, resulting in an infectious disease. The natural lines of defense by the body to combat infection are inflammation, phagocytosis by white cells, and production of antibodies. [Note the term phagocytosis means the condition (-osis) of cells (cyt-) eating (phago-); in this case, of body cells consuming the foreign invaders. **Opportunistic** infections result when the body's immune system is too weak to defend itself.

The federal government in order to protect workers requires that medical offices meet the guidelines of OSHA Bloodborne Pathogens Standards. These standards outline how to reduce exposure to disease-causing microbes as well as avoid exposure to chemicals. The standards also tell what measures to take when exposure has occurred.

150.

E. Dermatophytosis is any skin infection caused by pathogenic fungi. Fungi that cause diseases are often divided into two groups, those that infect only the skin (dermatophytes), and those causing systemic disease such as certain yeast. The term "dermatophytosis" comes from the word forms "derma-," skin; "phyton," plant; and "-osis," condition. Fungi are classified as a type of plant. Fungal diseases include yeast, jock itch, ringworm, and athlete's foot.

Referring to the other answer choices, viruses cause the diseases of measles, mumps, rubella, yellow fever, smallpox, chickenpox, influenza, hepatitis, AIDS, and the common cold among others.

151.

D. Viruses are the smallest of the microorganisms yet discovered and cause many devastating diseases. Viruses can only be seen by using the electron microscope while bacteria can be studied with an ordinary light microscope. Viruses multiply within other cells and are not affected by antibiotics although some antiviral medications are now being developed.

152.

B. Diplococci occur in pairs; hence, the use of the combining form diplo-, meaning double. Bacteria have **three basic forms**: round (or oval) known as **coccus** (plural, cocci); rod shaped known as **bacillus** (plural, bacilli); and spiral-shaped **spirillum** (plural, spirilla). Other terms combined with the -cocci suffix to describe round bacteria are streptococci, meaning twisted or chains of cocci, and staphylococci, meaning cocci that have an appearance like bunches of grapes due to their clustering together in groups. The two prefixes, strep-, and staph-, are often used alone by medical workers to describe the pathogens that cause many of the infections treated in the doctor's office.

153.

C. Streptococci appear in chains. Strepto- is a combining form meaning twist. Diseases caused by streptococci are "strep throat," scarlet fever, and rheumatic fever. The skin infection, impetigo, may be caused by either strep or staph bacteria.

154.

C. CLIA '88 (Clinical Laboratory Improvement Amendments of 1988) apply to laboratories that test for disease prevention, diagnosis, or treatment of humans. All clinical laboratories are assigned to a test category according to their test complexity. The lowest level, waived tests, include simple, stable tests that require little interpretation. The next level, moderate complexity, includes most clinical tests. The moderate complexity level requires proficiency testing, qualified personnel, and adequate record keeping to ensure documentation of adequate quality control and quality assurance. The highest level is high-complexity testing.

Proficiency testing tests unknown specimens in the laboratory which are submitted to a designated agency which tests their accuracy. The proficiency tests are scheduled four times per year.

155.

D. Viruses are different from bacteria (and other living organisms) in that they have only RNA or only DNA. They never have both RNA and DNA and, therefore, must reproduce within a living cell. Viruses can generally be treated only symptomatically (i.e., only the symptoms can be treated) although medicines that inhibit viruses are now beginning to appear on the market, for example, acyclovir. Tests are available for diagnosis of certain virus diseases.

156.

A. OSHA (Occupational Safety and Health Administration) issued standards of safety for all health facilities in its *OSHA Occupational Exposure to Bloodborne Pathogens Standards*. It mandates that employees receive information and training about AIDS and hepatitis. Employers must identify, in writing, tasks and procedures, as well as job positions, where occupational exposure to blood occurs and provide safety training. It recommends adhering to Universal Precautions Guidelines researched by the Centers for Disease Control and Prevention (CDC) which include engineering and work practice controls. Hand washing is emphasized, and procedures that minimize splashing and spraying of blood are defined.

Employers must offer employees the hepatitis B vaccination at no cost within 10 days of beginning occupational exposure. Post-exposure evaluation and follow-up must be provided to any employee who has had an exposure incident.

OSHA also provides guidelines for labeling and handling chemicals and maintaining a safe physical environment.

157.

A. Symbiosis is a term that describes the living together of two or more organisms. The three types of symbiosis in nature are commensalism, mutualism, and parasitism. With commensalism, neither party is harmed but neither benefits from the relationship. Mutualism (used as a synonym for symbiosis by some people) really means that both parties need each other. An example of mutualism is *Escherichia coli* in the human intestine, the human providing a home for the normal strains of *E. coli*, where it produces vitamin K needed by the human. In parasitism, one benefits and the other is harmed.

Disease organisms that harm humans are parasites living at the expense of the human body.

158.

C. In contrast to aerobic bacteria or anaerobic bacteria, facultative bacteria can adapt to an environment with or without oxygen. (The term facultative means capable.) Aerobic organisms live only in the presence of oxygen. Humans are aerobic. Anaerobic means in the absence of oxygen.

159.

D. Diseases that occur when the body fails to recognize its own constituents and begins to produce antibodies to fight them are autoimmune diseases. Examples of autoimmune diseases are rheumatoid arthritis (RA), which causes joint inflammation and bone and muscle deformity; rheumatic fever, which may damage the heart; and Grave's disease (hyperthyroidism). An autoimmune disease of connective tissue is systemic lupus erythematosus.

Hypersensitivity of the immune system to foreign substances results in allergies. Many laboratory tests depend on the reaction of the body's antibodies to antigens produced by bacteria and other microbes, which, of course, is a measure of the immune response of the body.

Opportunistic diseases occur when the body's immune system is weakened and the body cannot fight off infections, which ordinarily it would.

160.

A. Influenza is transmitted most commonly by droplets, but direct contact and fomites are two other methods. (Fomites are inanimate objects that carry disease-causing organisms.) There is no test that will confirm influenza, but immunization against common strains of the flu is available and is recommended for both old and young patients.

161.

E. Most rickettsial diseases (caused by tiny bacteria) are transmitted by arthropods, which include insects, ticks, lice, and mites. Rickettsial diseases are divided into groups. The most common are the spotted fever group and the typhus group.

162.

A. San Joaquin fever is the common name for coccidioidomycosis, which is caused by the fungus *Coccidioides immitis*. One form of the disease is an acute self-limiting disease that involves only the respiratory organs. The other form is progressive coccidioidomycosis, which is chronic and may involve almost any part of the body.

163.

E. An example of a pathogenic fungus that a medical assistant may see in a physician's office is ringworm. Ringworm is called tinea capitis. Athlete's foot is tinea pedis, and jock itch is tinea cruris. Yeast infections are fungal diseases. These are all dermatophytes, a term meaning literally that they eat skin. Regarding the other answer choices: fungi, bacteria, viruses, and protozoa are classes of organisms with pathogens that cause disease. *Trichomonas vaginalis*, sometimes seen in female urine specimens, is a pathogenic protozoa that is sexually transmitted. One cause of dysentery is a protozoa, although bacteria, viruses, parasitic worms, and irritating chemicals can also be the cause. Malaria is caused by a protozoan parasite that lives inside red blood cells during one stage of its life span. Tetanus is caused by a bacterium.

164.

C. The Celsius (centigrade meaning 100 gradations) has 100 divisions between the freezing and boiling points, hence the name. This scale is used in medical laboratory work. The body's normal temperature, 37°C, is the same as 98.6°F (on the Fahrenheit scale). This temperature is used extensively in the medical laboratory to grow bacterial cultures and in certain tests such as the prothrombin. Temperature readings of the refrigerator and freezer are also recorded in the laboratory to assure that reagents and stored specimens have the optimum temperature for preservation.

165.

C. The sensitivity test in microbiology tests the susceptibility of an organism to specific antibiotics. This is done by placing antibiotic disks of known strengths on the inoculated agar and letting the plate incubate overnight at 37°F (body temperature). The size of the inhibition (no growth) zone around each disk tells how effectively that antibiotic kills the organism.

166.

D. The Mantoux skin test is used to screen for tuberculosis, which is caused by acid-fast organisms (determined with a special stain). It can detect tuberculosis at an early stage. The Tine skin test may also be used although it is not as specific. Tuberculosis has become a resurgent disease in those with weak immune systems such as the AIDS population and in crowded conditions such as prisons and nursing homes. *Mycobacterium tuberculosis* causes tuberculosis; *M. leprae* causes leprosy. Tuberculosis must be reported to the public health officials.

167.

D. A persistent viral infection in which the symptoms come and go is called a latent infection. Cold sores (oral herpes simplex) and genital herpes are examples of this type of infection. The virus enters the body and remains dormant in a nerve cell until conditions in the body, such as fever, sunburn, or stress, allow it to leave the nerve cells and seek the surface again.

168.

A. A most important safety rule to follow when you work in the medical laboratory is to wash your hands frequently and thoroughly with disinfectant soap to prevent the transfer of pathogens from one source to another. It is necessary to wear gloves in the laboratory when handling various patient samples and reagents. You should never put things in your mouth and should not eat, drink, or smoke in the laboratory as this may provide a direct path to the mucous tissues of the eyes, nose, or mouth or provide entrance to the digestive tract.

169.

A. The Gram stain is widely used to classify and study bacteria. Without staining, bacteria are colorless and cannot be seen clearly under the microscope. Even with staining the bacteria are so small that they are visible only under the highest magnification (100X objective with immersion oil). The Gram stain is actually two stains. After first "fixing" (gluing) the bacteria on the slide with heat to prevent their washing away, the bacteria smear is stained with dark purple gentian or crystal violet. The bacteria on the smear are then decolorized with alcohol (or acetone) and counterstained with a pink stain (safranin). If the cell walls of the bacteria are thick, they retain the original dark purple dye through the decolorization and are, therefore, Gram positive. If the cell walls are thinner, they will not retain the purple dye and will have only the pink stain added afterward. These pink bacteria, which have only the color from the second stain, are Gram negative.

Most bacteria are classified as either Gram positive or Gram negative. Additional stains such as the acid-fast stain that identifies the tuberculosis bacterium are sometimes used.

170.

B. None of the glucose meters now being produced require that the blood sample be washed off of the reagent strip pad before reading. Both the Glucometer and the Accu-Chek glucose meters require that the blood be blotted or wiped from the reagent strip pad before the test is read. The One Touch blood glucose meter does not require that the blood sample be removed before it is read. All glucose meters can read a wide range of glucose concentrations (values). These range from 0–600 mg/dL. All systems require that periodic controls be performed. Several newer brands of glucose meters do not utilize strip pads.

171.

B. Prothrombin time is determined whenever the coagulation process is studied or when maintaining anticoagulant therapy such as heparin. The normal range of a "pro time" (PT) is from 11–13 seconds or within 2 seconds of the control. A prothrombin time is the time plasma requires to coagulate under a controlled test situation when a clotting agent, thromboplastin, is added.

172.

A. Computed tomography also known as CT or a CAT scan is a type of x-ray (radiograph = radiation writing) that produces numerous cross sectional images that are reconstructed by a computer to provide visualization of internal structures not available in conventional x-rays.

Regarding the other answer choices: an angiocardiogram is a radiograph (x-ray) of the heart using a contrast medium; a bronchogram uses an opaque x-ray contrast medium to reveal lung structures; a cystogram is a radiograph of the urinary bladder taken after a radiopaque (opaque) contrast medium has been injected; a hysterosalpingogram is an x-ray of the uterus and fallopian tubes after a radiopaque contrast medium has been introduced.

173.

D. Ultrasonography (ultra = beyond; sono = sound; graphy = written) uses high frequency sound waves to reveal soft tissue structure images. Obstetrical ultrasonography is used for a number of reasons: to diagnose abnormalities in the fetus; to confirm the age of the fetus; to confirm multiple births; and to reveal the position and size of the infant in late pregnancy.

The other answer choices are other types of imaging: magnetic reasonance imaging, which reveals structures not seen by other techniques such as tissue with high fat and water content; conventional x-ray used for a variety of imaging particularly bones and organs where high contrast can be provided; CAT scan, which uses x-ray images of body cross sections to provide images of organs; intraveous pyelography (IVP), which provides x-ray images of the kidney and urinary tract to help diagnose kidney stones and other abnormalities.

174.

E. Barium sulfate is a radiographic (radiopaque) contrast medium that is used in examination of the gastric tract because it provides contrast of the digestive organs and therefore an image on x-ray.

For gastric studies (upper GI series and lower GI series), the patient will be given detailed instructions to follow for one or two days before the exam concerning the medication and diet.

175.

A. The "chain of custody" is used to acknowledge each transfer of the specimen (usually urine) in the collection and testing procedure for illicit drugs in the workplace. In this way the results can be acknowledged as correct when they are obtained. Picture identification must be obtained and steps taken to prevent tampering with the specimen during collection. The specimen is sealed and initialized by both the employee-donor and medical worker upon collection. Each step thereafter is also protected from unauthorized tampering. The results of the tests are crucial because they may result in the loss of a job, labeling of persons as drug users, or the possible overlooking of a drug user whose employment may damage persons or property. The term "chain of custody" is a legal term that applies to any legal evidence. It guards the validity of the evidence by showing the path it traveled.

176.

E. Magnetic resonance imaging (MRI) does not use either x-rays or ionizing radiation of any kind. MRI uses an interaction of magnetism and radiowaves with body tissue to obtain its images. MRI cannot see the hard part of the bones; this requires the use of x-rays. It shows tissue with high water and fat content, which does not show on conventional x-rays and is therefore the choice to reveal soft tissue lesions and abnormalities.

177.

E. The sediment of a urine sample that is positive for occult (hidden) blood will give a green to dark blue reading on the test strip. Hemolyzed blood with hemoglobin residue from red cells that have disintegrated cannot be detected with the microscope. Large amounts may color the urine a dark brown. Green spots indicate nonhemolyzed (intact) erythrocytes. The presence of red blood cells in urine is known as hematuria. Hemoglobinuria really means hemoglobin in the urine, which is produced when red blood cells are lysed (destroyed).

Occult blood may also occur in stool specimens. When this occurs, the source of blood is generally higher up in the digestive system. It is an important finding that indicates lesions in the digestive system and therefore the possibility of cancer.

178.

D. A few leukocytes are present in normal urine, but if they are numerous, the cells are referred to as pus corpuscles and indicate pyuria. Pyuria usually indicates a bacterial infection in the urinary tract. The number of white cells in a urine specimen is an important indicator of infection.

179.

A. The reaction time on the urine test strip N-Multistix 10 SG ranges from 30 seconds to 2 minutes. The developed color is read by comparing the test strip to the color chart on the container at the recommended time. The glucose and bilirubin tests are read at 30 seconds. All others are read by 60 seconds except leukocytes, which are read at 2 minutes. It is important to adhere exactly to the recommended time for reading.

180.

E. Increasing intensities of pink to maroon on the ketone portion of a reagent dipstick indicate increasing amounts of ketone bodies in urine. Ketones in the urine result from inadequate carbohydrate in the diet and an increasing amount of metabolism of fatty acids. Ketones are found often in the urine of patients with uncontrolled diabetes mellitus. They also occur during starvation, carbohydrate-deprived diets, and excessive vomiting. Acetest reagent tablets provide an alternative for confirmatory testing.

181.

B. A female patient should be instructed to collect a urine specimen midstream in a sterile bottle if it is to be sent to a laboratory for a bacteriologic culture. When this container (and any other urine container) arrives in the laboratory, the outside should be wiped with disinfectant before it is labeled.

182.

B. The first morning urine specimen is the most concentrated and would give the best results. The test checks for the presence of human chorionic gonadotropin (hCG) hormone, which can be detected in early pregnancy. First morning specimens are also called overnight, early morning, or 8-hour specimens. They are the specimens collected at the first urination upon arising in the A.M. The ELISA pregnancy test is quick to perform and easy to read. Random tests are sometimes used simply because they are convenient during an office visit.

183.

B. A simple liver function test that tests urine for bilirubin uses Ictotest tablets. Bilirubinuria indicates the presence of hepatocellular disease or intra- or extrahepatic biliary obstruction. Ictotest tablets are used to confirm a positive dipstick bilirubin test. Bilirubin will appear in the urine early in the disease or disorder, so it is a useful diagnostic tool.

184.

A. Epithelial cells (both squamous and renal) are reported as number per high-power field (HPF) as are RBC and WBC. Casts are reported as number per low-power field (LPF). In the qualitative technique for examining urine sediment, a drop of the resuspended sediment is placed on the microscope slide and covered with a coverslip. Casts and other cellular elements that are present are first scanned and viewed with the low-power magnification, but the scope is changed to high power for the final observation and report. A squamous epithelial cell is a large flat cell with a small nucleus. A renal epithelial cell is smaller and more round and comes from further up the urinary system.

185.

B. The purpose of an Addis count is to determine the patient's urinary output of formed elements during a 12-hour period. It provides an important quantitative picture of the output of the urinary system. Average normal values for an Addis count include white blood cells 1,800,000; red blood cells 500,000; and casts (hyaline) 0–5000. Casts have the shape of renal tubules because they form from protein inside the tubules. They are important indicators of renal disease.

186.

E. A wound culture is taken to identify the cause of the infection, which may be one of many types of bacteria or a fungus. The culture specimen must be collected by swabbing with a Dacron swab (not cotton—because it may inhibit strep growth) or by withdrawing some material with a syringe and needle. The swab must be placed immediately into some type of media. The clinical laboratory that cultures the specimen will give directions as to the type of media and how transport is to be handled. Preferably cultures are taken on site at the laboratory.

187.

C. X-rays may be potentially dangerous to employees in a physician's office where they are taken because the effect of radiation is cumulative. The dose received tomorrow is added to the dose received today, which is added to the amount received yesterday, and so on.

188.

A. One way for a physician to be certain that the clinic employees are not receiving a dangerous amount of radiation is to subscribe to a film badge service. Such a service indicates the amount and type of radiation to which employees have been exposed. A dosimeter registers the radiation exposure.

189.

E. All of the above items should be included. Specimens for drug and alcohol analysis should be collected and handled carefully. Before collection you should explain the procedure and have the patient sign a consent/release form for the urine, blood, or both. The patient should list all medications, drugs, and alcohol consumed in the last 30 days. After collection, the medical assistant who collected the specimen attaches his or her signature certifying that the sealed specimen was received from the patient at the site.

190.

B. The direct roentgen (radiation) beam comes from the x-ray tube (head) of the x-ray machine and is necessary to photograph the areas that the physician wishes to analyze or study.

191.

A. Secondary radiation is emitted by a patient while being filmed, and the radiation is scattered in all directions. Some of the primary radiation bounces off the patient instead of going straight through to the film and becomes secondary radiation.

192.

E. Palpation is not used in the collection of sputum cultures. Palpation is the act of putting light pressure on the surface of the body for the purpose of diagnosis.

The other answer choices may be used in the collection of sputum. **Expectoration** attempts to collect sputum by coughing it up. (Saliva must not be substituted.) **Tracheal suctioning** is employed by passing a catheter through the nose to the trachea. It cannot be utilized if the patient has heart disease or esophageal abnormalities. Bronchoscopy is the insertion of a bronchoscope into the throat and then into the bronchus. The secretion is either aspirated or collected

with a bronchial brush. **Nebulization** (spraying with a heated aerosol spray) may be required.

Results of the culture may be available in 24 to 48 hours except for TB, which may take 2 months. TB is a slow-growing organism.

193.

B. The radiograph is a permanent record of the image produced by an x-ray. It may be preserved by different means such as film, computer, or tape. A similar term, roentgenography, means the imaging of internal structures of the body by passing x-rays through the body and onto specially sensitized film.

194.

D. In a retrograde pyelogram procedure, dye is inserted directly by way of the cytoscope and urethroscope. The area studied is the ureters, bladder, and urethra. X-rays are taken of the urinary tract during the procedure, which takes about 1 1/2 hours to complete.

195.

B. During the evening preceding an IVP, a patient should be instructed to eat a light meal, with no food or fluids after 9:00 P.M. both that evening and in the morning, until after the test. The patient will be instructed to use an enema and cathartic to empty the colon. The IVP is a radiograph of the kidneys and the urinary tract that assists in the diagnosis of kidney stones, blockage, narrowing, or growths within the urinary tract.

Iodine is a contrast medium used to visualize the structures.

196.

A. A cholecystogram is done to determine the presence of any gallstones in the gallbladder. The procedure uses oral contrast medium, which is taken the evening before the examination. The procedure takes about 15 minutes to perform.

197.

E. A patient who is having an upper gastrointestinal series of x-rays will drink a suspension of barium sulfate while the radiologist observes its passage down the esophagus and into the stomach and duodenum by fluoroscope. A number of radiographs are taken throughout the test to provide a permanent record and for more detailed study after the test is completed. This test is also known as an "upper GI."

198.

A. The metric system provides accurate units to measure very small quantities correctly. In the medical laboratory very small measurements are compared to normal values to assess the patient's condition. The metric system, based on the number 10 and its multiples and divisions, is very easy to calculate. Another clinical area using the metric system is medication dispensing. The metric system has largely replaced older and less accurate systems. However, some patient's lack of familiarity with the metric system necessitates the use of the household system of tablespoons, teaspoons, and drops. Another system of measurement used in medical clinics (but not laboratories) is the English system of weight (body weight is generally measured in pounds). The apothecary system of medication measurement, once widely used, has become obsolete.

199.

E. Epithelial cells are from the surface of either the interior or exterior surfaces of the body. The blood can be divided into two major divisions, (1) the liquid part that contains dissolved and suspended substances such as nutrients, antibodies, etc., and (2) the cellular part that is composed of erythrocytes (red cells), thrombocytes (platelets), and leukocytes (white cells). The white cells in turn consist of neutrophils, lymphocytes, basophils, eosinophils, and monocytes.

200.

A. In the AP (anterior posterior) position, the patient is positioned so that the anterior (front of the body) is facing the x-ray tube and the posterior (back of the body) is facing the film. Other positions are **posteroanterior** (x-rays are directed from back to front of the body); **lateral view** where the x-ray beam passes from one side to the opposite side; **supine position** (lies on back); **prone position** (lies face down with head to side); and **oblique** (at an angle or semi-lateral position). X-rays from several different views may be taken to provide a three-dimensional view of the organ.

201.

A. Platelets, also known as thrombocytes from the word thrombus, meaning clot, arise from large bone marrow cells called megakarocytes. As the cell's cytoplasm disintegrates the fragments migrate to the blood system, and are seen as small, azure-blue bodies. They are an important part of the body's clotting mechanism. To assess the blood's clotting ability, platelets are counted and other clotting factors such as Vitamin K and calcium are measured with a prothrombin time test. Therapeutic anticoagulant drugs such as heparin require assessment of clotting factors on a regular basis. These drugs are given to counteract a tendency of the body in certain diseases to form blood clots.

A number of other diseases such as hemophilia, liver, and bone marrow diseases inhibit the body's ability to form clots. These too, require assessment of the blood's clotting abilities. Surgery also requires routine assessment of platelets.

202.

A. Ivy bleeding times (also called template method) are performed by making a controlled incision in the forearm and timing the clotting process. It is a very good measure of the body's total ability to clot blood but it does not differentiate between the causes of prolonged bleeding.

The other answer choices are hematology tests performed or calculated on automated equipment. The clinical laboratory can perform automated versions of almost every test if the volume justifies it. Hematology machines may use diluted samples and count them by either electrical impedance or by the light beam scattering method. Tests may also be performed on undiluted samples using centrifugation. Regardless of the type of machine, operation procedures should be strictly adhered to for quality control. Calibration procedures are necessary.

The cell counts and cell indices performed on automated machines are far more accurate than manual methods. Cell indices derived from the different comparisons of hematology test parameters are also much more accurate. Cell indices give valuable information about different types of anemia.

203.

A. A normal erythrocyte (red blood cell) has a biconcave shape and no nucleus. The center of a red blood cell appears light because it is thinner than the sides or margin. A red blood cell has a nucleus as it develops in the bone marrow but loses it before it enters the peripheral or circulating blood. In some blood diseases, such as sickle-cell anemia, the shape of the red blood cell is distorted.

204.

B. A monocyte is a well-defined cell with a large nucleus that generally is centrally placed. It may be oval, indented, or horseshoe shaped. The cytoplasm has a fine granular appearance.

205.

B. In a blood cell differential smear, platelets appear as very small azure-blue bodies when stained with Wright's stain. The platelets, also known as thrombocytes, may contain small reddish purple granules and originate in the bone marrow as a large cell that disintegrates into platelets.

206.

D. All RBC pipettes are made so that if blood is taken to the 0.5 mark and diluted to the 101 mark, the dilution will be 1:200. If the blood is drawn to the 1.0 mark and diluted to the 101 mark, the dilution is 1:100.

207.

D. There are 9 square millimeters (mm^2) on one side of a hemocytometer counting chamber. In a manual white blood cell count, the area counted is 4 mm^2, the four corner areas. The manual red blood cell count usually uses only one-fifth of the center 1 mm^2 area.

208.

D. The correct answer is 6000 WBC/mm^3. The formula is cell/mm^3 = number of cells counted $\times$ dilution $\times$ depth/area in mm^2 counted = $120 \times 20 \times 10/4$ = 6000/mm^3.

209.

C. The normal WBCs per cubic millimeter for both men and women is 4,500 to 12,000. An increase in WBCs above normal levels is called leukocytosis. This is a normal physiologic response to a bacterial infection in the body. Leukopenia is a decrease in the WBC count and is caused by viral infections, radiation, and certain chemicals and drugs.

210.

A. The automated blood cell counters count larger numbers of cells in each sample compared to a manual method. This gives them greater precision and accuracy. Controls can be incorporated easily into the automated system and give good quality assurance to document the laboratory's performance. The blood sample must be handled only one time—to draw the sample, which may be used for several tests.

211.

B. The fibrometer, manufactured by BBL Microbiology Systems, is used for coagulation tests. Instruments, such as the fibrometer, have replaced the old manual tilt-tube method for performing prothrombin times to check coagulation levels of patients on "blood thinners," such as dicumarol (an anticoagulant drug). Quality control is part of every test performed on the fibrometer through the use of control plasma samples.

212.

D. The normal RBC count for men is 4.5 to 6.0 million cells/mm^3. For women, the range is 4.0 to 5.5 million cells/mm^3.

213.

E. A CBC consists of RBC count, WBC count, Hgb estimation, and a differential white cell count. A CBC usually includes a hematocrit determination and, in many laboratories, RBC indices will be part of the results. A sed rate is a separate test.

214.

E. Quality control testing does not check for hazards in the laboratory. However, the same careful workmanship and attitudes that build a good quality control program will also check for biohazards, chemical hazards, and physical hazards and take preventive steps. An unsafe clinical laboratory is also generally a laboratory in which quality control is not maintained. Quality control programs check the reliability of the test results and build the confidence of the laboratory worker.

215.

C. Urine usually becomes alkaline (basic) on long standing, which is caused by the decomposition of urea and the formation of ammonia (a basic substance) by bacteria.

216.

A. The most concentrated, and thus the urine with the greatest specific gravity, is urine voided first thing in the morning. The first morning specimen is best when testing for nitrite, protein, or microscopic examination.

217.

D. A 2-hour postprandial urine is one that is collected 2 hours after a person has eaten a meal. Glucose is the substance that the physician wants to check. A positive urine glucose on a 2-hour postprandial sample is an indicator that this patient may be a diabetic.

218.

D. Blood, either visible or occult, is not a normal constituent in urine, but it may be found as a contaminant in women with a vaginal discharge. Otherwise, it indicates a lesion somewhere in the urinary tract or perineum.

219.

C. The kidneys are capable of producing urine that ranges from a pH of 4.5 to 8.0. The letters "pH" refer to the hydrogen ion concentration present in a solution that determines the acid or base level. The complete pH scale ranges from 0 to 14 with 7 as the neutral point between acid and base readings. Readings above 7 are basic (alkaline), and those below 7 are acidic.

220.

C. The normal specific gravity of urine varies between 1.010 and 1.025. A specific gravity either below or above this range may be suggestive of disease and warrants further testing. Patients with diabetes insipidus will usually never produce urine with a specific gravity above 1.003.

221.

A. The specific gravity of a substance is expressed as the weight of that substance in relation to the weight of the same volume of water. Specific gravity of urine = weight of 1 mL of urine/weight of 1 mL of water. Specific gravity measures the concentration of urine, which becomes heavier with the addition of dissolved substances.

222.

C. When the oil immersion lens (100X) objective is used with an eyepiece that provides a magnification of 10 diameters (10X), an assistant may see an object 1000 times its actual size because the magnification of microscopes is the product of the eyepiece power times the objective power. ($100 \times 10 = 1000$.)

223.

E. It is important in the care of the microscope to remove all the excess oil from the oil immersion objective with lens paper before the microscope is stored. It is also important to leave the microscope set with the low power objective in place when the microscope is not in use. This prevents excess light in the body of the scope, which can damage the optics.

224.

A. The object or specimen is initially located by using the low power objective (10X) in combination with the coarse adjustment. After the specimen is located with low power, the revolving nosepiece that houses the objectives is rotated to the high power objective for greater magnification.

225.

C. To be examined, material is placed on slides. The slides are then placed on the stage and clipped or, if a mechanical stage is used, held in place by the stage.

226.

A. Universal precautions incorporated into OSHA's standards, and now a federal regulation, are guidelines followed by health care workers to prevent infection with AIDS, hepatitis, or other diseases transmitted through body fluids. Some specific guidelines are (1) take universal precautions with *all* blood and body fluids, not just those known to be contaminated; (2) use protective barriers such as gloves, gowns, and shields; (3) avoid injury from sharp objects, such as used needles; (4) wash hands as needed to prevent transferring disease microbes; (5) dispose of contaminated waste properly; and (6) disinfect work surfaces and equipment as recommended.

227.

D. The sputum should come from as deep within the respiratory tract as possible. Excretions from the lungs, bronchial tubes, or trachea are desirable. Saliva and mucous from the nose or mouth may interfere with the tests. Early morning specimens soon after waking are best. Sputum analysis in the laboratory can aid in the diagnosis of infectious organisms or cancer cells. The patient should be instructed as to why it is important to follow directions.

228.

D. In collecting a stool specimen for occult blood, a medical assistant should bear in mind that only a small amount of stool is required and that it need not be kept warm or examined immediately. It is not uncommon for patients to be given the supplies needed to collect a stool specimen for occult blood testing in the home. They are given a mailing container that is mailed back to the laboratory for analysis.

Other fecal tests are for ova and parasites of flat worms and round worms and occasionally cultures for bacterial infections. Most stool specimens will be sent to specialized laboratories, which will furnish instructions for collection and transport.

229.

A. Cancer of the cervix is diagnosed from the type of abnormal cell growth seen on Papanicolaou smears. They are taken during a vaginal examination and the procedure must be followed exactly in order for the Pap smear to be valid. It is either sprayed to preserve it or placed in an alcohol-ether solution for transport to the laboratory.

Pap smears, after having been properly collected and fixed by the clinical staff, are forwarded to a cytology laboratory directed by a pathologist. (Cytology = the study of cells.) At this laboratory, a report describing the adequacy of the specimen is issued by a pathologist. The specimen is rated as normal or abnormal, and a descriptive diagnosis, where the pathologist gives a detailed description of abnormal findings, is provided. This type of report has replaced the previous categories of five classes of cells.

230.

A. Normal bleeding time is from 1–3 minutes. Materials needed to determine bleeding time are sterile lancet, smooth filter paper, and a watch with a second hand. This procedure tests for a tendency to hemorrhage, since low platelet counts, hemophilia, and some other blood diseases cause a prolonged clotting time.

231.

C. A medical assistant should not squeeze out blood in drops after puncturing the finger because the tissue fluid will be expressed, diluting the blood, and test results will not be correct. It is very important to follow correct technique to obtain accurate results. Another puncture using a different finger should be made if enough blood cannot be obtained from the original puncture.

232.

E. The causative agent of gonorrhea is a Gram-negative diplococcus. Other Gram-negative organisms include typhoid bacilli, dysentery bacilli, whooping cough bacilli, and meningococci. Some antibiotics are effective against Gram-negative organisms, whereas others are most effective against Gram-positive organisms.

233.

C. *Staphylococcus aureus* is a common Gram-positive coccus that causes "staph" infections. Other Gram-positive organisms include pneumococci, streptococci, tubercle bacilli, and diphtheria bacilli. The Gram stain, the shape of the bacterium, its mobility, the medium required for growth, and chemical reactions are bacterial identification aids.

234.

E. The glucometer gives blood glucose values taken from a drop of blood obtained from a capillary puncture. A colorimetric strip test is also available that is designed to indicate blood glucose values by reading color development on the strip although the glucometer is more accurate. The test, which requires one large drop of whole blood from a finger puncture, may be read in exactly 1 minute following the application of the whole blood onto the reaction section of the strip. A quick, inexpensive, and accurate blood glucose test provides the information to help control the variations of diabetes.

A complimentary test, glucohemoglobin, which shows a modified form of hemoglobin to which glucose attaches, indicates how well the blood glucose level has been controlled over a period of the past two or three months.

235.

A. The normal Westergren ESR (erythrocyte sedimentation rate) for men is from 0–20 mm/hr if men older than 50 are included. For women, the normal Westergren ESR is 0-30 mm/hr if women older than 50 are included. The Wintrobe ESR values are lower: males, 0–7 mm/hr; and women, 0–15 mm/hr. The sedimentation rate provides useful information to differentiate a number of diseases in their early stages and is an important test. The Wintrobe ESR has similar but slightly different normal values from the Westergren ESR.

236.

B. Expressed as g/100 mL, the average range of hemoglobin values for women is 12.5 to 15. The average range of hemoglobin values for men is 14 to 18. Men have higher average values for hemoglobin and RBC counts than women. The hemoglobin value indicates whether a person is anemic, and further tests will distinguish the source of the anemia.

237.

A. In a WBC count, basophils and eosinophils may average less than 5%. Basophils range from 0–1%, and eosinophils range from 1–3%. These will rise dramatically in certain diseases and are, therefore, a diagnostic tool. Eosinophil rise is associated with allergies.

238.

D. In a WBC count, lymphocytes may average from 25–33%, with the average being about 26%. The number of lymphocytes will be increased in children. A 1-month-old baby may have 40–70% lymphocytes. An increase in lymphocytes is lymphocytosis, and lymphopenia is a decrease in lymphocytes.

239.

D. In a WBC count, neutrophils may average 50–70%, with the average being about 66%. Because both the total WBC count and counts of individual types of white cells decrease or increase predictably in certain diseases, the total WBC and differential counts are elementary diagnostic aids when compiled with information the doctor gathers from the physical examination and other sources.

240.

B. The normal hematocrit reading for men ranges from 40–52%. The normal hematocrit reading for women ranges from 37–47%. The hematocrit is obtained by centrifuging a microsample of blood and comparing the ratio of packed cells to the total volume of blood. The hematocrit, along with the hemoglobin value and RBC, provides much information about the red cell pathology and possible sources of anemia.

241.

A. Do not recap needles after you have used them. They should be disposed of in a container that is puncture resistant. Needles should not be broken after use, since this extra handling increases the chances of the medical assistant being stuck with the blood-contaminated needles. Recapping needles and improper disposal are frequent causes of needle sticks.

242.

E. Sodium hypochlorite (household bleach) is recommended as a disinfectant for working surfaces to kill the AIDS virus, since the AIDS virus has been shown to be sensitive to this chemical. Blood specimens pose the greatest risk for contact with the AIDS virus in the laboratory; therefore, all blood samples should be handled as if they are infected. All blood spills should be immediately soaked in bleach solution and then cleaned up immediately with paper towels by a gloved employee, who then again disinfects the area. At the end of the day, work surfaces should be wiped clean with a 10% bleach solution or similar approved disinfectant.

243.

C. The single most important objective to follow to prevent infection by pathogens such as HIV and HBV is to completely isolate the biological specimen so it cannot contaminate the laboratory or the persons working within it. Barring the ability to completely isolate the specimen, the workers should protect themselves and the work surfaces as much as possible and prevent any contamination spreading from one area to another. This is accomplished by safe work practices, the use of disinfectants, and frequent hand washing. Blood, semen, and vaginal secretions are known carriers of the AIDS virus. Proper hand washing after handling specimens is probably the single most important regular safety practice in the laboratory because it prevents contamination from one source to another.

244.

E. The quality control test results should be posted immediately after performing as mandated by CLIA regulations. Immediate (daily, in most cases) recording of both the normal and abnormal quality control results ensures that errors and trends are noted and corrected promptly. Levy-Jennings charts are often used to post quality control results because they make errors and trends quickly apparent.

245.

A. Quality control is essential to accurate patient test reporting. The Levy-Jennings chart makes the control test data easy to read over a period of days and makes errors and shifts away from normal in any direction easy to spot. It utilizes the mean and upper and lower

limits of statistical deviations on a chart with consecutive days. Errors due to operator fault or equipment failure can often be diagnosed by looking at the chart.

246.

A. Blood serum may be separated from clotted blood cells by centrifugation. It is always collected in red-top tubes or red/black-top tubes, and it is obtained from clotted blood that has not been mixed with an anticoagulant.

247.

B. Plasma is obtained from blood that has been mixed with an anticoagulant in the collection tube, and it contains albumin, globulin, and fibrinogen. Common anticoagulants used in the laboratory to prevent clotting are EDTA in a purple-stoppered tube, heparin in a green-stoppered tube, and sodium citrate in a blue-stoppered tube. Different colors of tube stoppers provide a quick, efficient identification method when collecting blood for serum, plasma, or anticoagulated (nonclotting) whole blood.

248.

E. In connection with blood collection tubes, if a vacuum tube is not filling properly, the medical assistant should substitute another tube; all tubes containing an anticoagulant or preservative must be allowed to fill to the exhaustion of the vacuum; and the medical assistant should verify the patient's identification. In addition, the venipuncture site should be selected by the feel, not the appearance, of the vein.

249.

B. To fully inform and prepare a patient for a blood glucose determination, the medical assistant should tell the patient to fast for 8–12 hours and to drink only water. The patient should be cautioned not to drink juices, coffee, and so on that might inadvertently add calories to the body.

250.

E. To perform a venipuncture, the medical assistant should take a position in front or slightly to the side of the patient, fasten the tourniquet, locate the vein, swab the puncture site with alcohol, and penetrate the skin about 1/4 to 1/2 inch below the point where the vein will be entered. The needle should be at a 15-degree angle, which is nearly parallel to the skin. The tourniquet should be released before the needle is removed from the venipuncture to prevent bleeding from the site and a resulting hematoma under the skin.

251.

E. When the medical assistant is preparing a blood smear he or she should place one-half of a drop of blood about 1/2 to 3/4 inch from the end of the slide. The spreader slide should be brought back into the drop to start the smear. The spreader slide should be held at a 35–40 degree angle, and the feathered edge, which is only one cell layer thick, should appear at the thin end of the smear.

252.

E. All of the four factors are needed in calculating a blood cell count using the hemocytometer. The dilution factor for white blood cell counts is usually 1:20, and for red blood cell counts 1:200. The depth between the coverslip and chamber that is filled with fluid from the pipette is always 0.1 mm; thus, to make this 1 mm, you must multiply by 10. The blood cells are reported in units of cubic millimeters or in some labs, as cells per liter.

253.

D. The hemoglobin determination is colorimetric. Both the WBC and the RBC counts are performed in most automated cell counters by passing the cells in their diluting solution through a special narrow opening in the machine. The cells in the fluid interrupt the electric current, and each interruption is counted. The diluting solution is a sodium chloride solution that conducts electric current.

254.

D. Cardiac, liver, general metabolism (thyroid), lipid, renal, and hepatic (liver) profiles are all common profiles ordered by physicians. A panel (profile) usually includes many blood tests. Studies of the skeletal system would require more radiologic work, with blood chemistries being secondary in importance. Some panels and profiles include 20 or more blood chemistry tests. They are almost always performed on automated equipment.

255.

A. The butterfly method of venipuncture is preferred when patients are hard to stick and multiple tubes of blood are needed for tests. An alternate method with a syringe may be used when less blood is needed. Children who of course have smaller veins, obese patients, elderly patients and adults with small veins all may benefit from a butterfly venipuncture.

A third method of venipuncture is the vacuum tube method. It is more difficult to perform and requires more experience. Capillary punctures are made when the amount of blood needed is small. When obtaining blood from a small infant or newborn, the heel and sole of the foot can be utilized. Otherwise capillary punctures are ordinarily made in the finger.

256.

C. The reagent strip method for occult blood usually is capable of detecting 0.015–0.06 mg/dL of free hemoglobin or 5–20 intact red cells/microliter. The normal value for a random specimen is negative for both hemoglobin and occult blood. A normal urine sediment report for red blood cells should not be more than 2 per high power field. Occult blood refers to blood that is not obvious. Blood in the urine is also referred to as hematuria.

257.

B. The condenser and the iris diaphragm regulate the light that strikes the object being viewed or studied. The condenser and the iris diaphragm are located below the stage. The condenser is adjusted up or down to change the light intensity, and the iris diaphragm is opened and closed.

258.

E. Agglutination test kits used to test for heterophil antibodies in plasma or serum of patients with infectious mononucleosis contain slides, reagents, and both positive and negative controls. The positive and negative controls must be run each time the test is performed. Visible clumps indicate positive tests. Commercial tests for mono include Monospot and Mono-Test. It is the lymphocytes, not the monocytes, which are affected by the Epstein-Barr virus (EBV), so the name of the disease is a misnomer. The abnormal lymphs were misnamed monocytes by the earliest researchers.

answers & rationales

259.

E. The VDRL is a screening test for syphilis (a sexually transmitted disease) as is the RPR (rapid plasma reagin). Because these tests sometimes give false-positive results in other diseases, positive results must be confirmed with the fluorescent treponemal antibody (FTA) test. Both use blood serum in the test.

Syphilis begins with a lesion at the source of entry (which develops into a chancre) in the primary stage, which is followed by the secondary stage of lesions in the skin and mucous membranes. The tertiary (third) stage, which may last many years, frequently involves the heart, other internal organs, and the central nervous system. It may result in insanity, heart disease, kidney disease etc. Because this disease is not apparent except in the early stages, a diagnostic test is very important to detect it before irreparable damage occurs.

260.

D. All of the four methods listed are ways of determining specific gravity in urine. The urinometer, refractometer, and dipsticks, such as N-Multistix SG, which includes a specific gravity segment, are the most common methods. The Ames Clinitek Auto 2000 uses the falling drop method. This method is very accurate, but the instrument is too expensive for physician's office laboratory use.

261.

E. A feathered edge is one of the marks of a good blood slide. Many factors will affect the quality of a blood smear. A drop of blood that is too large will produce thick smears. Thin smears occur when the drop of blood is too small. Grease on slides will produce holes in the smear. A spreader slide should be used only once, and it must not be chipped. Delays in application of blood drops to the slide and spreading will cause uneven distribution of cells on the smear. The wrong angle will produce a blood slide that is too thin or thick.

262.

E. Bleach should not be added as a preservative. Directions must be followed explicitly. Written instructions for 24-hour urine collections should include all of the other points mentioned in this question. Urinate into a small container and transfer to a larger collection bottle. Do not collect the first sample of initial day on arising in the morning but write down the time. Follow directions given by the laboratory that is supplying the container for preservation of the specimen. Void at exactly the same time the following morning, and add the sample to the collection container.

263.

A. The first part of the urine voided should be discarded and the midstream portion collected instead. The midportion is less likely to be contaminated with cells or bacteria. For a clean-catch specimen, a female patient should follow the directions provided regarding insertion of a fresh tampon if menstruating and keeping the skin folds apart while urinating.

264.

B. Pregnancy can be detected as early as 10 days after conception. A first morning urine sample is preferred because it will have a higher concentration of the hormone hCG. The specific gravity must be at least 1.010 because a reading below this would be too dilute and may cause a false-negative test result. Most test kits will detect pregnancy as early as the tenth day after conception.

265.

B. Glucose levels will NOT increase but they may decrease due to bacteria using the glucose as food if it is present as a resource. Samples that must be tested and read after a period of 1 hour after collection should be refrigerated to retard all four conditions listed. Urea in the urine may be converted to ammonia, giving a foul smell (along with bacteria) to the urine. Bilirubin is a very unstable pigment in urine.

266.

C. The record made by the diagnostic ultrasound is a sonogram or an echogram. The ultrasound uses high-frequency sound waves to create an image of the organ being studied. The technique has wide use in diagnosing conditions of fetuses while still in the womb. The diskogram is an x-ray record of the vertebral column after injection of a contrast medium. The urogram is the x-ray record of any part of the urinary tract after injection of a contrast medium.

267.

E. A test with a high urine protein concentration indicates that immediate action is needed, and the test results should be called to the doctor's attention at once. The other test results listed were within the normal range. Higher levels of protein in urine is an important indicator of renal disease in which there is glomerular or tubular damage.

Tests with action values indicate that the patient needs **immediate medical care**—that is, the patient is in a crisis. Very high blood glucose values, very low hemoglobin and hematocrit readings, very high readings of enzymes that indicate tissue (and heart) damage, very prolonged prothrombin times, very high sedimentation rates, very high or low red or white cell counts—all of these indicate that the patient needs immediate medical attention. The office physicians decide what test values indicate crises for their patients. A list should be drawn up and kept available to alert the medical assistant to call test results to the doctor's attention.

11 Medication and Pharmacology

chapter objectives

Major areas of knowledge/content included in this chapter are:

I. Pharmacology

➤ drug classification

➤ drug forms/actions/uses/side effects/adverse reactions

➤ emergency use

➤ substance abuse

➤ calculation of dosage

II. Routes and procedures for administering medications including immunizations

III. Prescriptions

➤ prescription parts

➤ safekeeping and recordkeeping

➤ controlled substances

IV. Top 50 most prescribed drugs

DIRECTIONS (Questions 268 through 371): Each of the numbered items or incomplete statements in this section is followed by answers or by completions of the statement. Select the ONE lettered answer or completion that is BEST in each case.

The following questions include the list of 50 most frequently prescribed drugs according to the April 1999 issue of *Pharmacy Times*. When both the trade name and generic name are written together, the trade name is capitalized, the generic name follows in parentheses.

268. Amoxil and Trimox are trade names for amoxicillin, a generic drug, which is a/an
    A. antibiotic
    B. diuretic
    C. antifungal
    D. hypnotic
    E. opiate

    (Gauwitz and Bayt, pp 113, 121; Physician's Desk Reference (PDR), pp 2969–2972; Kizior and Hodgson, pp 53–54)

269. Lanoxin (digoxin), which comes in tablets, injections, and pediatric elixir preparations, is one of the group of glycosides referred to as "digitalis" and is used to treat
    A. eczema
    B. coronary disorders
    C. vomiting
    D. hypertension
    E. organ transplant patients

    (PDR, pp 1228–1231; Rice #2, pp 372–373; Kizior and Hodgson, pp 321–323)

270. Xanax (alprazolam) and Klonopin (clonazepam) have which drug classification?
    A. vasoconstrictor
    B. antispasmodic
    C. antianxiety
    D. antiarrhythmic
    E. carminative agent

    (Gauwitz and Bates, p 322; PDR, pp 2492–2496, 2646–2648; Kizior and Hodgson, pp 26–27, 240–242)

271. Zantac (ranitidene) is a histamine blocker and, therefore, is useful in the treatment of
    A. hypertension
    B. ulcers
    C. vomiting
    D. hemorrhage
    E. asthma

    (PDR, pp 1310–1312; Rice #2, p 352; Kizior and Hodgson, pp 891–892)

272. The main body organ involved in drug metabolism is the
    A. kidney
    B. brain
    C. small intestine
    D. stomach
    E. liver

    (Gauwitz and Bayt, p 209; Hitner and Nagle, p 25)

273. Veetids (penicillin V potassium) is used to treat staphylococci, streptococci, and gonococci and as a prophylaxis for rheumatic fever. It is a/an
    A. antibiotic
    B. antihistamine
    C. antifungal agent
    D. antihypertensive
    E. none of the above

    (Gauwitz and Bayt, p 113; Kizior and Hodgson, pp 807–809)

274. To determine a child's dose (pediatric dose or pd) in a pediatrician's office, a medical assistant may use one of several rules: Young's Rule [adult dose × fraction (child's age in years over age of child plus 12) = pd]; Fried's Rule [adult dose × fraction (infant's age in months over 150 months) = pd]; Clark's rule [adult dose × fraction (child's weight in pounds over 150 pounds) = pd]. Use the appropriate rule to calculate how much streptomycin a child of 6 years should receive if the adult dose is 0.5 g?

    A. 0.10 g
    B. 0.13 g
    C. 0.15 g
    D. 0.17 g
    E. 0.25 g

    (Hitner and Nagle, p 52; Kinn and Woods, pp 1022–1023)

275. Premarin (conjugated estrogen), used as a hormone replacement and for other treatments, belongs to the chemical group

    A. emetics
    B. steroids
    C. opiates
    D. cholinergics
    E. miotic

    (Gauwitz and Bayt, p 260; Kizior and Hodgson, pp 258–261; PDR, pp 3302–3305)

276. Cardizem (diltiazem) is used to treat coronary circulation problems and acts as a

    A. digestant
    B. cholinergic
    C. sedative
    D. calcium ion influx inhibitor
    E. diaphoretic

    (Kizior and Hodgson, pp 325–327; PDR, pp 1358–1360)

277. Drug references do not usually include which of the following information?

    A. indications
    B. contraindications
    C. description composition
    D. dosage and administration
    E. cost of the drug

    (Gauwitz and Bayt, pp 5–6)

278. Ceclor (cefaclor) is an

    A. antitussive
    B. antispasmodic
    C. antifungal
    D. emetic
    E. antibiotic

    (Kizior and Hodgson, pp 162–164; PDR, pp 990–992; Rice #2, p 222)

279. Prednisone is the generic name for a drug sold under the product names Orasone, Deltasone, and Meticorten. These drugs are classified as

    A. bronchodilators
    B. corticosteroids
    C. beta blockers
    D. diuretics
    E. expectorant

    (Kizior and Hodgson, pp 840–843, 1145)

280. Synthroid and Levoxyl are two product names for the generic drug levothyroxine, which is a synthetic hormone replacement for the principal hormone secreted by the

    A. pancreas
    B. thyroid
    C. pituitary
    D. hypothalamus
    E. prostate

    (Kizior and Hodgson, pp 592–594; PDR, pp 1467, 1513–1516)

281. Accupril (quinapril hydrochloride) and Capoten (captopril) are used to treat

    A. diabetes
    B. vomiting
    C. neoplasms
    D. hypertension
    E. epilepsy

    (Kizior and Hodgson, pp 148–150, 880–882; Rice #2, p 378)

282. Acetaminophen with codeine is an
    A. antipruritic
    B. expectorant
    C. analgesic
    D. antiflatulent
    E. antidepressant
    (Kizior and Hodgson, pp 6–8)

283. Pepcid (famotidine) is a drug used in the treatment of
    A. depression
    B. emphysema
    C. constipation
    D. duodenal ulcer
    E. bacterial infection
    (Kizior and Hodgson, pp 402–403; PDR, pp 1852–1855)

284. Cephalexin (the generic name for Keflex) is an anti-infective used in the treatment of
    A. respiratory infections
    B. genitourinary infections
    C. skin infections
    D. bone infections
    E. all of the above
    (Kizior and Hodgson, pp 199–201; Rice #2, p 558)

285. Vasotec (enalapril)
    A. is an antihypertensive
    B. lowers blood pressure
    C. lessens resistance to blood flow
    D. has contraindications and precautions
    E. all of the above
    (Kizior and Hodgson, pp 361–363; PDR, pp 1909–1912)

286. Procardia (nifedipine) affects the
    A. coronary circulation
    B. ovaries
    C. digestive tract
    D. cerebral circulation
    E. adrenal glands
    (PDR, pp 2361–2365)

287. Furosemide and Triamterene/HCTZ reduce hypertension and act as
    A. diuretics
    B. demulcents
    C. deflatulents
    D. hematinics
    E. protectives
    (Gauwitz and Bayt, pp 240–241; Kizior and Hodgson, pp 455–457, 1026–1028)

288. Zoloft (sertraline hydrochloride) and Paxil (paroxetine hydrochloride) are prescribed as tablets and are drugs classified as
    A. antihypertensives
    B. antihistamines
    C. antihyperlipidemics
    D. anticonvulsants
    E. antidepressants
    (Gauwitz and Bayt, p 321; Kizior and Hodgson, pp 926–927; PDR, pp 2399–2404, 3027–3033)

289. Dilantin (phenytoin) is a medication used for the treatment of
    A. hyperglycemia
    B. hepatitis
    C. depression
    D. epilepsy
    E. nausea
    (Gauwitz and Bayt, p 311; Kizior and Hodgson, pp 821–823; PDR, pp 2242–2246)

290. Propoxyphene napsylate acetaminophen (N/APAP), sold under the trade (product) names of Darvocet N 100 and Propacet 100, is an analgesic prescribed for
    A. pain
    B. insomnia
    C. depression
    D. hypoxia
    E. hypertension
    (Kizior and Hodgson, pp 862–863; PDR, pp 1574–1576)

291. Zocor (simvastatin), Lipitor (atorvastatin calcium), Pravachol (pravastatin sodium), and Mevacor (lovastatin) are drugs classified as
    A. antihypertensives
    B. antihistamines
    C. antihyperlipidemics
    D. anticonvulsants
    E. antidepressants
    (Kizior and Hodgson, pp 616–618, 932–934; PDR, pp 1917–1920, 2254–2257, 846–849, 1833–1837)

292. Which of the following drugs is classified as an agent to suppress gastric acid secretion?
    A. Prilosec (omeprazole)
    B. Claritin (loratidine)
    C. Paxil (paroxetine hydrochloride)
    D. Relafen (nabumetone)
    E. Klonopin (clonazepam)
    (Kizior and Hodgson, p 778; PDR, pp 617–621)

293. The drug Biaxin (clarithromycin) and Zithromax (azithromycin) are classified as
    A. antihypertensives
    B. antibiotics
    C. antihistamines
    D. anticonvulsants
    E. antidepressants
    (Kizior and Hodgson, pp 233–234; PDR, pp 409–417, 2389–2396)

294. Glucophage (metformin hydrochloride), Glucotrol XL (glipizide), and Micronase (glyburide), oral medications in the form of tablets, are used to treat
    A. diabetes
    B. thrush
    C. asthma
    D. angina
    E. proctitis
    (Kizior and Hodgson, pp 473–475; PDR, pp 831–835, 2347–2349, 2466–2467)

295. Augmentin (amoxicillin clavulanate)
    A. is an antibiotic
    B. kills Gram-positive bacteria
    C. kills Gram-negative bacteria
    D. is related to penicillin
    E. all of the above
    (Gauwitz and Bayt, pp 113, 121; PDR, pp 2978–2980)

296. Hydrocodone bitartrate and acetaminophen, also written hydrocodone/APAP, is classified as a/an
    A. diuretic
    B. antiemetic
    C. analgesic
    D. antiseptic
    E. hemostatic
    (Kizior and Hodgson, pp 502–504)

297. K-Dur (potassium chloride) is prescribed for
    A. potassium replacement
    B. endocrine imbalance
    C. flu
    D. typhoid
    E. obesity
    (Kizior and Hodgson, pp 832–835; PDR, pp 1473–1474)

298. Ventolin (albuterol) and Proventil aerosol (albuterol) are two brand names (or trade names) of the same medicine, which are used as
    A. decongestants
    B. expectorants
    C. bronchodilators for asthma
    D. antitussives
    E. antihistamines
    (Kizior and Hodgson, pp 19–21; PDR, pp 1294–1300, 2834–2836)

299. Claritin (loratidine) and Zyrtec (cetirizine hydrochloride) have a drug classification of
    A. antihypertensive
    B. antihistamine
    C. anticonvulsant
    D. anti-inflammatory agent
    E. none of the above
    (Kizior and Hodgson, pp 610–611; PDR, pp 2781–2783, 2404–2406)

300. Relafen (nabumetone) has which drug classification?
    A. antihypertensive
    B. antihistamine
    C. anticonvulsant
    D. anti-inflammatory
    E. antihyperlipidemic
    (Kizior and Hodgson, pp 711–712, 1178; PDR, pp 3035–3037)

301. Drug classifications under the Controlled Substances Act of 1970 are divided into schedules. Which of the following does not require a prescription from a doctor to purchase?
    A. Schedule I
    B. Schedule II
    C. Schedule III
    D. Schedule IV
    E. Schedule V
    (Gauwitz and Bayt, pp 9–10; Hitner and Nagle, pp 3–4, 12)

302. Provera (medroxyprogesterone) is used in cases of
    A. amenorrhea and menopause symptoms
    B. mental depression
    C. senility
    D. Alzheimer's disease
    E. premenopausal syndrome (PMS)
    (Kizior and Hodgson, pp 634–636; PDR, pp 2481–2482)

303. Timoptic (timolol) reduces intraocular pressure and is used to treat
    A. conjunctivitis
    B. cataracts
    C. myopia
    D. ametropia
    E. glaucoma
    (Kizior and Hodgson, pp 994–996; PDR, pp 1891–1896)

304. Ery-Tab (erythromycin base) is the antibiotic used to treat and prevent
    A. measles
    B. staphylococcus infections
    C. streptococcal pharyngitis
    D. carbuncles
    E. neuritis
    (Kizior and Hodgson, pp 379–382; PDR, pp 441–443)

305. Advil, Motrin, and Nuprin are trade names of the generic medication ibuprofen. It has antipyretic and analgesic properties used to treat
    A. rheumatoid arthritis
    B. osteoarthritis
    C. pain
    D. primary dysmenorrhea
    E. all of the above
    (Kizior and Hodgson, pp 516–519; PDR, pp 1684–1686)

306. Prempro (conjugated estrogens/ medroxyprogesterone acetate) is a hormone replacement drug that belongs to the chemical group
    A. steroids
    B. cholinergics
    C. anesthetics
    D. antiarrhythmics
    E. opiates
    (Kizior and Hodgson, pp 259–261, 634–635; PDR, pp 3308–3312)

307. Humulin N (human insulin) is a hormone replacement used to treat
A. pituitary dwarfism
B. acromegaly
C. diabetes
D. hypothyroidism
E. Cushing's syndrome
(Kizior and Hodgson, pp 533–536; PDR, pp 1606–1610)

308. Ortho-Novum 7/7/7–28 (norethindrone/ mestranol) and Triphasil-21 and -28 (levonorgestrel and ethinyl estradiol) are prescribed for
A. hormone replacement
B. birth control
C. diabetes
D. hypothyroidism
E. endometriosis
(PDR, pp 2184–2191, 3328–3334; Rice #2, pp 481–482)

309. Coumadin (warfarin), commonly known as a "blood thinner," is an anticoagulant used in the treatment of
A. hemorrhagic diseases
B. blood dyscrasias
C. ulceration
D. venous thrombosis
E. hepatitis
(Kizior and Hodgson, pp 1067–1069; PDR, pp 969–974)

310. Calculate the pediatric dose (pd) of a drug for a 30 lb child from an adult dose of 50.0 mg. Choose between Young's Rule [adult dose × fraction (child's age in years over age of child plus 12) = pd]; Fried's rule [adult dose × fraction (infant's age in months over 150 months) = pd]; Clark's rule [adult dose × fraction (child's weight in pounds over 150 pounds) = pd].
A. 5.0 mg
B. 10.0 mg
C. 20.0 mg
D. 25.0 mg
E. 30.0 mg
(Hitner and Nagle, p 52; Kinn and Woods, pp 1022–1023)

311. Nitrostat (nitroglycerin) is a vasodilator and is used in the treatment of
A. anxiety
B. angina
C. hypertension
D. edema
E. hemophilia
(Gauwitz and Bayt, p 174; PDR, pp 2271–2272)

312. The medical assistant must be aware of the dangers associated with the administration of injections. Which danger or complication may be associated with injection?
A. injuring superficial nerves or blood vessels
B. breaking off a needle in a tissue
C. hitting a bone when injecting a very thin person
D. introducing an infection to the body by means of injection
E. all of the above
(Gauwitz and Bayt, p 338)

313. Drugs in amounts of 4 or 5 mL that are given intramuscularly are
A. divided into half
B. given in a large syringe
C. given in the middeltoid area
D. given with a larger needle
E. any of the four ways
(Pickar, pp 181–182; Zakus et al, p 278)

314. Which of the following letters is NOT used in the FDA's Use-in-Pregnancy rating system?
A. A
B. B
C. C
D. D
E. E
(PDR, p 345)

315. Injections for sensitivity (allergy) testing are given
    A. intramuscularly
    B. intravenously
    C. intradermally
    D. subcutaneously
    E. any of the four ways
    (Bonewit-West #1, pp 284–285)

316. The most preferred site in adults for an intramuscular injection in the amount of 3 mL is usually the
    A. middeltoid area
    B. upper, outer quadrant of the buttocks
    C. sartorius
    D. trapezius
    E. coracobrachialis
    (Bonewit-West #1, p 280; Thibodeau and Patton #1, p 126)

317. Injections are given only on order of a
    A. physician
    B. registered nurse
    C. medical assistant
    D. registered or licensed medical technologist
    E. pharmacist
    (Kinn and Woods, p 1040; Zakus, p 273)

318. The type of injection made almost at a parallel angle between the layers of skin is
    A. intramuscular
    B. intravenous
    C. intradermal
    D. subcutaneous
    E. needleless
    (Bonewit-West #1, pp 284–287; Kinn and Woods, pp 1057–1058; Zakus, pp 280–283)

319. In the subcutaneous injection, the needle is inserted at an angle of
    A. 45 degrees
    B. 60 degrees
    C. 75 degrees
    D. 5 degrees
    E. almost 180 degrees
    (Gauwitz and Bayt, p 346; Keir et al, p 677; Kinn and Woods, pp 1053–1055)

320. Sizes of 1/2 inch, 3/4 inch, and 1 1/2 inch are typical sizes of
    A. needle length
    B. gauge of lumen
    C. barrel
    D. plunger
    E. tip
    (Gauwitz and Bayt, pp 345–348; Zakus, pp 276–279)

321. For subcutaneous injections, the average length and gauge of needle would be
    A. 1/2 inch length, 20 gauge
    B. 5/8 inch length, 25 gauge
    C. 1 inch length, 20 gauge
    D. 1 1/2 inch length, 20 gauge
    E. 1 1/2 inch length, 25 gauge
    (Keir et al, p 673; Rice #2, p 162; Zakus, pp 276–277)

322. The Z-tract method of injection is a modified type of
    A. subcutaneous injection
    B. intravenous injection
    C. intradermal injection
    D. intramuscular injection
    E. syringe
    (Bonewit-West #1, p 284; Zakus, p 292)

323. For intramuscular injections, the average length and gauge of needle would be
    A. 1/2 inch length, 20 gauge
    B. 5/8 inch length, 25 gauge
    C. 1 inch length, 20 gauge
    D. 1 1/2 inch length, 22 gauge
    E. 1 1/2 inch length, 25 gauge
    (Bonewit-West #1, p 280; Rice #2, p 162; Zakus, pp 276–279)

324. The medication for injections should be verified at least
    A. one time
    B. two times
    C. three times
    D. four times
    E. five times
    (Bonewit-West #1, pp 265–266; Zakus, p 265)

325. The reason for aspirating the plunger when administering the injection is to
    A. verify quantity of medication
    B. check for appearance of blood
    C. reduce discomfort to the patient
    D. eliminate air bubbles
    E. provide better leverage
    (Bonewit-West #1, pp 279, 282–283; Keir et al, pp 677–679)

326. Which of the following are included in the FIVE RIGHTS for rules when giving medications?
    A. right patient
    B. right drug
    C. right dose
    D. right route
    E. all of the above
    (Bonewit-West #1, pp 265–266; Gauwitz and Bayt, pp 74–75; Zakus, pp 280–283)

327. Intramuscular injections are administered at an angle of
    A. 30 degrees
    B. 45 degrees
    C. 60 degrees
    D. 90 degrees
    E. almost 180 degrees
    (Bonewit-West #1, pp 282–284; Zakus, pp 280–283)

328. A physician has prescribed that a patient take medication buccally. The medical assistant should advise the patient to
    A. place the medication under the tongue
    B. place the medication outside the teeth in the lower portion of the mouth
    C. swallow the medication
    D. dissolve the medication in water and swallow it
    E. chew the medication and then swallow it
    (Gauwitz and Bayt, p 58; Rice #2, p 101)

329. If a medical assistant is called to administer eyedrops for a patient, he or she should
    A. drop the medication directly on the cornea
    B. drop the medication directly on the covering over the iris
    C. drop the medication directly on the pupil
    D. place the medication in the lower lid while the patient looks up
    E. place the medication in the upper lid with the patient in the recumbent position
    (Bonewit-West #1, p 316; Keir et al, pp 503–504)

330. If a medical assistant is asked to administer eardrops, he or she should avoid
    A. keeping the drops as close to the body surface temperature as possible
    B. allowing the drops to flow by gravity down the side of the canal
    C. having the patient lie still for 15 to 30 minutes
    D. using an ear plug whether ordered or not
    E. straightening the ear canal by manipulating the ear lobe
    (Kinn and Woods, pp 585–587; Zakus, pp 313–314)

331. If the physician requests that an infant be held in the upright position for an injection, the medical assistant will hold the infant
    A. in his or her lap, with the infant's head facing away
    B. cradled in his or her arms
    C. supporting the infant's head close to his or her own, with the infant facing the physician
    D. supporting the infant's head close to his or her own, facing the infant toward himself or herself
    E. none of the above

    (Bonewit-West #1, p 412; Zakus, p 153)

332. A medical assistant should practice all of the following precautions regarding subcutaneous injections EXCEPT
    A. administer medications only on a physician's order
    B. cleanse the skin thoroughly
    C. always aspirate on injections
    D. inject rapidly
    E. record immediately the medication given with strength and site

    (Bonewit-West #1, pp 277–279)

333. Sometimes the available dosage of medication on hand is not the same as that which the physician has ordered. The medical assistant must determine how much of the medication should be used. In the equation used for this calculation, the needed dosage is indicated by
    A. the numerator
    B. the denominator
    C. a whole number
    D. both the numerator and denominator
    E. numbers less than 10

    (Gauwitz and Bayt, pp 37–42; Pickar, pp 150–155)

334. Tablets and capsules are measured in metric units of
    A. grains
    B. milliliters
    C. cubic centimeters
    D. milligrams
    E. ounces

    (Gauwitz and Bayt, p 32)

335. Which of the following is a liquid type of medication given orally?
    A. lotion
    B. liniment
    C. elixir
    D. ointment
    E. cream

    (Gauwitz and Bayt, pp 147–150; Kinn and Woods, pp 1032–1033)

336. As a method of medication administration, instillation means
    A. proctoclysis
    B. inhaling the medication
    C. introducing a liquid by drops
    D. applying an ointment or lotion to the skin
    E. using a suppository

    (Bonewit-West #1, p 304)

337. For quickest results, the best method of administering medication generally is
    A. parenteral
    B. buccal
    C. inhalation
    D. sublingual
    E. oral

    (Gauwitz and Bayt, pp 57–59; Bonewit-West #1, p 266)

338. Opium and its derivatives are classified as
    A. depressants
    B. hallucinogens
    C. stimulants
    D. narcotics
    E. tranquilizers
    (Gauwitz and Bayt, p 9)

339. Infants should be actively scheduled and immunized for diphtheria, tetanus, and pertussis (DTP) at
    A. 1 month, 2 months, and 3 months
    B. 2 months, 4 months, and 6 months
    C. 3 months, 6 months, and 9 months
    D. 3 months, 6 months, and 1 year
    E. 6 months, 9 months, and 1 year
    (Keir et al, p 683; Kinn and Woods, p 654)

340. The vaccine TOPV or OPV provides active immunization against
    A. tetanus toxoids
    B. smallpox
    C. polio
    D. tetanus toxoids and pertussis
    E. tuberculosis
    (Bonewit-West #1, pp 428–429; Kinn and Woods, p 653)

341. Immunity resulting from antibodies produced externally and introduced into the body is called
    A. induced immunity
    B. active immunity
    C. cellular immunity
    D. passive immunity
    E. natural immunity
    (Kinn and Woods, pp 653–655; Zakus, p 174)

342. The drug commonly used to counteract the effects of anaphylactic shock is
    A. nitroglycerin
    B. epinephrine
    C. heparin sodium
    D. penicillin
    E. phenobarbital
    (Bonewit-West #1, pp 688–691; Kinn and Woods, pp 789–790; Zakus, p 556)

343. Which of the following factors will affect drug action?
    A. age
    B. size/weight
    C. sex
    D. emotional state
    E. all of the above
    (Gauwitz and Bayt, p 16; Kinn and Woods, pp 1006–1008)

344. The generic name is usually the same as the
    A. official name
    B. brand name
    C. chemical name
    D. trade name
    E. product name
    (Bonewit-West #1, p 253; Gauwitz and Bayt, pp 4–5; Zakus, p 250)

345. Ultram (tramadol hydrochloride) is classified as a/an _____ drug.
    A. analgesic
    B. anti-inflammatory
    C. cholinergic
    D. antihypertensive
    E. anti-anxiety
    (Kizior and Hodgson, pp 1014–1015; PDR, pp 2218–2220)

346. The study of the processes of drug absorption, distribution, metabolism, and excretion is
    A. pharmacodynamics
    B. pharmacokinetics
    C. pharmacotherapeutics
    D. pharmacy
    E. posology
    (Gauwitz and Bayt, p 2)

347. The study of diseases and disorders in the elderly is called
    A. pediatrics
    B. podiatry
    C. geriatrics
    D. genetics
    E. none of the above

    (Gauwitz and Bayt, p 363)

348. Norvasc (amlodipine besylate), Prinivil (lisinopril), and Zestril (lisinopril) are drugs used in the treatment of
    A. diabetes
    B. depression
    C. hypothyroidism
    D. hypertension
    E. Cushing's syndrome

    (Kizior and Hodgson, pp 49–51; PDR, pp 2359–2360, 1866–1870, 578–581)

349. A drug that may be prescribed for hypertension is
    A. Polycillin (ampicillin)
    B. Lanoxin (digoxin)
    C. prednisone
    D. Tetracyn (tetracycline)
    E. Hytrin (terazosin)

    (Kizior and Hodgson, pp 968–969; PDR, pp 454–457)

350. An example of an antibiotic is
    A. reserpine
    B. tetracycline
    C. nitroglycerin
    D. nicotinic acid
    E. digoxin

    (Gauwitz and Bayt, p 110; Hitner and Nagle, pp 559–560)

351. A sweetened, aromatic, alcoholic preparation used to administer an active medicine is called a/an
    A. stock solution
    B. suspension
    C. elixir
    D. emulsion
    E. extract

    (Gauwitz and Bayt, p 54; Kinn and Woods, p 1031)

352. A drug that stops or retards bleeding or discharge and shrinks tissue is classified as a/an
    A. astringent
    B. beta-adrenergic blocker
    C. cytotoxin
    D. diuretic
    E. emetic

    (Gauwitz and Bayt, p 147)

353. A medicine that increases the output of urine is a/an
    A. emetic
    B. vasoconstrictor
    C. cathartic
    D. astringent
    E. diuretic

    (Gauwitz and Bayt, pp 169–170; Kizior and Hodgson, pp 1148–1149)

354. The abbreviation that means every day is
    A. qod
    B. qid
    C. qs
    D. qn
    E. qd

    (Gauwitz and Bayt, p 64; Kinn and Woods, p 999)

355. A proper gauge needle for an intradermal injection is
    A. 18–20
    B. 21
    C. 22
    D. 23–25
    E. 26

    (Bonewit-West #1, pp 284–287; Keir et al, p 673)

356. To prepare a powdered drug for injection, use a diluent of
    A. 70% alcohol
    B. Zephiran
    C. sterile water
    D. milk
    E. oil
    (Gauwitz and Bayt, p 344; Pickar, p 193)

357. In the metric system, fractional quantities are expressed using
    A. lowercase Roman numerals
    B. uppercase Roman numerals
    C. decimals
    D. Arabic numbers in fractions
    E. percentages
    (Pickar, p 63; Zakus, pp 268–269)

358. In the storage of medications, the medical assistant should keep in mind that
    A. drugs for internal and external use should be integrated
    B. drugs should be stored alphabetically by name
    C. oils should be kept in a warm place
    D. antibiotics usually have to be refrigerated
    E. unused drugs should be kept locked up
    (Gauwitz and Bayt, pp 67–68)

359. If the medical assistant finds a container of medication without a label, the correct procedure to follow is
    A. report it at once to his or her physician-employer
    B. attach a new label
    C. discard the container
    D. lock it in the narcotics cupboard
    E. retain it for identification
    (Zakus, p 261)

360. Fosamax (alendronate sodium) is a drug used in the treatment of
    A. Parkinson's disease
    B. osteoporosis
    C. hypergastric acid
    D. orthostatic hypotension
    E. kidney failure
    (Kizior and Hodgson, pp 21–23; PDR, pp 1798–1802)

361. Cipro (ciprofloxacin hydrochloride) and Bactrim (trimethoprim and sulfamethoxazole) are classified as an
    A. anticholinergic
    B. antidepressant
    C. antispasmatic
    D. anti-inflammatory
    E. antibacterial
    (Gauwitz and Bayt, p 240; PDR, pp 678–683, 2614–2616; Rice #2, pp 228–229, 423–426)

362. Ambien (zolpidem tartrate) is classified as a/an
    A. antipsychotic
    B. sedative-hypnotic
    C. cathartic
    D. antibiotic
    E. anticholinergic
    (Kizior and Hodgson, pp 1076–1077; PDR, pp 2884–2888)

363. Prozac (fluoxetine hydrochloride) is a drug used in the treatment of
    A. hypertension
    B. depression
    C. arrhythmias
    D. tuberculosis
    E. diabetes mellitus
    (Gauwitz and Bayt, pp 316–317; PDR, pp 962–966)

364. Which medication(s) might be kept on an emergency tray along with other emergency supplies such as surgical supplies, sterile syringes, sponges, a tourniquet, and disinfectants?

A. adrenalin (epinephrine)

B. benadryl

C. digoxin

D. steroids

E. all of the above

(Zakus, p 261)

365. The process the body uses to convert drugs into harmless by-products is called

A. absorption

B. distribution

C. action

D. biotransformation

E. excretion

(Gauwitz and Bayt, p 18; Kinn and Woods, p 1007)

366. Which is the most common route for the elimination of drugs from the body?

A. kidneys

B. lungs

C. sweat glands

D. salivary glands

E. milk glands

(Hitner and Nagle, pp 25–26; Kinn and Woods, p 1007)

367. Transdermal patches contain time-released medication that enters the body through the

A. lungs

B. skin

C. muscle

D. veins

E. gut

(Gauwitz and Bayt, p 148; Keir et al, pp 260, 665–666)

368. Which of the following is/are parts of a prescription?

A. superscription

B. inscription

C. subscription

D. signature

E. all of the above

(Kinn and Woods, p 1000; Zakus, pp 252–256)

369. Which of the choices is NOT a formula used to calculate a dosage of medication?

A. West's nomogram

B. Clark's Rule

C. Young's Rule

D. Fried's Law

E. Blalock-Taussig procedure

(Kinn and Woods, pp 1022–1023; Hitner and Nagle, p 52)

370. The treatment of disease by medicines or drugs is known as a therapeutic process. Which of the following would constitute other uses of the drugs?

A. preventive

B. palliative

C. replacement

D. diagnostic

E. all of the above

(Gauwitz and Bayt, pp 3–4; Kinn and Woods, p 1004)

371. Which of the following instructions might be included in a patient education pamphlet to instruct patients in the wise use of medication?

A. give every physician you consult a list of all drugs you take

B. know the medication you are taking, name, dosage, and purpose

C. inform your physician of any allergies or drug reactions you have had

D. call your physician if you have any unusual reaction to the drugs

E. all of the above

(Zakus, pp 272–273)

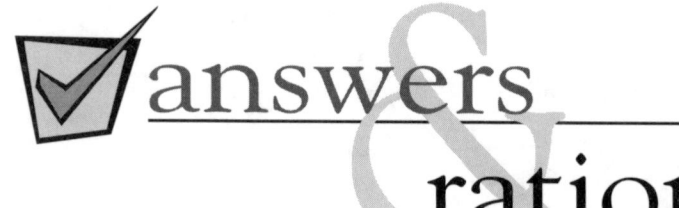

answers & rationales

268.

A. Amoxil and Trimox are trade names for the generic antibiotic, amoxicillin. It is bacteriolytic, which means that it gives results by killing the bacterial cell. Other types of antibiotics work by limiting reproduction, dissolving the bacterial cell membranes, or interrupting the metabolic process. Amoxil and Trimox are a type of penicillin, also sold under the generic name amoxicillin trihydrate amoxil. It comes in capsules, powder for oral suspension, and chewable tablets. Antibiotics belong to a larger class of drugs called anti-infectives, all of which in some way counter infections.

269.

B. Lanoxin (digoxin), used to treat certain coronary disorders, is extracted from the leaves of *Digitalis lanata*. It ameliorates symptoms characteristic of heart failure, dyspnea, edema, and cardiac asthma. Patients receiving Lanoxin (digoxin) must be closely monitored for digitalis intoxication as well as disturbances of the coronary disorder. Digoxin is a drug used to treat paroxysmal (suddenly recurring) tachycardia, as well as cardiac failure and atrial fibrillation and flutter. Digoxin acts in various ways to regulate the heartbeat. It belongs to the digitalis family and is classified as an anti-arrhythmic drug.

270.

C. Xanax and Klonopin are anti-anxiety drugs. Zanax is also classified as a sedative, which does not have the sleep-producing power of a hypnotic drug. It is prescribed for short-term anxiety relief and the management of anxiety disorders and may cause withdrawal symptoms if withdrawn abruptly.

Klonopin is also classified as an anticonvulsant drug. Anticonvulsant drugs are used for the control of chronic seizures and involuntary muscle spasms or movements characteristic of certain neurologic diseases. Anticonvulsant drugs are most frequently used in the therapy of epilepsy. Contraindications include patients with severe liver disease and acute narrow-angle glaucoma. Xanax and Klonopin may cause fetal harm in pregnant women, especially in the first trimester.

271.

B. Zantac is a histamine blocker used to treat stomach ulcers. It inhibits gastric acid secretions by blocking histamine, which regulates the flow of stomach acid.

272.

E. The main body organ involved in drug metabolism is the liver. The cells of the liver contain a group of enzymes that specifically function to metabolize foreign (drug) substances. These enzymes are referred to as the drug microsomal metabolizing system (DMMS). The main function of the DMMS is to take lipid-soluble (fat-soluble) drugs and change them chemically so that they become water-soluble compounds. Only water-soluble compounds can be excreted by the kidneys. Lipid-soluble compounds are repeatedly reabsorbed into the blood. Drug dosage is based on a person with normal liver function, which will result in part of the converted drug leaving the body by way of the kidney. If the liver is impaired, this conversion from lipid soluble to water soluble does not occur at the expected rate and the concentration of the drug in the body will build up if the dosage is not adjusted.

273.

A. Veetids is a brand name of penicillin V potassium, an antibiotic, which may be prescribed as tablets or oral solution. It is used in the treatment of staph, strep, gonococci, and other infections. It is also used to prevent rheumatic fever (a complication of strep infections) and bacterial endocarditis. It is of special concern that more and more strains of bacteria are becoming resistant to penicillin and other antibacterial agents. It should be noted that penicillins cause more severe and frequent allergic reactions than any other antibiotic.

274.

D. The medical assistant should substitute the amounts as follows in Young's Rule:

Adult dose × fraction of child's age (years) ÷ child's age + 12 = pediatric dose.

0.5 gram × 6 (child's age) ÷ 6 + 12 (child's age + 12) = 0.17 gram pediatric dose

Since the age of the child was given, the formula using age, not weight, was used. Mastery of calculating dosages comes in three steps: (1) mastery of the basic arithmetic, placement of decimals, and converting equivalents; (2) mastering the concepts of ratio and proportion for each type of calculation; and (3) practicing, double checking, and inspecting for units used until the skill is acquired.

275.

B. Premarin is an estrogen hormone replacement that is prescribed to treat a number of conditions—difficult menopause, osteoporosis, primary ovarian failure, and so on. Estrogen, along with the other male and female hormones and adrenocorticosteroids, is a powerful steroid.

276.

D. Cardizem is a calcium ion influx inhibitor. It is used to treat angina pectoris due to coronary artery spasm and other coronary circulation disorders, such as tachycardia and atrial flutter. Digoxin and digitalis are other medications used to treat heart problems.

277.

E. Drug references do not usually include the expected cost of the drug. Any good drug reference such as the *Physician's Desk Reference (PDR)* or *Nurses' Drug Reference (NDR)* would include a description of what the drug was made of or its composition. It should also explain how the drug works or its action. The indication tells the condition (disease or disorder) that the drug treats. Contraindication explains under what conditions the drug should not be used. Special conditions that may alter the drug's effects are listed under precautions. Dosage and administration tells the amount and which routes are available (oral, sublingual, topical, rectal, inhalation, or parenteral). The drug reference should tell how the drug is supplied or packaged, such as in tablet, liquid, capsule, or cream form.

278.

E. Ceclor is an antibiotic that destroys bacteria by interfering with their cell wall synthesis. Used to treat a number of different organisms, its effectiveness may be determined by testing the suspected microbe with disks impregnated with the antibiotic. Patients allergic to penicillin may also be allergic to Ceclor.

279.

B. Orasone, Deltasone, and Meticorten are all forms of the generic drug prednisone. Prednisone is a corticosteroid. These three trade name drugs are taken orally. They are used in replacement therapy in adrenal insufficiency including Addison's disease. They are used in the symptomatic treatment of multiorgan disease/conditions including rheumatoid and osteoarthritis, severe psoriasis, ulcerative colitis, and lupus erythematosus.

280.

B. Synthroid is a synthetic replacement for thyroxine, the principal hormone secreted by the thyroid gland. A deficiency of this hormone results in hypothyroidism. Overdosage will induce hyperthyroidism.

281.

D. Accupril and Capoten are used to treat hypertension. They are the first of a new type of antihypertensive. Hypertensives include several types of medications that reduce high blood pressure by acting in different ways on the mechanisms controlling blood pressure. These drugs may be used alone or in combination with thiozide diuretics.

282.

C. Acetaminophen with codeine, a stronger analgesic, relieves pain and lowers blood pressure by dilating the blood vessels. Acetaminophen often sold by the brand name of Tylenol is an antipyretic (anti-fever drug). Codeine is a narcotic that enhances the pain-relieving properties.

283.

D. Pepcid is a drug used in the treatment of short-term active duodenal ulcers. Famotidine is a competitive inhibitor of histamine H_2 receptors that leads to inhibition of gastric acid secretion. It is contraindicated with cirrhosis of the liver, impaired renal or hepatic function, and lactation.

284.

E. Cephalexin is an anti-infective agent used in the treatment of a wide range of Gram-negative and Gram-positive organisms. These include infections of the respiratory tract and genitourinary tract, as well as skin, bone, and ear infections. An anti-infective agent is defined as any drug used to kill microorganisms or to stop the reproduction of microorganisms. It may be prescribed in the form of capsules, tablets, or oral suspension. Dosage may be increased for severe infections or reduced in the case of renal impairment.

285.

E. Vasotec is an antihypertensive, which means that it lowers blood pressure, lessens resistance to blood flow, and, probably like all medications, has contraindications and precautions for certain patients. Some patients may have a hypersensitivity to the drug. These possibilities are outlined in the PDR.

286.

A. Procardia is an anti-anginal drug prescribed for the coronary circulation. It is a calcium ion influx inhibitor.

287.

A. Furosemide and triamterene HCTZ are diuretics that function as antihypertensives through their action as diuretics, removing water from the body, thereby reducing tissue edema. Other antihypertensives may act in various ways to reduce hypertension, such as vasodilators, sympathetic blocking agents, and centrally acting agents.

288.

E. The antidepressants Zoloft (sertraline hydrochloride) and Paxil (paroxetine hydrochloride) are believed to act by inhibiting central nervous system uptake of serotonin. One of the actions of serotonin in addition to its role of constricting blood vessels is that of a powerful neurotransmitter involved in sleep and sensory perception. These medicines are prescribed in the form of tablets and are used to treat depression, anxiety, and insomnia. The use of these drugs is being investigated in the treatment of obsessive-compulsive disorders. Contraindications of these drugs are as follows: they should not be used within 14 days of the discontinuation of monoamine oxidase inhibitors. Serious, even fatal, reactions may occur when these two types of drugs are used together. Drug interactions are also possible with other prescription drugs. In addition, alcohol should not be used by depressed patients.

289.

D. Dilantin is prescribed to prevent epileptic seizures. It is similar in chemical makeup to the barbiturates, and, therefore, the patient should be cautioned against the use of alcoholic beverages and other drugs.

290.

A. Propoxyphene napsylate acetaminophen (N/APAP), also sold under the trade name Darvocet-N-100, is a combination of two pain relievers (analgesics). (APAP stands for acetaminophen.) The two drugs combined are more effective than either administered alone. Patients should be advised about the risk of combining alcohol or other narcotic drugs with Darvocet.

291.

C. Mevacor (lovastatin) and Zocor (simva-statin) are drugs prescribed as tablets that are classified as antihyperlipidemics or antihypercholesteremic. Both Mevacor (lovastatin) and Zocor (simvastatin) inhibit an enzyme necessary as an early step in the biosynthesis of cholesterol. The levels of "bad" cholesterol (VLDL and LDL) and plasma triglycerides are reduced, while the plasma concentration of "good" cholesterol (HDL) is increased. These drugs are prescribed only after restricted diet and other measures have failed. Special caution with these drugs should be observed with patients who have liver disease and those who are known to consume large quantities of alcohol.

292.

A. Prilosec (omeprazole) is classified as an agent to suppress gastric acid secretion. A similar drug is Prevacid (lansoprazole). These drugs are believed to be a gastric pump inhibitor in that they block the final step of hydrochloric acid production. They are used to treat duodenal ulcers, erosive esophagitis, and gastroesophageal reflux disease. They may interact with a number of other drugs. Referring to the other answer choices: (1) Claritin is classified as an antihistamine drug, (2) Paxil has the classification of antidepressant, (3) Relafin is a nonsteroidal anti-inflammatory agent, and (4) Konopin is an anticonvulsant.

293.

B. Biaxin (clarithromycin) and Zithromax (azithromycin) are classified as antibiotics and also as anti-infectives. They are in the group of antibiotics known as macrolides, which includes azithromycin, clarithromycin, diuthromycin, and erythromycin. They are effective against both Gram-positive and Gram-negative microorganisms. These drugs are rapidly absorbed from the gastrointestinal tract after oral administration. Food does not affect the extent of bioavailability of the drugs. Food in the GI tract will slightly delay the onset of absorption of the drugs.

294.

A. Micronase (glyburide) Glucophage (metformin hydrochloride) and Glucotrol XL (glipizide) are prescribed for diabetes mellitus (II). They work indirectly by lowering the blood glucose, thereby stimulating the insulin cells of the pancreas to produce more insulin. The patient should understand that these drugs are in addition to diet restrictions and is not a substitute.

295.

E. Augmentin (amoxicillin clavulanate), which is related chemically to penicillin, is an oral, broad-spectrum antibiotic that kills both Gram-positive and Gram-negative organisms. Medical assistants should be aware that penicillin-related antibiotics have caused anaphylaxis in rare cases, and when anaphylaxis occurs, immediate emergency treatment with epinephrine, steroids, and airway management should be administered.

296.

C. Hydrocodone/APAP is classified as an analgesic or narcotic/analgesic combination drug. It produces its analgesic activity by an action on the central nervous system by way of the opiate receptors. It is contraindicated for persons with hypersensitivity to acetaminophen or hydrocodone and in patients who are lactating. Regarding the other answer choices; diuretics are drugs that increase urine output; anti-emetics are drugs that help prevent or stop vomiting; antiseptics are agents that prevent or inhibit the growth of microorganisms and are used widely in physicians' offices for control of microbe growth on instruments, furniture, etc; and a hemostatic drug is one that stops blood flow.

297.

A. K-Dur (potassium chloride) is a replacement for potassium, the most common intracellular cation (K+) of the body and also essential for life. Excess amounts of potassium may be lost through the kidneys because of diuretics or diseases such as diabetic ketoacidosis or through the intestinal tract because of diarrhea or because of disease, such as diabetic ketoacidosis. This lost potassium, because it is essential to life, must be replaced.

298.

C. Ventolin and Proventil are used as bronchodilators in the treatment of asthma. Antitussives are cough suppressants, such as codeine. Expectorants increase the secretions and mucus from the bronchial tubes and act in an opposite manner to antitussives. Decongestants relieve local congestion and often are combined with antihistamines.

299.

B. Claritin (loratidine) and Zyrtec (cetirizine hydrochloride) are classified as antihistamines. They are metabolized in the liver to active metabolites. Loratidine is excreted through both the urine and feces. Cetirizine is excreted primarily in the urine. They are used to relieve nasal and non-nasal symptoms of seasonal allergic rhinitis. The most common side effects are headache, fatigue, and dry mouth. Antihistamines are a class of drugs that oppose the action of histamine, a substance produced within the body cells. When cells are injured, they release histamine into the tissue and initiate a series of reactions finalized in local edema. Antihistamines are widely prescribed to treat allergies and rhinitis. These drugs cause drowsiness and increased sensitivity of skin to sun.

300.

D. Relafen (nabumetone) is classified as a non-steroidal anti-inflammatory drug (NSAID). It is prescribed in tablet form and is used to treat both acute and chronic osteoarthritis and rheumatoid arthritis. Chronic, long-term therapeutic use of this drug requires monitoring values of the complete blood cell count (CBC) as well as the liver and renal function values. The most common side effects of this drug, which affect the gastrointestinal (GI) tract, are peptic or duodenal ulceration and GI bleeding. NSAIDs have analgesic, anti-inflammatory, and antipyretic action similar to aspirin. Although they relieve some pain and discomfort, there is no evidence that they slow the disease progression of rheumatoid arthritis and osteoarthritis. Gastrointestinal irritation or hemorrhage is a common side effect.

301.

E. Schedule V drugs may be purchased without a doctor's prescription. These are over-the-counter (OTC) drugs and can be sold only by a registered pharmacist. The buyer must be 18 years old and show identification. Schedule I drugs are not prescribed. They are used only for research. They have a high potential for abuse. Examples of these drugs are heroin and lysergic acid diethylamide (LSD). Schedule II drugs are acceptable for medical use with restrictions. Examples of these drugs are cocaine, morphine, opium, and pentobarbital. They have a high potential for abuse. Schedule III drugs are acceptable for medical use.

Examples of these drugs include barbiturates and Tylenol with codeine. They have a moderate abuse potential. Schedule IV drugs are accepted for medical use. They have a lower potential for abuse than Schedule III drugs. Examples include phenobarbital and Darvon (propoxyphene).

302.

A. Provera (medroxyprogesterone) is a steroid hormone and is used to treat amenorrhea (absence of menstruation) and other disorders such as abnormal uterine bleeding and menopausal symptoms. Adverse reactions to this drug have included bleeding, rash, mental depression, and edema.

303.

E. Timoptic (timolol) is used to treat glaucoma by reducing the high intraocular pressure. It is an adrenergic blocking agent that is applied topically. Timoptic is well tolerated and produces fewer and less severe side effects than pilocarpine.

304.

C. Ery-Tab (erythromycin base) is the antibiotic of choice to treat or prevent streptococcal pharyngitis. It is also the antibiotic of choice to prevent rheumatic fever, a complication of streptococcal infections, such as strep throat. Strep throat infections should always be treated with antibiotics. This usually prevents the later development of rheumatic fever, an autoimmune reaction to the strep infection. Anaphylaxis from the use of erythromycin is rare. Erythromycin belongs to the macrolide group of antibiotics.

305.

E. Advil, Motrin, and Nuprin are trade (brand) names for the generic drug, ibuprofen, which is an NSAID used to treat the symptoms of various types of arthritis and also primary dysmenorrhea. The exact mode of action is not known.

306.

A. Prempro (conjugated estrogens/medroxyprogesterone) is classified as a steroid. It is single tablet therapy, unlike Premphase therapy, which utilizes two separate tablets. Prempro is used in the treatment of moderate to severe vasomotor symptoms associated with menopause. It is also used in the treatment of vulvar and vaginal atrophy and in the prevention of osteoporosis. It is contraindicated for patients known to be or suspected to be pregnant. It is not recommended to persons with liver dysfunction or disease.

307.
C. Humulin N is a hormone replacement used to treat diabetes. A medication that is the result of genetic engineering, it is manufactured by a nonpathogenic, special laboratory strain of *Escherichia coli* into which the human gene for insulin production has been inserted.

308.
B. Ortho-Novum 1/35–28 and Ortho-Novum 7/7/7–28 are combination oral contraceptives prescribed for birth control. The contraindications and adverse reactions associated with oral contraceptives should be relayed through patient education to the patient. Women using oral contraceptives should be strongly advised not to smoke.

309.
D. Coumadin (warfarin) is used in the prophylaxis and treatment of venous and pulmonary thromboses and circulatory disorders. It inhibits the synthesis in the liver of several necessary clotting factors and must be closely regulated with prothrombin time tests. The use of Coumadin is contraindicated in any hemorrhagic dyscrasia because the patient's clotting abilities are impaired, and a serious hemorrhage is possible.

310.
B. Using Clark's Rule, the medical assistant should substitute in the rule as follows:

$$30/150 \times 50.0 \, mg = pediatric \, dose$$

$$1/5 \times 50.0 \, mg = 10.0 \, mg$$

It is crucial that a child receives the correct dosage of medication since a too large or too small dose might have a very detrimental effect on a critically ill child. Two approaches to figuring medication for children are to figure the ratio of child weight to adult weight or the ratio of the child's age to an adult age. Neither of these

approaches works in all cases since a child might be very over- or underweight. A third method, West's nomogram, which calculates dosage by using a ratio of the child's body surface area to that of an adult, may be used.

311.
B. Nitrostat, a sublingual tablet better known by its generic name, nitroglycerin, is a vasodilator that treats angina by relaxing the vascular smooth muscle of both arteries and muscles, thus removing stress from the heart muscles. Nitrostat is administered sublingually (under the tongue). It acts extremely fast (in 1 to 3 minutes) and may be repeated three times at 5-minute intervals.

312.
E. Using the next larger syringe that could hold more medication does not matter as long as the proper needle gauge and length are used. Other dangers associated with injection include introducing an infection due to improper sterilization of the injection site, needle, or syringe and the possibility of the injection material causing an allergic reaction. Injection sites must be chosen carefully so that they are in muscle tissue able to absorb the medication and away from major nerves, blood vessels, and bones. Sudden movement by small children should be guarded against since this might conceivably cause injury.

313.
A. Large doses of drugs, in amounts of 2 mL or more, are given intramuscularly. If the volume of dosage ordered is 3 to 5 mL, it should be divided and injected into two or more sites. Unabsorbed medicines can cause damage to the tissues. The condition of the patient must be considered.

314.
E. The letter "E" is not used in the FDA's pregnancy rating system. The categories in the system utilize the letters A, B, C, D, and X as follows: A—controlled studies show no risk; B—no evidence of risk in humans; C—risk cannot be ruled out; D—positive evidence of risk; X—contraindicated in pregnancy.

315.

C. Diagnostic tests, such as the Dick test, Schick test, or Mantoux test, are conducted by the administration of an intradermal injection. The Tine test employs a multipuncture, four-pronged lancet and is also a type of intradermal injection used to detect tuberculosis.

316.

B. The upper, outer quadrant of the buttocks is often preferred because of the depth of muscular tissue (gluteus maximus and gluteus medius), which permits the injection of large amounts of drugs without danger of trauma to tissues. To be safe, the injection must be made away from large blood vessels, large nerves, and bones. The sites must be located by sight and also by touch, using prominent bones as landmarks. The four most common sites are the deltoid muscle of the upper, outer arm, the dorsogluteal and ventrogluteal areas of the buttocks, and the vastus lateralis muscle of the upper leg. In infants, the gluteal muscles are not well developed and there is more danger of damaging the sciatic nerve. Therefore, other sites are used such as the vastus lateralis muscle of the upper leg.

317.

A. A medical assistant should give injections only on direct, written orders of the physician. The written order will complete the communication cycle and allows for no error in the order. There are many ethical considerations concerning drug administration, and the medical assistant cannot risk giving incorrect medications.

318.

C. The intradermal injection is made with the needle inserted at practically a parallel angle between the layer of skin just under the corneum layer of the epidermis. Little or no bleeding should occur. Bleeding would indicate that the injection was given into the dermis, which would denote an imperfect test. The angle for the intradermal injection is 10 to 15 degrees.

319.

A. Subcutaneous injections are used to administer small doses of medication ranging from 0.5 to 2.0 mL into the subcutaneous tissue. They are administered at a 45-degree angle of insertion. The subcutaneous injection is most often given in the upper, outer part of the arm (deltoid area) or the upper thigh (midvastus lateralis).

320.

A. Needle length is measured in inches or fractions of inches (e.g., 1/2, 3/4, 1, 1 1/2). The gauge of the lumen refers to the diameter or size of the hole. The smaller the gauge, the larger the hole or lumen. A needle that is 26 or 27 gauge makes a very small hole in the skin.

321.

B. A subcutaneous injection is given with a needle of about 1/2 to 3/4 inches in length and a gauge of between 25 and 27. Medications, such as allergy and insulin injections, are administered using the subcutaneous injection method.

322.

D. The intramuscular injection by the Z-tract method is used when medications are given that contain materials that would cause tissue discoloration and irritation if they got into the subcutaneous tissue by leakage occurring through the path made by the needle. This is prevented by pulling the skin/tissue to one side and inserting the needle at a 90-degree angle.

323.

D. For intramuscular injections, needles are somewhat longer—possibly 1 1/2 inches—and the gauge would be between 20 and 23. They are injected deep in the muscle tissue, where the medication will be absorbed quickly by the rich blood supply present.

324.

C. The medication for injections should be verified three times. The medication order and the drug label should be checked when the medication is removed from the shelf, before it is withdrawn into the syringe, and before it is returned to the shelf or its proper storage place.

325.

B. The plunger should be aspirated to verify that the needle has not entered a blood vessel. If blood appears, the needle must be withdrawn immediately and a new site has to be prepared for injection.

326.

E. The five rights for proper drug administration are the right patient, right drug, right dose, right route, and right time. These rules are brief ways of stating what must be checked for in every instance of administered medication. Some authors list a sixth right, the right documentation—that is, the proper entry with initials in the patient's record. It is the patient's right to receive these rights.

327.

D. Intramuscular injections are administered at approximately a right angle to the skin or in other words at a 90-degree angle.

328.

B. Buccal medications are placed between the cheek and gum (outside the teeth). The mucous membranes in this area have a rich blood supply that can absorb the drug rapidly (e.g., nitroglycerin administered for angina pectoris). Some medications are administrated by the buccal method because, if swallowed, they would be destroyed by digestive juices.

329.

D. The lower lid should be pulled outward gently while the patient looks upward, and the drops permitted to fall into the lower portion of the eye (conjunctival sac). The tip of the dropper should not touch the eye (to prevent contamination). The solution and dropper should be sterile to prevent infection. The solution should be at room temperature for the comfort of the patient. Patients may sit up and tilt the head back although some may prefer to lie down. After instilling the drops, ask the patient to blink to distribute the medication but caution against rubbing the eye. The excess medication should be wiped away from the cheek with a sterile gauze. The usual precautions common to most medication administrations are followed to prevent mistakes. Use precautions for preventing the spread of disease (e.g., wash hands before and afterward and wear latex gloves). (Eyedrops are often used to treat infections as well as eye irritations.) The medication should be verified before and after the instillation and before being returned to its storage, according to the usual procedures for administering medication. Out-of-date medication should not be used. The patient should be identified and the procedure explained to the patient. The necessary patient education procedures should be explained. Record the details of the procedure on the patient's chart and initial (date, name and strength of medication, number of drops, any significant observations, and the patient's reaction).

330.

D. A medical assistant should follow the instructions of the physician and not use an ear plug unless ordered by the physician. If a cotton ball is inserted, it should be coated with petroleum jelly or moistened as directed by the physician. The petroleum jelly will prevent absorption of the medication by the cotton ball. The patient should sit or lie with the affected ear upward so that gravity will cause the medication to run into the ear canal and remain there. The dropper should be used to place the prescribed medication in the ear canal. The medication should bear the word "otic," indicating it is used for insertion in the ear. The patient should remain leaning for 2 to 3 minutes in a position that enables the medication to remain in the ear. (See Answer 329 for a list of the usual procedures of medication verification, infection prevention, patient identification and education, and charting. These also apply to ear instillation and ear irrigation.) Ear irrigation is the washing of the external auditory canal with a flowing solution for the purposes of removing cerumen (ear wax), discharge, or a foreign body. The ear canal should be examined with an otoscope before and after the irrigation. If the tympanic membrane (ear drum) is perforated, the irrigation should not be performed since this could infect or irritate the middle ear.

331.

D. For the upright position, the medical assistant should hold the child upright with its head facing his or her body. Its head should be supported with one of his or her hands. The physician can then approach the child. There are three basic positions for handling infants: the upright position just described; the cradle position, where the infant is cradled in the adult's arms next to the body; and the football position, where the infant is held horizontally and straight out in front of the adult with the infant's head and body supported. The position chosen is the one needed for the medical procedure underway. The infant should feel safe and comfortable in whatever position is chosen; most prefer to be held upright.

332.

D. The medical assistant should not administer the medication rapidly when giving a subcutaneous injection because it can be painful. After the needle has been removed, pressure should be applied to the injection site for several seconds.

333.

A. The dosage to administer is indicated by the numerator of the equation. (The numerator is the top number of the fraction; the denominator is the bottom number of the fraction.) The equation is

$$\frac{Desired\ Dosage}{Dosage\ Available} = Dosage\ Given$$

Example: If you have tetracycline on hand that is labeled 200 mg/tablet and the doctor orders a 600 mg dosage, you would give 3 tablets.

$$\frac{600\ mg}{200\ mg\ tablet} = 3\ tablets$$

334.

D. Fractions of milligrams are used to make up tablets and capsules. Tablets may be scored. Tablets that are scored are marked with indentations that make it possible to break them into halves or quarters for proper dosage.

335.

C. The elixir is not a topical skin medicine. Elixirs are liquid oral dosage forms of medicine such as cough syrups. Lotions are commonly used to control itching. Liniments contain high levels of oil and are used to protect dried or cracked skin. Ointments also help dry skin conditions. These terms are used in the classification of drugs based on preparation into liquid or solid preparations.

Other terms for liquid preparations are aerosol (a mist or cloud), emulsion (mixture of fat and water), solution (contains dissolved substance), spirit (an alcoholic solution that evaporates easily), suspension (solid insoluble particles in liquid), syrup (drug in a sugar and water solution), and tincture (drug in alcohol solution). Solid preparations are capsules (drug in a gelatin capsule to prevent tasting), cream (drug in a nongreasy base), lozenge (drug in a candy-like base), ointment (drug with oil base), suppository (drug with a firm base such as cocoa butter for insertion into body cavity such as vagina or rectum), tablet (discs), and transdermal patch (drug contained in a patch applied to the skin).

Another classification of drugs is based on the action they have on the body. Examples belonging in this classification are analgesics (pain relievers), anorectics (appetite depressants), antibiotics (drugs that inhibit or kill disease-producing bacteria, antitussives (prevent coughing), cathartics and laxatives (promote defecation), and sedatives (drugs that calm and quiet). Obviously, this list is incomplete; consult a textbook for further information.

336.

C. Instillation means introducing a liquid by drops, and this is a frequent method of administering medication in the eyes and ears. Eye instillations may be performed for the purpose of soothing an irritated eye or to treat an eye infection with medication.

337.

A. Parenteral administration of drugs brings a more prompt and complete effect of the drug. Methods of parenteral administration include subcutaneous, intramuscular, intrasternal, and intravenous injections.

338.

D. Drugs derived from opium include morphine, codeine, and meperidine and are known as narcotics. They produce sound sleep, stupor, and relief of pain. They also are addictive and are, therefore, included among the controlled drugs in Schedule I to V of the Drug Enforcement Agency (DEA).

339.

B. Infants should be actively scheduled and immunized for DTP (or DPT) at 2 months, 4 months, and 6 months. DTP is commonly used as an abbreviation for diphtheria and tetanus toxoids combined with pertussis (whooping cough) vaccine. The medical assistant should be sure to record the information on the patient's chart.

340.

C. TOPV provides active immunization against poliomyelitis. TOPV is recommended by the American Academy of Pediatrics to be suitable for both breast-fed and bottle-fed infants. Other diseases against which infants receive immunization include diphtheria, tetanus, and whooping cough (pertussis).

341.

D. Immunity that is the result of antibodies produced externally and introduced into the body is known as passive immunity. This can be achieved by antibodies crossing the placenta from the mother to the child or by the inoculating process. The passive immunity will last only for a short period and then will gradually fade. The infant must receive immunizations to stimulate active production of his or her own antibodies against specific communicable diseases such as polio and whooping cough.

342.

B. The drug most commonly used to counteract the effects of anaphylactic shock is epinephrine. Injectable epinephrine (adrenalin) should be available at all times on an emergency or crash tray in a physician's office. Oxygen is also administered during anaphylactic shock because the patient's breathing is impaired.

A stocked emergency cart will also have a variety of other medications useful in an emergency. Some of these are local anesthetics and painkillers such as lidocaine and xylocaine; syrup of Ipecac to instigate vomiting in cases of oral poisoning or drug overdose; nitroglycerin, used to treat anginal attacks; isotonic saline for IVs; insulin (kept in refrigerator) and instant glucose for use in diabetic and insulin shock; and diazepam used as an antipanic drug and anti-anxiety agent.

343.

E. Age, size/weight, sex, and emotional state are all factors that affect drug action. Drugs affect people in different ways because no two persons are exactly the same. Other factors affecting drug action are genetic variation in individuals, disease conditions, route of administration, time of day, and the drug-taking history of the person. Has the individual previously taken doses of the same or another drug? Environmental conditions such as extremes in weather conditions affect the action of the medication because body functions are influenced by heat and cold. If the patient has a positive attitude and believes that the drug or treatment will help his or her condition, this can affect outcomes due to the placebo effect. The placebo effect may be observed in medical studies when the expected effect of the drug is achieved by an inactive substance such as a sugar pill given in place of the active drug.

344.

A. The generic name is usually the same as the official name. The official name is the one under which the drug is listed in the book *The United States Pharmacopeia/National Formulary (USP/NF)*. The USP/NF is recognized by the U.S. government as the official list of drug standards. These standards are enforced by the U.S. Food and Drug Administration. The USP/NF is regularly updated and a new edition is published every 5 years. Chemical names of drugs describe the structure of the drug compound. Brand name, trade name, and product name are all the same. They are the drug name owned by the manufacturer. They are registered names.

345.

A. Ultram (tramadol hydrochloride) is classified as an analgesic. It is used in the management of moderate to moderately severe pain. Tramadol has been found to inhibit reuptake of norepinephrine and serotonin in vitro, as have some other opioid analgesics. It is absorbed rapidly, almost completely, following oral administration. It can be given without regard to meals and starts to work in less than one hour. The effect lasts for up to 6 hours. Ultram can interact with alcohol. It should not be given to opioid-dependent patients. Patients taking Ultram should not drive a car or operate machinery because the drug may impair mental or physical abilities.

346.

B. The study of the processes of drug absorption, distribution, metabolism, and excretion is called pharmacokinetics. Pharmacodynamics is the study of the action of a drug on living tissue. Pharmacotherapeutics is the study of the use of drugs in treating diseases. Pharmacy is the science of preparing and dispensing medicines. Posology is the study of the amount of a drug that is required to produce therapeutic effects.

347.

C. The study of diseases and disorders in the elderly is called geriatrics (geri = old age; atric = medical treatment). As people age, a decrease in organ function is normal. Therefore, elderly patients become more prone to disease. The elderly, because of more disorders, tend to receive a larger number of drugs than younger adults. Over-the-counter products are geared toward the elderly. The elderly patient is also more prone to side effects from all categories of medications.

348.

D. Norvasc, the brand name for the generic drug amlodipine, and Prinivil and Zestril, two brand names for one generic drug, lisinopril, are used in the treatment of hypertension (high blood pressure). They are classified as antihypertensives and are prescribed as tablets. Lisinopril, the compound found in both Prinivil and Zestril, is an angiotensin-converting enzyme (ACE) inhibitor. Both the supine (lying on one's back) and standing blood pressure are reduced. Norvasc (amlodipine) is an anti-anginal (calcium channel blocking agent) and increases myocardial contractibility. Food does not alter the bioavailability of lisinopril but only 25% of an oral dose is absorbed. Both are prescribed in tablet form. Patients should report any side effect that they believe is due to the medication.

349.

E. Hytrin (terazosin) is a drug that may be prescribed for hypertension. This antihypertensive drug is used alone or in combination with diuretics or beta-adrenergic blocking agents to treat high blood pressure. It is also used to treat benign prostatic hyperplasia.

350.

B. Tetracycline is a broad-spectrum antibiotic that is used systemically as well as topically. An antibiotic may be a narrow-spectrum drug that kills only selective organisms, or it can be a broad-spectrum type. Broad-spectrum antibiotics will destroy a wide range of microorganisms. Tetracycline absorption in the gastrointestinal tract is interfered with by milk and antacids commonly taken for stomach upset. Certain foods and other drugs may interact with a prescribed drug to interfere with the intended use. These should be pointed out to the patient as part of patient education.

351.

C. "Elixir" is a term used for a sweetened, aromatic, alcoholic preparation used to administer an active medicine. Elixirs are liquid preparations of medication to be taken orally. An example of an elixir is liquid phenobarbital.

352.

A. A drug that stops or retards bleeding or discharge is called an astringent. Alum and zinc oxide are commonly used. Astringents are used in the treatment of dermatitis.

353.

E. Medicines or beverages that increase the output of urine are called diuretics. Diuretics act on the renal tubules in the kidneys by limiting their water reabsorption, which results in increased urine output. Caffeine is a diuretic.

354.

E. The abbreviation that means "every day" is qd. "Every night" is abbreviated qn. The abbreviation qs means "as much as is required." "Every other day" is abbreviated qod. "Four times a day" is abbreviated qid.

355.

E. For intradermal injections of medications, needles of 26 to 27 gauge should be used. The length of the needle used in intradermal injections is short, usually 3/8 to 5/8 inch. The tuberculin syringe often is used because it is easy to measure the very small amounts of medication to be administered.

356.

C. To prepare a drug for injection, a powdered drug may be dissolved in a diluent, which might be either sterile water or sterile normal saline solution. Medications that are stable for only a short period of time in liquid form are stored in powdered form. Adding the liquid to the powdered drug is known as reconstitution.

357.

C. Fractional quantities in the metric system are expressed as decimals. For example, 1/10 mL or 1/10 cc should be written 0.1 mL or 0.1 cc, and 1/2 gram should be written 0.5 g. Be sure to review the different units of the metric and household system of drug measurement.

358.

D. The medical assistant should be aware that some medications should be refrigerated (e.g., antibiotics). Reconstituted penicillin G potassium is stable in the refrigerator for 1 week. Other drugs requiring refrigeration include insulin, suppositories, eye drops, and tetanus vaccines. Other medications may also require special storage (i.e., some drugs are sensitive to light). Controlled substances must always be stored in locked cabinets due to the possibility of theft. All medications must be stored in their original containers to avoid mix-ups. The medical assistant should read medication labels and follow the instructions necessary to ensure that all medications are stored so that they retain their potency until their expiration dates.

359.

C. Labeling is not a task for the medical assistant, and any container of medication that lacks a label should be discarded. When you are discarding a drug or medicine, it should be poured down the sink to make sure that no one will administer it to themselves or dispense it to others.

360.

B. Fosamax (alendronate sodium) is a drug used in the treatment and prevention of osteoporosis. It inhibits normal and abnormal bone resorption without retarding mineralization. This leads to a significant increase of bone mineral density and mass. This helps prevent fractures of the vertebra, hips, and wrists, which are most vulnerable to fracture. It is also used in the treatment of Paget's disease.

361.

E. Cipro is a synthetic broad-spectrum antibacterial agent for oral administration. It is designated as a broad-spectrum antibiotic because it is effective against a large number of both Gram-positive and Gram-negative organisms. It is contraindicated for patients that have hypersensitivity to quinolones. A narrow-spectrum antibiotic would be so called because it is effective against only a small portion of the many types of bacteria. For instance, it might be effective against only Gram-negative gas producers, not the other Gram-negative organisms and not any of the Gram-positive organisms.

362.

B. Ambien is classified as a sedative hypnotic drug. It is used to treat short-term insomnia and is safe to use in pregnant women (Category B). Ambien is included in Schedule IV of controlled substances and requires a doctor's prescription. Sedatives decrease activity and excitement. They have a calming effect on the patient. Hypnotics produce drowsiness which will bring about sleep as well as the maintenance of sleep. Sleep caused by hypnotics tends to resemble natural sleep. This drug will reduce the number of nocturnal awakenings, increase length of sleep and improve sleep quality.

363.

B. Prozac is an antidepressant for oral administration in the treatment of depression and obsessive-compulsive disorders. The drug action inhibits serotonin re-uptake. Side effects and adverse reactions include anxiety, insomnia, weight loss, sexual dysfunction, nausea, and headaches.

364.

E. All of the above listed drugs would be included. A special tray or cart should be accessible at all times for use with emergencies. The tray should be checked frequently and supplies should never be borrowed from it. Among the drugs used during emergencies are adrenalin (epinephrine) used for anaphylactic shock; aminophylline, a bronchodilator; benadryl, an antihistamine; dextrose 50% for hypoglycemia; insulin for hyperglycemia; digoxin for heart failure and arrhythmia; nitroglycerin for angina pectoris; steroids for anti-inflammatory action; and tranquilizers for hysteria and depression. Individual physicians may have a checklist of drugs and supplies for the emergency tray or cart that is tailored to the specific needs of the medical practice.

365.

D. The process by which drugs are broken down into harmless by-products is biotransformation. Most breakdown of drugs occurs in the liver by enzymatic activity. Absorption is how the drug is absorbed into the body's circulation, also known as administration routes including oral and parenteral (injection). Distribution is the process by which the circulatory system transports drugs to the area in the body that it will affect. Drugs can attach to plasma proteins and then be freed to pass from the blood into the site of action. Drug action is the change the drug makes in the body. There are many types of drug actions, which include (1) those that combine with body chemicals on the cell surface or within specific cell receptors, (2) those that affect the enzyme functions of the body, and (3) anti-infective drugs that have a selected toxicity for pathogens or parasites that have invaded the body. Penicillin works because it poisons or interferes with the life processes of bacteria without affecting normal human cells. The study of drug excretion is concerned with the route of excretion and the amount of time the process requires.

366.

A. Most drugs are filtered out of the blood by the kidneys. The liver is responsible for breaking down most drugs by enzymatic action. If a patient has kidney disease or malfunction, the drug therapy must be carefully monitored to make sure that drug levels are not building up in the blood. Drugs are also eliminated through the lungs, sweat glands, salivary glands, and in the intestine (bile). Drugs also may be eliminated through milk glands so nursing mothers must be extremely careful about taking medications.

367.

B. Transdermal patches ("trans-", across, "-dermal", skin) release timed medication dosages to the skin where it is absorbed into the underlying tissues. From there it enters the circulatory system and travels to all parts of the body. These small patches release medication such as nitroglycerin to treat the pain of angina pectoris, scopolamine to prevent nausea, and estrogen for relief of menopause symptoms. Transdermal patches are popular with smokers trying to quit who wish to receive diminishing time-released amounts of nicotine. Medical assistants applying transdermal patches should take care to avoid getting the medication on their hands. The medication can either be absorbed into the medical assistant's body or transferred to another patient. The hands should be washed immediately after applying a patch to remove any possible medication.

368.

E. All of the above are parts of a prescription. The superscription includes the patient's name, address, the date, and the symbol "Rx" (Latin word for "take"). The inscription lists the name and quantity of the drug. The subscription lists directions for compounding. However, most drugs today are ready to use when purchased. The signature lists directions for the patient, which are put on the label of the medication. The doctor may use standardized abbreviations when writing a prescription. While only the doctor writes prescriptions, the medical assistant should know prescription terms and abbreviations in order to follow written orders and communicate with the physician and druggist about medications. Prescription blanks have the physician's Drug Enforcement Administration number printed on them. All prescription pads must be kept safe and out of the public view. Some drug addicts are adept at stealing prescription blanks and forging prescriptions for scheduled substances.

369.

E. The Blalock-Taussig procedure is a surgical procedure for "blue babies" born with a malformed heart (tetralogy of Fallot). The other selections are methods of calculating medical dosages for children. Fried's Law compares the child's age in months to a child 12 1/2 years old (150 months). Young's Rule compares the child's age in years to an adult (the child's age in years + 12). West's nomogram calculates the body surface area of infants and children. (A nomogram is a chart that shows the relationship between numerical variables.) Clark's Rule bases the medication dosage on the weight of the child compared to a normal adult's weight. When a child is critically ill or extremely over- or underweight, special care must be used to calculate the medication dosage. These rules make possible a more accurate dosage than taking a simple fraction of an adult dosage.

370.

E. All four choices are uses of drugs. Drugs are used to prevent a condition, such as motion sickness. Palliative refers to the use of drugs to relieve the symptoms of disease, such as pain. Drugs are used as a replacement or supplement to the body, such as insulin for diabetes, and for diagnostic purposes (e.g., the dyes used in radiographic examinations).

371.

E. All of the listed instructions should be included in patient education, possibly as a pamphlet. In addition to these precautions, patients should understand when and how drugs are to be taken, where to store the drugs, the dangers of alcohol and drug combinations, the dangers of dependency from certain drugs, and when to check back with the physician.

12 Emergencies and First Aid

chapter objectives

Major areas of knowledge/content included in this chapter are:

I. Preplanned action

➤ policies and procedures

➤ documentation and legal implications of actions

➤ equipment including CPR and crash cart and supplies

II. Assessment and triage

III. Injuries, symptoms, and types of first aid treatments

➤ bleeding/pressure points

➤ burns

➤ cardiac and respiratory arrest/CPR

➤ airway checklist; choking and Heimlich maneuver

➤ diabetes mellitus

➤ fractures and wounds

➤ syncope, seizures, and shock

➤ poisoning

IV. Recognizing signs and symptoms in an emergency

V. Management

DIRECTIONS (Questions 372 through 445): Each of the numbered items or incomplete statements in this section is followed by answers or by completions of the statement. Select the ONE lettered answer or completion that is BEST in each case.

372. Preplanning by medical assistants for emergencies in the clinic should include
  A. a clear understanding of the doctor's familiarity with emergency equipment and medications and also guidelines
  B. posting telephone numbers of hospitals, emergency medical services and rescue units, the Poison Control Center, other local physicians, taxi companies, etc.
  C. keeping a crash tray or cart up to date and ready for emergencies
  D. acquiring a thorough background in first aid and CPR and keeping current by taking refresher courses
  E. all of the above
  (Frew et al, pp 670–671)

373. The primary assessment of the patient in an emergency includes all of the following EXCEPT
  A. is the patient cold
  B. is the patient responsive
  C. does the person have an open airway
  D. is the patient breathing
  E. does the patient have a pulse
  (Bonewit-West #1, p 694)

374. The OSHA Blood-borne Pathogens Standards, which apply the Universal Precautions, mandate that medical workers protect themselves in treatment of emergencies by using precautions. All of the following are safety precautions EXCEPT
  A. assess the ABCs (airway, breathing, and circulation) of the patient
  B. wear gloves and other protective clothing when in contact with blood
  C. do not allow blood or other body fluids of the patient to splash, spatter, or generate droplets

  D. wash hands and any other body surface that comes in contact with blood
  E. when providing emergency care, do not touch near or on the surfaces of your face, nose, eyes, or mouth
  (Bonewit-West #1, pp 597–598)

375. People particularly susceptible to heat reactions are
  A. chronic invalids
  B. alcoholics
  C. obese persons
  D. small children
  E. all of the above
  (American Red Cross, pp 299–362)

376. In treating for suspected brain injury, which of the following should NOT be done?
  A. keep the victim lying down
  B. give the victim fluids by mouth
  C. control hemorrhage
  D. record extent and duration of unconsciousness
  E. administer artificial respiration when necessary
  (Zakus, p 567)

377. In mouth-to-mouth artificial respiration in CPR, air should be blown into the victim's mouth at the rate of
  A. 5 per minute
  B. 8 per minute
  C. 12 per minute
  D. 16 per minute
  E. 21 per minute
  (American Red Cross, p 93)

378. An acceptable emergency or first aid treatment for open wounds of the abdomen is to

   A. replace protruding intestines or abdominal organs
   B. apply dressing and bandage so as to cause constriction
   C. give fluids
   D. give solid foods
   E. cover protruding intestines or abdominal organs with a sterile dressing, clean towel, plastic, or metal foil

   (American Red Cross, p 283; Frew et al, p 676)

379. First aid for a penetrating injury to the eye is to

   A. remove the object
   B. wash the eye
   C. cover both eyes with a sterile or clean dressing
   D. cover only the affected eye with a sterile dressing
   E. keep the victim in a standing position

   (American Red Cross, pp 268–269; Frew et al, p 675)

380. Patients can have severe allergic reactions to an insect sting. Which insect leaves the stinger in the skin?

   A. wasp
   B. hornet
   C. mosquito
   D. yellow jacket
   E. honeybee

   (Keir et al, p 703)

381. A diabetic coma may be caused by

   A. too much sleep
   B. too much insulin
   C. convulsions
   D. too high a level of glucose in the blood
   E. none of the above

   (Bonewit-West #1, pp 723–725; Keir et al, pp 692–693)

382. Which of the following is correct about a patient suffering anaphylactic shock?

   A. develops a rash
   B. has tight feeling in chest and throat
   C. has difficulty in breathing
   D. has swelling of neck, face, and tongue
   E. all of the above

   (Tuttle-Yoder and Fraser-Nobbe, p 151)

383. An acceptable procedure for treating frostbite is to

   A. apply a heat lamp
   B. rub the affected part
   C. rewarm the frozen part quickly
   D. break blisters
   E. have the victim bring the affected part near a high heat source

   (American Red Cross, p 367)

384. During which period of time will ultraviolet (UV) rays be most harmful?

   A. 8 A.M.–12 noon
   B. 9 A.M.–1 P.M.
   C. 10 A.M.–2 P.M.
   D. 11 A.M.–3 P.M.
   E. 12 noon–4 P.M.

   (American Red Cross, p 365)

385. Of the following, which is NOT an appropriate first aid procedure for prolonged exposure to the cold?

   A. remove wet or frozen clothing
   B. rewarm the victim slowly
   C. give hot liquids by mouth if conscious
   D. give artificial respiration if indicated
   E. dry the victim thoroughly if water is used to rewarm him or her

   (American Red Cross, p 186; Frew et al, p 681)

386. When skin is scraped against a hard surface, the type of wound resulting is probably a/an
    A. abrasion
    B. avulsion
    C. incision
    D. laceration
    E. puncture

    (American Red Cross, p 186; Frew et al, p 677)

387. A cut from a knife or a sharp edge of metal is what type of wound?
    A. abrasion
    B. avulsion
    C. incision
    D. laceration
    E. puncture

    (American Red Cross, p 187; Frew et al, p 678;
    Tuttle-Yoder and Fraser-Nobbe, p 134)

388. Which of the following statements does NOT apply to splinting?
    A. splints decrease the likelihood of shock
    B. splints may be held in place by strips of cloth
    C. after splinting, help the patient to use the injured part
    D. splints should extend past the joints on either side of a suspected fracture
    E. splints should be adequately padded between the splint and the skin

    (American Red Cross, pp 232–233)

389. The Rule of Nines classifies third-degree burns by assigning a percentage value to different body surfaces. In the case of a small child, which of the following is given a value of 18%?
    A. head
    B. each lower limb
    C. each arm
    D. genitalia
    E. both palms

    (Keir et al, pp 704–705; Kinn and Woods, pp 696–698)

390. If the wounding object is still in place in a sucking wound of the chest
    A. remove the object as soon as possible and cover the opening with a sterile dressing
    B. remove the object as soon as possible and apply direct pressure to the wound
    C. remove the object and send the victim to the hospital
    D. leave the object undisturbed
    E. partially withdraw the object and anchor it in place

    (American Red Cross, pp 195–196)

391. In treating a laceration or puncture wound of the neck, a medical assistant should NOT
    A. exert direct pressure over the wound
    B. apply a circular bandage around the neck
    C. seek medical attention without delay
    D. apply pressure continually until the victim is seen by a physician
    E. keep airway open

    (American Red Cross, pp 270–271)

392. Apoplexy is a term meaning
    A. heart attack
    B. stroke
    C. fainting
    D. epilepsy
    E. convulsions
    (Keir et al, p 699)

393. The cells most sensitive to lack of oxygen are those of the
    A. lungs
    B. heart
    C. larynx
    D. brain
    E. esophagus
    (American Red Cross, p 87)

394. Which of the following warning sign(s) of stroke indicate that the patient needs immediate medical care?
    A. unconsciousness
    B. paralysis in part of the body
    C. slurring of speech
    D. unequal pupil size
    E. all of the above
    (Kinn and Woods, p 800)

395. Which of the following would NOT be characteristic of injuries to the genital organs?
    A. great pain
    B. marked swelling
    C. unawareness of injury
    D. considerable bleeding
    E. possible shock
    (American Red Cross, pp 284–285)

396. Which blook vessel is too deep to serve as a site for a pressure point?
    A. radial artery
    B. carotid artery
    C. femoral artery
    D. vena cava
    E. temporal artery
    (Bonewit-West #1, pp 708–709; Frew et al, pp 674–675)

397. To stop severe bleeding, the first step for a medical assistant should be to
    A. elevate the body part
    B. apply direct pressure
    C. apply pressure over the supplying artery
    D. apply a tourniquet
    E. treat for shock
    (American Red Cross, p 159)

398. Appropriate first aid for treating an alkali burn of the eye (caused by drain cleaner or a detergent) is to
    A. irrigate with a soda solution
    B. apply alternating hot and cold packs
    C. flood the eye thoroughly with water for 15 minutes
    D. apply a clean bandage over the affected eye
    E. apply a clean bandage over both eyes
    (American Red Cross, p 269)

399. An acceptable procedure for treating second-degree burns is to
    A. immerse in cold water for 1 to 2 hours
    B. break blisters
    C. remove tissue
    D. use an antiseptic preparation
    E. apply a sterile dressing
    (American Red Cross, pp 200–201; Frew et al, p 681; Tuttle-Yoder and Fraser-Nobbe, p 48)

400. Fluids should be withheld from victims in shock because
    A. the victim is likely to require surgery
    B. the victim appears to have a brain or abdominal injury
    C. the victim is likely to vomit
    D. it interferes with oral medication
    E. none of the above
    (American Red Cross, pp 176–177)

401. First aid measures for a heat stroke victim might include
   A. sponging bare skin with water
   B. undressing the victim
   C. placing the victim in a tub of cold water
   D. applying cold packs continuously
   E. all of the above

   (American Red Cross, pp 364–366)

402. First aid for the aspiration of fluids and objects in the larynx or lower air passages includes
   A. remove the object with fingers
   B. give cough syrup
   C. give crackers
   D. encourage the victim to cough
   E. give a laxative drug

   (American Red Cross, pp 99–105; Frew et al, p 100)

403. The leading cause of accidental deaths is
   A. poisoning
   B. fires and burns
   C. motor vehicle accidents
   D. falling accidents
   E. suicide

   (American Red Cross, p 457)

404. All of the following may be symptoms of asphyxia caused by choking EXCEPT
   A. violent coughing
   B. cyanosis of the face
   C. unconsciousness
   D. cessation of breathing
   E. normal inhalation

   (Frew et al, p 680; Kinn and Woods, pp 796–798)

405. If a victim is having epileptic seizures, the first aid treatment involves all of the following EXCEPT
   A. loosen tight clothing
   B. restrain the victim
   C. do not put anything in the victim's mouth

   D. protect victim from self-injury by removing objects
   E. if seizure is prolonged, call EMS

   (American Red Cross, p 299)

406. The immediate physical effects of smoking one or more marijuana cigarettes are as follows EXCEPT
   A. throat irritation
   B. decreased heart rate
   C. increased appetite
   D. sleepiness
   E. reddening of eyes

   (American Red Cross, p 350)

407. Suddenly discontinuing barbiturates to a person who is dependent on the drug will produce all of the following withdrawal symptoms EXCEPT
   A. restlessness
   B. nausea and vomiting
   C. muscular relaxation
   D. convulsions
   E. delusions and hallucinations

   (Red Cross, pp 351–355)

408. In treating shock, which of the following steps should be avoided?
   A. keep the victim lying down
   B. get medical help as soon as possible
   C. raise the feet 8 to 12 inches
   D. cover victim so that body temperature will become elevated
   E. cover victim just enough to prevent loss of body heat

   (Frew et al, pp 676–680)

409. Which of the following are causes of breathing emergencies?
   A. poisoning by drugs
   B. obstructed airway
   C. circulatory collapse (shock)
   D. heart disease
   E. all of the above

   (Keir et al, p 697; Red Cross, p 87)

410. Symptoms of head injury may include all of the following EXCEPT
    A. skull deformity and/or unconsciousness
    B. unequal pupils of the eyes
    C. extreme thirst
    D. bleeding from nose, mouth, or ears
    E. vomiting and convulsions
    (Kinn and Woods, pp 806–807; Zakus, p 567)

411. Which one of the following first aid procedures would be acceptable in treating an injured ear with a perforated eardrum?
    A. place a small pledget of gauze loosely in outer ear
    B. clean the ear
    C. stop the flow of cerebrospinal fluid from the ear
    D. assist the victim to hit himself or herself on the side of the head to restore hearing
    E. use a syringe to insert liquid into the ear canal
    (American Red Cross, pp 269–270)

412. An acceptable procedure for treating a sprain is to
    A. keep the injured part flat for at least 24 hours
    B. pack the joint in ice
    C. immerse the injured limb in ice water
    D. apply hot, wet packs
    E. apply cold, wet packs
    (American Red Cross, p 247; Kinn and Woods, p 870)

413. Which of the following is NOT a type of shock?
    A. hypovolemic
    B. cardiogenic
    C. antigenic
    D. anaphylactic
    E. psychogenic
    (Bonewit-West #1, pp 706–707)

414. In victims of heat cramps, the muscles likely to be affected first are those of the
    A. chest
    B. arms
    C. legs and abdomen
    D. neck
    E. back
    (American Red Cross, p 362; Tuttle-Yoder and Fraser-Nobbe, p 39)

415. Bandaging a wound
    A. holds the dressing in place
    B. assists in controlling bleeding
    C. offers support
    D. promotes restraint of movement
    E. all of the above
    (American Red Cross, pp 191–192)

416. An injury to muscle that results from stretching is called a
    A. dislocation
    B. strain
    C. sprain
    D. laceration
    E. fracture
    (American Red Cross, p 223; Frew et al, p 435; Keir et al, p 274)

417. Subnormal body temperature is most typical of victims of
    A. heatstroke
    B. heat cramps
    C. heat exhaustion
    D. all of the above
    E. none of the above
    (American Red Cross, p 364; Frew et al, p 482; Tuttle-Yoder and Fraser-Nobbe, p 39)

418. The outstanding signs and symptoms of shock are denoted by the five Ps. Which of the following is NOT one of the five Ps?
    A. perspiration, cold clammy skin
    B. pulse—weak, rapid, irregular

C. pulmonary deficiency, shallow and fast breathing

D. prostration or extreme weakness

E. palpation

(Zakus, p 555)

419. A type of open wound where a piece of soft tissue is torn loose or left hanging as a flap is called a/an

A. abrasion

B. avulsion

C. incision

D. laceration

E. puncture

(Kinn and Woods, p 1136; Tuttle-Yoder and Fraser-Nobbe, p 135)

420. The body temperature of a victim of heat-stroke may be as high as or higher than

A. 98.6°F

B. 99°F

C. 102°F

D. 104°F

E. 106°F

(American Red Cross, p 366; Frew et al, p 682)

421. A characteristic of second-degree but not first-degree burns is

A. redness

B. discoloration

C. development of blisters

D. swelling

E. pain

(American Red Cross, p 198; Frew et al, p 681; Zakus, pp 560–561)

422. The following first aid procedures for a fainting (syncope) victim are all acceptable EXCEPT

A. loosen tight clothing

B. pour water over the victim's face

C. examine the victim for injuries

D. seek medical assistance unless the recovery is prompt

E. leave the victim lying down

(American Red Cross, pp 293–294; Frew et al, pp 672–673)

423. When administering artificial respiration to a laryngectomee, air should be blown into

A. the mouth

B. the nose

C. both the mouth and nose

D. the stoma

E. none of the above—use another method

(American Red Cross, p 96)

424. The best first aid procedure to follow in treating blisters is to

A. leave them unbroken

B. apply dressing

C. wash area and then apply dressing

D. treat all blisters as open wounds

E. treat all blisters as closed wounds

(American Red Cross, p 201)

425. Skin contact with poisonous plants is characterized by all of the following EXCEPT

A. itching

B. nausea

C. redness

D. rash

E. headache and fever

(Frew et al, p 682)

426. After an animal bite, the first step should be to

A. kill the animal

B. treat for shock

C. get medical attention as soon as possible

D. cleanse the wound and apply dressing

E. determine whether the animal has rabies

(Bonewit-West #1, p 721; Tuttle-Yoder and Fraser-Nobbe, p 36)

427. Because it is caused by an anaerobe, most likely tetanus develops in a wound of which type?
    A. abrasion
    B. contusion
    C. incision
    D. laceration
    E. puncture
    (American Red Cross, p 188–189; Frew et al, p 676; Kinn and Woods, p 944)

428. The first aid treatment for most tick bites is to
    A. administer artificial respiration
    B. induce vomiting
    C. make an incision above the bite
    D. cover the tick with a heavy oil
    E. apply hot packs
    (American Red Cross, pp 327–328; Tuttle-Yoder and Fraser-Nobbe, p 35)

429. Internal bleeding is possible with a/an
    A. abrasion
    B. avulsion
    C. incision
    D. laceration
    E. puncture
    (American Red Cross, pp 161, 164)

430. Air leaving the body contains
    A. 0.04% oxygen
    B. 4% oxygen
    C. 16% oxygen
    D. 21% oxygen
    E. no oxygen
    (American Red Cross, p 92)

431. A medical instrument that prevents many deaths from cardiac arrest is the
    A. spirometer
    B. automated external defibrillator
    C. sphygmomanometer
    D. electrocardiograph
    E. MRI
    (American Red Cross, pp 732–733)

432. Displacement of a bone end from the joint, particularly at the shoulder, elbow, thumb, or fingers, is known as a dislocation. Which of the following is NOT a sign of dislocation?
    A. swelling
    B. obvious deformity
    C. numbness (senseless) to touch
    D. loss of normal motion
    E. painful when moved
    (American Red Cross, pp 220–221)

433. A break or crack in a bone is called a
    A. dislocation
    B. sprain
    C. fracture
    D. strain
    E. laceration
    (American Red Cross, p 220; Keir et al, pp 276–278)

434. A chronic condition characterized by episodes of spasmodic constrictions of the bronchi resulting in wheezing, choking, and shortness of breath is
    A. pleurisy
    B. CVA
    C. asthma
    D. shock
    E. epilepsy
    (Kinn and Woods, p 802)

435. A wallet card, bracelet, or necklace that warns of a medical condition would most likely be worn by most individuals with which of the following diseases?
    A. Graves' disease
    B. Cushing syndrome
    C. diabetes mellitus
    D. osteoporosis
    E. synovitis
    (Bonewit-West #1, p 724)

436. A universal choking distress signal is
    A. clapping hands
    B. calling for help
    C. stamping foot
    D. clutching neck with thumb and fore-
       finger of hand(s)
    E. waving arms above the head
    (Kinn and Woods, p 796)

437. An acceptable first aid procedure for treat-
    ing third-degree burns of the feet or legs
    is to
    A. keep burned feet or legs elevated
    B. remove adhered particles of charred
       clothing
    C. apply ointment, grease, or other
       home remedy
    D. apply ice water
    E. induce vomiting
    (American Red Cross, pp 200–201; Frew et al, p 681;
    Tuttle-Yoder and Fraser-Nobbe, p 49)

438. The sign or symptom NOT indicative of
    the presence of an infection is
    A. redness
    B. heat
    C. pain
    D. swelling
    E. the absence of pus
    (American Red Cross, p 189)

439. Cocaine is classified as a
    A. depressant
    B. hallucinogen
    C. stimulant
    D. hormone
    E. tranquilizer
    (American Red Cross, p 344)

440. Which of the following is an effect of
    hallucinogenic abuse such as LSD?
    A. dilated pupils
    B. decreased heart rate

C. lowered blood pressure
    D. decreased body temperature
    E. decrease in activity through action on
       central nervous system
    (American Red Cross, p 345)

441. A patient is obviously suffering with
    epistaxis, and the physician is unavailable.
    A medical assistant should
    A. refer the patient to a specialist
    B. send the patient to the nearest hospital
    C. apply cold packs or cotton moistened
       with cold water
    D. have patient place the head between
       the knees
    E. apply artificial respiration
    (Kinn and Woods, p 805)

442. A medical assistant who suspects that a
    patient is suffering from syncope (fainting)
    should
    A. apply hot packs
    B. have patient lie down with feet and
       legs elevated
    C. apply artificial respiration
    D. give patient a drink of water
    E. take vital signs
    (Keir et al, p 693)

443. In poisoning emergencies, in order to
    gather information for the Poison Center
    and treatment of the victim, you should
    determine
    A. what type of poison was taken
    B. when the poison was taken
    C. how much of the poison was taken
    D. under what circumstances the poison
       was taken
    E. all of the above
    (Kinn and Woods, pp 800–801)

444. A type of wound in which the skin is not broken is called a closed wound. An example of a closed wound is
    A. an incision
    B. a contusion
    C. an abrasion
    D. an animal bite
    E. a gunshot wound
    (Kinn and Woods, p 1136)

445. All of the following actions for office emergencies should be preplanned EXCEPT
    A. contact fire and police departments before emergencies occur to find out what services they offer
    B. post phone numbers of fire and police department and emergency services on the emergency supply cart and by each phone
    C. know the clinic's policy on procedures that medical assistants can perform in emergencies
    D. keep the emergency supply cart equipped with all needed supplies and unexpired medications
    E. lay out on a sterile towel, the sterile gloves, syringe and needle, scissors, hemostats, sponges, sutures, and needle holder needed for an emergency
    (Zakus, p 548)

answers & rationales

372.

E. All of the answer selections were correct. It is important for the medical assistant to have a clear understanding of the restrictions and expectations that the doctor requires of him or her. The entire clinic staff should have an understanding with each other of the role each is to assume in an emergency so that they act as a team and valuable time is not lost. A medical assistant should have a background of courses in first aid and cardiopulmonary resuscitation so that the procedures are familiar. The staff should be familiar with back-up services of other medical facilities and the police and fire departments. Telephone numbers should be posted by all phones and also on the crash cart for quick access.

In the case of multiple demands, there must be a priority assessment with immediate attention given to those victims of respiratory or circulatory collapse, those with severe bleeding, poisoning, or severe allergic reactions, and those in shock or suffering from burns.

Competent emergency care depends on (1) the assessment of the situation and the patient, (2) administration of the correct first aid procedures, (3) arrangement of transportation to medical facilities, and (4) obtaining prompt follow-up patient care from EMS or hospital services. The family may also require notification.

373.

A. Although the patient should be covered with a blanket if he or she is cold, this is not one of the primary assessment goals. The primary assessment includes first determining if the patient is responsive. If there is no response, the patient may be unconscious. If responsive, the patient also must have an open airway, be breathing, and have a pulse. The medical worker should check to see if there is an open airway, if the patient is breathing, and if there is a pulse. Is the patient hemorrhaging?

374.

A. Although necessary in an emergency situation, making an ABC assessment (airways, breathing, and circulation) is not a safety precaution. Safety precautions implemented to avoid exposure to blood-borne pathogens and other infectious agents include the following: (1) Make sure that personal protective equipment is on hand during an emergency on the crash cart or emergency kit. (2) Wear waterproof gloves in particular but also masks and face shields if indicated whenever contact and exposure to blood, mucous membranes, nonintact skin, and contaminated articles is anticipated. (3) Make every effort to minimize splattering, spraying, or the creation of blood droplets or other infectious material. (4) Wash your hands after wearing gloves or handling infectious material (even with gloves). (5) Avoid eating, drinking, or touching your face, eyes, nose, or mouth while providing medical care or before you have washed your hands. (6) If you have cuts or open skin areas, cover them before working with emergencies. (7) Avoid unnecessary touching of objects contaminated with blood or other infectious agents. (8) If there is accidental exposure of your skin to infectious fluids such as blood, wash the area with soap as soon as possible. If your mucous membranes are exposed to blood or other infectious agents, rinse well with water. (9) If you do have an exposure to blood or other potentially infectious material, you must report it to your supervisor so that a post-exposure workup can be initiated.

375.

E. Among persons particularly susceptible to heat reactions are the elderly, small children, chronic invalids, alcoholics, and obese people. This is especially true during heat waves in areas where a moderate climate usually prevails.

376.

B. In treating for a suspected brain injury, an assistant should not give the victim fluids by mouth. The assistant should not place a pillow under the victim's head because this could result in head flexion and in airway obstruction. The victim's head should not be positioned lower than the rest of the body, either.

377.

C. In administering artificial respiration, one breath should be given every 5 seconds (or 12 per minute). It is very important that the volume of air be sufficient to make the victim's chest rise. To administer cardiopulmonary resuscitation, the victim should be placed in a supine position. Artificial respiration is administered along with external chest compression. See a textbook or American Red Cross book for complete details on how to administer cardiopulmonary resuscitation (CPR). Medical assistants should take refresher courses in CPR to stay in training.

Cardiac arrest may occur during a heart attack necessitating CPR. The signs and symptoms of a heart attack include (1) severe pain in midchest region possibly radiating to neck, jaw, or left shoulder and arm; (2) nausea; (3) profuse perspiration; (4) ashen skin; (5) cyanosis; and (6) weak pulse. First aid for heart attacks consist of the following: If the physician is not present, call an ambulance or rescue team. If the patient takes medication for chest pain such as nitroglycerin, administer this medicine. If patient becomes unconscious and breathing ceases, work to restore breathing with mouth-to-mouth resuscitation. If no pulse is present, begin CPR including chest compressions. If the physician is present in the office, call him or her at once and follow his or her orders. Prepare medication and administer oxygen according to the physician's orders.

378.

E. Protruding intestines or abdominal organs should be covered with a sterile dressing, a clean towel, plastic, or metal foil. If there is a delay in obtaining medical attention, the dressing should be dampened with sterile water or cool, boiled water, if it is available.

379.

C. For a penetrating injury to the eye, both eyes should be covered with clean dressings to eliminate movement of the affected eye. A penetrating injury to the eye is extremely serious and should receive medical attention by an eye specialist as soon as possible to improve the chances of saving the victim's sight. Foreign objects may be removed from the inner eyelids by pulling or folding the eyelids back and touching the object with a sterile moistened pledget of gauze.

380.

E. The honeybee leaves the stinger in the skin. It is important that the stinger be removed immediately. The stinger should be removed by scraping it out carefully with a sharp object. Do not remove the stinger with your fingers or a pair of tweezers, as this can result in the release of additional venom. Wasps, hornets, yellow jackets, and mosquitoes do not leave their stingers and can sting repeatedly. Insect stings can cause anaphylactic shock.

381.

D. A diabetic coma is caused by a very high level of glucose in the blood. This may be the result of a diabetic eating too much sugar or not taking sufficient insulin. However, other factors such as emotional crisis or infections also may contribute to diabetic coma. The patient may be confused, dizzy, weak, or nauseated with intense thirst. The patient's breath may have a sweet or fruity odor and the skin may be dry and flushed. If not treated, the patient may lose consciousness and die. The physician should be alerted if he or she is in the office, and the patient should be taken by ambulance to the nearest hospital for immediate care.

The opposite condition of insufficient blood glucose can produce insulin shock or reaction, caused by too much insulin or oral hypoglycemic drug, not enough to eat, or an unusual amount of exercise. The patient's pulse is generally full and bounding, his or her skin is moist and pale, and his or her behavior is often excited. This condition also is life threatening if not treated promptly. The physician should be alerted and the patient transported to the nearest hospital immediately. The antidote for insulin shock is some form of sugar such as sweetened orange juice or tubes of glucose.

382.

E. Anaphylactic shock is characterized by the development of a rash, a tight feeling in the chest and throat, difficulty in breathing, and the feeling of swelling in the neck, face, and tongue. This condition can be life threatening and requires immediate attention. Anaphylactic shock can be brought on by a reaction to many things including insect bites, food reaction, medicine, or allergy shots. For this reason, patients receiving allergy, antibiotic, and other shots should be requested to remain in the clinic's waiting room for 15 minutes. Adrenalin (epinephrine) should be immediately available whenever vaccines are being administered that are made from horse serum or when allergy shots or antibiotics are being administered. Patients may suffer anaphylaxis, a severe allergic reaction, from these products. Shock and death can follow quickly as a result.

383.

C. In the case of frostbite, the frozen part should be rewarmed quickly by immersing it in water that is warm but not hot. Water temperature can be tested by pouring over the inner surface of the assistant's or rescuer's forearm.

384.

C. A person should avoid exposure to the sun between 10:00 A.M. and 2:00 P.M. because ultraviolet (UV) rays are most harmful during this period. Both alpha and beta ultraviolet rays harm the skin. Beta rays are the burn-producing rays; however, alpha rays (sometimes called "safe rays") more readily penetrate the deeper layers of the skin. This increases the risk of skin cancer, skin aging, and eye damage. Both the American Academy of Dermatology and the Food and Drug Administration (FDA) recommend that people exposed to the sun protect themselves by using sun protection factor (SPF) sunscreens.

385.

B. For prolonged exposure to the cold, the victim should be rewarmed quickly by wrapping in warm blankets or by placing the victim in a tub of warm water. The treatment for prolonged exposure to the cold is similar to that for frostbite.

386.

A. An abrasion, which damages the outer layers of the protective skin, usually occurs when the skin is scraped against a hard surface. This type of wound is also called a brush burn and is treated by cleansing with soap and water. Apply an antiseptic solution.

387.

C. A cut on a knife or a smooth, sharp edge of metal is an incision type of wound. Incised wounds also result from cuts on broken glass and other sharp objects. Bleeding from this type of wound may be rapid and heavy.

388.

C. The very purpose of splinting is to prevent motion of the injured part. Do not test for a fracture by having the victim move the part in question. A feeling of numbness or tingling sensations is a signal to loosen the ties of the splint to avoid nerve damage.

389.

A. The head of a small child is rated as 18% because it is relatively larger than an adult's head. Each lower limb of a small child is adjusted to 14%; the back and front torso are 18% each. Each arm is 9%. The palms and genitalia are 1% each. In adults, the body surface is divided into areas of 9% and 18%. The head is 9%, each leg is 18%, and each arm is 9%. The genitalia is 1%. These divisions are known as the Rules of Nines for third-degree burns. Hospitalization usually is required for adults who have suffered third-degree burns of 15% of the body surface and for children with burns of 10% of the body surface, wherever located. (Third-degree burns are the most severe.)

390.

D. With sucking wounds of the chest, the wounding object or instrument should be left undisturbed. Attempting to remove such an object could result in fatal bleeding. A deep, open wound through the chest wall that lets air flow in and out with breathing is a sucking wound.

391.

B. A circular bandage should never be applied around the neck. Lacerations or puncture wounds of the neck may involve the jugular veins, which are located on the sides of the neck. This type of wound is dangerous, and bleeding is difficult to control. Pressure is applied over the wound and pressure points may be applied on the blood vessel feeding the hemorrhage. Emergency medical assistance should be summoned as soon as possible.

392.

B. Apoplexy is another term meaning stroke. It usually involves a spontaneous rupture of a blood vessel in the brain, which results in interference of the blood supply to a part of the brain. It may also result from a blood clot in the brain. This condition is also known as a cerebrovascular accident (CVA). It is serious, may result in instant death, and requires immediate hospitalization for further tests and treatment.

393.

D. The cells most sensitive to lack of oxygen are those of the brain. Irreversible damage to the brain is probable if a period of 4 to 6 minutes elapses after breathing has stopped.

394.

E. All of the listed symptoms are included as warning signs for stroke. It is most important that the seriousness of the situation be recognized and the patient be directed to a hospital. Harvard Heart Letter, Feb. 1994 (Keir et al) lists the following: "Strokes are emergency situations where care such as administering medication can dramatically change the outcome." "Time Is Brain" emphasizes the nature of the emergency.

395.

C. Injuries to the genital organs are accompanied by great pain, marked swelling, and possibly considerable bleeding. The first aid treatment for this type of injury may include treatment for shock.

396.

D. Pressure cannot be applied to the vena cava since it is inaccessible to outside pressure. Generally, pressure points are applied to arteries since the hemorrhaging is more life threatening from an artery. Pressure may be applied above a bleeding point on the blood vessel feeding the hemorrhage. Pressure also may be applied where an artery passes over a bone. Several well-known pressure points are recognized on the body. These include pressing the common carotid artery of the neck toward the spine 2 inches above the clavicle; the temporal artery at the side of the face in front of the ear; the radial artery, thumb side of the wrist toward the radius; femoral artery by bending leg, bringing head of femur into groin, and pressing artery against it; and the brachial artery is pressed above the bend of the elbow.

397.

B. The first technique that should be used by a medical assistant to control severe bleeding is the application of direct pressure. The preferred method is direct pressure by a gloved hand over a dressing. This will prevent loss of blood without interfering with normal blood circulation. Pressure may be applied at pressure points toward the source of the blood circulation if application of pressure over the wound is not sufficient. The medical assistant should follow Universal Precautions guidelines (e.g., wearing gloves and other protective clothing) when controlling hemorrhaging. HIV, HBV, and other diseases are blood borne and can be transmitted during hemorrhage if proper precautions are not followed.

398.

C. The appropriate first aid treatment for an alkali burn of the eye is to flood the eye thoroughly with water for 15 minutes. Loose particles of dry chemicals floating on the eye should be gently removed using a sterile gauze or a clean handkerchief.

399.

E. In treating second-degree burns (partial thickness burns that penetrate into the dermis of the skin and have blisters), a medical assistant rendering first aid might immerse the burned part in cold water or apply a sterile cloth moistened with cool water until the pain subsides. Then blot dry gently and apply a dry, sterile gauze or clean cloth as a protective bandage. Do not break the blisters or attempt to remove any of the burned area.

On a third-degree burn (a full thickness burn that destroys all layers of skin), the patient should be checked for breathing, especially if the burn resulted in smoke inhalation or was near the face. Then remove any burning agent present and all clothing or jewelry that might retain heat. Cut away the clothing. Keep burned limbs above the level of the heart. Cool the wound with cool (not ice-cold) water or saline and cover. Wrap the person and arrange transport to a medical center. Separate layers of burned flesh that may adhere together such as fingers and toes. Inform the patient that he or she is being transferred to a treatment center. Keep the patient warm and give emotional support.

First aid treatment for a chemical burn is to flood the affected body area with water (if the chemical is known and will not react with water) and when the chemical has been washed from the skin, cover it with a sterile dressing. Acid burns that are caused by phenol (carbolic acid) should be washed with ethyl alcohol before flooding with water because phenol is not water soluble. A hose is helpful and should be used as quickly as possible and for at least 5 minutes. Chemical burns of the eye should be flooded with water for 15 minutes.

Some "don'ts" when treating burns include: (1) don't contaminate the burn by blowing on it; (2) don't apply unclean dressings; (3) don't pull clothing across the burned area, cut it off; (4) don't use absorbent cotton on a burn; and (5) don't use any kind of medication or ointment on a burn or change dressings that were initially applied unless directed to do so by the physician.

400.

A. Do not give shock victims drink or food without the doctor's permission even if they are thirsty. If they are accident victims and require surgery, the stomach should be empty to prevent nausea. You should minimize blood loss in the patient by controlling any external bleeding. Keep the person lying down and quiet. A person in shock requires life support as soon as possible.

Shock can result from many different kinds of injuries and seriously depresses the vital body functions. The decreased cardiac output of blood causes a decreased blood volume, which in turn creates a low blood pressure, a weak rapid pulse, rapid breathing, ashen color, cold clammy skin, and dilated pupils. The victim should be placed in a recumbent position with the feet elevated. If the victim has a head injury or has difficulty breathing, keep the patient flat. Maintain body heat (with a blanket) but do not overheat.

Anaphylactic shock sometimes occurs after an allergy shot or medication such as penicillin. Oxygen and epinephrine should be available for use by the physician or under his or her direction.

401.

E. All of the listed procedures may be used because they all are directed toward cooling the body as quickly as possible. Heat stroke victims have a thermoregulatory system malfunction in the body that permits the body temperature to climb dangerously high (106–113°F). At these temperatures, brain, liver, and kidney cells are destroyed, and a variety of physiologic systems are disrupted. The patient may be unconscious.

402.

D. As soon as the spasm of the larynx subsides, a victim should first be encouraged to cough. No one should attempt to remove the object with fingers or to give cough syrup, medicines, crackers, or bread. If coughing is not effective, other first aid procedures for choking should be implemented and the EMS should be called.

403.

C. Motor vehicle accidents are the leading cause of accidental deaths, followed by falls, and fire and burn fatalities. Medical personnel who treat accidents will need to know the procedures required for these victims.

404.

E. Victims of choking usually make alarming attempts at inhalation. The victim can exhale, but the inhalation process is blocked. Exhalation without inhalation quickly empties the lungs. They are not capable of normal inhalation and immediate urgent action is necessary. Shout for help and begin first aid procedures. The person who is choking should be encouraged to cough. If this is not possible, begin abdominal thrusts (also known as the Heimlich maneuver). The procedure must be modified for infants, the unconscious person, and pregnant women. The distress signal for choking is made by gesturing and clutching the neck between the thumb and forefingers.

If the patient can talk, he or she is not choking. Severe coughing can also produce symptoms of asphyxia (insufficient oxygen intake) and blueness of the face. However, the victim can talk somewhat.

405.

B. Rather than restraining patients who are suffering epileptic seizures, position them in such a way that they will not injure themselves by knocking against furniture or other objects. The patient should be rolled to a side-lying position to prevent aspiration in case of vomiting. Call for assistance, but do not leave the victim.

406.

B. Immediate physical effects of smoking one or more marijuana cigarettes are increased heart rate, throat irritation, reddening of the eyes, occasional dizziness, incoordination, sleepiness, and an increased appetite. The dependence on marijuana is not physical, it is psychological. Discontinued use does not produce withdrawal symptoms.

407.

E. Drug-related emergencies may mimic other medical emergencies such as diabetic emergencies or accidental poisonings. Therefore, remember you do not have to have a diagnosis to treat the patient. It should be considered a poisoning emergency if the cause is unknown. If a physician is not in the office for consultation, call the Emergency Center or Poison Control Center and follow the instructions given for treatment.

408.

D. The purpose of covering a victim of shock is to keep him or her from losing body heat, not to elevate the body temperature. The victim should be kept warm enough to avoid chilling. Additional blankets and clothing may be used if the victim is exposed to cold or dampness. Shock is a serious condition that may result in death. It occurs as a result of the heart providing inadequate circulation and the blood vessels dilating. The symptoms include reduced blood pressure, a weak rapid pulse, ashy color, cool clammy skin, rapid shallow breathing, and dilated pupils. The doctor should be alerted immediately and his or her directions followed regarding medication. The brain suffers from lack of blood circulation and therefore treatment is aimed at re-oxygenation of the brain by lying the patient down and elevating the feet (unless an injury interferes).

409.

E. Respiratory failure may be caused by drug poisoning, electrocution, circulatory collapse, heart disease, drowning, disease or injury to the lungs, compression of the chest, and external strangulation (such as hanging). Respiratory failure also may result when blood accumulates in the chest cavity from hemorrhage. Breathing must be restored quickly so that oxygen can be circulated to the cells of the body. Otherwise permanent brain damage and/or death will result.

410.

C. Extreme thirst is not a symptom of severe head injury. Included among the symptoms of severe head injury are (1) skull deformity; (2) unequal or poorly reacting pupils of the eye; (3) convulsions; (4) respiratory difficulty; (5) vomiting; (6) paralysis; or (7) blood flowing from eyes, ears, or nose. One or more of these may be present. First aid includes following the physician's orders to administer oxygen, to maintain an open airway, to minimize movement of the head and neck, and to telephone for an ambulance.

A concussion, the most common form of head injury, results in injury to the brain, which may result in loss of consciousness, loss of vision, memory loss, or vomiting. Symptoms may disappear soon or last for several hours. Immediate hospitalization is necessary for more severe brain injuries, such as bleeding into the brain and skull fractures.

411.

A. In treating an ear injury, a small pledget of gauze or cotton placed loosely in the outer ear canal provides protection. However, the physician's individual directions for the treatment of such cases must be followed. Eardrums may be perforated (ruptured) as a result of a loud blast, a blow to the head, diving, or a disease of the middle ear.

412.

E. Cold, wet packs may be applied to the affected area. A small bag of crushed ice could also be used over a thin towel to protect the victim's skin. First aid treatment of a mild sprain is to keep the injured part raised for at least 24 hours.

413.

C. Antigenic is not a type of shock but instead refers to a substance capable of causing the production of antibodies in defense of the body.

Types of shock are: (1) hypovolemic (low blood volume) shock due to loss of volume of blood or other body fluids, which occurs from severe hemorrhaging, plasma loss from severe burns, or dehydration from vomiting or diarrhea; (2) psychogenic from an unpleasant experience, the mildest type; (3) cardiogenic shock resulting from injury to the heart (it has a high fatality rate); and (4) anaphylactic shock, a life-threatening reaction to an allergen. Epinephrine is the medication used to reverse the reaction.

414.

C. Muscles of the legs and abdomen are likely to be affected first in victims suffering from heat cramps. The first aid treatment for these symptoms is to exert firm pressure with your hands on the cramped muscles or to gently massage to help relieve the muscle spasm. Sips of salt water may also be used as a treatment.

415.

E. Bandaging accomplishes the objectives described in the other choices. It holds the dressing that covers the injury in place, assists in controlling bleeding, offers support, and promotes restraint of movement. It also protects against contamination.

Bandages are of various types and materials suited to the purpose at hand. They may hold a dressing in place over the injury, apply pressure, aid in checking hemorrhaging, or immobilize or support a body part. Bandages may be elastic, adhesive, impregnated (as with Plaster of Paris), stockinet, or roller. They may consist of cotton, synthetic material, rubber, and combinations thereof.

The many types of bandages include the following types. Figure eight bandages have turns that cross each other like the figure 8. They are used to retain dressings, to immobilize splints, for sprains, and for hemorrhages. Butterfly adhesive strips are used to hold the edges of a wound together. Triangular bandages are often used in first aid and may be fashioned into other bandages such as a cravat (like a necktie) to fasten around the head or other body part, a kerchief for a head injury, or a sling for the arm. A spiral bandage can be either open or closed and is created from a long roll of gauze or similar material.

416.

B. An injury to a muscle that results from overstretching is a strain, and it may be associated with a sprain or fracture.

417.

C. One of the symptoms of heat exhaustion is that victims have subnormal body temperature. Victims of heatstroke, however, may have a temperature as high as 106°F or higher. Victims of heat exhaustion have symptoms that include skin that is cool and clammy, with profuse diaphoresis (profuse perspiration).

418.

E. Palpation is not one of the five Ps. It is an examination method that uses different parts of the hand to locate and feel all accessible body parts. Regarding the other answer choices, the five outstanding signs and symptoms of shock are: (1) pallor of the skin, denoting pale, cold, and moist skin; (2) prostration or extreme weakness and exhaustion, occasionally excited or anxious; (3) perspiration, with moist skin; (4) pulse is weak, rapid and irregular; and (5) pulmonary deficiency with rapid and shallow breathing. In addition to these symptoms, the systolic blood pressure is lower than 90 mm, and the patient may be bluish (cyanotic), with the face and eyes expressionless and pinched. Although the patient may be moaning, there is little reaction to pain.

Shock is a serious condition. If untreated, the patient may become unconscious, vital signs may drop, and he or she may die. Call the physician or hospital immediately if a patient is going into shock. Follow the physician's previous instructions for such emergencies.

The first aid procedures for shock include the ABCs of emergencies: Airway open, breathing and circulation checked. CPR may be necessary. Control severe bleeding when present and keep the patient warm. Lie the patient down unless it is painful, or the patient is vomiting or has a head injury. Do not give anything by mouth or move the patient unless the surroundings would cause further harm.

419.

B. Avulsions result when tissue is forcibly separated or torn from a victim's body. (If fingers, toes, or hands are completely torn away, they may be successfully rejoined if prompt, expert surgical care is given.) All of the answer choices are examples of types of open wounds. Open wounds are those in which the skin and mucous membranes are broken. Abrasions occur when a portion of skin or mucous membrane is scraped away. An incision ("incise," cut) occurs from some type of cut. A laceration is an irregular tear of the body tissue (lacerate means to tear). A puncture is a hole or wound made with a sharp, pointed object. (A nail stuck into the foot is a puncture wound and so is a venipuncture.) Tetanus antitoxin is usually given in case of severe puncture wounds to prevent tetanus (lockjaw).

420.

E. Victims of heatstroke may have an extremely high body temperature; it may be 106°F or higher. Other signs and symptoms of heatstroke may include hot, red, and dry skin because the sweating mechanism is blocked. The patient may be unconscious.

421.

C. Although some of the symptoms of second-degree burns may resemble those of first-degree burns, they differ in the development of blisters, which are associated with second-degree burns. Another difference is the wet appearance of the surface of the skin, which is due to the loss of plasma through the damaged layers of the skin.

First-degree burns penetrate only to a minimal depth in skin, damage being to the outer layer of the epidermis without blisters. Second-degree burns penetrate to deeper layers of the skin causing blisters but the skin is still capable of regenerating. Third-degree burns include the full thickness of the skin plus some tissue below the skin. Tissue may be charred or seared. Burns, especially large ones, are serious even when they are first degree. In this event, the patient should be transferred immediately to a burn center. The doctor's orders should be followed in emergency burn cases and preferably there are standing instructions for such emergencies.

The first aid for burns consists of three Bs and three Cs. The Bs stand for burn, breathing, and body examination. Stop the burning, check the breathing, and determine where and how extensive the burn is. The three Cs are cool, cover, and carry. Cool the burn, cover the burn, and carry the burn patient to the nearest medical facility.

422.

B. Water should not be poured over a victim's face because of the danger of aspiration. You may give liquid to the victim only after he or she has revived. It is important to maintain an open airway so that the victim can breathe.

423.

D. The same general procedures should be followed for laryngectomees in administering artificial respiration, but air should be blown into the victim's stoma. The stoma is an opening in the windpipe (trachea) in the front of the neck. The laryngectomee cannot use the nose or mouth for breathing.

424.

A. Blisters are best left unbroken if all pressure can be relieved until the fluid is absorbed. If it is necessary to drain the blister, a small puncture is made at the base of the blister after the area has been cleaned with soap and water. A sterile needle is used for this purpose.

425.

B. Characteristic reactions following skin contact with such poisonous plants as poison ivy, poison oak, and poison sumac are headache and fever, itching, redness, and a rash but not nausea. The reaction also may produce blisters and intense burning.

426.

C. Following an animal bite, the first step should be to obtain immediate medical attention. The patient should be told that, if feasible, a suspected rabid animal should be restrained, and the animal should not be killed unless absolutely necessary. However, risk or time should not be taken to capture wild animals. Before the physician takes charge, thoroughly wash the wound with soap and water, flush the bitten area, and apply a dressing. Human bites are a special type because they are likely to be contaminated with bacteria and they also tend to be on higher risk areas of the body.

427.

E. Tetanus (lockjaw) most likely develops with puncture wounds caused by such objects as bullets, pins, nails, and splinters. A puncture wound usually produces a small opening to the outside, and external bleeding is usually quite limited, resulting in limited flushing action of the wound by the blood. Tetanus is caused by an anaerobic, spore forming, toxin-producing bacillus, Clostridium tetani, which finds a fertile ground to grow in deep puncture wounds not exposed to air. Other species of the same genus produce deadly toxins that cause botulism, gas gangrene, and diptheria.

428.

D. To disengage a tick, it should be covered with heavy oil, such as mineral, salad, or machine. If the tick must be removed using tweezers, it is very important that all parts (including the head) are removed. After the tick is removed, the area should be thoroughly but gently scrubbed with soap and water because disease germs may be present. The longer a tick remains attached, the greater the possibility of contacting Lyme disease, tularemia, or several other tick-borne diseases.

429.

E. External bleeding is quite limited with puncture wounds, but damage may have occurred to internal organs. Severe and even life-threatening internal hemorrhaging requiring immediate attention may not be apparent except by clinical examination. This hemorrhaging may only be revealed by clinical tests such as low blood pressure and weak pulse, and laboratory tests such as CBCs and blood enzyme tests, and x-rays.

430.

C. Air leaving the body contains 16% oxygen and 4% carbon dioxide. Oxygen makes up 21% of the air that enters the body. All cells in the body require a continuous supply of oxygen for life processes because the body cannot store oxygen. Oxygen is carried by the hemoglobin in the red blood cells to the body cells. Carbon dioxide, the waste product of oxidation, is then transported back to the lungs to be exchanged for more oxygen in the never-ending lifetime cycles of respiration.

431.

B. The automated external defibrillator has prevented many deaths during cardiac arrests by stopping ventricular fibrillation so that the heart can then resume its regular rhythm. It can be operated by even an ordinary citizen. However it must be available immediately when the cardiac arrest occurs.

It has two electrodes that are placed on the chest and two buttons to push. The first button analyzes the heart rhythm and the need for shock. The second button administers the shock.

432.

C. Dislocations are not numb or senseless but instead exhibit a tenderness to touch, swelling, and discoloration of the area. The displacement (dislocation) of a bone occurs usually as a result of a fall or a direct blow. A dislocation is an injury to the capsule and ligaments of a joint.

433.

C. A fracture is a break or crack in a bone and can be either an open (compound) or a closed (simple) fracture. A closed fracture is one where the broken end of the bone does not come through the skin. An open fracture is one where the broken end of the bone protrudes through the body surface (skin).

434.

C. Asthma attacks result in emergencies when breathing is severely restricted due to spasmodic narrowing of the bronchi of the lungs. Respiratory inhalators are commonly used by patients. The drugs, epinephrine and aminophylline, may be prescribed to dilate the bronchi. Mucus thinners may also be prescribed.

435.

C. Most diabetics carry medical identification that indicates they have diabetes. There is a likelihood that they might pass into a coma or stupor and be unable to communicate the cause for their illness. In this way they may receive the treatment they need.

436.

D. Clutching the neck with the thumb and forefinger of the hand(s) is universally recognized as a distress signal for choking. It should generate immediate response from those nearby. The choking victim cannot make sounds or talk because sounds must be made by expelling air through the airway.

437.

A. In treating a victim of a third-degree burn, the burned legs or feet should be elevated, and the victim should not be permitted to walk. Nothing is applied to a burn without the physician's order and examination.

438.

E. The presence of pus along with redness, heat, pain, and swelling are common signs and symptoms of infection. A throbbing sensation at the wound site, pus, and fever often accompany infection. Common pathogenic organisms causing wound infections are staphylococci; streptococci; and bacillus found in the colon such as *E. coli*, tetanus bacilli, and gas bacilli (Clostridium), which produce gangrene.

439.

C. Cocaine is a stimulant and affects the central nervous system. Cocaine can be used medically as a local anesthetic. It is also abused by drug addicts and is legally a narcotic because it is habit forming.

440.

A. Some of the physical effects of hallucinogens are dilated pupils, increased heart rate, blood pressure, and body temperature, and increased activity through action of the drug on the central nervous system. Although the most important hallucinogen is LSD, other hallucinogens include mescaline, psilocybin, morning glory seeds, and a number of synthetic substances. They have no accepted medical use and are Schedule I drugs.

441.

C. Epistaxis is the medical term for nosebleed. The medical assistant, in the absence of the physician, may issue first aid by applying cold packs or cotton moistened with cold water. External pressure may be applied to the affected side by pinching the nostril.

442.

B. Syncope, or fainting, indicates a sudden lack of circulation of blood to the brain. A medical assistant should have the patient increase the circulation to the head by lying down with feet and legs elevated or place the patient's head between the knees to increase blood flow to the brain. Paleness, perspiration, cold skin, dizziness, and nausea are some of the usual symptoms that may precede a fainting attack. Syncope (fainting) may be difficult to distinguish from the symptoms of many diseases such as diabetes, heart disease, epilepsy, or stroke. Therefore, the physician should be notified of these cases. Other first aid management may include ensuring the person's airway is open, loosening tight clothing, observing the person closely, applying cold cloths to the face, and having the person lie flat with head slightly lowered.

443.

E. All of the answers are important in poisoning emergencies. What type of poison, when the poison was taken, and how much was taken are important to determine the proper treatment. The circumstances under which the poisoning occurred may also be important. For example, was it a suicide attempt, or was it an industrial poisoning?

The telephone number and location of the local Poison Control Center should always be available so callers can be directed to the best source of help. The medical assistant when dealing with a poisoning emergency should first contact the Poison Control Center or the physician and follow their directions. The type of poison will need to be ascertained before the proper antidote can be known. Vomiting may be induced with ipecac or large amounts of warm water if the poison is safe to dilute or to vomit. Patients ingesting petroleum products, alkali, or acid should not have vomiting induced.

Different types of poisoning include those ingested; those inhaled, such as carbon monoxide or cleaning sprays; those injected as a result of drug abuse; contact poisons, such as poison ivy and chemicals; and insect stings, which can cause anaphylactic shock and result in the death of sensitive persons.

444.

B. Contusions and hematomas are closed wounds. Internal bruising is a contusion, and internal bleeding is a hematoma. In either case, there is not a break in the skin.

Avulsions, incisions, puncture wounds, and abrasions are examples of open wounds. These will require first aid treatment for pathogens that may have contaminated the wound. Animal bites should be seen by the physician. The animal may be tested for rabies and a series of rabies shots may be required. Gunshot wounds and stabbings may require the patient to be treated for shock and have treatment for hemorrhage. If a lung puncture is suspected, do not remove the object but instead send the patient immediately to an emergency treatment center. In the case of a snakebite, an ice pack may be used to slow down circulation along with a tourniquet that is not applied too tightly. The patient should be seen by the physician immediately.

445.

E. One should not lay out a sterile setup for suturing or surgery until actually needed because it would be contaminated beforehand. Pre-planned actions would include knowing the policy of the office concerning the responsibilities and the procedures that the physician has given permission for the medical assistant to perform. Telephone numbers that could assist in emergencies especially when the physician is not available should be posted by every phone and on the emergency cart. The emergency cart should be equipped with all needed instruments, supplies, and medications in up-to-date working condition. The fire and police departments should be contacted beforehand to learn what services they offer in medical emergencies.

Another possibility that requires forethought in a physician's office is the death of a patient without the physician being present. The medical assistant should know whom to call and how the body will be removed. (The deceased person should not be taken from the office through the waiting room.)

13 Visual Aids

chapter objectives

Major areas of knowledge/content included in this chapter are:

I. Illustrations

➤ hand-held instruments commonly used in diagnosis and treatment

➤ abdominal regions and body cavities

➤ positions for physical examination of the body

➤ microscopic views of various microbe smears and urine slides

➤ digestive tract, heart, and spine

➤ types of bone fractures

➤ EKG tracing and limb leads

DIRECTIONS Match the lettered illustrations on this page with the numbered items.

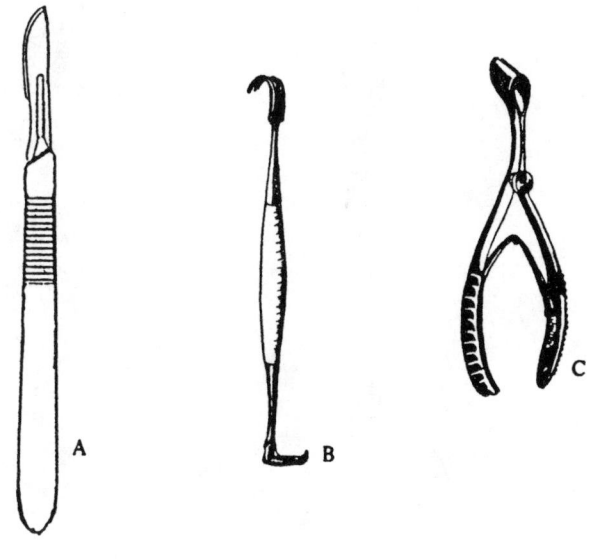

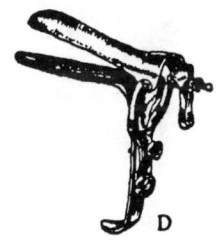

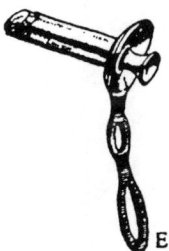

446. Senn retractor
(Bonewit-West #1, p 201)

447. Scalpel
(Bonewit-West #1, p 198; Keir et al, p 644)

448. Hirschmann anoscope
(Bonewit-West #1, p 478)

449. Nasal speculum
(Frew et al, p 608; Kinn and Woods, p 481)

450. Graves vaginal speculum
(Bonewit-West #1, p 202)

DIRECTIONS Match the lettered illustrations on this page with the numbered items.

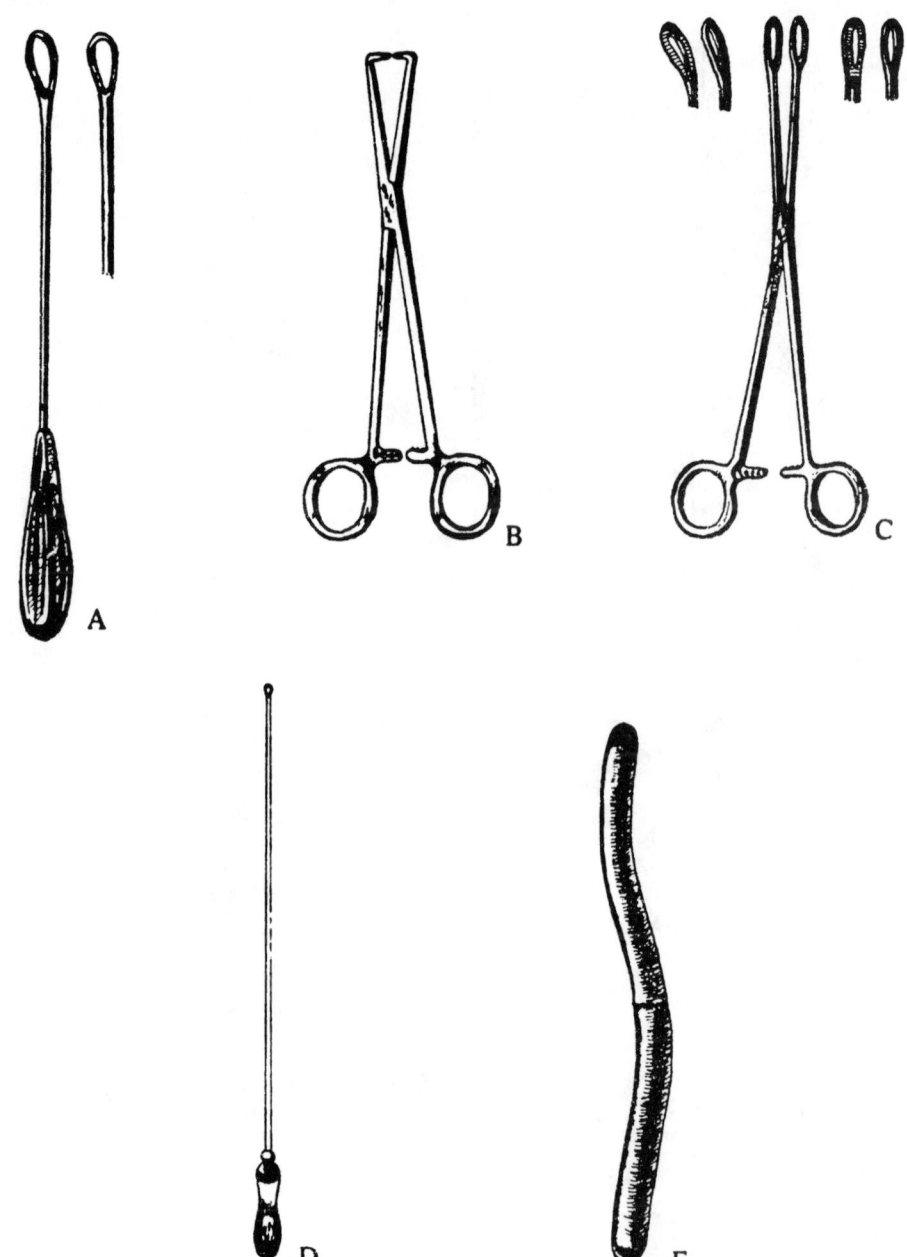

451. **Sims uterine sound**
(Bonewit-West #1, p 202; Kinn and Woods, p 1075)

452. **Sims uterine curette**
(Bonewit-West #1, p 202)

453. **Hegar uterine dilator**
(Kinn and Woods, p 1075)

454. **Uterine dressing forceps**
(Kinn and Woods, p 1075; Keir et al, pp 642, 644)

455. **Schroeder uterine tenaculum forceps**
(Kinn and Woods, p 1075)

DIRECTIONS Match the lettered illustrations on this page with the numbered items.

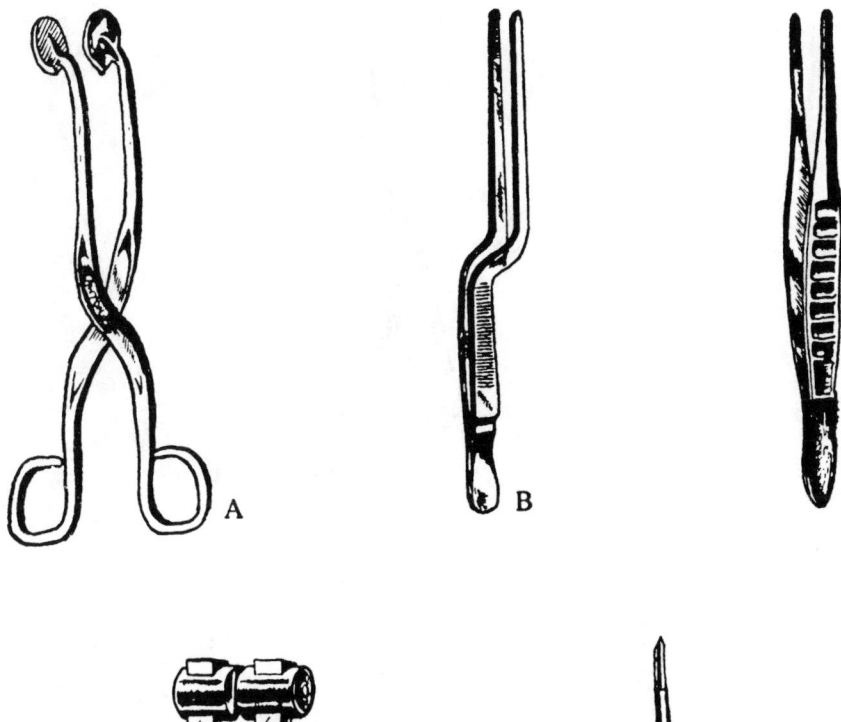

A

B

C

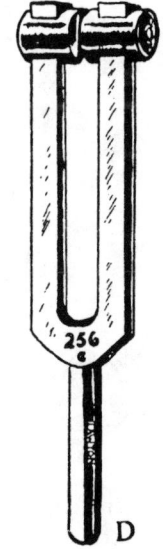

D

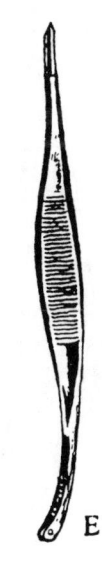

E

456. Bayonet forceps
(Keir et al, pp 642, 644; Kinn and Woods, p 1072)

457. Long transfer forceps
(Kinn and Woods, p 1072)

458. Comedone (blackhead) extractor
(Frew et al, p 607)

459. Tuning fork
(Bonewit-West #1, p 321)

460. Plain thumb forceps
(Bonewit-West #1, p 199; Keir, pp 642, 644)

DIRECTIONS Match the lettered illustrations on this page with the numbered items.

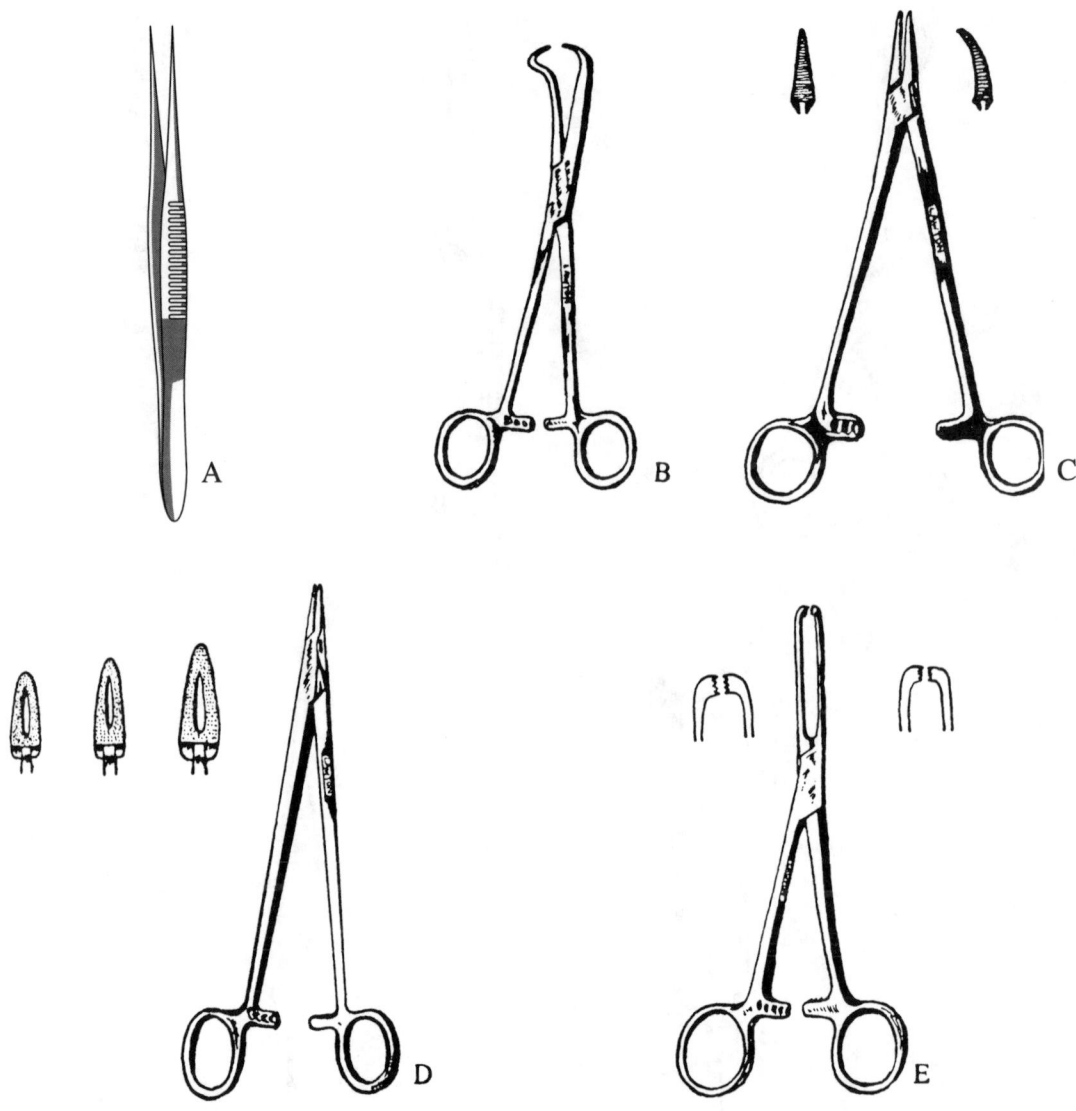

461. Allis tissue forceps
(Kinn and Woods, pp 1071–1072; Keir et al, p 642)

462. Backhaus towel clamp
(Bonewit-West #1, p 201; Keir et al, pp 642, 644)

463. Splinter forceps
(Bonewit-West #1, p 199; Kinn and Woods, p 1071)

464. Plain mosquito hemostat
(Bonewit-West #1, p 200; Keir et al, pp 642–643)

465. Needle holder
(Bonewit-West #1, p 200; Keir et al, pp 642, 644)

DIRECTIONS Match the lettered illustrations on this page with the numbered items.

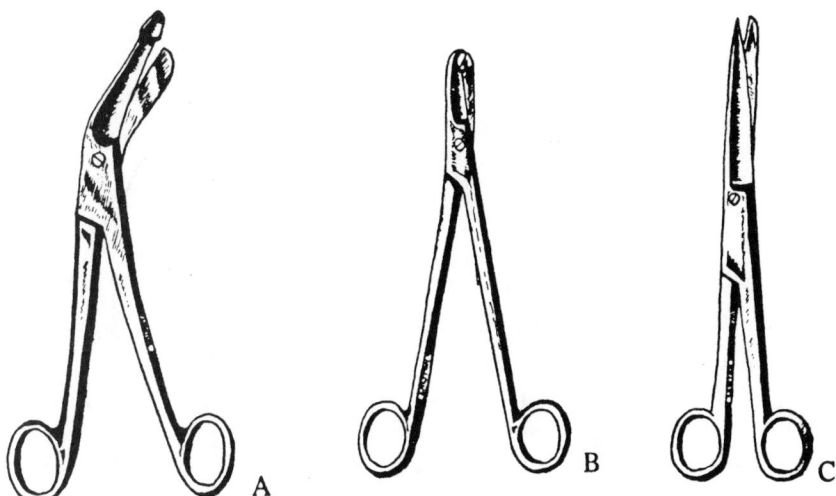

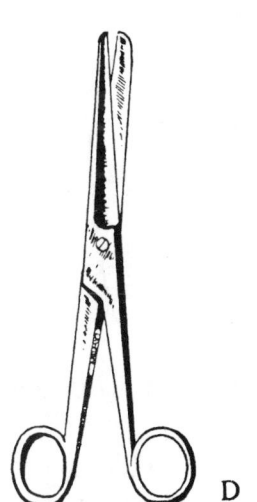

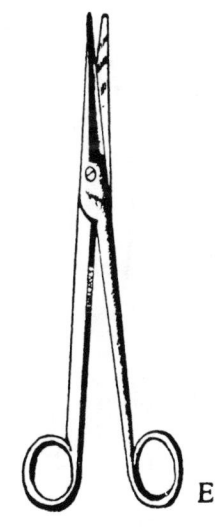

466. Lister bandage scissors
(Bonewit-West #1, p 198; Keir et al, p 643)

467. Blunt-sharp operating scissors
(Bonewit-West #1, p 198; Frew et al, p 605)

468. Littauer suture scissors
(Bonewit-West #1, p 198; Frew et al, p 605)

469. Mayo dissecting scissors
(Frew et al, p 605; Bonewit-West #1, p 199)

470. Blunt-blunt operating scissors
(Bonewit-West #1, p 198; Frew et al, p 605)

DIRECTIONS Match the lettered illustrations on this page with the numbered items.

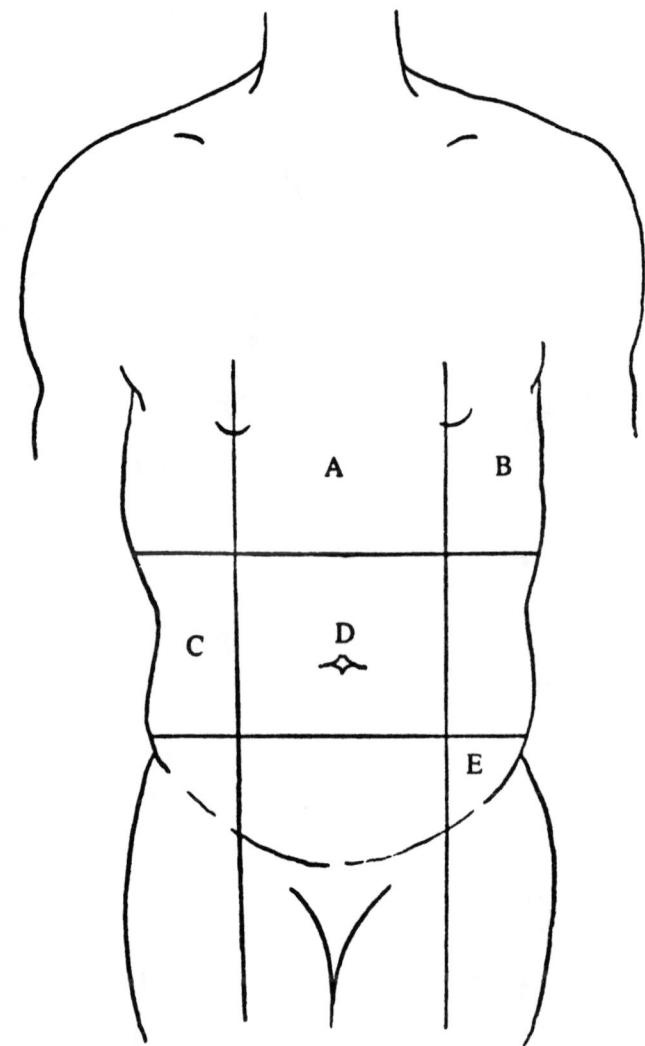

471. Left hypochondriac region
(Keir et al, p 211; Rice #1, p 43; Zakus, p 581)

472. Right lumbar region
(Keir et al, p 211; Rice #1, p 43; Zakus, p 581)

473. Epigastric region
(Keir et al, p 211; Rice #1, p 43; Zakus, p 581)

474. Left iliac region
(Keir et al, p 211; Rice #1, p 43; Zakus, p 581)

475. Umbilical region
(Keir et al, p 211; Rice #1, p 43; Zakus, p 581)

DIRECTIONS Match the lettered illustrations on this page with the numbered items.

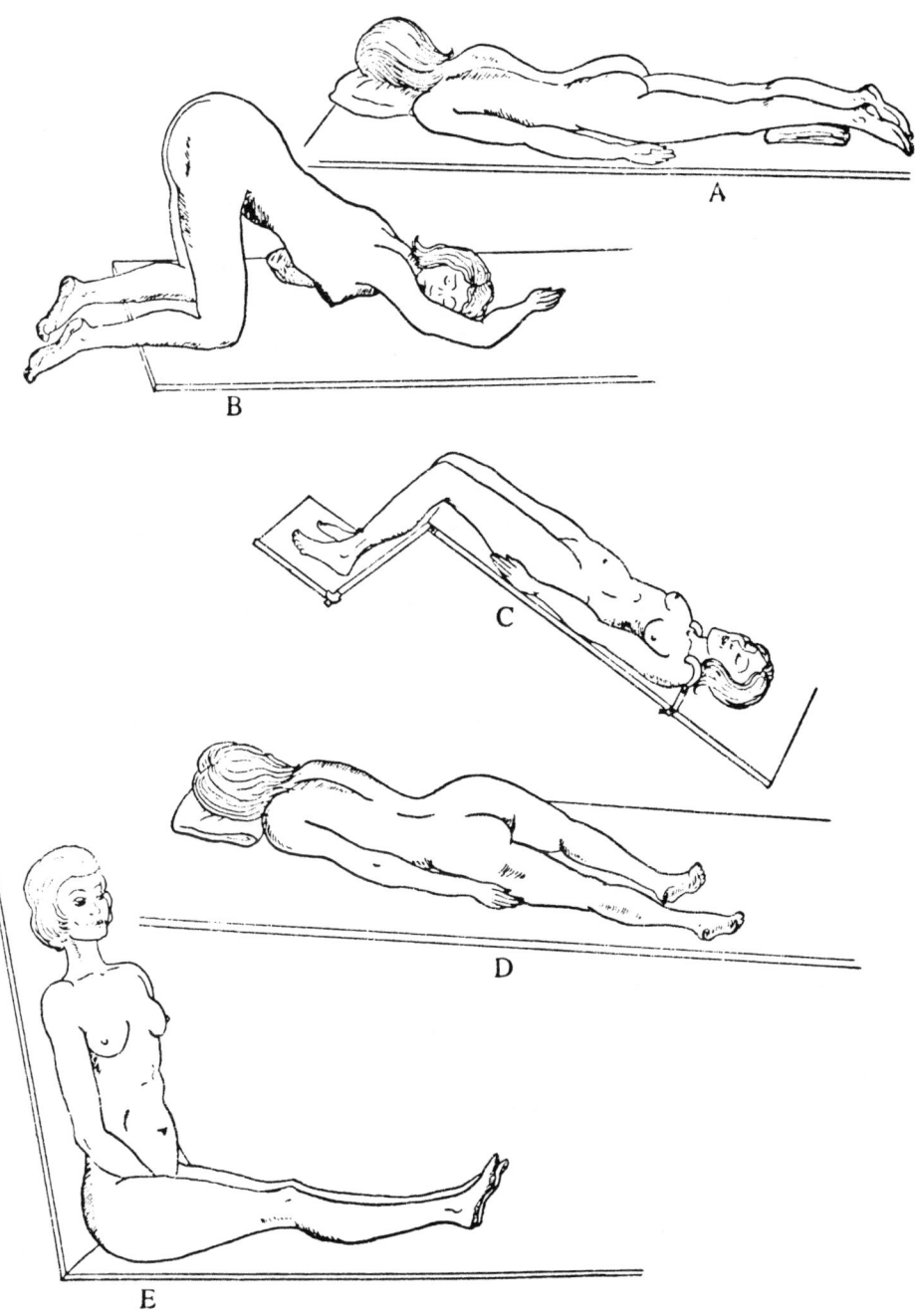

476. Prone position
(Bonewit-West #1, p 136; Frew et al, p 388; Keir et al, p 515)

477. Knee-chest position (genupectoral)
(Bonewit-West #1, pp 140–141; Frew et al, p 388)

478. Fowler's position
(Bonewit-West #1, p 142; Frew et al, p 388; Keir et al, p 518)

479. Trendelenburg (shock or fainting) position
(Keir, p 519)

480. Sims position
(Bonewit-West #1, pp 139–140; Frew et al, p 388; Keir et al, p 516)

DIRECTIONS Match the lettered illustrations on this page with the numbered items.

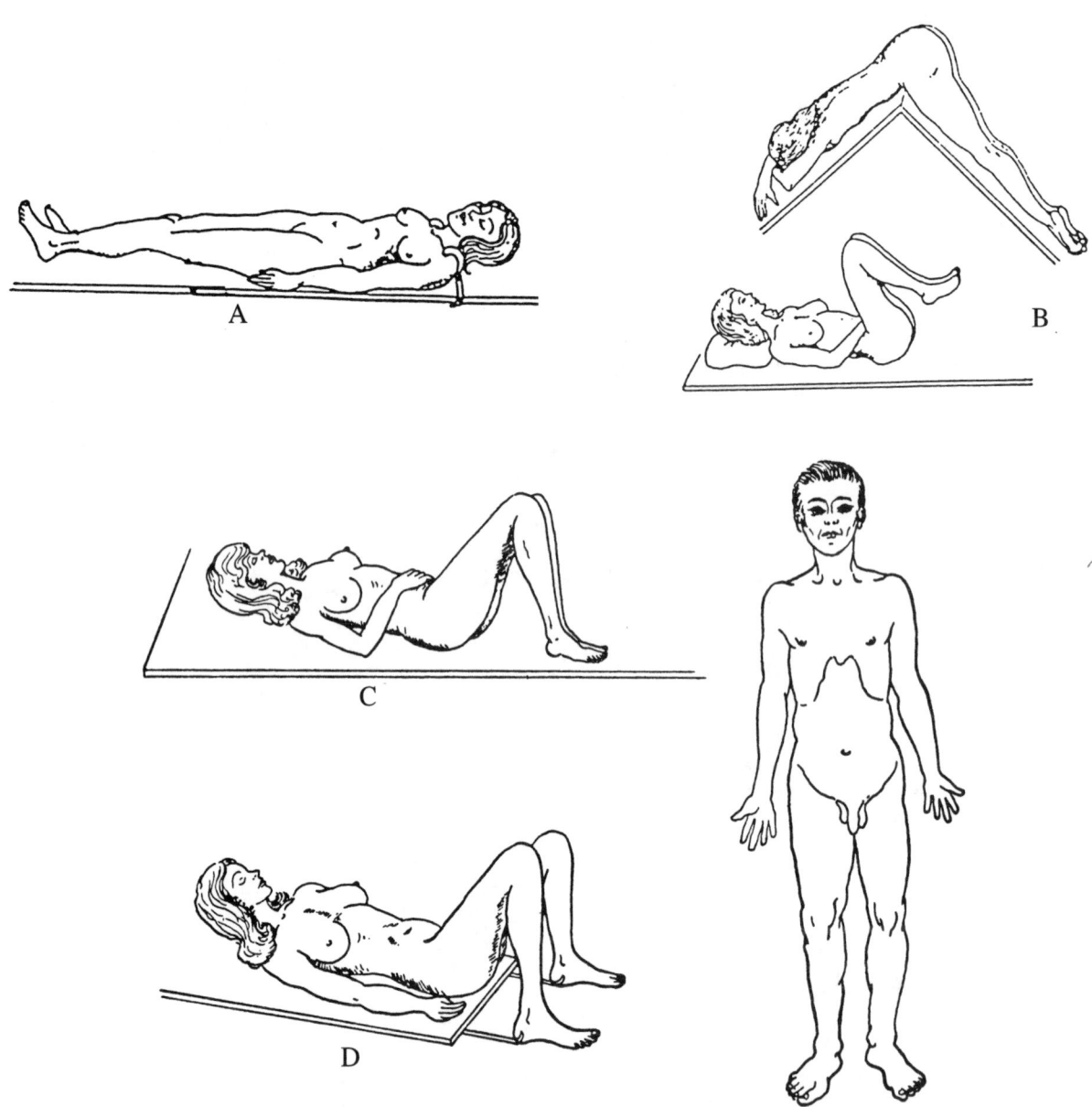

481. Anatomic position
(Thibodeau and Patton #1, p 3; Keir et al, p 209)

482. Supine (horizontal recumbent) position
(Bonewit-West #1, p 135; Kinn and Woods, pp 486–487)

483. Dorsal recumbent position
(Bonewit-West #1, p 137; Frew et al, p 388; Keir et al, p 514)

484. Lithotomy position
(Bonewit-West #1, p 138; Frew et al, p 388)

485. Jackknife positions
(Keir et al, p 520)

DIRECTIONS Match the lettered illustrations on this page with the numbered items.

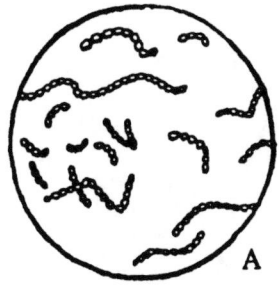 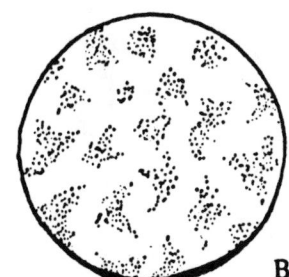 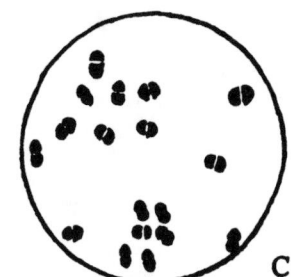

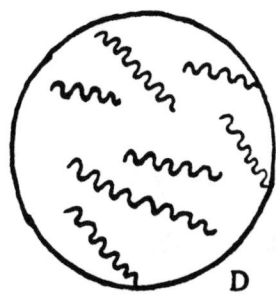 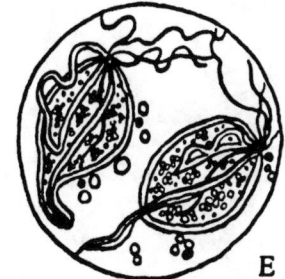 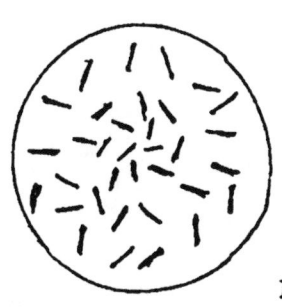

486. Spirochetes
(Bonewit-West #1, p 664; Palko and Palko, pp 486–487)

487. Diplococci
(Keir et al, p 596; Palko and Palko, p 664)

488. Trichomonas vaginalis
(Keir et al, p 596; Palko and Palko, p 493)

489. Streptococci
(Keir et al, p 596; Memmler et al, p 60)

490. Staphylococci
(Keir et al, p 596; Memmler et al, p 60)

491. Rod-shaped bacteria
(Keir et al, p 596; Memmler et al, p 61)

DIRECTIONS Match the lettered illustrations on this page with the numbered items.

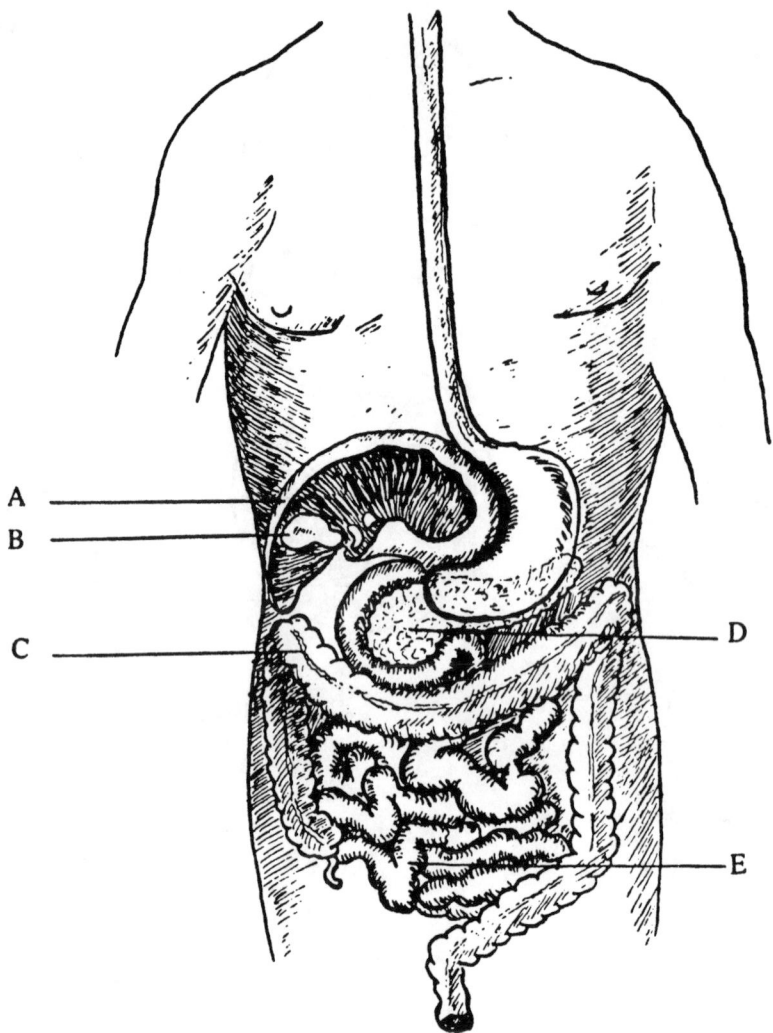

492. A medical assistant has made an appointment for a patient to see the doctor in a follow-up visit after recuperating from a cholecystectomy. Indicate which organ was involved.
(Bonewit-West #1, p 747; Keir et al, p 211; Memmler et al, pp 306, 315)

493. A patient had surgery that rendered him diabetic. Indicate which organ was involved.
(Bonewit-West #1, p 747; Keir et al, p 211; Memmler et al, pp 306, 315)

494. Indicate the organ that may be affected with such diseases as cirrhosis and infectious hepatitis.
(Bonewit-West #1, p 747; Keir et al, p 211; Memmler et al, pp 306, 314)

495. The small intestine consists of the duodenum, jejunum, and ileum. Locate the ileum.
(Bonewit-West #1, p 747; Keir et al, p 211)

496. The colon may be broken down into the ascending, transverse and mesial, descending, and sigmoid colon. Locate the transverse colon.
(Bonewit-West #1, p 747; Keir et al, p 211; Memmler et al, p 306)

DIRECTIONS Match the lettered illustrations on this page with the numbered items.

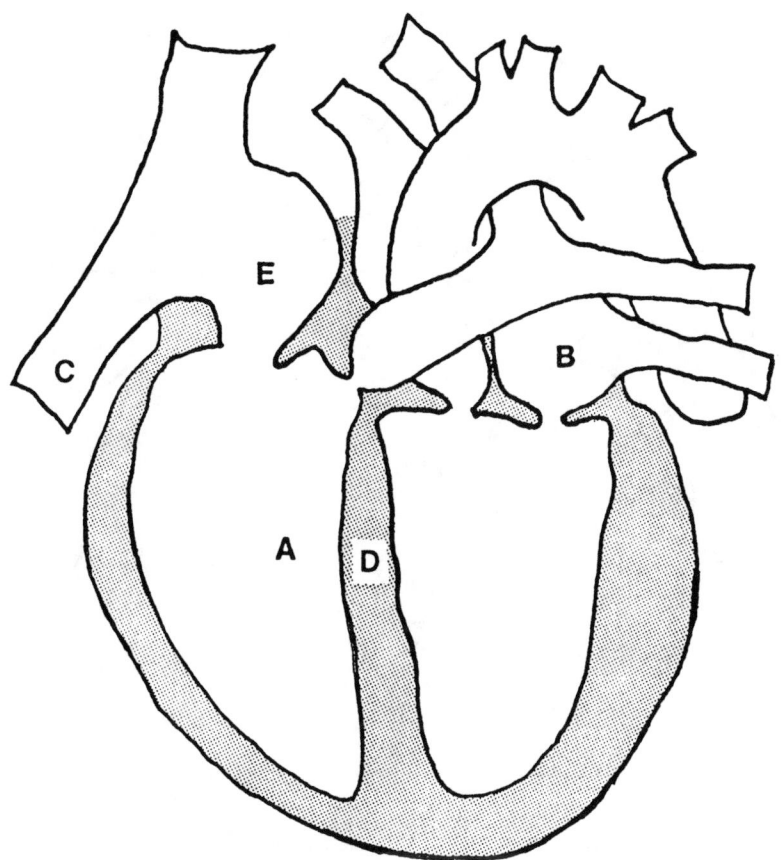

497. Right atrium
(Frew et al, p 839; Keir et al, p 309; Thibodeau and Patton, p 237)

498. Right ventricle
(Frew et al, p 839; Keir et al, p 309; Thibodeau and Patton, p 237)

499. Ventricular septum
(Frew et al, p 839; Keir et al, p 309; Thibodeau and Patton, p 237)

500. Left atrium
(Frew et al, p 839; Keir et al, p 309; Thibodeau and Patton, p 237)

501. Inferior vena cava
(Frew et al, p 839; Keir et al, p 309; Thibodeau and Patton, p 237)

DIRECTIONS Match the lettered illustrations on this page with the numbered items.

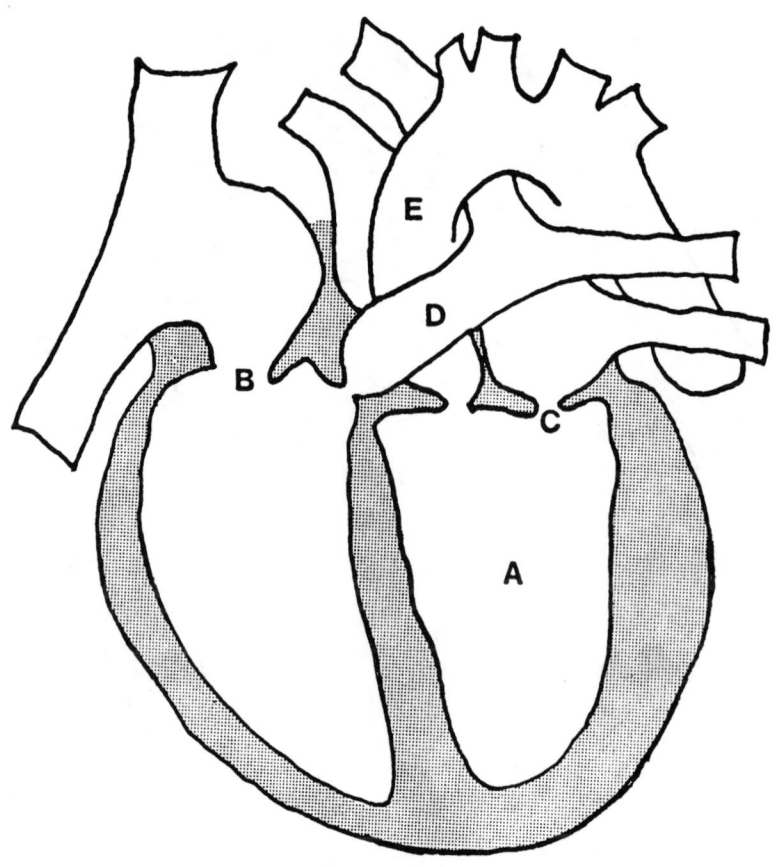

502. Tricuspid valve
(Frew et al, p 839; Keir et al, p 309)

503. Pulmonary artery
(Frew et al, p 839; Keir et al, p 309; Memmler et al, p 221)

504. Aorta
(Frew et al, p 839; Keir et al, p 309; Memmler et al, p 221)

505. Left ventricle
(Frew et al, p 839; Memmler et al, p 221)

506. Bicuspid valve
(Frew et al, p 839; Memmler et al, p 221)

DIRECTIONS Match the lettered illustrations on this page with the numbered items.

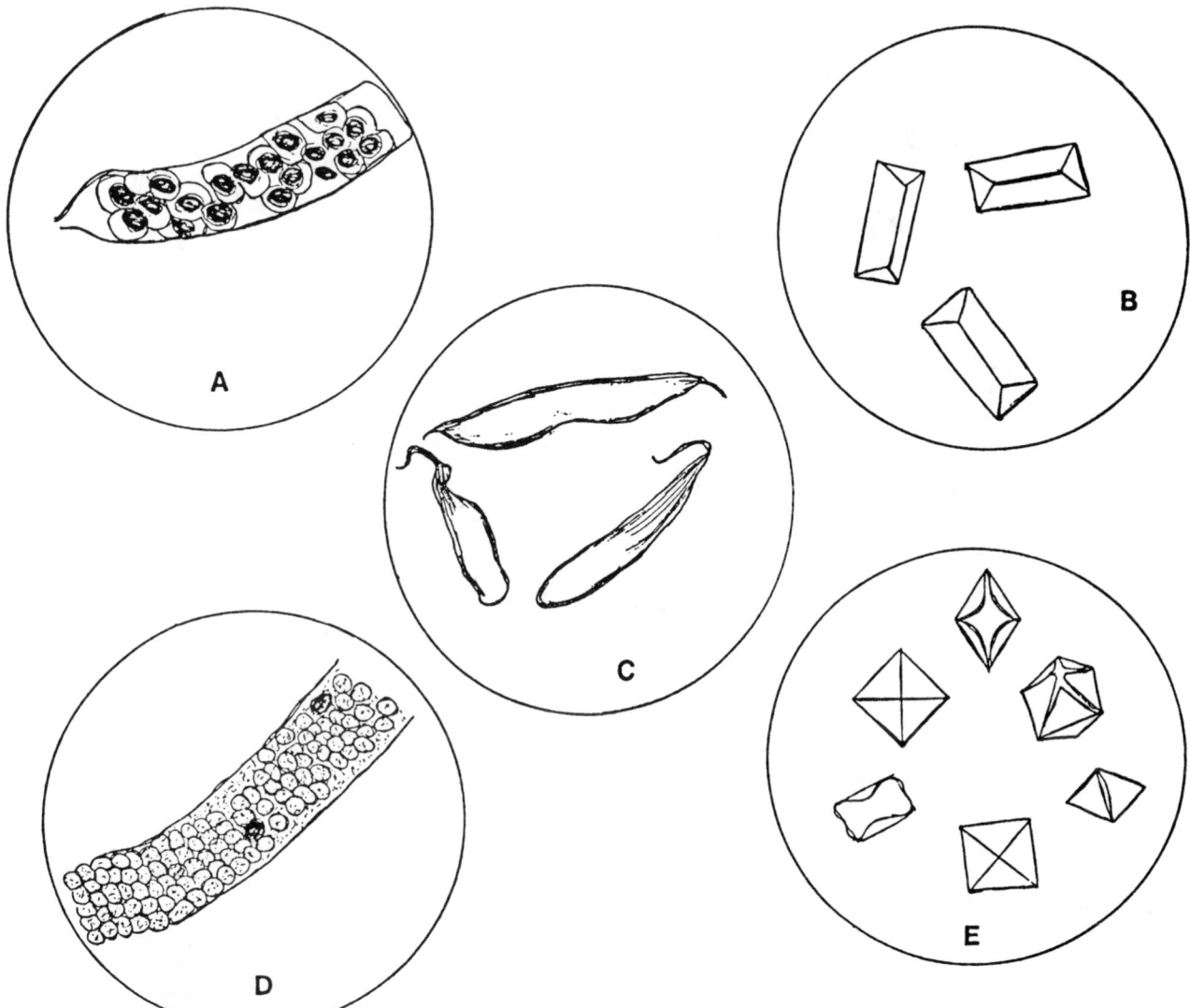

507. Calcium oxalate crystals in urine
(Bonewit-West #1, p 553; Palko and Palko, p 202)

508. WBC cast in urine
(Bonewit-West #1, p 548; Palko and Palko, pp 199, 202)

509. RBC cast in urine
(Bonewit-West #1, p 552; Palko and Palko, pp 199, 202)

510. Triple phosphate crystal in urine
(Bonewit-West #1, p 554; Palko and Palko, p 202)

511. Cylindroids in urine
(Bonewit-West #1, p 548; Palko and Palko, p 199)

DIRECTIONS Match the lettered illustrations on this page with the numbered items.

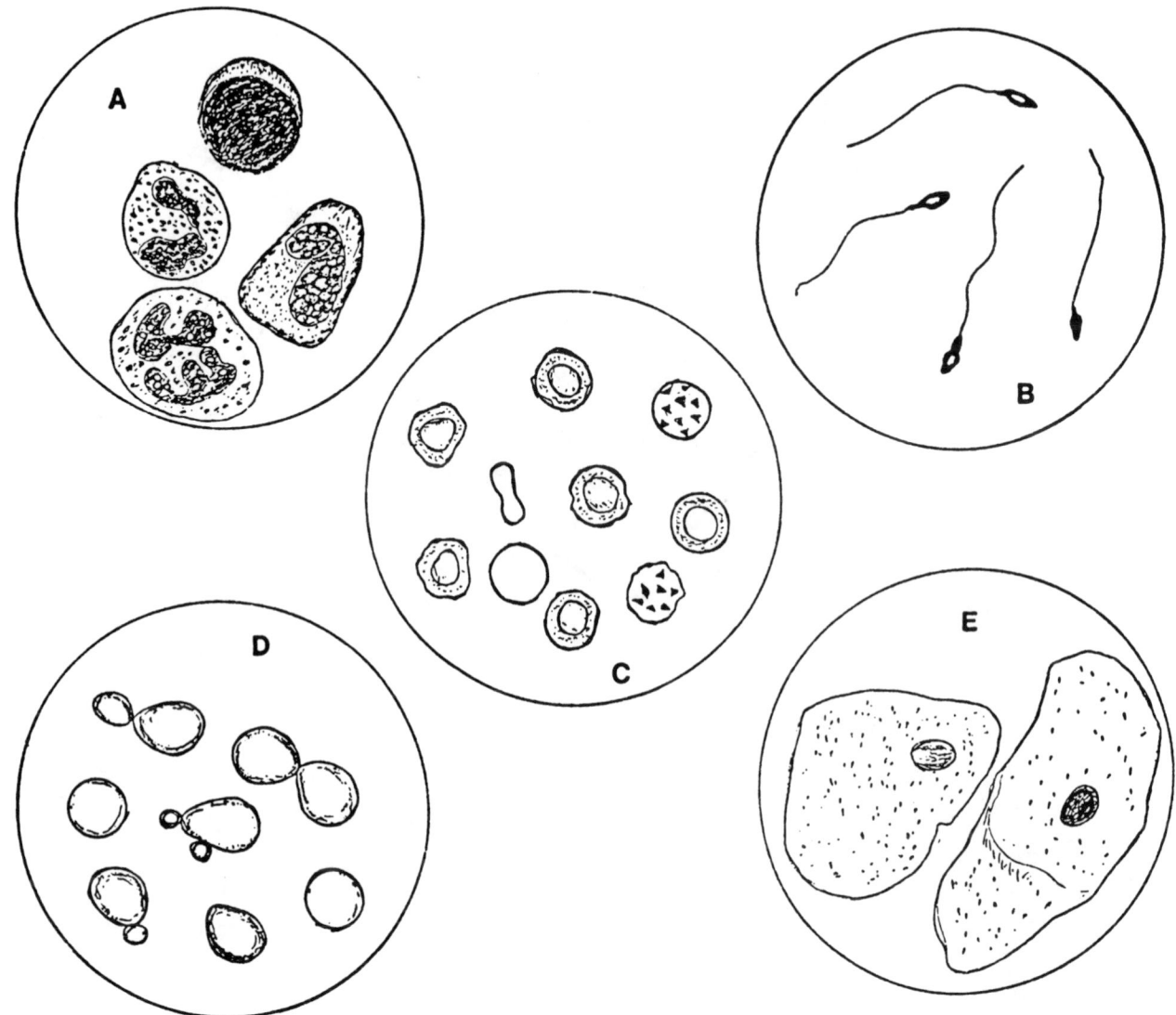

512. Epithelial cells in urine
(Bonewit-West #1, p 550; Palko and Palko, p 202)

513. RBCs in urine
(Bonewit-West #1, p 550; Frew et al, p 766)

514. WBCs in urine
(Bonewit-West #1, p 550; Palko and Palko, p 202)

515. Spermatozoa
(Bonewit-West #1, pp 548; Kinn and Woods, p 747)

516. Yeast
(Bonewit-West #1, pp 548, 558; Palko and Palko, p 202)

DIRECTIONS Match the lettered illustrations on this page with the numbered items.

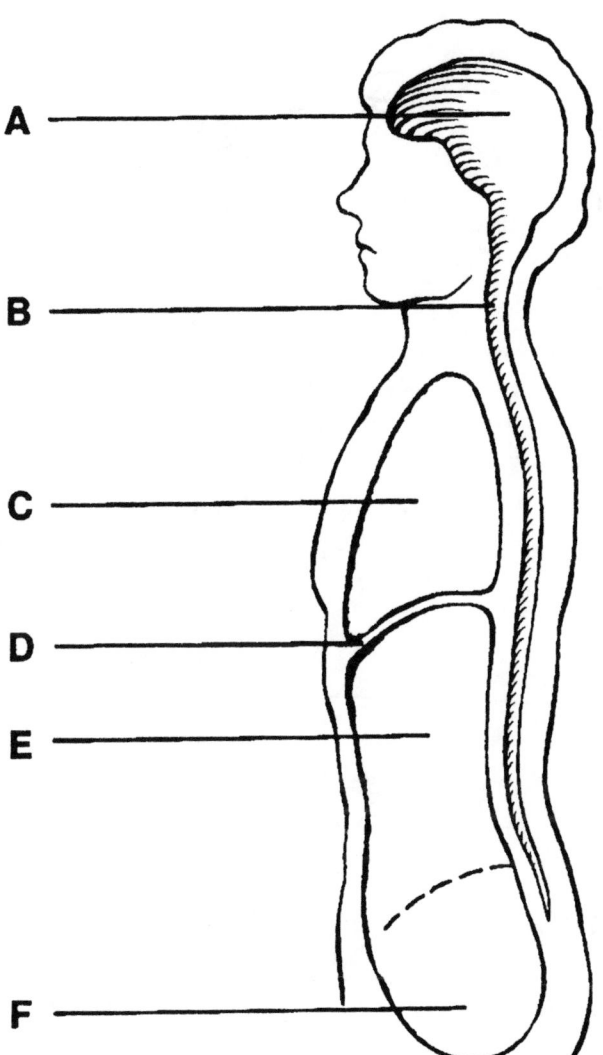

517. Abdominal cavity
(Keir et al, p 210; Thibodeau and Patton #1, p 5; Zakus, p 580)

518. Cranial cavity
(Keir et al, p 210; Thibodeau and Patton #1, p 5; Zakus, p 580)

519. Thoracic cavity
(Keir et al, p 210; Memmler et al, p 9; Zakus, p 580)

520. Spinal (vertebral) cavity
(Keir et al, p 210; Memmler et al, p 9; Zakus, p 580)

521. Diaphragm
(Keir et al, p 210; Memmler et al, p 9; Zakus, p 580)

522. Pelvic cavity
(Keir et al, p 210; Memmler et al, p 9; Zakus, p 580)

DIRECTIONS Match the lettered illustrations on this page with the numbered items.

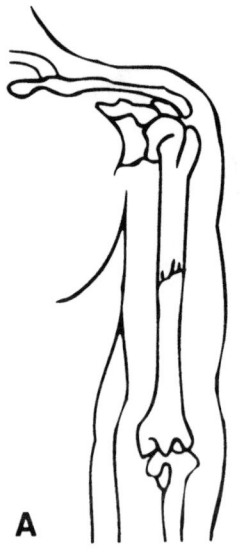

A

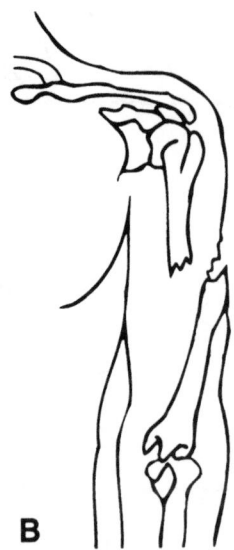

B

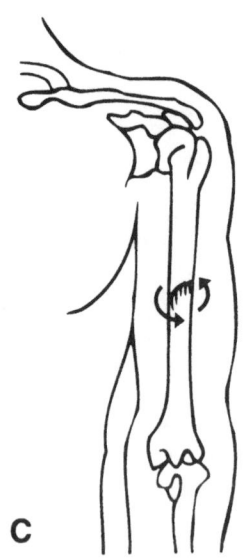

C

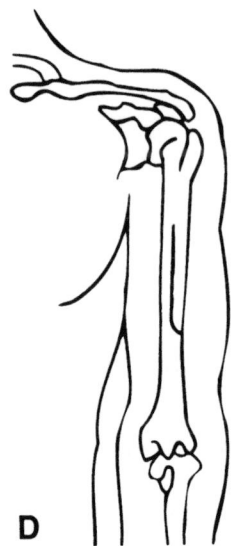

D

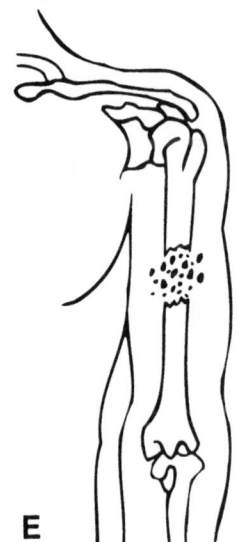

E

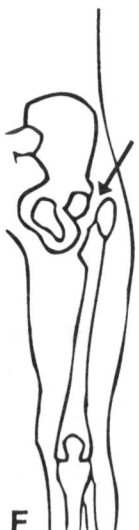

F

523. Longitudinal fracture
(Kinn and Woods, pp 720–721)

524. Compound (open) fracture
(Kinn and Woods, pp 720–721; Zakus, p 566)

525. Comminuted fracture
(Kinn and Woods, pp 720–721; Zakus, p 566)

526. Simple (closed) fracture
(Kinn and Woods, pp 720–721; Zakus, p 566)

527. Extracapsular fracture
(Kinn and Woods, pp 720–721)

528. Spiral fracture
(Kinn and Woods, pp 720–721; Zakus, p 566)

DIRECTIONS Match the following questions with the correct stage of the ECG pattern.

ECG PATTERN

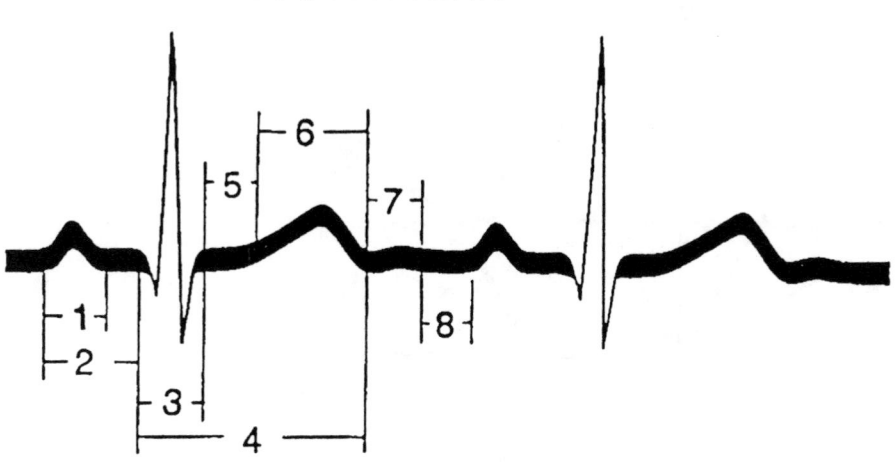

529. QRS complex

530. P wave

531. ST segment

532. PR interval

533. QT interval

534. U wave

535. Baseline

536. T wave

(Burdick, pp 5–8; Kinn and Woods, pp 508–510)

DIRECTIONS Match the correct number with the correct lead that indicates the direction of the electrical output of the heart.

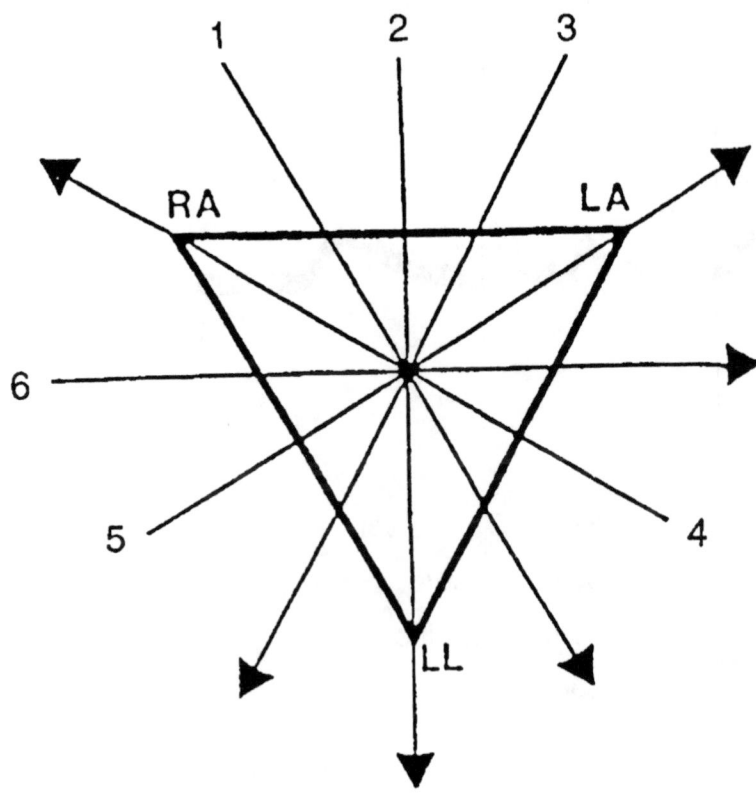

537. Standard limb lead I

538. Standard limb lead II

539. Standard limb lead III

540. AVF (augmented lead)

541. AVR (augmented lead)

542. AVL (augmented lead)
(Bonewit-West #1, pp 447–448; Burdick, pp 10–12; Keir et al, p 612)

DIRECTIONS Match the lettered illustrations on this page with the numbered items.

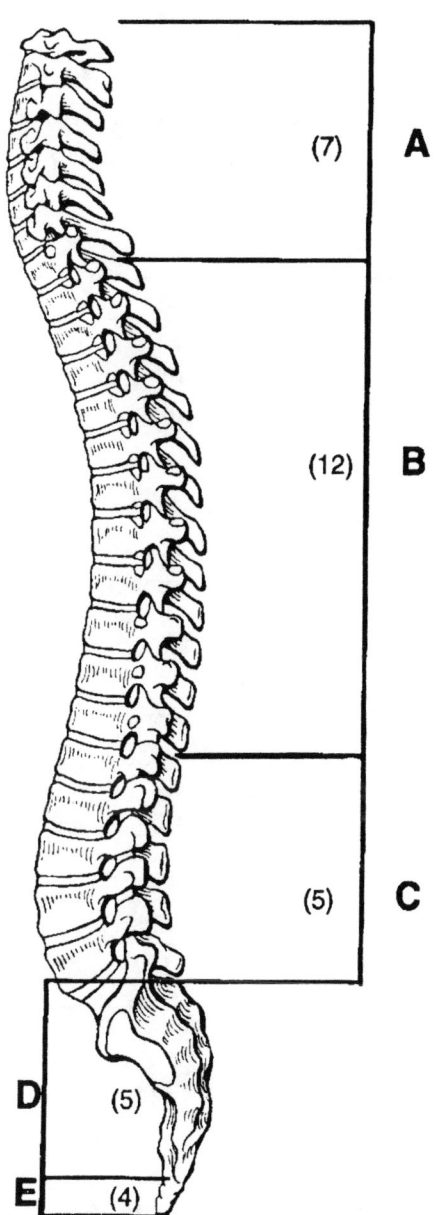

543. Lumbar vertebrae

544. Cervical vertebrae

545. Thoracic vertebrae

546. Coccyx

547. Sacral vertebrae

(Memmler et al, p 96; Thibodeau and Patton #1, p 93; Zakus, p 586)

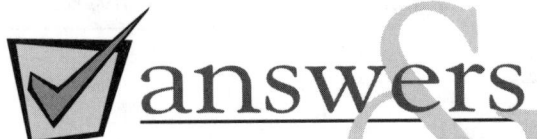

answers & rationales

446.

B. The Senn retractor is used to hold open small incisions by retracting their edges.

447.

A. The purpose of a scalpel, a small, surgical knife with a convex edge and thin, sharp blade, is to make surgical incisions. Different blades are specialized for specific tasks.

448.

E. The Hirschmann anoscope, which is not illuminated, enables the physician to examine the anal area and the lower rectum.

449.

C. This nasal speculum, which is not illuminated, is used to spread the nares *(nostrils)* for examination of the nasal cavity. Some physicians may use an illuminated bivalve nasal speculum.

450.

D. The Graves vaginal speculum, which is available in different sizes, is used in vaginal examination.

451.

D. The Sims uterine sound is used by the physician to determine the size and shape of the uterus.

452.

A. The Sims uterine curette is available in different sizes and is used to remove foreign matter, such as secretions, bits of afterbirth, or minor polyps. The curette is also used to obtain uterine specimens.

453.

E. The Hegar uterine dilator illustrated is one of a set of eight sizes and is used to dilate the cervix in examinations and before D & Cs.

454.

C. Sponge holding forceps are used to hold either sponge or dressing, and they also may be used to apply medication.

455.

B. Schroeder uterine tenaculum forceps are designed to hold tissue during the obtaining of a specimen or biopsy, particularly of the cervix.

456.

B. The shape of bayonet forceps provides a better field of vision when used in the ear or nose.

457.

A. Transfer forceps, which come in different sizes and lengths, are used to retrieve instruments and other items from a sterilizer or autoclave. If sterile, they may be used to arrange items on a sterile tray.

458.

E. The comedone (blackhead) extractor is available in various sizes and styles. The type illustrated has both a blunt and a lance end.

459.

D. The tuning fork, which is available in various frequencies or wavelengths, is used to test hearing sensations of each ear and also bone conduction.

460.

C. Plain thumb forceps, which are used primarily to grasp dressings, have tips that are finely serrated. Thumb forceps are in lengths from 4 to 12 inches.

461.

E. Allis tissue forceps may serve both to grasp tissue, such as muscular or epithelial, and sponges or bandages. Forceps vary in design, and construction depends on their use.

462.

B. The Backhaus towel clamp is used to hold sterile drapes around an operation site or to hold various layers of drapes or towels in place.

463.

A. As their name implies, Virtus splinter forceps are used to remove splinters or foreign bodies that are embedded in the skin or under the fingernails.

464.

C. The Halsted mosquito hemostat, which may be curved or straight, is used to clamp off small blood vessels and bleeders.

465.

D. The needle holder is used to grasp a needle, which is then employed to pass through the skin flaps near the incision.

466.

A. Lister bandage scissors are used to remove bandages, a procedure that is facilitated by the probe point.

467.

C. Blunt-sharp operating scissors are made with one blunt tip and one sharp tip. They may be straight or curved and of varying lengths from 4 1/2 to 6 1/2 inches.

468.

B. Littauer suture scissors contain a hook or a beak that makes it possible to get under a suture.

469.

E. Mayo dissecting scissors are used to expose vessels from surrounding tissue or to expose bone or cartilage, or to separate layers of tissue.

470.

D. Blunt-blunt operating scissors contain two blunt tips. As with other operating scissors, which may be blunt-sharp or sharp-sharp, these scissors may be straight or curved and of varying lengths.

471.

B. Physicians often locate internal organs by topographic anatomy, either by quadrants or regions. Represented in the region identified by B is the left hypochondriac region.

472.

C. The right lumbar region is located between the right hypochondriac and the right iliac regions.

473.

A. The epigastric region is located directly above the umbilical region.

474.

E. The left iliac region is located directly below the left lumbar region and just above the femoral region.

475.

D. The umbilical region is located in the vicinity of the umbilicus and is surrounded by the other abdominal regions.

476.

A. The patient lies face down on the ventral surface of the body in the prone position, the opposite of the supine position.

477.

B. In the knee-chest or genupectoral position, patients rest on their knees and chest. This position is used for proctologic, rectal, sigmoidoscopy, and some vaginal examinations. The position is difficult to achieve and to maintain. The patient must have the medical assistant's support and assistance during the entire exam.

478.

E. The high Fowler's position where the patient is sitting at almost a 90-degree angle enables patients with breathing difficulties to breathe more easily. The semi-Fowler's position is a modification of the Fowler's position, in which the back is raised to a 45-degree angle and the knees can be flexed with the aid of the hospital bed. This position may be used when the patient has a headache or high fever to examine the frontal area. Most examination tables can facilitate this position.

479.

C. The Trendelenburg, or shock, position places the patient on his or her back on an incline, with the head lower than the rest of the body. The knees may be flexed over the lower end of the table. This position may be used for specialized procedures such as varicose vein studies and abdominal surgery.

480.

D. In the Sims (lateral) position, the patient is placed on the left side, and the left leg is fairly straight. The right leg is flexed sharply upward, the left arm and shoulder are drawn back, and the right arm is placed forward for support. This position is used primarily for rectal examinations and temperature, and enemas because the rectal ampulla drops down into the abdomen, making the exam easier. It is also sometimes used for pelvic or perineal exams.

481.

E. In the anatomic position, the patient stands erect, with the palms turned forward. This position is used to describe the direction and position of different body areas so there is not confusion about the directions.

482.

A. The supine (horizontal-recumbent) position has the patient lying flat, back down, with face up. This position is used to examine the frontal portion of the body including breast, heart, and abdominal organs. The patient is gowned with the front open. A drape is placed over the areas not examined.

483.

C. In the dorsal recumbent position, the patient lies on the back and flexes the knees so that the soles of the feet rest on the examination table. It allows the abdominal muscles to relax and is used to examine the rectal, vaginal, and perineal areas.

484.

D. The lithotomy position is sometimes called the stirrups position or dorsosacral position. The patient lies on the back with buttocks at the extreme edge of the table and with the feet supported in stirrups. This position is used for vaginal and rectal examinations.

485.

B. In the jackknife positions, the patients lie in either of two positions: (1) The first position is on the abdomen with the body flexed sharply at the hips so that the thighs are at right angles to the abdomen. This may be achieved by bending over a table bent upward in the middle and is used for proctologic examinations. (2) An alternate position is with the patient on his back on a table with his knees at right angles. (3) A table that is folded down at right angle in the buttocks area and upward to the knees allowing them to bend at a right angle provides another position. This position is used for examination of the male urethra.

486.

D. Spirochetes are bacteria that are spiral in shape.

487.

C. Diplococci are round bacteria that appear in groups of two.

488.

E. *Trichomonas vaginalis* causes trichomoniasis, a sexually transmitted disease. Symptoms may be persistent burning and itching of the vulvar tissue, associated with a white frothy discharge.

489.

A. Streptococci are round bacteria that appear in chains.

490.

B. Staphylococci appear as grapelike bunches.

491.

F. Many bacteria are rod shaped. They may be either Gram positive or Gram negative. The Gram stain is an important aid in distinguishing types of bacteria. Gram-positive bacteria are purple, while Gram-negative bacteria are pink. Bacteria are distinguished by their shape, their Gram stain and other stains, their ability to grow on different media, and their reactions to various chemical tests.

492.

B. The organ involved is the gallbladder.

493.

D. The surgery that rendered the patient diabetic would have been a total pancreatectomy. The pancreas, indicated by the letter D, contains scattered clumps of cells called the islets of Langerhans. These islets function as endocrine glands and produce insulin, a hormone necessary for the metabolism of glucose.

494.

A. The liver is affected with such diseases as cirrhosis and infectious hepatitis.

495.

E. The ileum is the distal portion of the small intestine.

496.

C. The transverse colon is the portion that runs transversely across the upper part of the abdomen, from the right to the left colic flexure.

497.

E. The right atrium is the chamber of the heart that receives all of the blood from the body. The sinoatrial (SA) node is located in the upper portion of the right atrium. The SA node is known as the pacemaker of the heart.

498.

A. The right ventricle, which receives the blood from the right atrium, pumps blood into the pulmonary artery. The wall of the right ventricle is not as muscular as the wall of the left ventricle.

499.

D. The ventricular septum is the partition that separates the blood in the right ventricle from the blood in the left ventricle.

500.

B. The left atrium receives blood that is returning from the lungs, where it has taken on a new oxygen supply and has given up its carbon dioxide. The pulmonary veins empty into the left atrium.

501.

C. The inferior vena cava is one of two blood vessels that return the body's blood supply back to the heart. The inferior vena cava collects its blood from the legs and lower trunk of the body. The superior vena cava is the other blood vessel that returns blood to the heart. This blood comes from the arm and head and upper part of the trunk. Both the inferior and superior vena cava empty into the right atrium.

502.

B. The tricuspid valve is the structure that opens to let the blood pass from the right atrium to the right ventricle. When valves of the heart become defective, they sometimes permit blood to leak back from the ventricle to the atrium. This condition is called a murmur.

503.

D. The pulmonary artery carries blood from the right ventricle to the lungs. The valve that controls this flow is the pulmonary semilunar valve.

504.

E. The aorta is known as the main artery of the body because it receives all of the blood from the heart. The aorta has many branches, which convey the oxygenated blood to all parts of the body.

505.

A. The left ventricle is the chamber that must pump hard enough to supply all of the body with blood. The wall of the left ventricle is more muscular than that of any other chamber in the heart.

506.

C. The bicuspid valve is the structure that permits blood to flow from the left atrium to the left ventricle.

507.

E. Calcium oxalate crystals are normally seen in acid urine (pH of less than 7). They are "envelope shape" in appearance. The ingestion of certain foods, such as cabbage and asparagus, may cause calcium oxalate crystals to appear in the urine.

508.

A. WBC casts are more commonly called "pus" casts. They usually indicate an infection, most commonly pyelonephritis.

509.

D. RBC casts in the urine indicate a diseased condition. They are usually a sign of severe injury to the glomerulus. Both acute glomerulonephritis and bacterial endocarditis will cause RBC casts to form.

510.

B. Triple phosphate crystals are seen in basic (alkaline) urine. They have a "coffin lid" shape and are colorless. Some fruits in the diet will cause triple phosphate crystals to appear in the urine.

511.

C. Cylindroids appear in the urine as long, ribbon-like formations that resemble hyaline casts. Differences between the two are that cylindroids are much longer and are often tapered at one end.

512.

E. Epithelial cells are seen in urine sediment as three types: tubular, transitional, and squamous. The appearance of a few epithelial cells in urine is normal. Squamous epithelial cells are very large and have a prominent nucleus.

513.

C. RBCs, when present in urine in large quantities, suggest infection, trauma, or even renal calculi. The presence of one or two RBCs per high power field (HPF) of urine sediment is within normal limits. If there are more than three RBCs per HPF, an abnormal condition exists.

514.

A. WBCs are seen more commonly in the urine of females or children. Large numbers of WBCs per HPF in a urine sediment may suggest infection, cystitis, or pyelonephritis.

515.

B. Spermatozoa may be seen in urine sediment. They appear as oval bodies with long delicate tails. The sperm may be mobile or stationary.

516.

D. Yeasts (one-celled fungi) are sometimes seen in urine sediment. The common yeast organism is Candida albicans. Yeast cells are ovoid, not round, and frequently are seen budding, which is their method of reproduction. Yeast may cause infections such as vaginitis, particularly in immunocompromised individuals or diabetic patients.

517.

E. The abdominal cavity holds most of the digestive system (the stomach, most of the intestines, the kidneys, the liver, the gallbladder, the pancreas, and the spleen). (The word "abdominal" refers to abdomen, the Latin word for "belly." Therefore, the abdominal cavity is the belly cavity.) It is separated from the thoracic cavity by the diaphragm. The pelvic cavity, considered part of the abdominal cavity, holds the urinary bladder, rectum, and internal parts of the reproductive system. The thoracic, abdominal, and pelvic cavities are ventral cavities because they are located on the underside of most animals.

518.

A. The cranial cavity contains the brain, and the spinal cavity contains the spinal cord. Although referred to as two cavities, they form one continuous space. They are the dorsal cavities because they are located on the upper side of most animals.

519.

C. The thoracic cavity contains the heart, the lungs, and the large blood vessels that enter these organs. The word "thoracic" refers to "thorax," the Greek word for chest.

520.

B. The spinal (vertebral) cavity contains the spinal cord enclosed within the vertebra of the backbone. It is a dorsal cavity.

521.

D. The diaphragm is a muscular, membranous partition between the chest and the abdomen. It contracts with each inspiration of breath downward into a flatter shape and expands with each expiration into a higher dome shape. Spasms of the diaphragm result in hiccups.

522.

F. The pelvic cavity lies at the bottom of the abdominal cavity and contains the reproductive organs, the urinary bladder, and the rectum. It is a ventral cavity.

523.

D. Longitudinal fractures are breaks that are parallel with the bone. There are many types of fractures depending on the location and type. They are generally named according to the appearance of the fracture. Another type, the greenstick fracture, is common in children because their bones are more flexible and less brittle. The bone is broken with several fractures like a stick of green wood might break when bent. While the bone is broken and bent, it is still hinged on one side of the bone.

524.

B. Compound (open) fractures are among the worst types of fractures because the skin is broken allowing infection to penetrate the tissues. They must receive prompt treatment to control the infection.

525.

E. Comminuted fractures have more than one fracture line with several fragments resulting. (The word "comminute" means "to break into pieces.") A blow to a limb can produce this type of fracture.

526.

A. A simple (closed) fracture does not have a break in the skin. Neither is it broken into fragments. Some other names for types of fractures are pathologic fracture—caused by the bone's weakening from disease such as osteoporosis; oblique fracture—break runs in a slanting direction on the bone; transverse fracture—break is across the bone; depressed fracture—broken skull bone is driven inward; and impacted fracture—bone is broken and wedged into the other break.

527.

F. An extracapsular fracture occurs just outside the capsule of a joint. An intracapsular fracture occurs inside the capsule of a joint. A fracture dislocation consists of both a fracture and a bone that is out of joint.

528.

C. A spiral fracture is common in skiing accidents. The bone has been twisted apart.

529.

3. The three words that describe the activity of the heart are polarization, depolarization, and repolarization. The QRS complex is the electrical activity generated by the heart muscle when the ventricles contract (depolarize). The ventricles make up the largest mass of the cardiac muscle, which accounts for the large QRS complex. The QRS is really a combination of three waves, which include the Q wave, R wave, and S wave.

530.

1. The P wave is the first electrical activity produced during a cardiac cycle. It represents atrial depolarization (contraction). It is not as large as the QRS complex because of the reduced amount of heart muscle that makes up the atria (plural for atrium). The cardiac cycle is initiated by the sinoatrial (SA) node, which is located in the upper, right-hand corner of the right atrium. The SA node is called the "pacemaker."

531.

5. The ST segment is a transition period between the end of the ventricular contraction (brought on by depolarization) and the beginning of electrical recovery (repolarization) of the ventricles, which is represented by the T wave.

532.

2. The PR interval is the period of time between the beginning of atrial contraction (depolarization) and the beginning of ventricular contraction (depolarization).

533.

4. The QT interval represents the period of time from the Q wave to the end of the T wave. The Q wave is the beginning of ventricular depolarization to the end of ventricular repolarization. After the ventricle has been repolarized, it returns to the baseline, which represents zero electrical activity state. This baseline represents no current flowing in the heart. The baseline is also called an isoelectric line.

534.

7. The U wave is a very small mound that occasionally appears on an electrocardiogram (ECG) after the T wave. This small wave appears on the ECG of patients with a low serum potassium level. Remember that the electrocardiograph is the instrument used to produce the ECG, which is the tracing of the heart's electrical activity.

535.

8. This part of the ECG is known as the baseline, which indicates that no electrical activity is being generated by the heart.

536.

6. The T wave represents that electrical activity produced by the ventricles when they are repolarized. The atria also undergoes repolarization but this electrical activity is covered up by the contraction (depolarization) and the repolarization of the ventricles. The heart is now ready for the next cardiac cycle.

537.

6. The standard 12-lead electrocardiograph records electrical activity from the frontal and horizontal planes of the body. The 12-lead includes three standard leads, three augmented leads, and six chest leads. Line number 6 represents the standard limb lead I. The standard limb leads are bipolar leads. Standard limb lead I records the voltage through the heart from right arm to left arm.

538.

1. This line represents the standard limb lead II. This lead records voltage down through the long axis of the heart from right arm to left leg.

539.

3. This line represents the standard limb lead III. This lead records voltage from the left arm to the left leg.

540.

2. This line represents the AVF lead. The augmented leads are designated by AVR, AVL, and AVF. (AV stands for "augmented voltage" and the last letter corresponds to Right, Left, and Foot.) All leads are taking "electrical pictures" of the heart. The last letter in the augmented leads indicates the direction toward which the "picture" is aimed. Augmented leads are unipolar limb leads. The AVF is the recording made from the midpoint between Right Arm and Left Arm to Left Leg. You should note that the Right Leg sensor does not provide cardiac information for use in the actual ECG recording. It serves as an electrical reference point. It is called the "ground" or "reference electrode."

541.

4. This line represents the AVR lead. The AVR lead is the recording made from the midpoint between the Left Arm and Left Leg to the Right Arm.

542.

5. This line represents the AVL lead. The AVL lead is the recording made from the midpoint between Right Arm and Left Leg to the Left Arm.

543.

C. The lumbar vertebrae are the five vertebrae between the thoracic (chest) vertebrae and the sacrum. They are designated as L 1 through L 5.

544.

A. The cervical vertebrae are the seven vertebrae of the neck.

545.

B. The thoracic vertebrae are the 12 vertebrae that connect the ribs and form part of the posterior wall of the thorax (chest).

546.

E. The coccyx (coccygeal vertebrae) consists of four fused vertebrae. It is also called the tailbone.

547.

D. The five fused sacral vertebrae form the sacrum.

Practice Test

CHAPTER 14 Practice Test

14 Practice Test

chapter objectives

Major areas of knowledge/content included in this chapter are:

I. Sections of practice test

➤ general

➤ administrative

➤ clinical

II. Answer sheets for practice test

➤ general

➤ administrative

➤ clinical

GENERAL QUESTIONS

DIRECTIONS (Questions 1 through 100): Each of the numbered items or incomplete statements in this section is followed by answers or by completions of the statement. Select the ONE lettered answer or completion that is BEST in each case.

1. Directional terms are used in describing relative positions of body parts. Which of the following terms means "toward the head"?
   A. superior
   B. inferior
   C. anterior
   D. posterior
   (Thibodeau and Patton #1, p 3)

2. Which term is used in medical terminology to describe "front" or "in front of"?
   A. superior
   B. inferior
   C. anterior
   D. posterior
   (Thibodeau and Patton #1, p 3)

3. What word in medical terminology is used to mean "toward the feet"?
   A. superior
   B. inferior
   C. anterior
   D. posterior
   (Thibodeau and Patton #1, p 3)

4. What term is used in anatomy and physiology to mean "back" or "in back of"?
   A. superior
   B. inferior
   C. anterior
   D. posterior
   (Thibodeau and Patton #1, p 3)

5. The word used in medical terminology to mean "toward the midline of the body" is
   A. medial
   B. lateral

C. ventral
D. dorsal
(Thibodeau and Patton #1, p 3)

6. What word means toward the side of the body or away from the midline?
   A. medical
   B. lateral
   C. ventral
   D. dorsal
   (Thibodeau and Patton #1, p 3)

7. What word is utilized in medical terminology to mean "toward or nearest the trunk of the body"?
   A. proximal
   B. distal
   C. superficial
   D. deep
   (Thibodeau and Patton #1, p 3)

8. To indicate that something lies nearer the surface, we would use the term
   A. proximal
   B. distal
   C. superficial
   D. deep
   (Thibodeau and Patton #1, p 3)

9. The word used in anatomy and physiology to mean farther away from the body surface is
   A. proximal
   B. distal
   C. superficial
   D. deep
   (Thibodeau and Patton #1, p 3)

10. What word means farther away or farthest from the trunk or the point of origin of a body part?
    A. proximal
    B. distal
    C. superficial
    D. deep
    (Thibodeau and Patton #1, p 3)

11. The body is divided into subdivisions or smaller segments to facilitate the study of the body as a whole or individual organs. What plane divides the body into two equal halves?
    A. midsagittal plane
    B. frontal plane
    C. transverse plane
    D. crosswise plane
    (Thibodeau and Patton #1, pp 4–5)

12. The plane that divides our body into anterior and posterior portions is called the
    A. sagittal plane
    B. frontal plane
    C. midsagittal plane
    D. transverse plane
    (Thibodeau and Patton #1, pp 4–5)

13. Which plane of the body is synonymous with a horizontal or crosswise plane?
    A. sagittal plane
    B. frontal plane
    C. midsagittal plane
    D. transverse plane
    (Thibodeau and Patton #1, pp 4–5)

14. Which part of the circulatory system is not a completely closed vessel?
    A. arteries
    B. veins
    C. capillaries
    D. lymphatic vessels
    (Thibodeau and Patton #1, pp 52–53)

15. Which of the following is NOT part of bone formation and growth?
    A. periosteum
    B. chondrocytes
    C. erythropoiesis
    D. osteocytes
    (Thibodeau and Patton #1, pp 82–86)

16. Which one of the endocrine glands produces epinephrine and norepinephrine?
    A. thyroid
    B. adrenal
    C. pituitary
    D. thymus
    (Thibodeau and Patton #2, pp 193–194)

17. Which of the endocrine glands is divided into anterior and posterior lobes?
    A. thyroid
    B. adrenal
    C. pituitary
    D. thymus
    (Thibodeau and Patton #2, pp 193–194)

18. Which endocrine gland requires iodine to produce its hormone?
    A. thyroid
    B. thymus
    C. gonads
    D. parathyroid
    (Thibodeau and Patton #2, pp 200–201)

19. The islets of this endocrine gland regulate the levels of glucose in our blood. This gland is the
    A. parathyroid gland
    B. thyroid gland
    C. pineal gland
    D. pancreatic gland
    (Thibodeau and Patton #2, pp 200–201)

20. In the conduction system of the heart, which of the following is responsible for initiating a heart beat?
    A. Purkinje fibers
    B. Bundle of His
    C. atrioventricular node
    D. sinoatrial node
    (Thibodeau and Patton #2, pp 236–238)

21. The signal from the sinoatrial (SA) node is then picked up by which of the following?
    A. atrioventricular node
    B. aorta
    C. Purkinje fibers
    D. Bundle of His
    (Thibodeau and Patton #2, pp 236–238)

22. The part of the conduction system of the heart that wraps around in the outer walls of the ventricular is the
    A. Bundle branches
    B. Purkinje fibers
    C. Bundle of His
    D. aorta
    (Thibodeau and Patton #2, pp 236–238)

23. The main trunk of the respiratory system is the
    A. pharynx
    B. trachea
    C. primary bronchi
    D. bronchioles
    (Thibodeau and Patton #2, pp 287–289)

24. The exchange of carbon dioxide and oxygen with the blood occurs in the
    A. bronchi
    B. bronchiole
    C. alveolar ducts
    D. alveolar sacs
    (Gauwitz and Bayt, pp 183–184; Thibodeau and Patton #2, pp 287–289)

25. Which of the following refers to slow and shallow respiration?
    A. eupnea
    B. dyspnea
    C. hypoventilation
    D. apnea
    (Thibodeau and Patton #2, p 299)

26. Which of the following is NOT a part of the colon?
    A. ileum
    B. ascending
    C. descending
    D. sigmoid
    (Thibodeau and Patton #2, p 306)

27. The first part of the small intestine where food enters from the stomach is the
    A. plicae
    B. duodenum
    C. jejunum
    D. ileum
    (Thibodeau and Patton #2, pp 314–315)

28. Which part of the urinary system is responsible for transporting urine from the kidneys to the bladder?
    A. proximal convoluted tubule
    B. distal convoluted tubule
    C. collecting tubule
    D. ureters
    (Thibodeau and Patton #2, pp 341–345)

29. Which of the following words refers to scanty amounts of urine production?
    A. glycosuria
    B. anuria
    C. oliguria
    D. polyuria
    (Thibodeau and Patton #2, pp 347–349)

30. Which of the following refers to the passage of urine from the body?
    A. micturition
    B. urination
    C. voiding
    D. all of the above
    (Thibodeau and Patton #2, p 353)

31. A nerve that carries impulses away from the brain is a/an
    A. efferent nerve
    B. afferent nerve
    C. neurotransmitter
    D. receptor
    (Rice #1, p 395)

32. The body is arranged in levels of organization. Which of the following is the third level of organization?
    A. cell
    B. tissue
    C. organ
    D. system
    (Rice #1, pp 34–37)

33. A disease that results in the enlargement of bones of the hands, feet, jaws, and cheeks is
    A. acroarthritis
    B. acromegaly
    C. arthralgia
    D. gigantism
    (Keir et al, pp 386–387)

34. A word meaning pain in a joint is
    A. arthralgia
    B. arthritis
    C. arthrocentesis
    D. arthroplasty
    (Brooks and LaFleur, pp 202–203)

35. A surgical puncture of a joint to remove fluid is called
    A. arthrodesis
    B. arthroplasty
    C. arthrocentesis
    D. arthrogram
    (Brooks and LaFleur, pp 202–203)

36. The word that means the study of the skin is
    A. dermatitis
    B. dermatology
    C. dermopathy
    D. dermal
    (Brooks and LaFleur, p 28)

37. The word intradermal means
    A. pertaining to "upon the skin"
    B. pertaining to "under the skin"
    C. pertaining to "below the skin"
    D. pertaining to "within the skin"
    (Brooks and LaFleur, p 28)

38. When a person has a surgical repair of the nose it is called
    A. rhinoplasty
    B. rhinorrhea
    C. rhinorrhagia
    D. rhinomycosis
    (Brooks and LaFleur, p 44)

39. A word meaning the surgical removal of the larynx is
    A. laryngoscopy
    B. laryngoplasty
    C. laryngectomy
    D. laryngopharyngeal
    (Brooks and LaFleur, p 44)

40. Inflammation of the kidney is
    A. nephrectomy
    B. nephritis
    C. nephroplasty
    D. nephrostomy
    (Brooks and LaFleur, p 66)

41. The surgical repair of the renal pelvis is
   A. pyeloplasty
   B. pyelitis
   C. pyelonephritis
   D. ureteropyelonephritis
   (Brooks and LaFleur, p 66)

42. Which of the following word forms means breast?
   A. gynec-
   B. mast-
   C. mamm-
   D. both B and C
   (Brooks and LaFleur, pp 93, 110–111)

43. The word for a stone in the prostate gland is
   A. prostatitis
   B. prostatocystitis
   C. prostatolith
   D. prostatectomy
   (Brooks and LaFleur, pp 110–111)

44. Which of the following drug classifications generally used in blood and lymphatic diseases and disorders would best describe aspirin?
   A. hematinic drug
   B. antiplatelet drug
   C. thrombolytic agent
   D. hemastatic agent
   (Rice #1, p 278)

45. A word that means an enlargement of the heart is
   A. cardiomegaly
   B. cardiopathy
   C. cardiac
   D. cardiology
   (Brooks and LaFleur, pp 122–123)

46. When the physician performs a visual examination of the stomach, this procedure is a
   A. gastroenteritis
   B. gastrectomy
   C. gastroscope
   D. gastroscopy
   (Brooks and LaFleur, pp 144–145)

47. A word that means pain in the gums is
   A. gingivitis
   B. gingivalgia
   C. gingivoglossitis
   D. stomatitis
   (Brooks and LaFleur, pp 144–145)

48. A condition of gallstones is
   A. cholelithiasis
   B. cholecystitis
   C. cholecystogram
   D. cholecystectomy
   (Brooks and LaFleur, pp 154–155)

49. An instrument used to measure the muscle (power) of vision is an
   A. ophthalmoscope
   B. optometer
   C. ophthalmometer
   D. optomyometer
   (Brooks and LaFleur, pp 176–177)

50. Inflammation of the eardrum is called
   A. myringectomy
   B. myringoplasty
   C. myringitis
   D. myringotomy
   (Brooks and LaFleur, pp 186–187)

51. Which of the following means inflammation of the gray matter of the spinal cord?
    A. meningitis
    B. poliomyelitis
    C. meningocele
    D. meningomyelitis
    (Brooks and LaFleur, pp 234–236)

52. The medical term that means a condition of difficulty in speaking is
    A. dysphasia
    B. dysphagia
    C. bradyphagia
    D. bradyphasia
    (Brooks and LaFleur, pp 234–236)

53. Which of the following words means pertaining to the head and to the tail?
    A. anterolateral
    B. dorsocephalad
    C. cephalocaudal
    D. anteroposterior
    (Brooks and LaFleur, pp 252–254)

54. Which of the following is not considered to be one of the three layers in the integumentary system?
    A. epidermis
    B. dermis
    C. hair papilla
    D. subcutaneous
    (Thibodeau and Patton #1, pp 66–69)

55. The part of the integumentary system containing fat as a stored energy source is the
    A. sebaceous glands
    B. epidermis
    C. dermis
    D. subcutaneous
    (Thibodeau and Patton #1, pp 65–66)

56. A nerve (neuron) that transmits impulses to the spinal cord and brain from all parts of the body is a/an
    A. efferent nerve
    B. afferent nerve
    C. motor neuron
    D. neurotransmitter
    (Thibodeau and Patton #1, pp 137–138)

57. Our body is arranged in levels of organization. Which of the following is the second level of organization?
    A. cell
    B. tissue
    C. organ
    D. system
    (Rice #1, pp 374–377)

58. Which of the following could be classified as a type of tissue?
    A. epithelial
    B. connective
    C. nervous
    D. all of the above
    (Thibodeau and Patton #1, pp 31–32)

59. Which endocrine gland stimulates synthesis and dispersion of melanin pigment in the skin?
    A. anterior pituitary
    B. parathyroid
    C. thyroid
    D. hypothalamus
    (Thibodeau and Patton #1, p 193)

60. Which endocrine gland regulates electrolyte and fluid homeostasis?
    A. thyroid
    B. parathyroid
    C. cortex of adrenal glands
    D. pancreatic islets
    (Thibodeau and Patton #1, pp 193–194)

61. An abnormal posterior thoracic spinal curvature is called
    A. spondylitis
    B. kyphosis
    C. scoliosis
    D. lordosis
    (Thibodeau and Patton #1, p 144)

62. An anterior lumbar curvature of the spine that becomes abnormally exaggerated is known as
    A. spondylitis
    B. kyphosis
    C. scoliosis
    D. lordosis
    (Thibodeau and Patton #2, p 144)

63. There are four types of skeletal muscle contractions. Which type results in a quick, jerky response to a stimulus?
    A. twitch contraction
    B. tetanic contraction
    C. isotonic contraction
    D. isometric contraction
    (Thibodeau and Patton #1, p 117)

64. What type of skeletal muscle contraction do we find when the muscle shortens and the insertion end moves toward the point of origin?
    A. twitch contraction
    B. tetanic contraction
    C. isotonic contraction
    D. isometric contraction
    (Thibodeau and Patton #1, pp 117–118)

65. What type of skeletal muscle contraction is named from the Greek words that mean "equal measure"?
    A. twitch contraction
    B. tetanus contraction
    C. isotonic contraction
    D. isometric contraction
    (Thibodeau and Patton #1, pp 117–118)

66. There are several terms used in anatomy and physiology to describe body movements. Which of the following is commonly described as bending?
    A. flexion
    B. extension
    C. abduction
    D. adduction
    (Thibodeau and Patton #1, pp 117–118)

67. A type movement that results in moving a part away from the midline of the body is
    A. rotation
    B. extension
    C. abduction
    D. adduction
    (Thibodeau and Patton #1, pp 127–129)

68. To avoid abandonment charges a physician should notify active patients by letter that the practice is being discontinued. If a patient has been discharged or has not received medical care for some time, it is not necessary to send a notice. What time limit distinguishes active from inactive patients?
    A. 2 years
    B. 4 years
    C. 6 years
    D. 8 years
    (Kinn and Woods, pp 392–393)

69. The primary concern of the attending physician must always be
    A. what is best for the patient
    B. the burden placed on caregivers
    C. cost to society of illness
    D. proper allocation of health resources
    (Kinn and Woods, p 54)

70. If a physician accidentally removed the right kidney from a patient instead of the left kidney which was diseased, this malpractice suit would be based on which legal concept?

A. *res gestae*

B. *res ipsa loquitur*

C. *res judicata*

D. criminal law

(Flight, pp 92–93; Taber's, p 1660)

71. The ethical use of computer technology to store patient records requires

A. media communication

B. respect for patient confidentiality

C. professional courtesy

D. public domain

(Kinn and Woods, p 56)

72. The written form of defamation, which damages an individual's character, is known as

A. forgery

B. libel

C. slander

D. battery

(Becklin and Sunnarborg, pp 48–49)

73. Within a physician-patient contract, both parties have certain rights. It is within the realm of physician rights to

A. set up practice outside the boundaries of his or her license to practice medicine

B. set fees for procedures independent of any other agency or group regardless of who pays

C. set up an office without regard to ADA requirements

D. set up an office where he or she chooses and to select the hours it is open

(Judson and Hicks, p 64)

74. Information that is to be held in confidence between the patient and physician only is referred to as

A. disclosure

B. interrogatory

C. consideration

D. privileged communication

(Judson and Hicks, pp 78–80; Flight, pp 214–216)

75. The legal order that directs that certain records or documents be brought to court is the

A. subpoena

B. interrogatory

C. deposition

D. subpoena duces tecum

(Kinn and Woods, p 69; Flight, p 188)

76. Faxing of confidential patient information is acceptable when following approved guidelines such as

A. discard all fax copies in the nearest trash container

B. leave faxes in the fax machine until the end of each day

C. do not fax confidential material if other unauthorized persons in the room can observe the material

D. confidential material may be faxed to anyone asking for the documents

(Judson and Hicks, p 116; Flight, pp 180–181)

77. In which of the following situations is prosecution for billing fraud most likely to occur?

A. repetitious overbilling of procedures and/or diagnostic tests

B. cases resulting in malpractice

C. patients with chronic illnesses

D. pediatric patients

(Flight, p 48)

78. Should a medical professional fail to act in a medical situation, thereby causing harm to the patient, he or she would be guilty of
    A. malfeasance
    B. misfeasance
    C. nonfeasance
    D. disfeasance
    (Judson and Hicks, p 82; Kinn and Woods, p 67)

79. What medical report is based on analysis of tissue or fluid removed in surgery?
    A. history and physical
    B. progress notes
    C. pathology
    D. consultation
    (Kinn and Woods, p 174)

80. A division of the Department of Labor that sets standards and protocols for the health and safety of workers is
    A. OSHA
    B. CLIA
    C. DEA
    D. ADA
    (Kinn and Woods, pp 73–74)

81. Which of the following is a diagnostic procedure for prostatic cancer?
    A. palpation of the testes
    B. urine culture
    C. orchidectomy
    D. prostatic-specific antigen test
    (Tamparo and Lewis, pp 107–108)

82. A normally nonpathogenic bacteria found in the large intestine which in some mutant forms causes traveler's and infantile diarrhea and severe food poisoning is
    A. E. coli
    B. hepatitis
    C. periodontitis
    D. scurvy
    (Tamparo and Lewis, pp 32–33)

83. Diverticulitis, pancreatitis, and pyloric stenosis are disorders of which body system?
    A. respiratory system
    B. reproductive
    C. urinary system
    D. digestive system
    (Hurlbut, pp 36–37)

84. Myasthenia gravis, rheumatoid arthritis, and hiatal hernia are conditions or diseases that affect the
    A. musculoskeletal system
    B. reproductive
    C. central nervous system
    D. endocrine system
    (Hurlbut, p 35)

85. An aneurysm of a cerebral artery may result in
    A. a heart attack
    B. thrombophlebitis
    C. arteriosclerosis
    D. paralysis
    (Scanlon and Sanders, p 169)

86. Cor pulmonale is hypertrophy (excessive growth) and failure of the right ventricle of the heart. It may be caused by a disorder of the
    A. kidneys
    B. lungs
    C. spleen
    D. pancreas
    (Tamparo and Lewis, pp 173–174)

87. A disease that primarily affects youth and usually follows an upper respiratory or viral infection is
    A. lymphosarcoma
    B. Reye's syndrome
    C. Hodgkin's disease
    D. monoblastic leukemia
    (Tamparo and Lewis, pp 212–213)

88. Which of the following is a medical term for what is commonly called "hives"?
    A. psoriasis
    B. urticaria
    C. acne
    D. alopecia
    (Tamparo and Lewis, pp 287–288)

89. Birth defects are included in which of these categories of disease?
    A. infectious
    B. deficiency
    C. congenital
    D. degenerative
    (Thibodeau and Patton #2, p 548)

90. Which of the following molecules is formed and stored in the liver and muscle cells?
    A. monosaccharide
    B. glucose
    C. glycogen
    D. disaccharide
    (Thibodeau and Patton #1, pp 434–435)

91. Dialysis is used to treat a failure within the
    A. reproductive system
    B. urinary system
    C. respiratory system
    D. circulatory system
    (Tamparo and Lewis, pp 86–88; Thibodeau and Patton #2, pp 472–473)

92. PID, PMS, and endometriosis are disorders of the
    A. reproductive system
    B. circulatory system
    C. endocrine system
    D. central nervous system
    (Thibodeau and Patton #2, pp 527, 551–553)

93. Which of the following medical terms contains a silent letter *within* it?
    A. vermiform
    B. crysotherapy
    C. phlegm
    D. apnea
    (Rice #1, p 7)

94. Which of the following persons formulated the hierarchy of needs, which illustrates motivating forces for human behavior?
    A. Jean Piaget
    B. Abraham Maslow
    C. Elizabeth Kubler-Ross
    D. B. F. Skinner
    (Tamparo and Lindh, pp 95–105, 108–109, 118–121)

95. Elizabeth Kubler-Ross is known for the classic theory that identifies the five stages of grief and loss. Which of the following is usually considered to be the last stage?
    A. acceptance
    B. denial
    C. anger
    D. depression
    (Milliken, pp 404–409)

96. In protecting the confidentiality of patient records maintained on the computer, all of these guidelines should be followed EXCEPT
    A. make sure the monitor is located in an area not seen by unauthorized viewers
    B. avoid sending confidential patient information via e-mail
    C. never leave a computer unattended, allowing others access to confidential information
    D. do not block use of computer with passwords
    (Judson and Hicks, p 117; Kinn and Woods, p 56)

97. Diabetes mellitus is known as an endocrine system disease. Which of the following parts of the endocrine system fails to function?
    A. thyroid glands
    B. adrenal glands
    C. pancreatic islets
    D. thymus

    (Thibodeau and Patton #1, pp 198–209)

98. Cerebrovascular accident (CVA) is due to a disorder of the blood vessels that supply blood to the brain. A CVA is commonly called a stroke. Which of the following may be symptom(s) of a minor stroke?
    A. headache
    B. confusion
    C. slight dizziness
    D. all of the above

    (Kinn and Woods, p 800)

99. Dialysis is used to treat a failure within the
    A. reproductive system
    B. urinary system
    C. respiratory system
    D. digestive system

    (Keir et al, p 376)

100. Which organ in the body is responsible for the metabolism and detoxification of drugs?
    A. liver
    B. kidney
    C. lungs
    D. intestine

    (Gauwitz and Bayt, p 18)

ADMINISTRATIVE QUESTIONS

DIRECTIONS (Questions 101 through 200): Each of the numbered items or incomplete statements in this section is followed by answers or by completions of the statement. Select ONE lettered answer or completion that is BEST in each case.

101. A telephone call that is operator assisted and includes several doctors at separate offices is a
    A. conference call
    B. message-unit call
    C. international call
    D. referenced call

    (Fordney and Follis, p 92)

102. Which of the following types of phones can be used to signal or access other office extensions while placing calls on hold?
    A. voice mail
    B. cellular phone

    C. call director
    D. six-button touch-tone telephone

    (Fordney and Follis, p 77)

103. Which of the following can be used to keep a record of incoming telephone calls so that no message is overlooked?
    A. conference call
    B. pager
    C. telephone log
    D. voice mail

    (Fordney and Follis, p 83)

104. A system that selects the order of patients to receive urgent medical treatment is often referred to as
   A. triage
   B. selection
   C. streamlining
   D. matrixing
   (Fordney and Follis, p 104)

105. Which of the following scheduling practices would help to avoid an audit by a managed care organization that operates the medical facility?
   A. Keep a close watch and analyze telephone and office delays and other problems.
   B. Do not schedule emergency slots during the day.
   C. Make sure to follow the same guidelines as in the past.
   D. If an urgent appointment cannot be given to an established patient, have the patient come in the next day.
   (Fordney and Follis, p 105)

106. Which of the following would NOT be part of scheduling a patient for outside appointments such as x-ray and laboratory appointments and hospital admission?
   A. check patient identification and certification numbers
   B. schedule laboratory and other diagnostic procedures
   C. log arrangements in the appointment books and patient chart
   D. visit the patient in the hospital
   (Fordney and Follis, p 106)

107. How may patient records and other documents that are computer generated be authenticated?
   A. by electronic signature
   B. by manual signature
   C. by notarizing the records
   D. by patient registration
   (Fordney and Follis, p 128)

108. When the doctor asks the patient oral questions designed to reveal information about the present illness and begins at the head and continues through the body, the doctor is compiling a
   A. complete inventory
   B. complete physical analysis
   C. an organic profile
   D. a Review of Systems
   (Fordney and Follis, p 134)

109. Which type of patient record stores similar reports and forms together?
   A. POMR
   B. juvenile
   C. SOMR
   D. accredited
   (Humphrey, p 244)

110. A type of clinic record that permits quick identification of a type or group of patients (for example, those having a certain disease) is known as a
   A. spreadsheet
   B. database
   C. inventory
   D. index
   (Humphrey, p 246)

111. A list of medical services the doctor performs and the corresponding charges are found on a
   A. assignment of benefits
   B. benefits list
   C. fee schedule
   D. none of the above
   (Becklin and Sunnarborg, p 153)

112. How often should checks and cash from a medical practice be deposited in the bank?
    A. daily
    B. bi-weekly
    C. weekly
    D. monthly
    (Humphrey, p 269)

113. Which type of organization has the lowest administrative and medical expenses?
    A. private hospitals
    B. fee-for-service medical clinics
    C. health maintenance organizations
    D. none of the above
    (Humphrey, pp 286–287)

114. Which type of medical service would a large corporation likely select for its employees?
    A. HMO
    B. private individual insurance policies
    C. preferred provider organization
    D. Medicaid
    (Humphrey, p 287)

115. Which program provides medical services to the age group with the highest medical expenses per individual?
    A. Medicaid
    B. Blue Cross-Blue Shield
    C. HMOs
    D. Medicare
    (Humphrey, pp 288–289)

116. To protect the confidentiality of patient records maintained on the computer, which of these guidelines should be followed?
    A. make sure the monitor is located in an area not seen by unauthorized viewers
    B. avoid sending confidential patient information via e-mail or fax
    C. never leave a computer unattended, allowing others access to confidential information
    D. all of the above
    (Judson and Hicks, p 117; Kinn and Woods, p 56)

117. What is the percentage of patients that never intend to pay their medical bill?
    A. 30%
    B. 20%
    C. 10%
    D. fewer than 5%
    (Kinn and Woods, p 290)

118. A new employee has been given a new job of filing. What reference can be checked to find filing guidelines for that office?
    A. employee handbook
    B. office policy manual
    C. CPT book
    D. office procedures manual
    (Fordney and Follis, pp 188–189; Kinn and Woods, pp 365–368)

119. In order for the employees of a clinic to give standard answers over the telephone as authorized by the physician, they should
    A. have a session and discuss the answer
    B. let one employee answer the telephone
    C. keep a phone triage manual by the phone for reference
    D. develop a good telephone personality
    (Keir et al, p 102)

120. Telephone triage is the eliciting of a caller's _____, which will decide when to schedule the patient.
    A. condition
    B. debt profile
    C. insurance status
    D. none of the above
    (Keir et al, p 102)

121. A necessary identification number for all employees in a physician's office is the
    A. driver's license number
    B. social security number
    C. health insurance number
    D. bank account number
    (Keir et al, p 199)

122. Which government form must be on file before the employee can be paid for the employment?
    A. W-2
    B. W-4
    C. Form I-9
    D. social security
    (Keir et al, p 199)

123. A good method for keeping an office in good working order is to
    A. maintain a separate maintenance file and inspect equipment as needed
    B. assess the level of supplies each day, week, and month as needed
    C. maintain separate inventory cards for all major items
    D. all of the above
    (Keir et al, pp 202–203)

124. Which of the following is used to make sure that all office computer programs and data are secure in case of a mishap, fire, or natural disaster?
    A. RAM
    B. microprocessor
    C. write-protection
    D. backup policy
    (Keir et al, p 69)

125. Which of the following is not a part of the hardware of a computer system?
    A. disk drive
    B. monitor
    C. hard copy
    D. printer
    (Keir et al, pp 67–69)

126. The science that studies how to increase human efficiency and well-being at the workplace is
    A. traumatic medicine
    B. occupational medicine
    C. psychology
    D. ergonomics
    (Taber's, p 665; Keir et al, pp 74–78)

127. The procedure that determines beforehand if a patient is eligible for coverage for the expenses of medical care is called
    A. precertification
    B. single booking
    C. precaution
    D. preliminary premium
    (Keir et al, p 114)

128. Which of the following is not a logical step in filing?
    A. inspect
    B. index
    C. code
    D. proofread
    (Keir et al, pp 144–145)

129. Magnetic tape reels, cartridges, magnetic disks, and microforms are known as
    A. alphabetical files
    B. numbered files
    C. paperless files
    D. administrative files
    (Keir et al, pp 147–148)

130. The filing system requiring a cross-index or cross-reference in order to access the data is the
    A. electronic filing system
    B. numerical filing system
    C. alphabetical filing system
    D. chronological filing system
    (Keir et al, p 149)

131. A much-used system of bookkeeping that lines forms up exactly in numeric sequence and makes all entries at one time is
    A. double-entry bookkeeping
    B. accounting
    C. computer billing
    D. pegboard
    (Keir et al, pp 161–162)

132. In managed care delivery systems the "gatekeeper" is responsible for coordinating all care for the patient and is generally
    A. the primary care physician
    B. the specialist
    C. the insurance agent
    D. the independent practice association
    (Keir et al, p 174)

133. The type of insurance in which the employer pays the premium is
    A. Medicare
    B. Easter Seal/Crippled Children
    C. Workers' Compensation
    D. Medicaid
    (Keir et al, pp 174–175)

134. An area of the applicant's background, which might be checked by a prospective employer, is
    A. record of chemical abuse
    B. hobbies
    C. religion
    D. ethnic background
    (Keir et al, p 758)

135. A chart of procedures or an order of business to be followed in conducting a meeting is a/an
    A. proposal
    B. agenda
    C. minutes
    D. resolution
    (Fordney and Follis, pp 182–188)

136. Important permanent information about the patient including name, birthdate, responsible party, social security number, address, and telephone and driver's license numbers would be included on the
    A. referral slip
    B. letter of recommendation
    C. registration form
    D. clinical diagnosis
    (Kinn and Woods, pp 94–96)

137. If a patient has been referred to your office by another doctor, which of the following statements are true?
    A. a thank you note should be sent to the referring physician
    B. the referring physician should notify your office physician as to the reason for referral
    C. a release form should be signed by the patient before any records are sent to another medical practice
    D. all of the above are true
    (Becklin and Sunnarborg, pp 127–128)

138. Medicare coverage is available to
    A. persons over age 65
    B. disabled worker adults
    C. disabled before the age of 22
    D. all of the above
    (Fordney, p 294)

139. Supplemental insurance plans usually
    A. cover the deductible
    B. cover the copayments or coinsurance of the primary policy
    C. cover additional benefits not included in the primary policy
    D. all of the above
    (Rowell, p 234)

140. Common errors that delay insurance claims processing include all of the following EXCEPT
    A. typographical errors
    B. staples or other defacement of the bar code area of the claim form
    C. omission of data
    D. attachments to the claim
    (Rowell, p 235)

141. Insurance coverage that covers all or part of the physician's fees for nonsurgical services and sometimes diagnostic laboratory, x-ray, and pathology fees is referred to as
    A. major medical
    B. HMO
    C. basic medical
    D. PPO
    (Kinn and Woods, p 305)

142. A committee that reviews cases for managed care plans to make sure medical care services are medically necessary and studies how providers use medical care resources is
    A. the claims department
    B. provider relations
    C. utilization review
    D. member services
    (Kinn and Woods, p 315)

143. Health plans of various types developed to provide health services at a low cost are called
    A. HMOs
    B. PPOs
    C. managed care
    D. capitation
    (Kinn and Woods, p 311)

144. How many levels of HCPCS are there?
    A. 4
    B. 3
    C. 6
    D. 2
    (Kinn and Woods, p 324)

145. In CPT coding, what does a star (*) by a procedure indicate?
    A. changed code
    B. new code
    C. surgical package concept does not apply
    D. none of the above
    (Kinn and Woods, p 324; CPT 2000, pp 47, 51)

146. What is the major factor in determining the assignment of a DRG?
    A. the principal diagnosis
    B. the patient's age
    C. the disposition of the patient
    D. complications and comorbidities
    (Kinn and Woods, p 336)

147. The major advantage of electronic claims is
    A. time saved
    B. decreased rejected claims
    C. increased payment
    D. none of the above
    (Sanderson, p 23)

148. Each of the following is considered an output device EXCEPT
    A. printer
    B. scanner
    C. monitor
    D. both A and C
    (Gylys #2, pp 6–7)

149. Formatting a disk
    A. makes it usable
    B. organizes disks into tracks and sectors
    C. both A and B
    D. none of the above
    (Gylys #2, p 8)

150. Auxiliary storage devices include all of the following EXCEPT
    A. hard disk drive
    B. modem
    C. CD-ROM drive
    D. Zip drive
    (Gylys #2, pp 7–10)

151. All of the following are advantages to using laser printers EXCEPT
    A. expense
    B. speed
    C. quality of printing
    D. efficiency
    (Gylys #2, p 7)

152. Microcomputers perform which of the following functions?
    A. input
    B. storage
    C. processing
    D. all of the above
    (Gylys #2, p 3)

153. Repetitive strain injury (RSI) accounts for approximately what percentage of all job-related illness?
    A. 40%
    B. 10%
    C. 25%
    D. >50%
    (Gylys #2, p 11)

154. Which of the following is internal memory that cannot be overwritten and is not erased when the computer is turned off?
    A. RAM
    B. ROM
    C. CPU
    D. hard disk
    (Kinn and Woods, p 183)

155. An application program is software that is designed to
    A. perform a variety of tasks such as word processing, database functions, and patient billing
    B. provide the computer with a set of basic instructions for executing other programs
    C. interpret the program instructions
    D. all of the above
    (Kinn and Woods, p 186)

156. Which of the following are advantages of a computerized office database?
    A. All information about providers, patients, insurance carriers, diagnosis and procedure codes, charges, and payments are together and easily accessible.
    B. It can be used by more than one person at the same time if networked.
    C. It has the ability to link related pieces of information to process insurance claims.
    D. all of the above
    (Sanderson, p 18)

157. A graphical user interface (GUI) is
    A. the computer language of DOS (disk operating system)
    B. a type of computer-operating system in which commands are carried out by responding to visual information on the screen
    C. a computer application designed to perform billing and scheduling for the medical office
    D. none of the above
    (Sanderson, p 30)

158. A dialog box in Windows 95 is
    A. a box used to turn options on and off
    B. a window that appears requesting more information from the user
    C. a standard value used by the software
    D. a location on screen in which files are stored
    (Sanderson, p 38)

159. A series of computers that are linked together allowing them to share information is a(n)
    A. database
    B. clearinghouse
    C. network
    D. Internet
    (Sanderson, p 23)

160. An insurance claim that is sent by computer over a telephone line using a modem is an
    A. electronic media claim
    B. electronic funds transfer
    C. electronic remittance advice
    D. electronic mail
    (Sanderson, p 23)

161. Which kind of printer would be most beneficial for printing multi-part insurance claim forms?
    A. laser
    B. inkjet
    C. dot matrix
    D. bubble jet
    (Kinn and Woods, pp 184–185)

162. A computer system that operates as an answering device is
    A. automatic routing
    B. voice mail
    C. conference call
    D. electronic mail
    (Kinn and Woods, p 115)

163. If a worker is injured on the job, which type of insurance will likely pay the medical expenses?
    A. Medicare
    B. Medicaid
    C. Champus
    D. Workers' Compensation Insurance
    (Humphrey, pp 290–291)

164. If physicians agree to accept the amount offered by Medicare as the payment in full for services, they are accepting
    A. a claims register
    B. usual and customary fees
    C. CPT-4
    D. assignment of benefits
    (Rowell, p 405; Kinn and Woods, pp 327, 330)

165. A superbill has the following code listed on it: 99213. This indicates
    A. hypertension
    B. a Level III Office Visit
    C. insurance I.D.
    D. patient Medicare I.D.
    (Humphrey, p 295)

166. An insurance claim has the code 401.0, which indicates
    A. surgery
    B. emergency room service
    C. physician's I.D. number
    D. hypertension
    (Humphrey, pp 295–296)

167. A continuing insurance forms log in the medical office exists for the purpose of tracking outstanding insurance claims and is called a
    A. audit trail
    B. claims register
    C. insurance diary
    D. claims processor
    (Humphrey, pp 302–304)

168. A chronological file that reminds the staff that an insurance claim has not yet been paid is a
    A. account file
    B. insurance file
    C. audit file
    D. tickler file
    (Humphrey, p 303)

169. A universal health insurance claim form developed by the AMA and most used in the health industry is
    A. OWCP - 1500
    B. RRB - 1500
    C. HCFA - 1500
    D. none of the above
    (Humphrey, p 299)

170. Which is the easiest and least expensive type of billing for a health service facility?
    A. cycle billing
    B. ledger card billing
    C. computerized mailout statement
    D. superbill at time of visit
    (Humphrey, pp 312–318)

171. A collection letter to insurance companies is not considered effective until after
    A. 30 days
    B. 60 days
    C. 90 days
    D. 120 days
    (Humphrey, p 320)

172. A federal law that requires lenders who provide installment credit to clearly state the terms and express the interest in annual terms is known as the
    A. Truth-In-Lending Act
    B. Consumers' Bill of Rights
    C. Patients' Bill of Rights
    D. SOAP formula
    (Fordney and Follis, p 277)

173. Which of the following is legal to ask a prospective employee who is applying for a position?
    A. Will your family obligations prevent you from performing the tasks we expect of you?
    B. What is your religion?
    C. Are you married?
    D. Have you been arrested?
    (Humphrey, p 374)

174. The "challenge of change" may best be coped with by
    A. staying with one employer and one position
    B. cultivating political alliances
    C. upgrading skills and knowledge
    D. none of the above
    (Humphrey, p 375)

175. Revalidation of a professional medical assistant provides
    A. continuing certification
    B. formal recognition of continuing professional learning
    C. utilizes CEUs
    D. all of the above
    (Humphrey, p 376)

176. Which of the following is a document to inform employers of a job candidate's qualifications for a position?
    A. diploma/certificate
    B. resume
    C. reference letters
    D. letter of referral
    (Humphrey, pp 365–366)

177. If you need a similar or opposite term to better express your thought, what feature on the word processor would you use?
    A. spell checker
    B. thesaurus
    C. table menu
    D. format menu
    (Fordney and Follis, pp 20–24, 213)

178. The process of combining a form letter with a list of names and addresses is known as
    A. justifying
    B. formatting
    C. mail merge
    D. text-editing
    (Fordney and Follis, p 215)

179. The general outline of a letter or document that includes margins, headings, columns, etc., is
    A. editing
    B. formatting
    C. filing
    D. print preview
    (Fordney and Follis, p 408)

180. When indexing alphabetical files how would hyphenated names such as Ross-David be indexed?
    A. by the other remaining name
    B. by the address
    C. as one combined name and one indexing unit
    D. as two separate names and indexing units
    (Fordney and Follis, pp 168–169)

181. When the names of two different patients are identical, how are they indexed?
    A. by date of entry into system
    B. by sex
    C. by birthdate
    D. by address
    (Becklin and Sunnarborg, p 111; Fordney and Follis, p 169)

182. The employment eligibility verification form I-9 is for the purpose of
    A. authorization to work by citizens and noncitizens
    B. for withholding federal unemployment tax
    C. for verifying Workers' Compensation eligibility
    D. for verifying the social security number of an employee
    (Fordney and Follis, p 392)

183. Which of the following can help to trace a check from a patient after it is deposited?
    A. signature card
    B. warrant
    C. voucher
    D. ABA transit number
    (Fordney and Follis, p 355)

184. Which of the following is the best instrument with which to write a check?
    A. permanent ink
    B. erasable ball point
    C. pencil
    D. correctable typewriter
    (Fordney and Follis, p 357)

185. The process of ascertaining that the bank statement agrees with the in-house financial record of the bank balance is
    A. counter checking
    B. drafting
    C. reconciliation
    D. endorsement
    (Fordney and Follis, pp 360–362)

186. How often must a wage and tax statement, W-2, be given to an employee?
    A. annually in January
    B. semiannually
    C. quarterly
    D. weekly
    (Fordney and Follis, p 399)

187. Which of the following methods might be used to record information from the doctor's hospital visits with patients?
    A. index cards carried by the doctor
    B. patient information on computer printouts from the hospital
    C. voice recorder or telephone call where information is dictated
    D. all of the above
    (Becklin and Sunnarborg, p 87)

188. If a patient slips and falls in the office and sustains an injury, what type of insurance carried by the medical practice will cover the accident?
    A. malpractice
    B. personal liability
    C. catastrophic
    D. none of the above
    (Becklin and Sunnarborg, p 223)

189. Information about the medical practice such as the physician's license and narcotic registration would be stored
    A. in a personal file in a locked drawer
    B. with the employees' files
    C. with the building maintenance file
    D. with the patient files
    (Becklin and Sunnarborg, p 222)

190. An outline and description of the work duties along with examples is included in the
    A. maintenance manual
    B. office personnel manual
    C. office procedures manual
    D. administrator's file
    (Becklin and Sunnarborg, pp 215–221)

191. Information such as office hours, facts about the doctors, services, and facilities, and instructions for obtaining emergency care would be included in the
    A. personnel manual
    B. procedures manual
    C. patient education brochure
    D. medical journal
    (Becklin and Sunnarborg, p 214)

192. When the doctor writes a paper, what may be used to refer the reader to sources of information?
    A. endnotes
    B. drafts
    C. quotations
    D. reprints
    (Becklin and Sunnarborg, p 231)

193. The best way to handle emergencies called in over the telephone is to
    A. tell the patient you will find a doctor to talk to them
    B. have ready a prepared chart about handling specific emergencies
    C. use your best judgment—emergencies are unpredictable
    D. direct all emergencies to the nearest emergency room

    (Becklin and Sunnarborg, p 231)

194. The official record of a meeting and its transactions and business is called the
    A. agenda
    B. quorum
    C. order of business
    D. minutes

    (Becklin and Sunnarborg, pp 240–241)

195. Which of the following is NOT a duty performed when the doctor is away on a trip?
    A. notifying patients that their appointments during the absence are canceled
    B. scheduling new appointments for when the doctor returns
    C. placing the covering doctor's name, address, and telephone number by your phone
    D. disregarding daily logs of phone calls, payments, and important business

    (Becklin and Sunnarborg, pp 245–247)

196. The code system that includes units based on the median charges of all physicians is the
    A. CPT
    B. ICD-9-CM
    C. RVS
    D. HCPCS

    (Fordney and Follis, p 325)

197. If the physician needs to see emergency patients during the same office hours as other patients, which type of scheduling might be used?
    A. double column scheduling
    B. modified wave
    C. advanced booking
    D. wave

    (Becklin and Sunnarborg, p 88)

198. Which patient with the listed conditions asking for an appointment over the telephone should be seen "stat"?
    A. vaginitis
    B. blood in stools
    C. dermatitis
    D. breathing difficulty

    (Becklin and Sunnarborg, p 90)

199. Which would be included in the follow-up record of a telephone call from a patient?
    A. patient's name
    B. date and time of call
    C. reason for call
    D. all of the above

    (Becklin and Sunnarborg, pp 76–77)

200. If an error is discovered in a medical record, which of the following is NOT permissible?
    A. draw a line in ink through the error in the medical record
    B. carefully erase the error, insert it into the typewriter, and correct it
    C. write your initials next to the correction with the date
    D. carefully write or type the correct information into the medical record

    (Becklin and Sunnarborg, p 140)

CLINICAL QUESTIONS

201. Which portion of the vertebral column contains twelve vertebrae?
    A. cervical
    B. thoracic
    C. lumbar
    D. sacral
    (Thibodeau and Patton #2, pp 92–93)

202. Which part of the vertebral column is made up of five vertebrae, which are fused together?
    A. cervical
    B. thoracic
    C. lumbar
    D. sacral
    (Thibodeau and Patton #2, pp 92–93)

203. In a standard 12-lead ECG, the measurement of current the heart muscle produces between the right arm electrode and left arm electrode is known as the
    A. standard limb lead I
    B. standard limb lead II
    C. standard limb lead III
    D. augmented lead—AVL
    (Bonewit-West #1, pp 444–449)

204. The greatest deflection from the baseline on the electrocardiogram is the
    A. P wave
    B. T wave
    C. ST segment
    D. QRS complex
    (Bonewit-West #1, p 444)

205. Which deflection from the baseline represents the repolarization of the ventricles?
    A. P wave
    B. T wave
    C. ST segment
    D. QRS complex
    (Bonewit-West #1, p 444)

206. What part of the ECG complex represents the atrial depolarization?
    A. P wave
    B. T wave
    C. ST segment
    D. QRS complex
    (Bonewit-West #1, p 444)

207. In mouth-to-mouth artificial respiration in CPR, air should be blown into the victim's mouth at the rate of
    A. 4/min
    B. 8/min
    C. 12/min
    D. 16/min
    (American Red Cross, p 93)

208. Which of the following is NOT a sign or symptom of a heart attack?
    A. profuse perspiration
    B. cyanosis
    C. weak pulse
    D. thirst
    (American Red Cross, pp 93–94)

209. Claritin™ (loratidine) is classified as an antihistamine and used in the treatment of
   A. hypertension
   B. vomiting
   C. allergies
   D. hemorrhage
   (Kizior and Hodgson, pp 1121–1122)

210. An acceptable procedure in treating of frostbite is to
   A. rewarm the frozen part quickly
   B. rewarm the frozen part very slowly
   C. place the affected part in cold water
   D. rub the affected part
   (American Red Cross, p 367)

211. The type of deep wound that may result from a bullet is a/an
   A. laceration
   B. puncture
   C. abrasion
   D. avulsion
   (Kinn and Woods, p 1136)

212. Pressure points used to stop or slow bleeding include all of the following blood vessels EXCEPT the
   A. carotid artery
   B. radial artery
   C. pulmonary artery
   D. femoral artery
   (Thibodeau and Patton #2, pp 241–242)

213. A fracture or break in a bone that runs parallel with the bone is known as a/an
   A. compound (open) fracture
   B. longitudinal fracture
   C. intracapsular fracture
   D. spiral fracture
   (Kinn and Woods, pp 720–721)

214. A type of fracture or break in a bone in which the broken bone is inside a joint is known as a/an
   A. compound (open) fracture
   B. longitudinal fracture
   C. intracapsular fracture
   D. spiral fracture
   (Kinn and Woods, pp 720–721)

215. When taking an oral temperature with a standard oral thermometer, it should be left in place for
   A. 1 minute
   B. 3 minutes
   C. 5 minutes
   D. 10 minutes
   (Bonewit-West #1, pp 92–93)

216. If the pulse is taken at the side of the neck, the artery used is the
   A. radial artery
   B. temporal artery
   C. femoral artery
   D. carotid artery
   (Bonewit-West #1, pp 92–93)

217. If the pulse is taken back of the knee, the pulse site is the
   A. brachial
   B. popliteal
   C. femoral
   D. apical
   (Bonewit-West #1, p 99)

218. Which of the following types of pulse is always taken using a stethoscope?
   A. radial
   B. femoral
   C. apical
   D. temporal
   (Bonewit-West #1, p 99)

219. A patient having a Pap smear should be placed in the
    A. lithotomy position
    B. supine position
    C. anatomical position
    D. prone position
    (Bonewit-West #1, p 364; Zakus, pp 84–85)

220. What method used in the physical examination involves the art of observation to detect significant physical features?
    A. percussion
    B. manipulation
    C. inspection
    D. palpation
    (Kinn and Woods, pp 485–486)

221. The method of physical examination that uses the sense of touch is called
    A. palpation
    B. percussion
    C. auscultation
    D. mensuration
    (Kinn and Woods, pp 485–486)

222. The method of physical examination that uses a stethoscope to listen to sounds arising from the body is known as
    A. percussion
    B. auscultation
    C. manipulation
    D. inspection
    (Kinn & Woods, p 26)

223. The method of physical examination that involves tapping or striking the body to elicit sounds or vibratory sensations is known as
    A. auscultation
    B. manipulation
    C. palpation
    D. percussion
    (Kinn and Woods, pp 485–486)

224. A method of examination that involves measuring is known as
    A. manipulation
    B. mensuration
    C. inspection
    D. palpation
    (Kinn and Woods, pp 485–486)

225. A type of examination used especially by orthopedists and neurologists is
    A. manipulation
    B. percussion
    C. inspection
    D. palpation
    (Kinn and Woods, pp 485–486)

226. Which of the following drugs is classified as a broad-spectrum antibiotic?
    A. Prilosec™
    B. Biaxin™
    C. Zocor™
    D. Claritin™
    (Kizior and Hodgson, pp 233–234, 1099–1100)

227. In the drug classification under the Controlled Substance Act of 1970, which schedule of drugs does not permit refills without a new written prescription by a physician?
    A. Schedule V drugs
    B. Schedule IV drugs
    C. Schedule III drugs
    D. Schedule II drugs
    (Gauwitz and Bayt, p 9)

228. Which type of injection involves the displacing of the upper tissue laterally before the needle is inserted?
    A. intradermal
    B. subcutaneous
    C. intramuscular
    D. Z-track intramuscular
    (Kinn and Woods, pp 1050–1053)

229. Which type of injection uses the smallest angle between it and the skin?
    A. subcutaneous
    B. intradermal
    C. intramuscular
    D. Z-track intramuscular

    (Gauwitz and Bayt, pp 345–348, 351–352)

230. Penicillin V potassium is used to treat staphylococci and streptococci infections. This drug is classified as an
    A. antibiotic
    B. antihistamine
    C. antifungal agent
    D. antihypertensive

    (Kizior and Hodgson, pp 53–54, 1101–1103; Rice #2, p 219)

231. Tylenol w/codeine, a Schedule III drug, is an
    A. antipuritic
    B. expectorant
    C. analgesic
    D. antidepressant

    (Kizior and Hodgson, pp 253–255; Rice #2, pp 456–457)

232. A drug prescribed to control abdominal gas is called a/an
    A. cathartic
    B. antiflatulent
    C. emetic
    D. demulcent

    (Gauwitz and Bayt, pp 215–217)

233. Nitroglycerin is a vasodilator used in the treatment of
    A. anxiety
    B. hypertension
    C. edema
    D. angina

    (Gauwitz and Bayt, p 169; Kizior and Hodgson, pp 755–757)

234. Insulin is most often given by
    A. intramuscular injection
    B. subcutaneous injection
    C. intravenous injection
    D. intradermal injection

    (Gauwitz and Bayt, pp 280–281; Rice #2, p 193)

235. Which of the following denotes the smallest lumen (space within) of a hypodermic needle?
    A. 20 gauge
    B. 21 gauge
    C. 25 gauge
    D. 26 gauge

    (Gauwitz and Bayt, pp 340–341; Rice #2, p 159)

236. When the medication for injection is being prepared, it should be checked at least
    A. one time
    B. two times
    C. three times
    D. four times

    (Bonewit-West #1, pp 265–266; Rice #2, p 122)

237. Which of the following is not one of the four parts of a prescription?
    A. superscription
    B. inscription
    C. signature
    D. cost

    (Kinn and Woods, p 1000)

238. In the reading of a Mantoux test for tuberculosis only the area of induration should be measured and reported in millimeters (mm). Which of the following is reported as negative?
    A. 10 mm
    B, 8 mm
    C. 7 mm
    D. less than 5 mm

    (Bonewit-West #1, p 289)

239. The abbreviation that means four times a day is
    A. qd
    B. qod
    C. qm
    D. qid
    (Gauwitz and Bayt, p 64; Kinn and Woods, p 1001)

240. The abbreviation that means every other day is
    A. qn
    B. qod
    C. qm
    D. qid
    (Gauwitz and Bayt, p 64; Kinn and Woods, p 1001)

241. A type of medication tablet that is placed outside the teeth in the lower portion of the mouth is known as a/an
    A. enteric-coated tablets
    B. buccal tablets
    C. sublingual tablets
    D. layered tablets
    (Rice #2, pp 101–102)

242. Which of the following FDA pregnancy-rating category is used to denote that risk cannot be ruled out?
    A. A
    B. B
    C. C
    D. D
    (PDR, p 345)

243. An anti-inflammatory agent used in treating rheumatic arthritis and rheumatic fever is
    A. phenobarbital
    B. paregoric
    C. prednisone
    D. reserpine
    (Kizior and Hodgson, pp 843–845)

244. Triphasil-21 and Triphasil-28 are drugs that are classified as an
    A. antibiotic
    B. antiparasitic
    C. oral contraceptive
    D. antacid
    (PDR, pp 3333–3334; Rice #2, pp 481–483)

245. Both Polymox and Trimox are trade names for the drug
    A. amoxicillin
    B. levodopa
    C. hydrochlorothiazide (HCTZ)
    D. propranolol
    (Kizior and Hodgson, pp 53–54)

246. Sterile gloves have the tops turned down to form a cuff. The reason is
    A. the gloves are sterile. The inside surface will touch your skin and become nonsterile.
    B. the gloves' cuffs provide a means to slip on the gloves without contaminating them.
    C. sterile areas of the glove must touch only other sterile areas.
    D. all of the above
    (Bonewit-West #1, pp 203–205; Kinn and Woods, pp 1094–1096)

247. All of the following rules are important in cases of emergencies treated in the doctor's office EXCEPT
    A. keep a prominent list of telephone numbers of trauma centers, other physicians, fire, police, and EMS rescue units
    B. keep a well-stocked and up-to-date cart or kit of medical supplies for emergencies
    C. staff should have a good general knowledge of first aid
    D. be innovative and make your own guidelines for an emergency
    (Zakus, p 548)

248. Which type of breathing pattern frequently precedes death?
    A. hyperventilation
    B. Cheyne-Stokes
    C. rales
    D. bradypnea
    (Keir et al, pp 486–487)

249. Calculate the correct pediatric dose (pd) for a child that is two years and one month old, if the average adult dose of this medicine is 40.0 mg. Choose between Young's Rule [adult dose × fraction (child's age in years over age of child plus 12) = pediatric dose (pd)]; Fried's Rule [adult dose × fraction (infant's age in months over 150 months) = pd]; and Clark's Rule [adult dose × fraction (child's weight in pounds over 150 pounds) = pd].
    A. 8.7 mg
    B. 7.7 mg
    C. 6.7 mg
    D. 5.7 mg
    (Hitner and Nagle, p 52; Kinn and Woods, pp 1022–1023)

250. The chronic condition where seizures recur is known as
    A. a stroke
    B. epilepsy
    C. auras
    D. Reye's syndrome
    (American Red Cross, pp 298–300)

251. The medical assistant should use open-ended questions when gathering information about the chief complaint from a patient. Which of the following would be close ended and an INCORRECT question for the medical assistant to ask?
    A. What seems to be your problem?
    B. How can we assist you today?
    C. What can we do for you today?
    D. Did you have this problem last week?
    (Bonewit-West #1, p 65)

252. Remember that in the preparation of hinged instruments, such as hemostats, for sterilization in the autoclave, they should always be
    A. oiled first
    B. left closed
    C. opened
    D. none of the above
    (Kinn and Woods, p 431; Zakus, p 188)

253. Which solution of alcohol commonly used for cleansing injection sites is most effective?
    A. 100%
    B. 90%
    C. 80%
    D. 70%
    (Bonewit-West #1, p 171)

254. The autoclave is usually operated at approximately 15 pounds of pressure per square inch (psi) at a temperature of
    A. 400°F
    B. 350°F
    C. 250°F
    D. 150°F
    (Bonewit-West #1, pp 174–175)

255. The exposure time for instruments that may be disinfected by boiling water (moist heat) should not be less than
    A. 15 minutes
    B. 30 minutes
    C. 45 minutes
    D. 60 minutes
    (Kinn and Woods, p 428)

256. The timing for the autoclave starts when the
    A. instruments are being wrapped
    B. instruments are placed inside the autoclave
    C. door is closed and sealed
    D. gauges show proper temperature and pressure
    (Kinn and Woods, pp 436–437)

257. Articles cannot be partially sterile; therefore objects should be categorized as either sterile or
    A. clean
    B. disinfected
    C. nonsterile
    D. fumigated
    (Frew et al, p 611)

258. Which of the following principles DOES NOT apply to maintaining a sterile surgical environment?
    A. touch only the outside of a sterile wrapper
    B. when in doubt consider an object nonsterile
    C. avoid talking and sneezing over a sterile field
    D. hold gloved hands at your side
    (Bonewit-West #1, p 197)

259. The leads I, II, and III in a routine ECG require the use of
    A. two arms and two legs
    B. two arms and one leg
    C. one arm and one leg
    D. one arm and two legs
    (Kinn and Woods, pp 512–513)

260. Which of the vital signs taken in the office requires a stethoscope to perform?
    A. blood pressure
    B. pulse
    C. respiration
    D. temperature
    (Kinn and Woods, p 442, 467; Keir et al, p 470)

261. An electrocardiograph lead designated as a VL is a type of
    A. limb lead
    B. unipolar lead
    C. precordial lead
    D. bipolar lead
    (Burdick, p 11; Kinn and Woods, pp 512–513)

262. The position of the second standard chest lead V2 is the
    A. third intercostal space, left sternal margin
    B. third intercostal space, right sternal margin
    C. fourth intercostal space, left sternal margin
    D. fourth intercostal space, right sternal margin
    (Bonewit-West #1, p 449; Kinn and Woods, p 511)

263. A ventricular contraction that occurs too early in the ECG cycle is abbreviated as
    A. PAT
    B. APC
    C. PVC
    D. none of these
    (Bonewit-West #1, pp 461–464)

264. When performing a Snellen eye chart test, the distance where the patient stands away from the chart should be
    A. 10 feet
    B. 20 feet
    C. 30 feet
    D. 40 feet
    (Bonewit-West #1, pp 306–307; Kinn and Woods, p 575)

265. Persons that are nearsighted have a condition called
    A. myopia
    B. hyperopia
    C. presbyopia
    D. conjunctivitis
    (Bonewit-West #1, pp 304–305)

266. Which of the following is NOT correct about ear irrigations?
    A. They are performed to wash the external auditory canal.
    B. They are used to relieve inflammation by applying antiseptic solution to the external auditory canal.
    C. They are used to remove cerumen from the external auditory canal.
    D. They may be performed if the tympanic membrane (eardrum) is perforated.
    (Bonewit-West #1, p 323)

267. Otitis media is a middle ear infection. Which of the following is NOT a common symptom?
    A. pain
    B. improved hearing acuity
    C. fever
    D. feeling of fullness in the ear
    (Bonewit-West #1, p 319)

268. Mammography uses what level of x-rays?
    A. low doses
    B. moderate doses
    C. moderately high doses
    D. high doses
    (Bonewit-West #1, pp 488–489)

269. Mammography can be used to detect a breast tumor when the growth is less than _____ cm in diameter.
    A. 0.2
    B. 1.0
    C. 2.0
    D. 3.0
    (Bonewit-West #1, pp 488–489; Kinn and Woods, p 638)

270. Which of the following best describes the sorting out and classification of patients to determine priority of need and treatment?
    A. assessment
    B. interview

C. triage
D. review of symptoms
(Keir et al, pp 468–469)

271. A fever that remains elevated, hovering slightly above 101°F for a period of two days, is described as
    A. remittent
    B. crises
    C. lysis
    D. constant
    (Frew et al, p 348; Kinn and Woods, pp 442–443)

272. A type of fever that comes and goes or spikes and then returns to average range is a/an
    A. remittent fever
    B. intermittent fever
    C. lysis fever
    D. crisis fever
    (Frew et al, p 348; Kinn and Woods, pp 442–443)

273. A fever that has great fluctuations but never gets back into the average range is called a/an
    A. remittent fever
    B. crisis fever
    C. lysis fever
    D. intermittent fever
    (Frew et al, p 348; Kinn and Woods, pp 442–443)

274. An elevated, 102°F or more, suddenly drops to subnormal or normal body temperature. Most of the time after the sudden drop, the temperature will be subnormal. What type is it?
    A. remittent fever
    B. crisis fever
    C. lysis fever
    D. intermittent fever
    (Frew et al, p 348; Kinn and Woods, pp 442–443)

275. A difference between the apical pulse and the radial pulse is called
    A. collapsing pulse
    B. pulse pressure
    C. low-tension pulse
    D. pulse deficit
    (Kinn and Woods, pp 460, 465)

276. The difference between the systolic and diastolic blood pressures is referred to as
    A. fibrillation
    B. pulse pressure
    C. low-tension pulse
    D. pulse deficit
    (Kinn and Woods, pp 460, 465)

277. There are four important characteristics to note when taking a pulse. Which one of the following is NOT a characteristic to note?
    A. rate
    B. rhythm
    C. volume of the pulse
    D. consideration of pulse site
    (Kinn and Woods, pp 460–461)

278. Therapeutic ultrasound uses high-frequency sound waves as a deep heating agent. Which of the following would NOT be recommended for therapeutic ultrasound treatment?
    A. areas of inadequate circulation
    B. areas of edema
    C. scar tissue
    D. synovitis
    (Bonewit-West #1, pp 341–342)

279. When fitting a patient with crutches, many factors must be considered. Which is a correct assumption when measuring for axillary crutches?
    A. Have the patient stand with a slight bend.
    B. Position the crutches with the tips 4 to 6 inches in front and 2 inches to the side.

C. Adjust the crutch length so that the distance between the axilla and the top of the crutch is approximately 1 1/2 to 2 inches (about two fingers' width).
    D. Adjust the handgrips so that the patient's elbow is flexed at an angle of 50 degrees.
    (Bonewit-West #1, pp 352–354)

280. Pregnancy tests detect the presence of
    A. human chorionic gonadotropin (hCG) hormone
    B. heterophile antibodies
    C. febrile agglutinations
    D. autoimmune antibodies
    (Palko and Palko, pp 459–460; Wedding and Toenjes, p 366)

281. The laboratory urinalysis test that can confirm the ability of the body to concentrate urine measures
    A. glucose
    B. ketone bodies
    C. protein
    D. specific gravity
    (Keir et al, p 580; Palko and Palko, pp 164–165, 197)

282. Clinitest is a test used in the laboratory to detect
    A. hematuria
    B. ketonuria
    C. glucosuria
    D. proteinuria
    (Keir et al, pp 583–584; Palko and Palko, p 186)

283. When performing a venipuncture it is important for the medical assistant to not leave a tourniquet in place for longer than
    A. 30 seconds
    B. 1 minute
    C. 2 minutes
    D. 3 minutes
    (Estridge et al, p 115; Palko and Palko, p 234)

284. Bacilli bacteria are found in which of the following shapes?
    A. spiral
    B. rod
    C. spherical
    D. curved
    (Bonewit-West #1, pp 441–442; Palko and Palko, p 486)

285. When a medical assistant is performing a venipuncture, which of the following would NOT be a rule to follow?
    A. instruct the patient to hold the arm straight and stiff
    B. apply the tourniquet just above the elbow
    C. swab the area of the puncture site with alcohol
    D. insert the needle with the bevel facing down
    (Palko and Palko, pp 236–237, 248)

286. The smallest microorganisms are the
    A. viruses
    B. rickettsiae
    C. protozoa
    D. fungi
    (Kinn and Woods, pp 946–947)

287. Which federal regulation mandates the clinical laboratory guidelines that define quality control and quality assurance?
    A. OSHA
    B. CLIA '88
    C. CDC
    D. FDA
    (Bonewit-West #1, pp 517–518; Palko and Palko, pp 76–77)

288. A pathogenic fungus commonly encountered in a physician's office is
    A. pinkeye
    B. staph
    C. strep throat
    D. ringworm
    (Kinn and Woods, p 946; Palko and Palko, pp 492–493)

289. Which temperature scale is utilized by the medical laboratory?
    A. Fahrenheit
    B. absolute
    C. centigrade or Celsius
    D. Kelvin
    (Palko and Palko, pp 54–55)

290. The stain most utilized in the medical laboratory to study bacteria is the
    A. Gram stain
    B. acid-fast stain
    C. Wright's stain
    D. Quick stain
    (Estridge et al, p 461; Palko and Palko, p 487)

291. A contrast media used to study the gastric tract in radiographic diagnostic procedures is
    A. carbon dioxide
    B. air
    C. iodine
    D. barium sulfate
    (Bonewit-West #1, p 487; Keir et al, p 629)

292. Numerous leukocytes in the urine are referred to as
    A. polyuria
    B. pyuria
    C. leukocytopenia
    D. leukocytosis
    (Palko and Palko, p 184)

293. The type of urine specimen that would be best to use for a pregnancy test is a
    A. random specimen
    B. 2-hour postprandial specimen
    C. first morning specimen
    D. 24-hour specimen
    (Palko and Palko, pp 459–460)

294. A glucose tolerance test (GTT) is used to diagnose
  A. diabetes mellitus
  B. liver function
  C. kidney function
  D. bone marrow function
  (Palko and Palko, p 409)

295. A cholecystogram is performed to examine the
  A. colon
  B. small intestine
  C. kidneys
  D. gallbladder
  (Bonewit-West #1, pp 492–493)

296. What system of scientific measurement is used in the medical laboratory?
  A. English system
  B. metric system
  C. apothecary system
  D. household system
  (Palko and Palko, p 73)

297. The normal WBC per cubic millimeter for both men and women is
  A. 2,500–5,500
  B. 4,500–6,000
  C. 4,500–12,000
  D. 6,000–11,000
  (Palko and Palko, p 278)

298. To adjust the level of light on a light microscope which of the following can be used?
  A. rheostat
  B. condenser
  C. diaphragm
  D. all of the above
  (Palko and Palko, p 31)

299. The best way to disinfect work surfaces and equipment in the medical laboratory is to use
  A. soap and water
  B. 70% alcohol
  C. household bleach
  D. ammonia
  (Palko and Palko, pp 8, 12)

300. Which of the following could NOT occur if a urine specimen without a preservative stands longer than one hour at room temperature?
  A. urea may be converted to ammonia
  B. glucose levels will increase
  C. bilirubin will undergo change
  D. bacteria will multiply rapidly
  (Palko and Palko, p 151)

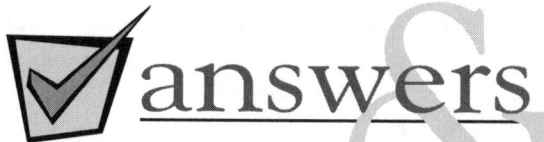

answers & rationales

GENERAL

1.

A. Superior is used to mean toward the head when giving relative positions of body parts in an anatomy and physiology class.

2.

C. The term anterior is used in medical terminology to mean "front" or "in front of." In animals such as humans that walk in an upright position the word ventral (toward the belly) can be used interchangeably with the word anterior.

3.

B. Inferior is a word in medical terminology used to mean "toward the feet." Inferior also is used to mean "lower" or "below." For example, the stomach is inferior to the diaphragm.

4.

D. In anatomy and physiology the word posterior means "back" or "in back of." In animals that walk upright the word dorsal (toward the back) can be used instead of the word posterior.

5.

A. The term medial is used in medical terminology to mean "toward the midline of the body." The big toe, for example, is at the medial side of the foot while the little toe is at the lateral side.

6.

B. The word lateral means toward the side of the body or away from the midline. An example would be that the lungs lie lateral to the heart.

7.

A. The word used in medical terminology to mean toward or nearest the trunk of the body or nearest the point of origin of one of its parts is proximal. For example in a kidney, the tubules of the nephron that lie closest to Bowman's capsule are called the proximal tubules of the nephron.

8.

C. The word superficial is used to describe something nearer the surface. A superficial wound is one that is not very deep. The skin of the arm is superficial to the muscles below it.

9.

D. The word used to describe farther away from the body surface is deep. A cut that extends a couple of inches into the body would be referred to as a deep wound.

10.

B. The word distal is used in medical terminology to mean away from or farthest from the trunk or the point of origin of a body part. For example, the foot is distal to the hip.

11.

A. The plane that divides the body into two equal halves is called the midsagittal plane. It cuts the body lengthwise from front to back. This cut illustrates bilateral symmetry.

12.

B. The plane that divides our body into anterior and posterior portions is called the front plane. This plane is also called the coronal plane. It is a lengthwise plane running from side to side.

13.

D. The transverse plane is a horizontal or crosswise plane of the body. It divides the body or any of its parts into upper and lower portions.

14.

D. The lymphatic vessels are open-ended vessels that collect fluid from around cells and return it to the circulatory system through ducts. The fluid in the lymphatic vessels is called lymph. Lymph does not contain red blood cells. Arteries and veins are connected by capillaries and the fluid in these vessels circulate in a loop fashion.

15.

C. Erythropoiesis is concerned with the formation of red blood cells. Chondrocytes are cartilage cells and osteocytes are bone cells, both of which are involved in bone formation. Periosteum is the tissue covering the bone.

16.

B. Epinephrine and norepinephrine are hormones produced by the adrenal glands. These hormones are used to prolong and intensify the sympathetic nervous responses during stress.

17.

C. The pituitary gland is divided into anterior and posterior lobes. The two lobes are really two endocrine glands. Because of the control of the pituitary over other glands, it is often referred to as the master gland.

18.

A. The thyroid gland produces a hormone that requires iodine as a part of its chemical makeup. The lack of iodine in the diet of adults will result in a painless enlargement of the thyroid gland called simple goiter.

19.

D. The islets in the pancreatic gland are too tiny to see without a microscope. There are two different kinds of cells in the pancreatic islets. The alpha cells produce the hormone glucagon, which increases blood glucose levels by stimulating the liver to convert glycogen to glucose. The beta cells secrete insulin, which helps cells pick up and absorb glucose. This process lowers blood glucose levels.

20.

D. The sinoatrial node (SA node) is responsible for initiating a heart beat. It is also called the pacemaker. It is located in the upper right atrium of the heart.

21.

A. The signal from the sinoatrial (SA) node spreads across the atria, which causes them to contract. It also travels to the atrioventricular (AV) node. This AV node is connected to the Bundle of His located in the ventricular septum of the heart.

22.

B. The Purkinje fibers wrap around in the outer walls of the ventricles. They are responsible for the contraction of the muscles of the ventricles. The ventricular contraction starts at the apex of the heart squeezing the blood in the right ventricle, forcing it into the pulmonary artery. The blood in the left ventricle is at the same time being forced through the aortic semilunar valve into the aorta where it is distributed to the entire body.

23.

B. The main trunk of the respiratory system is the trachea. The trachea is also called the windpipe. It is joined at the anterior end by the larynx and posteriorly by the bronchi. The trachea is composed of C-shaped pieces of cartilage that keep it firm to prevent it from collapsing.

24.

D. The exchange of gases, carbon dioxide, and oxygen with the blood (capillaries) occurs in the alveolar sacs (alveoli). The alveoli appear as clusters of grapes on stems called alveolar ducts.

25.

C. Hypoventilation describes slow and shallow respiration. Labored or difficult breathing refers to dyspnea. It is often associated with hypoventilation. Eupnea is normal breathing while apnea has periods where breathing ceases.

26.

A. The ileum is not part of the colon. It is the last part of the small intestine just before the colon begins. The colon consists of the ascending, transverse, descending, and sigmoid segments.

27.

B. The first portion of the 20 feet long small intestine is called the duodenum. The other two parts of the small intestine are the jejunum and ileum, arranged in this order. The most common ulcer occurring in humans is the duodenal ulcer. Ulcers in the GI tract also occur in the stomach (gastric ulcers).

28.

D. The ureters, one from each kidney, take the urine after it collects in the renal pelvis and conveys it to the bladder. The movement of urine through the ureters is not by gravity flow. It is moved along by peristalsis-type muscular contractions.

29.

C. Oliguria means scanty amounts of urine being produced by the kidney. Anuria means the absence of urine, while polyuria means an unusually large amount of urine production.

30.

D. Micturition, urination, and voiding are words that all refer to the emptying of the bladder. Urine is held in the bladder by two sphincters or rings of muscles. The emptying reflex is set into the process by (1) the bladder wall stretching that (2) stimulates the second, third, and fourth sacral segments of the spinal cord and (3) the spinal cord nerves signalling relaxation of the sphincter muscles.

31.

B. Efferent nerves are nerves that conduct impulses to muscles, organs, and glands. Conduction is away from the brain.

32.

C. The third level of organization is the organ. The lowest level of organization is the cell, followed by the tissue, then by the organs, and then by the system. Organs are groups of tissues working together. Examples are brain, skin, or heart.

33.

B. A disease that results in adult enlargement of bones of the hands, feet, jaws, and cheeks is acromegaly. A prominent forehead and large nose are characteristic of the disease. The mandible grows in length causing separation of the lower teeth. It results from overproduction of the growth hormone of the anterior lobe of the pituitary. Gigantism, which results in very large, tall individuals, occurs when there is an overproduction of growth hormone during childhood. Dwarfism results when there is insufficient production during childhood.

34.

A. Arthralgia means pain in a joint. It comes from the word root "arthr-" which means joint and the suffix "-algia" meaning pain. Arthritis comes from the word root "arthr-" meaning joint and "-itis" meaning inflammation. Arthritis means inflammation of the joint.

35.

C. Arthrocentesis is a surgical puncture of a joint to remove fluid. It comes from the word root "arthr-" meaning joint and the suffix "-centesis" which means surgical puncture. It uses the combining vowel "o."

36.

B. Dermatology means the study of the skin. It is from the Greek word derma, which means skin, and the suffix "-ology," which means "the study of." Dermatitis means inflammation of the skin.

37.

D. The word intradermal means pertaining to "within the skin." Remember that in medical terminology we start from the end. "Intra/dermal" is read as "-al" which is a suffix meaning "pertaining to," "intra-" which means within, and "derm-" which means skin.

38.

A. A surgical repair of the nose is called rhinoplasty. Excessive discharge from the nose is rhinorrhea. Rhinorrhagia is hemorrhaging of the nose and rhinomycosis is a fungal infection of the nose. Remember that the prefix "rhin-" means nose and is combined with the different suffixes to give different conditions. "Rrhea" means flow or discharge.

39.

C. Laryngectomy means the surgical removal of the larynx. Remember that the larynx is the organ of voice, the voice box. Laryngopharyngeal means pertaining to the larynx and pharynx.

40.

B. Nephritis is inflammation of the kidney. Nephroplasty is the surgical repair of the kidney. Nephrostomy means making an artificial opening into the kidney. Note the use of the prefix "nephr/o" meaning kidney, which combines with various suffixes to describe conditions or surgical procedures of the kidney.

41.

A. The surgical repair of the renal pelvis is pyeloplasty. Remember that "-plasty" is a suffix that means molding or surgically forming. The word root "pyel" means renal pelvis. Ureteropyelonephritis means inflammation of the ureter, renal pelvis, and the kidney.

42.

D. There are two word roots that mean breast. They are "mast-" and "mamm-." The word root "gynec-" means woman. Therefore, gynecology is the study of women. Mammoplasty is the surgical repair of the breast.

43.

C. Prostatolith refers to a stone in the prostate gland. Prostatocystitis means inflammation of the prostate gland and the urinary bladder.

44.

B. Aspirin is an antiplatelet drug. It is frequently recommended by physicians to reduce the risk of a second heart attack. It is also recommended that a person take an aspirin daily to reduce the risk of having a first heart attack and/or stroke. Aspirin makes the platelets slippery.

45.

A. Cardiomegaly means an enlargement of the heart. Cardiac means pertaining to the heart. Cardiopathy means disease of the heart.

46.

D. The visual examination of the stomach is called a gastroscopy. A gastroscope is the instrument used in the process of visual examination of the stomach.

47.

B. Gingivalgia means pain in the gums. Gingivitis means inflammation of the gums. Stomatitis is inflammation of the mouth and gingivoglossitis means inflammation of the gums and tongue.

48.

A. Cholelithiasis is a condition of gallstones. Cholecystectomy is the surgical removal of the gallbladder.

49.

D. An optomyometer is an instrument used to measure the muscle (power) of the eye. This word is made up of two word roots, two combining vowels, and a suffix. "Opt-" is a word root meaning vision; "my-" is a word root meaning muscle; and the suffix "-meter" is an instrument used to measure.

50.

C. Myringitis means inflammation of the eardrum. Myringoplasty is the surgical repair of the eardrum. Myringotomy means an incision into the eardrums.

51.

B. Poliomyelitis refers to inflammation of the gray matter of the spinal cord. Poliomyelitis is a viral disease that sometimes causes paralysis. Immunization is the recommended method to control this disease.

52.

A. Dysphasia is a condition of difficulty in speaking. A condition of difficulty in swallowing is dysphagia. Bradyphagia means slow eating. Note the similarity in -phasia and -phagia, which are suffixes with different meanings.

53.

C. Cephalocaudal means pertaining to the head and to the tail. Anterolateral means pertaining to the front and one side. Dorsocephalad means toward the back of the head.

54.

C. The hair papilla is not considered to be one of the integumentary layers. It is a structure lying deep in the dermis at the base of the hair follicle. The hair papilla is a cap-shaped cluster of cells from which hair growth begins.

55.

D. The subcutaneous tissue contains fat. This fat layer insulates the body from extremes of heat and cold. It also serves as a stored source of energy, which can be used as a food source by the body.

56.

B. Nerves, or neurons, that transmit impulses to the central nervous system (spinal cord and brain) are called sensory neurons or afferent nerves. Many sensory neurons are found associated with the dermis of the skin. They are specialized to detect different types of sensations. The efferent or motor nerves have just the opposite function.

57.

B. The second level of organization in our body is the tissue level. Tissues are defined as a group of similar cells working together to perform a common function. An example is muscle tissue.

58.

D. There are four main kinds of tissues that compose the body's many organs. These are epithelial, connective, muscle, and nervous tissues.

59.

A. The anterior pituitary produces melanocyte-stimulating hormone (MSH). This MSH stimulates synthesis and dispersion of melanin pigment in the skin.

60.

C. The adrenal cortex produces the hormone aldosterone, which regulates electrolyte and fluid homeostasis. The aldosterone causes the renal tubes to increase their secretion of potassium so that more of this mineral will be lost in the urine. At the same time it causes the tubules to speed up the reabsorption of sodium back into the blood. In other words, aldosterone increases blood sodium and decreases blood potassium.

61.

B. An abnormal posterior thoracic curvature of the spine is kyphosis. This type of spinal curvature is known as "hunchback." This type of abnormality limits lung capacity, therefore affecting breathing.

62.

D. A lumbar curvature of the spine that becomes abnormally exaggerated is known as lordosis. This condition is also called swayback. Scoliosis is an abnormal side-to-side spinal curvature. The traditional scoliosis treatment is to wear a supportive brace called the Milwaukee brace for 23 hours each day. This brace is worn on the upper body and the treatment is continued for several years.

63.

A. The type of skeletal muscle contraction that results in a quick, jerky response to a stimulus is the twitch contraction. This type of contraction can be seen in isolated muscles during research. These contractions play a minimal role in normal muscle activity.

64.

C. Examples of isotonic contractions include walking, running, breathing, and lifting. The muscle shortens, and the insertion end moves toward the point of origin. The tetanic contraction is a more sustained and steady response than a twitch contraction. Tetanic contraction is the result of a series of stimuli bombarding the muscle in rapid succession.

65.

D. Isometric means equal measure (iso = equal; meter = measure; -ic = adjective form). In an isometric contraction the muscle pulls forcefully against a load but the muscle does not shorten and no movement results. Repeated isometric contractions make muscles grow larger and stronger. This is the basis for the popular isometric exercises.

66.

A. The common word used to describe flexion is bending. The angle between the bones at their joint is smaller after the movement than it was at the beginning of the movement. An example would be bending your lower arm at the elbow.

67.

C. A type of movement that results in moving a part away from the midline of the body is called abduction. (Memory crutch—when someone is abducted, it can be said that they are moved away from their usual place of belonging.) If you move your arm from your side at a 180-degree angle so it is above your head, this movement is called abduction. Adduction moves a part toward the midline.

68.

C. To avoid abandonment charges a physician should notify active patients by letter that the practice is being discontinued.

There is no obligation to send a closing notice if the patient has been discharged or has not been given medical care by the physician for at least 6 years. In addition to sending a mail notice to active patients, the doctor should first tell his patients in the clinic. About one month after patients are being informed, an announcement should appear in a local paper(s) giving the date of closing. Hospital affiliations should be informed early. The patients should be informed that a copy of their record can be transferred to another doctor's office but the request must be in writing and signed.

69.

A. The attending physician is the patient's advocate in health matters and therefore must have the patient's welfare as the primary consideration. The other considerations such as allocation of medical resources (for example, insufficient transplant organs) must be decided in a fair, impartial manner by the involved institutions such as hospitals. The cost to society and the burdens of caretakers are also valid concerns that must be addressed by government, family, and society.

70.

B. The legal concept used in the malpractice suit would be based on *res ipsa loquitur*, which is translated as "the thing speaks for itself." In malpractice suits this concept is used in cases where an injury occurs to the plaintiff (patient) in a situation solely under the control of the defendant (physician).

71.

B. Respect for patient confidentiality must have primary consideration in computerized information storage systems. Massive amounts of information can be compiled and stored and later accessed by persons or organizations that gain access to the computer storage. This dilemma is being studied. Current ways to protect the records include assigning security levels to the information and controlling who has access to the information. Disclosure of the level of access should be made in advance to the patient.

Regarding the other answers: Media communication (TV, newspapers, radio, etc.) has specific rules to protect the patient's privacy. The physician may release only the types of news considered in the public domain such as births, deaths, accidents, and police cases. Professional courtesy is the practice rooted in long tradition of treating other physicians and/or their families free of charge or for a reduced charge. The term professional courtesy should be distinguished from professional ethics, which defines right and wrong for a profession.

72.

B. Written statements that are untrue and damage a person's reputation are considered libel, while spoken statements of this nature are called slander. It is best to keep these thoughts and suppositions about others to yourself. True statements may also be considered slander or libel if they were confidential and injured the person's reputation. In divulging statements of this type to others you are disproving your professionalism as well as putting yourself in jeopardy of being sued.

73.

D. Physicians do have the right to practice within the boundaries of their licenses, whether as a general practitioner or in a specialty area. Additionally, they have the right to choose where their office will be located as well as the hours it will be open. It is also the right of the physician to determine the services that will be provided to patients as well as the manner in which they will be provided. However, there are restrictions. State laws occasionally dictate that service cannot be refused to certain emergency or charity cases. Insurance companies, Medicare agencies, and hospitals dictate terms of practice and payment regarding their clients and the physician can either accept these terms or practice independently of the affiliation. The ADA (Americans with Disabilities) Act must be complied with. Finally the physician is restrained by professional ethics.

74.

D. Privileged communication is the term used. This means of communication is meant to protect the patient. It is felt that patients will not be hindered to seek needed treatment knowing that their information will be held in the strictest of confidence. There are certain exceptions to the rule of privileged communication. These include infectious diseases, which must be reported to health departments, and matters of public record such as crimes and deaths.

75.

D. As "custodian of the records" the medical assistant may at times be involved in appearing in court with a record. The physician should always be made aware of the order (subpoena). It is best to make photocopies of the record, to take along with the original. If possible, ask the court to accept the photocopy in lieu of the original. If this is not acceptable to the court, have the court clerk sign a statement of receipt of the original and keep this statement as an explanation along with the copy.

76.

C. Caution must always be exercised when faxing confidential information. Beyond being careful about others in the room, confidential faxes should be shredded. Other guidelines include verifying the receiver's telephone number before sending and making sure faxes are not unattended on a fax machine. It is also imperative that proper authorization is received before any information is released, whether faxed or in other forms. It is best to reserve the faxing of information for emergency situations.

77.

A. Patterns of a physician showing either consistent overbilling or billing for nonexistent procedures may flag an investigation by authorities. It is estimated that health care fraud costs the government and private insurance companies in the billions of dollars every year. Hotlines have been set up for the reporting of any suspected fraud, with reward money to those that turn in reports that are found to be true.

78.

C. Nonfeasance is the failure to perform a needed act. Malfeasance refers to performing a totally wrongful or inappropriate act, while misfeasance is the performing of a lawful act in an improper manner. Nonfeasance as well as malfeasance and misfeasance are all considered forms of malpractice (professional negligence). Negligence is the performing of an act a reasonable health professional would not perform, or the failure to perform an act a reasonable health professional would perform. The standard of acceptable (prudent) conduct is left for the jury to decide.

79.

C. Pathology reports are made from the pathologist's examination of tissue taken during surgery. If malignancy is suspected, the completion of surgery may be delayed until the report is received. Its parts include a usual heading, a gross description (macroscopic—as seen by the eye alone), a microscopic description, and the pathologic (disease) diagnosis. It is dictated in the present tense and like other reports becomes a permanent part of the medical record. Other reports (answer choices here) are history and physical (H & P) for the new patient, progress notes after each patient visit, a consultation report (by consultants) with the same general form as H & P. An operation report is dictated immediately after surgery by the surgeon.

80.

A. OSHA (Occupational Safety and Health Act) sets standards, rules, and practices (protocols) to protect workers in workplaces. All health care facilities, including doctor's offices, are covered. The most important regulations include (1) hazard communication plans (notifying workers of workplace hazards), (2) an exposure plan, (3) medical waste management, (4) housekeeping, (5) personal protection, (6) fire and general safety, and (7) training and education for the staff. All offices are subject to OSHA inspections at any time during work time.

The other answer choices are all other government acts or agencies that concern medical assistants. CLIA (clinical laboratory improvement amendment) requires all medical laboratories to perform at established levels. Laboratory inspections are conducted by HCFA and state agencies. DEA (Drug Enforcement Administration) enforces the Controlled Substances Act of 1970. Physicians must register every three years. Regulations also apply to administering, prescribing, or dispensing drugs. The ADA (Americans with Disabilities Act) of 1990 covers employers with fifteen or more employees and prohibits discrimination in hiring, job training, compensation, firing, or any other aspect of employment. Qualified persons must satisfy the ADA prerequisites for a position such as training, skills, and licenses. Public access is required of public service establishments including wide doors, handicap parking, elevators, doors to accommodate wheelchairs, etc.

81.

D. A blood test for the level of prostatic-specific antigen is used for detection of prostatic cancer along with a biopsy of the prostate for confirmation. A CT (computed tomography) scan may help in locating the tumor and estimating its size. Enlargement of the prostate is common among older men, as is cancer of the prostrate.

Palpation of the testes is a procedure useful in diagnosing testicular cancer because a lump or mass can be detected. It is recommended as a periodic self-examination. (Palpation is the examination of the outside surface of the body by applying the hands or fingers and may be used along with a CT scan or MRI to help in diagnosis.) Orchidectomy (removal of the testis) along with radiation and chemotherapy provides the treatment for malignant neoplasms (cancer) of the testes.

Urine cultures are not useful in diagnosing prostatic disease although they may reveal bacterial infections of the urinary system, which may be secondary to prostate disease.

82.

A. E. coli *(Escherichia coli)* is a Gram-negative bacteria commonly found in the alimentary tracts of humans and other animals and is normally harmless. However, it may mutate into toxin-producing strains, which cause illness and pose a death threat particularly to children and individuals with compromised immune systems. Even the usual strains may produce disease when entry is gained to the urinary tract or wounds.

Exposure to these bacteria is most common from raw or partially cooked meat, water, from food contaminated with sewage or animal products, or from another person who has handled contaminated material such as diapers. Therefore prevention consists of (1) heating meat, hamburger in particular, to 160 degrees F; (2) thorough hand washing after using the toilet or changing diapers; (3) preventing contamination of food and water; and (4) pasteurizing juices. (Commercial hamburger is a mixture of meat from many cattle and more likely contaminated.)

Regarding the other answer choices: hepatitis (hepat = liver; itis = inflammation) is as the name indicates, liver inflammation. It may be due to viral infections, autoimmune disease, or alcoholism. Periodontitis (peri/ = around; donti/ = teeth; and -itis = inflammation) is a disease of the supporting tissues of the teeth. The most common symptom is bleeding gums. Eventually as the disease progresses, bone is reabsorbed and the teeth fall out. It is preventable with good dental hygiene such as regular brushing, flossing, and dental care. Scurvy is a deficiency of vitamin C and can usually be corrected with a diet of fresh vegetables and fruit.

83.

D. The digestive system's colon is the site of diverticulitis, which is inflammation of small sacs (diverticuli), which form abnormally in the colon walls. The sacs trap food material or feces, which cause stagnation of the feces and pain. Other disorders of the large intestine (colon) include diarrhea, constipation, flatulence, colitis from other causes, and cancer of the colon.

The digestive system is complex and each area may have disorders. Pancreatitis means inflammation of the pancreas. It is a serious disorder that probably involves autodigestion of the pancreatic tissue by pancreatic enzymes and results in intense pain, nausea, and possibly collapse. Pyloric stenosis (stenosis is the narrowing of any passage or valve) is the narrowing of the pyloric valve between the stomach and duodenum

and prevents normal emptying of the stomach. Gastroenteritis is inflammation of the stomach and small intestine. Malabsorption syndrome results from failure (from different causes) of the small intestine to absorb food nutrients properly.

84.

A. The musculoskeletal system is necessary for the support, movement, and protection of the body's soft tissue. Many diseases may affect the muscles and bones.

Myasthenia gravis (my\a = muscle; asthenia = weakness) is an autoimmune disease that results in muscle weakness and abnormal fatigue because it attacks the synaptic junction between the muscles and nerves.

Rheumatoid arthritis is a type of joint inflammation due to an autoimmune disease that attacks the entire body. Severe crippling and deformation of the joints may occur.

Hiatal hernia (hiatus = opening) is the protrusion of the stomach up through the esophageal hiatus of the diaphragm and is due to a muscle weakness.

85.

D. Paralysis results from brain hemorrhage or obstruction of blood flow that deprives the brain of vital oxygen and nutrients. This damage is referred to as a cerebral vascular accident or stroke. A cerebral aneurysm (a localized ballooning of a blood vessel) is a weak area of the blood vessel that may hemorrhage massively into the brain when it breaks. In turn this may cause loss of speech, paralysis, or death. Early treatment is critical. Mini-strokes are so named because they produce only minor damage of disorientation, speech loss, and paralysis. However, they are serious especially because they often precede larger strokes and should receive treatment immediately.

86.

B. Lung disease is a major cause of cor pulmonale because the right heart ventricle must work so hard to supply blood to the lungs (cor = Latin for heart; pulmonale = the lungs). Eventually the stress weakens the right ventricle. The treatment is first of all to remove the primary cause of the stress (if possible). Fluids and salt may be restricted, and medications given (such as digitalis) for the heart, anticoagulants to prevent clots, and diuretics to remove excess fluid. Oxygen may be necessary.

Other disorders of the lower respiratory tract include obstructive disorders such as (1) emphysema, which reduces the total absorption surface within the lung; (2) asthma, which causes recurring spastic contractions, edema, and inflammation; and (3) chronic bronchitis, which is inflammation of the bronchi and bronchioles. Asbestos, coal dust, and other pollutants may scar the lungs. The lungs are also subject to different infections such as TB and pneumonia. Lung cancer destroys the ability to breathe and also metastasizes to other body systems.

Different types of breathing are (1) eupnea, which is normal; (2) dyspnea, which is difficult breathing; (3) orthopnea is difficult breathing relieved by moving into a sitting position; (4) apnea, which is stopping breathing for a brief period; and (5) Cheyne-Stokes (CSR), a combination of apnea and hyperventilation found in certain critical diseases. Oxygen therapy is often used to treat hypoxia (hypo = less; oxia = oxygen condition).

87.

B. Reye's syndrome is a life-threatening illness that results from a disruption in the body's urea cycle. It results in severe brain edema, high intracranial pressure, and hypoglycemia. Because the use of aspirin to treat fever has been implicated as a cause, children should be given analgesics and antipyretics, which do not contain salicylates (the active ingredient in aspirin and some other drugs).

88.

B. Urticaria (from Latin, meaning nettle) is also called "hives." It results from inflammation of the subsurface capillaries and produces severe itching and raised wheals on the skin. While often caused by allergies, it may also be caused by an adverse reaction to heat, cold, dampness, and sunlight.

Regarding the other terms, (1) psoriasis is a chronic noninfectious disease of unknown causes, which develops lesions that progress into silvery yellow-white scales. (2) Acne, especially acne vulgaris, is common among teenagers and results from inflammation of the sebaceous glands. Antibiotics, a restricted diet, cleansing and peeling agents, avoidance of sunlight, vitamin A acid, or other drugs may be prescribed. (3) Alopecia is the absence of hair and is most noticeable as baldness on the head. The drug monoxidil is often prescribed for the most common type, male pattern baldness related to aging.

89.

C. Congenital diseases are present at birth although they may not be obvious. They may be inherited, caused by nonhereditary agents (teratogens) such as pollutants, poisons, microbes, and drugs such as alcohol or food deficiencies, or a combination. For convenience they may be classified by the body system most affected. Examples are metabolic errors, musculoskeletal, genitourinary, or digestive system diseases, etc.

The other answer choices are (1) infectious diseases caused by invasions of the body by pathogenic agents such as bacteria, viruses, etc.; (2) deficiency diseases, the result of a lack of an essential element in the diet such as vitamins, minerals, amino acids, etc.; (3) degenerative diseases, which have as their chief symptom the deterioration of some part of the body and are further classified by the type of degeneration. The various types of arthritis are examples.

90.

C. Glycogen is formed and stored in the liver and muscle cells as a source of energy. Glycogen is commonly called liver starch because it is a polysaccharide that is in the same group of carbohydrates as other starches. When a person's blood glucose level begins to drop below a safe mark, the alpha cells in the pancreatic islets release glucagon into the blood stream. This glucagon converts stored glycogen in the liver to glucose, which is released into the blood and the glucose level goes up. Remember that the body can only use sugar in the form of glucose.

91.

B. The urinary system contains the kidneys, which may fail, resulting in the need for dialysis to assume their function. Dialysis is the process of removing toxic waste from the blood by filtration through a semipermeable membrane. The term, dialysis, can be dissected into its component parts as follows: dia = through; lysis = destruction—in this case by removing waste through a membrane. Proper fluid, electrolyte, and acid-base balances can also be maintained through dialysis. Dialysis is necessary when renal failure has occurred and the kidneys no longer perform their necessary task of waste removal.

Disorders commonly associated with the urinary system are: (1) infectious diseases such as cystitis, urethritis, and pyelonephritis; (2) congenital diseases such as polycystic kidney disease and childhood hydronephrosis; (3) renal calculi (uroliths or kidney stones) which have a number of causes; (4) neoplasms (cancers) such as adenocarcinoma, Wilms tumor, and tumors of the bladder; and (5) secondary disorders resulting from other diseases. These include chronic renal failure and other conditions often the result of diabetes, toxins, or cancers. (6) Chronic neurogenic bladder is due to damage to nerves.

92.

A. PID (pelvic inflammatory disease), PMS (premenstrual syndrome), and endometriosis are different disorders of the female reproductive system. Pelvic inflammatory disease is due to disease and may involve the uterus, fallopian tubes, or ovaries. Premenstrual syndrome due to unknown cause results in a number of symptoms causing discomfort or pain. At this time efforts are directed toward relieving the symptoms. Endometriosis results when the type of tissue lining the uterus also grows outside the uterus in various parts of the body. It reacts the same as uterine tissue to hormonal changes and causes pain during menstruation.

Other disorders of the female system are (1) tumors such as benign fibromyomas (fibroids), ovarian cysts (usually benign); (2) cancers of the breast, ovaries, uterus, cervix, and vagina; (3) hormonal imbalances causing amenorrhea (absence of menstruation), dysmenorrhea (painful menstruation), or PMS; and (4) infections from sexually transmitted diseases (STDs), toxic shock syndrome from staph infections of the vagina, and vaginitis from yeast infections.

Disorders of the male system include (1) disorders of the testes—oligospermia (low sperm production), cryptorchidism (undescended testes), and testicular cancer; (2) disorders of the prostate including enlargement (hypertrophy) and prostate cancer, a leading cause of death in men over 50; and (3) disorders of the penis and scrotum including phimosis (tight foreskin), impotence (failure to achieve erection), hydrocele (accumulation of fluid in scrotum), and inguinal hernia.

93.

C. Phlegm, which means thick mucus especially from the respiratory tract, is pronounced without the "g." Medical terms that have Greek origins may have silent letters either at the beginning or within the word, making them difficult to spell. Other examples are knuckle, knees, pneumonia, and psychiatry.

94.

B. All of the above individuals made important contributions to our understanding of how we learn and develop. Abraham Maslow was a Russian-Jewish immigrant to Brooklyn, New York, who founded the area of humanistic psychology. He is best known for his hierarchy of needs, which illustrates motivating forces. B. F. Skinner is also well recognized for his work in learning behaviors. Dr. Elizabeth Kubler-Ross is noted for writing about the process of dying as a series of growth and spiritual changes.

95.

A. Acceptance is usually the final or fifth stage of grief and loss. The order often listed for the five stages are denial, anger, bargaining, depression, and acceptance. Kubler-Ross's research found that there was no set order to the stages. Some persons might pass through all the stages several times. Others never made it through all five stages.

96.

D. Patient information should be safeguarded in all instances, whether in paper or electronic format. This is done through use of cautious measures. Never allow access to anyone not authorized. It is a good practice to use passwords at each level and change them often. Never allow anyone else use of your password.

97.

C. Diabetes mellitus is a disease caused by the lack of function of the pancreatic islets or islets of Langerhans. One kind of cells in the pancreas is known as the beta cells. These cells secrete one of the most famous of the hormones, insulin. Insulin is responsible for moving glucose across the cell membranes, thereby lowering the levels of glucose in the blood.

98.

D. The symptoms of a mini-stroke include headache, confusion, slight dizziness, and ringing in the ears (tinnitus). Symptoms of a major stroke include unconsciousness, paralysis on one side of the body, difficulty in breathing and swallowing, loss of bladder and bowel control, and slurring of speech.

99.

B. The function of the urinary system can be replaced by dialysis, a mechanical life-saving process that passes blood through thin membranes. Dialysis is used when the kidneys are greatly impaired and must be continued either for life or until a kidney is transplanted. It filters out toxic waste and maintains an appropriate level of sodium, bicarbonate, and other substances in the blood. Two basic types of dialysis are (1) hemodialysis where the blood is filtered by an external unit and (2) peritoneal dialysis where the peritoneal membrane of the abdomen serves as the filter. Hemodialysis requires either a fistula (an opening between an artery and vein) or a graft of one's own vein between an artery and vein to connect the dialysis unit to the body. In peritoneal dialysis, a catheter connects the abdomen to an exterior bag by which a fresh solution is introduced to the abdomen and waste containing solution is removed. In both types of dialysis, the entrance site must be guarded against damage and meticulous care taken to avoid infection.

100.

A. The liver is the most important organ in the body to carry on metabolism and detoxification/biotransformation of a drug. Some metabolism of drugs also occurs to some extent in the lungs, kidney, and intestines. However, the condition of the liver will dictate the dosage of the drug the doctor will prescribe. Patients with impaired liver damage can easily develop drug toxicity.

ADMINISTRATIVE QUESTIONS

101.

A. A conference call, also referred to as teleconferencing, may be necessary for consultation with several specialists at one time. The telephone operator must assist with such calls and each telephone station is treated as a separate call. Therefore such calls are expensive.

102.

D. A six-button touch-tone telephone can be used to put callers on hold and signal other offices. It is connected to several phone lines. It can also be used to set up conference calls. The call director is a desktop switchboard that permits handling calls on as many as sixty extensions. A cellular phone is portable and therefore very convenient but also expensive and not as private. A pager is a one-way communication device that signals that a telephone call is waiting so the person can go and call a prearranged number.

103.

C. A telephone log (another name for a diary) may be used to keep a record of all calls with the time they were received, caller, reason, etc. Other methods may also augment the log, such as preparing post-it notes for the doctor as a reminder to return calls. Colors may be used to highlight different types of messages such as those from pharmacies or to the doctor. Another color may be used to indicate the action needed has been taken and the business of the call is closed.

104.

A. Triaging is selecting the patients to receive medical treatment not in the order they arrive but according to their need for immediate attention. Flexible appointment systems allow for triaging. These include true wave, modified wave, and appointments made in blocks by categories of patients.

105.

A. The way to avoid an audit from the home office is to avoid or solve the problems as they arise. If there are telephone delays, consider getting better telephone equipment or personnel. Make sure that the person making appointments is capable of managing an appointment schedule based on the realities of the office.

106.

D. The medical assistant's responsibility is ended once she has notified the patient of the schedule of appointments that have been arranged, given needed instructions to the patient, and completed the necessary paperwork.

107.

A. Electronic signatures provide a way of authenticating documents that are computer generated. A number of ways can be used to accomplish this such as identification numbers and letters entered on the computer keyboard, writing on an electronic board, voice, or fingerprinting.

108.

D. A Review of Systems (ROS), also known as Systemic Review (SR), Functional Inquiry, or Inventory by Systems, is an organized, systematic review of the body's systems beginning at the head and proceeding through the body. It is based on oral questions to the patient and is for the purpose of finding symptoms that may reveal insight into the present illness.

109.

C. The SOMR (source-oriented medical record) stores all laboratory reports together by shingling them one on top of another. All doctors' notes, consultation reports, etc., are stored in their own section of the report. It is often less convenient than the POMR record.

110.

B. Databases maintained on computers will quickly identify patients having a particular disease or treatment if they are kept up to date. They are especially useful for research and when patients need to be notified quickly.

111.

C. A fee schedule is a list of medical services the doctor performs and the corresponding charges. This schedule should be posted where it is easily accessed by the medical assistant when completing the superbill.

112.

A. All checks and cash (with the exception of petty cash) should be deposited in the bank daily. All checks should be stamped for "deposit only" as soon as they are received. The payment should also be entered into the daily journal (log).

113.

C. Health maintenance organizations have the lowest administrative and medical expenses. Since they charge one yearly fee to all their patients, they do not have to fill out insurance forms, which requires a great deal of time. They also hold down the number of medical tests to two-thirds the number of fee-for-service medical clinics.

114.

C. A preferred provider organization provides insurance to a large block of people such as employees of a company at a competitive rate. They provide a choice of medical providers for their clients by offering a large volume of patients to fee-for-service medical facilities if they agree to accept the agreed upon payment. Therefore by dealing with large volumes they are attractive to both clients and health service providers.

115.

D. Medicare provides service to persons over 65 years of age. They have the largest medical expenditures per person as a group. They also comprise a sizeable segment of the total population. Therefore, the medical profession's percentage of patients that are over 65 is a large one.

116.

D. Patient information should be safeguarded in all instances, whether in paper or electronic format. This is done through use of cautious measures. Never allow access to anyone not authorized. It is a good practice to use passwords at each level and change them often. Never allow anyone else use of your password.

117.

D. Most patients are honest and intend to pay their medical bill. It is estimated that probably fewer than 5% do not intend to pay. The American Medical Association (AMA) lists the three most common reasons for patients not paying their bills as (1) negligence, (2) inability to pay, and (3) unwillingness to pay.

118.

D. The guidelines used for filing in the office should be listed in detail in an office procedures manual. The guidelines for an employee's grooming, proper dress, vacation time, sick leave, etc., are found in the office policy manual. In some offices this is called the employee handbook.

119.

C. In order for the office staff to give consistent, standard answers to patients over the phone, a phone triage manual should be kept nearby for reference. The medical assistant needs to know how to proceed through a standard set of questions and answers to elicit the best responses from patients and decide how soon patients should be seen. This is known as telephone triage.

120.

A. Telephone triage is the skill of talking to a patient over the phone and eliciting responses that will correctly schedule the patient according to the patient's needs. It is a skill that is gradually developed through experience and also by following guidelines set forth by the physician and office staff.

121.

B. All employees of a physician's office are required to have a social security number in order to report the employee's work to the governmental agencies such as the Social Security Administration, and the Internal Revenue Service. It also serves as a convenient identification for many other purposes.

122.

C. The Employment Eligibility Verification, Form I-9, is required before a person can be hired or paid. It is for the purpose of verifying that all employed persons are either U.S. citizens or aliens who have complied with the law. Other forms that should be filed are the Employee's Withholding Exemption Certificate, which shows how much income tax should be withheld from the paycheck (if the employee does not wish to pay as though there were no exemptions). The social security number must also be on file.

123.

D. All of the listed suggestions are necessary for maintaining a well-kept office that can give good quality medical care to patients. The equipment must be maintained with periodic servicing either by the clinic staff or by having it serviced. The supplies must be maintained at a sufficient level by maintaining an inventory and checking each category of supplies as often as needed. Linen supplies must be kept current. The facility must be inspected for needed cleaning and upkeep.

124.

D. A "backup policy" must be established and followed faithfully to guarantee that records are safe. All important material and programs must be recorded on "floppy" disks or tapes that are stored away from the site of the computer. This material must be updated daily. In addition to the backup policy, security measures such as passwords must be in place and used to prevent tampering with or destruction of data.

125.

C. The hard copy is the printout of information used for reading, editing, etc. The hardware is the actual equipment of the computer system. The software is the program used to direct the computer and process the output. Software that is specialized for the medical office is available and in widespread use. Medware is an example.

126.

B. Ergonomics (erg = work; /o/; nomics = law) is the science that attempts to fit the human body to the workplace and insure the worker's well-being by studying the anatomical, physiological, and psychological elements of an occupation. If computer work is awkward or too repetitious, the operator may develop carpal tunnel syndrome. If the microscope's height is wrong, the lab technician may eventually develop a neck injury. If a worker stands for long periods of time in one position, a back injury may develop. Examination rooms and other areas should be analyzed for efficient work patterns.

127.

A. Precertification is the procedure whereby a patient submits an intention to submit to a medical procedure along with coverage information such as insurance or HMO identification. The HMO or insurance company then decides prior to the medical service if the patient will be covered financially and what percent of expenses will be paid.

128.

D. Proofreading is not a logical step. The physician should have already inspected and released the document for filing by placing his or her initials or a check mark on the form. The logical steps to follow are (1) inspect to see if the document is released and ready to file; (2) indexing, which is a decision about what caption the document will be filed under; (3) coding is marking the index caption on the document so that it can be noted; (4) sorting, which puts the papers in order for filing making the process more efficient; and (5) the last step is storage. Inspect the folder and document to see if they agree. Place the heading on the documents to the left and put the most recent material on top. Follow the filing procedure of the office so the filing will be uniform.

129.

C. Paperless files are means of storage such as magnetic tape reels, cartridges, magnetic disks, and microforms, which do not use paper. These files can store a huge amount of material in a very small space but accessory viewing devices are required to access the information. Anyone working with these files will have to be shown how to use the devices.

130.

B. A numerical filing system requires a cross-index or cross-reference to access the alphabetical files stored in it. However, this cross-index provides a maximum amount of patient privacy. Most offices use the same number of digits for filing and a zero before another number is disregarded when filing. In some systems the digits are divided into groups of two and are sorted two digits at a time.

131.

D. The pegboard system uses a system of forms that must be lined up exactly in numerical order so that all entries may be made at once. It is efficient and easier to learn than the more complicated systems of bookkeeping. Another widely used system is computer billing, which permits great flexibility in filing insurance claims, and analyzing the practice finances.

132.

A. In managed care delivery systems, the primary care physician is the doctor a patient sees first. It is his responsibility to determine if the patient needs to consult a specialist. The managed care provider corporation determines the amount of copayment at the time of service, and the needs of patients for specialty tests such as mammograms and checkups with specialists.

133.

C. Workers' Compensation insurance has premiums based on job risk and is paid by the employer. Regarding the other answers: Easter Seal/Crippled Children is a program for children under age 21 operated with federal support. Medicaid is a government program under the operation of states to aid those needing medical services and unable to pay. These include low-income families, families with children, the blind, the elderly, and others. States determine eligibility. ID cards must be checked to see if they are up to date so that the medical office will be assured of payment. All patients should receive quality care, regardless of their financial ability to pay.

134.

A. The legal records that reveal chemical abuse may be checked as well as police records and credit records. You may be asked to produce documents or authorize the prospective employer to search records. Many factors are considered when a prospective employee is analyzed. However, they are all important to one central fact—the employer is searching for the most worthwhile, profitable employee. Character defects, ineligibility to work in the U.S., inefficient work patterns, poor public image—all of these adversely affect the employee's contribution.

135.

B. An agenda is a list of procedures or an order of business to be followed in conducting a meeting. An agenda usually includes such items of business as the reading of minutes, treasurer's report, committee reports, unfinished business, new business, and adjournment. Meetings of organizations generally follow Robert's Rules of Order in conducting business.

136.

C. The registration form is obtained as the first step in interviewing a new patient. It includes information that might be needed for later billing (and tracing unpaid bills) such as address, telephone number, employer, social security number, and driver's license number. It should also include other useful information such as insurance carrier, numbers and type of coverage, and names of referring physicians.

137.

D. All of the statements are true. The referring physician should be sent a note of thanks for a referral. The physician should have the patient sign a release form and send any pertinent records or exam results along with the reason for referral. If a referral letter is received in your office but the patient does not make an appointment or come in, you should do the following. After a reasonable period of time has passed, send a letter to the referring doctor explaining that the patient did not ask for treatment.

138.

D. All of the above are eligible for Medicare. Medicare is available to several groups of citizens: those 65 years of age or older who retired from the civil service or the railroad; individuals who are blind or disabled; other individuals eligible for social security benefits because they are disabled workers; disabled widows of workers insured through the federal government, Social Security Administration, Supplemental Security Income, or the Railroad Retirement Act, and those disabled before age 18 whose parents are eligible or retired on social security benefits. Individuals with chronic kidney disease requiring dialysis or kidney transplant, and kidney donors (expenses related to kidney transplantation only) are also eligible.

139.

D. Supplemental insurance plans may cover all of the above. However, they will vary according to price. The best-known, Medigap plans, are supplemental insurance plans designed by the federal government and sold by private commercial insurance companies to "close the gaps" in Medicare.

140.

D. Attachments to the claim can be added if they are identified with the patient and policy on each page. The most common errors on insurance claims are: (1) typographical errors or incorrect information; (2) omitting data; (3) staples or other defacement near the bar code area that prevents its correct reading; (4) not lining up the claim form in the printer so that each item fits within its space; (5) handwriting or messages on the claim other than required signatures; and (6) failing to link each procedure with the correct diagnosis.

141.

C. Basic medical covers the usual expenses not related to surgery. Another type of insurance coverage, major medical (formerly called catastrophic coverage) provides protection against especially heavy medical bills due to catastrophic or prolonged illnesses. An HMO (health maintenance organization) should provide specific services to every enrolled member for a prepaid fee. A PPO (preferred provider organization) preserves the fee-for-service concept, but relies on a group of providers (physicians) who agree to accept the charges of a predetermined list for all services.

142.

C. In the process of utilization review, a committee reviews cases for managed care plans. This committee reviews all the physician's referrals, emergency department visits, and urgent care in order to either approve or deny the referral. Regarding other answer choices: The claims department processes the medical claims. Provider relations assists the physicians' offices with inquiries about capitation, contract, credentialing, physician appeals, formularies, etc. Member services department assists the member/patients with inquiries and concerns that arise.

143.

C. Under managed care with the purpose of providing low-cost health care, a medical group such as an HMO (health maintenance organization) or IPA (independent practice association) is contracted by an insurance company. Claims processing, provider relations, members services, utilization review, and eligibility are some of the services contracted for. An HMO provides agreed upon services to enrolled members for a pre-paid fee. A PPO (preferred provider organization) preserves the fee-for-service concept, and uses a group of providers who accept agreed upon charges for all services. Capitation reimburses a health care provider at a fixed amount per member during a given time period.

144.

B. The HCPCS (Health Care Finance Administration's Common Procedure Coding System) has three levels of codes. (1) Level I—the current edition of CPT (5-digit numeric code), (2) level II—national codes (5-digit alphanumeric codes assigned by HCFA for services not in the CPT system), and (3) level III—local codes (5-digit alphanumeric codes assigned by the local fiscal intermediary).

145.

C. When a star (★) follows a procedure code number, it indicates there are variable preoperative and postoperative services and the usual "package" concept cannot be applied. (The "package" concept includes local infiltration, metacarpal/digital block or topical anesthesia, and normal uncomplicated follow-up care integral to the operation itself, which prevents these items

from being coded separately). In CPT, a changed code is indicated by a triangle (▲) in front of the code, and a new code is indicated by a bullet (•).

146.

A. The principal diagnosis is the major factor in determining the assignment of a DRG. The DRG (diagnosis related group) is based on five components: (1) the principal diagnosis, (2) treatment procedures performed, (3) the patient's age, (4) the patient's sex, and (5) the patient's disposition status. The DRG is derived by placing all possible diagnoses in the ICD-9-CM system into twenty-five major diagnostic categories, then further subdividing them into 495 DRGs.

147.

A. The time saved is the major advantage. Electronic claims can be filled out and processed faster than paper forms and requires fewer staff members. Although the chance for error or omission is reduced because information is entered once, not twice, it does not necessarily decrease the number of rejected claims. The amount of reimbursement is the same in electronic filing; however, the costs for nonelectronic filing—paper forms, envelopes, and postage—are much higher than the costs of filing over phone lines.

148.

B. A scanner is an input device because it works by converting text, drawings, or special symbols to digital data that can then be processed by a computer. Monitors work on the same principle as a television. They provide instant feedback from a computer by displaying information on the screen. A printer produces a hard copy (paper printout) of the information.

149.

C. A disk must be formatted to hold data. A track is a narrow recording band in a full circle around the disk. Each track is divided into sectors, forming the basic storage of a floppy disk. Floppy disks are convenient in that they can be stored away from a computer for safety and security and can be transported from one computer to another. They do require some basic care, however, since they are sensitive to stray magnetic waves and heat.

150.

B. The modem is a device that translates computer signals for the transfer of information via telephone lines. Hard disks are rigid disks built into the drive for extensive storage of data and they cannot be removed. They allow both reading and writing of data. Floppy disks are thin, flexible plastic disks coated with a magnetically sensitive material and facilitate reading and writing of data. CD-ROMs store more data than floppy disks but ordinarily do not permit writing data to them.

151.

A. Laser printers are usually much faster than dot matrix, ink jet, and letter-quality printers and have a high-quality output; however, they are considerably more expensive than the other three types of printers.

152.

D. Microcomputers perform four basic functions: input (typing, scanning, etc.), processing (formatting, calculating, etc.), output (hard copies of print and graphics, faxing, transmitting signals via modem to phone), and storage (on disks, tapes, etc.).

153.

D. Repetitive strain injury accounts for more than half of the job-related illnesses (>50%). The term RSI refers to a cluster of painful medical conditions caused by repeatedly straining the same muscles, tendons, nerves, and connective tissue. Therefore any job should be analyzed for the repetitive motions involved, especially the awkward or stressful ones. If they cannot be eliminated, they should be alternated with other tasks that are dissimilar on a regular basis so that muscle or skeletal fatigue does not occur.

154.

B. Read-only memory (ROM) is internal memory that contains the entire operating system and a computer language. Random access memory (RAM) can be thought of as a computer scratch pad. It holds the program instructions and the data that it is currently processing. It is generally erased when the power is shut off. The central processing unit (CPU), memory consisting of electronic and magnetic cells, facilitates the instructions from a program. A hard disk is a storage device enclosed within the computer.

155.

A. An application program is designed to perform a variety of tasks such as word processing, database functions, and patient billing. Many software applications programs can be purchased for complete medical practice management. An operating system such as DOS or Windows provides the computer with a set of basic instructions for executing other programs. The central processing unit (CPU), the "brain of the computer," actually carries out the program instructions.

156.

D. With a computer database, all the information is located in one place instead of different file cabinets in the office. In addition to the above advantages, the computer database provides simplicity of conducting a search for information. Instead of having to look in different file cabinets and folders, a search can be conducted by just entering a few keystrokes.

157.

B. Windows 95 uses a graphical user interface (GUI) so that "clicking" (with a mouse) on visual prompts carries out commands. Most users find programs that use a GUI very easy to use.

158.

B. A dialog box appears on the screen and asks for more information. Answer **A.** is the definition for a "check box." Answer **C.** is the definition for "prompt." Answer **D.** is the definition of "folders."

159.

C. A network of computers consists of computers linked together allowing them to share information. A database is a collection of related facts. A clearinghouse is a service bureau that collects electronic insurance claims and forwards them to the appropriate insurance carrier. The Internet is a worldwide computer/telephone network through which information and electronic mail is exchanged.

160.

A. The electronic media claim allows insurance forms to be filed from a computer. Electronic funds transfer allows payments for electronically filed claims to be deposited directly into the provider's bank account. The electronic remittance advice is an electronic explanation of benefits sent to the provider. Electronic mail (e-mail) is the electronic exchange of information via telephone lines through the use of a computer and modem.

161.

C. The dot matrix is an impact printer using an inked ribbon. Laser and inkjet printers use ink cartridges and cannot produce multiple copies with carbon sets or multiple copies.

162.

B. Voice mail operates much like the answering machines that we have in our home telephone systems. By dialing a personal code, a message can be recorded, sent, or received.

163.

D. Workers' Compensation Insurance will most likely pay the medical expenses of a worker injured on the job. There are some exceptions in some states with not all occupations covered. The states determine the benefits and they vary from state to state.

164.

D. An assignment of benefits occurs when physicians are willing to accept the amount offered by an insurance company or Medicare as payment in full for their services (except for the Medicare deductible and 20% co-insurance). Some physicians may decline to accept this agreement. The medical assistant must know whether assignment of benefits was accepted before filing a claim.

165.

B. A Level III Office Visit is indicated by this particular five-digit code without a decimal. The five-digit code indicates that it belongs to the CPT (Current Procedural Terminology) group of codes and is some

type of medical procedure, treatment, or service. If the code had had three digits followed by a decimal and one or two additional digits, a diagnosis would be indicated. The diagnosis, of course, is based on a disease or disorder.

166.

D. The three-digit code followed by a decimal and zero in this case indicates hypertension. It belongs to the ICD-9-CM codes (International Classification of Diseases, 9th edition, Clinical Modification).

167.

B. A claims register keeps the vital information needed to trace outstanding insurance claims through to their final disposition. It consists of pages of vertical columns that list vital information such as claim number, patient name, insurance carrier, date filed, etc.

168.

D. A tickler file means by its name that it tickles the memory to check on an item. In this case it reminds the staff that payment is outstanding and approximately when it should be expected. If it is not received by the expected date, the follow-up procedure must be started to trace the claim and find out why it has not been paid.

169.

C. The HCFA 1500 form is the universal form used by many private insurance carriers as well as many government health programs. There are exceptions, however, such as the Workers' Compensation program and some private insurance carriers.

170.

D. The superbill given to the patient at the time of the visit with encouragement to pay the bill is the easiest in terms of time, labor, and postage and also the best opportunity to collect. Other means of billing range from copies of the ledger card showing the balance to computerized mail out statements. The billing may be divided over a month's time if this works better in the schedule, or an external billing service may be contracted to manage patient accounts. In any case the bills must be paid in order to pay the expenses of the practice and keep the practice in business.

171.

B. The insurance claims process is lengthy so 60 days is considered a reasonable time to allow before following up on unpaid insurance claims.

172.

A. A federal law known as the Truth-In-Lending Act, and also The Consumer Credit Protection Act of 1968 requires that consumers be informed of the terms of their credit by providers of installment payment. This applies only when payments are divided into installments and are due "on time." The service is generally utilized by those who have large bills, are unable to pay, and do not have insurance to assist them.

173.

A. The interviewer may legally ask you if your family obligations, religion, or cultural beliefs will interfere with your job. The interviewer has no legal right to ask you if you have been arrested but you could be asked legally if you had ever been convicted of a crime (although it is unlikely). The prospective employer does have a right to ask that you submit to drug testing as part of a pre-employment physical examination.

174.

C. The best way to cope with the "challenge of change" brought on by the rapid introduction of new knowledge and technology and administrative changes into the medical field (as well as society in general) is to upgrade skills and knowledge on a day by day basis by accessing available resources. These may include community college courses, Internet courses, published articles, and professional conventions and workshops.

175.

D. Revalidation is achieved by completing courses, workshops, and study courses, which are accepted as continuing education units by the medical assistant agency. This provides a formal recognition of continued professional learning and therefore a means to increase job competence.

176.

B. The resume is a summary of the various items that show an individual is qualified for working in a particular field. It should be approached honestly but from a persuasive standpoint of selling the person's strong points to an employer. It may be chronological if the applicant has a strong employment background that should be emphasized. However, for the student just out of school, a functional resume that highlights qualifications and marketable skills may be preferable. The resume may be part of a portfolio that includes supporting documents for the resume. These include transcripts, letters of reference, etc.

177.

B. A thesaurus (treasury in Greek) is a dictionary of synonyms (words that mean the same) and antonyms (words that mean the opposite) and is found on most word-processing programs. It can provide variety in writing professional letters and articles and also can tickle the memory when a word is not quite right.

178.

C. Mail merge is the process of having a word processor automatically insert names and addresses from a list into letters and onto envelopes. It is a very useful tool for mass mailings.

179.

B. The format of a document or letter greatly affects its general appearance and readability. In word processing it includes the delineation of margins, headings, columns, etc., to make the document pleasing to the eye and readable. In such documents as resumes it can catch the attention of a busy employer, stress the most desirable features, and leave the impression of a capable and organized applicant.

180.

C. The hyphenated name is treated as one name and one indexing unit. The same applies to surnames with prefixes. Remember everyone must file the same way using the same indexing rules in order to maintain a useable file system.

181.

D. When names are identical, the address is used to distinguish the patients. The address is broken into different indexing units representing the state, city, street, and street number.

182.

A. The form I-9 is for the purpose of verifying that employees have met the requirements of the law and have a legal right to work in this country.

183.

D. The ABA (American Bankers Association) transit number identifies each bank. This when written on the deposit slip along with the patient's name, check amount, and date of deposit will permit tracing a bounced check.

184.

A. The best writing instrument listed for checks is handwriting with permanent ink unless a check writing machine is available with anti-forgery features. Writing with a ballpoint pen or pencil may be erased or altered. Typewriting can also be altered or erased. When a check is written, a number of precautions should be followed to prevent alterations. The amount when written out should begin at the far left and a line drawn at its finish to the word "dollars." The figures should be written close to the dollar sign.

185.

C. The bank statement is "reconciled" with the amount shown as the correct checkbook balance by (1) comparing the two documents for discrepancies, (2) comparing the ending balance on the previous statement with the beginning balance of the most recent statement, (3) subtracting service charges from the checkbook record, adding recent deposits or withdrawals not shown to the bank deposit, and subtracting outstanding checks. A written list of steps in the procedure helps until the task becomes memorized.

186.

A. A W-2, wage and tax statement, must be furnished by each employer every year in the month of January as a statement of the employee's earnings the past year. A similar report, Form W-3, Transmittal of Wage and Tax Statements, must be filed by the end of February that shows a summary of all the income taxes collected and shown on W-2 forms along with the income tax withheld and reported on the four quarterly Forms 941.

187.

D. All of the above methods might be used depending on the preference of the physician and medical office policies.

188.

B. Personal liability covers accidents and personal injuries. It may be attached to property insurance or sold separately. Malpractice insurance is professional insurance and covers only acts that are connected to the practice of medicine. Catastrophic insurance is a type of medical insurance that covers catastrophic illnesses such as cancer.

189.

A. The physician's personal file would contain information about his license, narcotic registration number, and social security number, along with affiliations in different organizations, medical societies and continuing education requirements. It should be kept secure and not comingled with other files.

190.

C. The office procedures manual would contain descriptions of work duties with examples so that work can always proceed. It may be used to help temporary workers fill in when the regular workers are out of the office or when a replacement or new employee is trained.

191.

C. The patient education brochure should contain items about the practice and personal medical care the patient may need. Items might be included about the office, personnel, phone numbers, address, office hours, insurance forms, medication, etc.

192.

A. Endnotes and footnotes refer the reader to sources of information the author has referenced or the reader may wish to explore further. Endnotes come at the end of the article, while footnotes are printed at the bottom of the page. Refer to a secretarial manual to find examples and use the style preferred by your employer for printing the footnotes or endnotes. Bibliographies list books that were used in the article or are of interest to the reader.

193.

B. The best way for a medical assistant to field phone questions about emergencies is to have a prepared chart with responses the doctor has given her for specific situations. Among these will be listed those emergencies that require her immediate attention and those which should be directed immediately to the nearest emergency room. The medical assistant must avoid (1) being unprepared and (2) anticipating the doctor's reply and assuming the role of a doctor.

194.

D. The minutes of the meeting are the official record of the business that transpired at a meeting. It includes such items as date, place, time, why the meeting was held, names of the presiding officer and attendees, motions made, and summaries of discussions. The minutes are kept by the secretary and copies may be sent to members or distributed before the next meeting.

195.

D. Obviously daily logs of phone calls, payments, and important business WILL NEED to be kept. Appointments will need to be restructured to fit the doctor's absence. Patients must have another doctor to refer to. Otherwise they would be abandoned. Mail, reports, and finances must proceed as agreed upon with the doctor before he or she left on the trip. The extra time may permit some tasks such as housecleaning and restructuring files, etc.

196.

C. RVS is the code system used that incorporates the medical charges made by physicians during the period the code was published. CPT has codes for medical procedures and treatments. ICD-9-CM has codes for diseases and diagnoses. HCPCS codes are used in Medicare.

197.

A. Double column scheduling is used to integrate emergency and other sick patients into the schedule after schedules have been filled.

198.

D. The patient with breathing difficulty needs to be seen immediately. The word "stat" means immediately. Stat cases are patients with life-threatening or serious illnesses. Note, however, that the medical assistant could elicit more information about the patient than is included in the above question and could therefore make a better decision. The critical point here is that a correct decision allows the most critical patient to see the doctor immediately. Pre-determined guidelines provide help for the medical assistant.

199.

D. All of the above information would be included in the telephone log for future reference. The telephone call is not completed until the reason for the phone call had been acted upon. A message might also be forwarded to another person if required.

200.

B. A medical record should never be erased since it is a legal document that may be inspected in court as well as a record to enable better treatment of the patient. Corrections should be neat and identified as to the person and date.

CLINICAL QUESTIONS

201.

B. The thoracic portion of the vertebral column consists of twelve vertebrae. The thoracic portion contains more vertebrae than any other part of the column.

202.

D. The sacral region contains five vertebrae that are fused. The lumbar region of the vertebral column is made up of five vertebrae that are not fused together.

203.

A. The standard limb lead I is a bipolar lead that records the heart's voltage difference between the right and left arms. It appears as the first recording on the standard 12-lead ECG. The AVL records the heart's voltage difference between the electrode of the left arm and a central point between the right arm and left leg. This lead is a unipolar lead.

204.

D. The greatest deflection from the baseline on the electrocardiogram is the QRS complex. This deflection represents the depolarization of the ventricles or ventricular depolarization. The T wave shows the repolarization of the ventricles.

205.

B. The T wave represents the repolarization of the ventricles or ventricular repolarization. The P wave shows the amount of voltage generated by the atria during depolarization.

206.

A. The P wave represents the atrial depolarization phase of the heart. It is the first deflection from the baseline noted on the ECG cycle. It precedes the QRS complex and is much smaller than either the QRS complex or the T wave.

207.

C. In mouth-to-mouth artificial respiration, one breath should be blown into the victim's mouth every 5 seconds, which equals 12 per minute. Remember CPR may pose a threat of infection to the caregiver unless precautions are taken.

208.

D. Signs and symptoms of a heart attack include profuse perspiration, cyanosis, weak pulse, and nausea. The victims would not crave food or water. In addition to these symptoms, the victim will often suffer severe pain in the midchest region possibly radiating to the neck, jaw, or left shoulder and arm.

209.

C. Claritin™ is classified as an antihistamine and is used in the treatment of allergic reactions. It is used in the relief of nasal and non-nasal symptoms associated with seasonal allergic rhinitis (hay fever). It is also used in the treatment of idiopathic chronic urticaria (hives). It is best given on an empty stomach because food delays absorption.

210.

A. In the case of frostbite, the affected part should be rewarmed quickly by placing it in water that is warm but not hot. Water temperature can be tested by pouring it over the inner surface of the assistant's or rescuer's forearm. Rubbing the affected part can cause damage to vulnerable tissues.

211.

B. The type of wound that is a result of a bullet is called a puncture wound. In a puncture wound the skin is pierced by a pointed object such as a pin, nail, splinter, or bullet.

212.

C. The pulmonary artery is located deep in the body near the heart so it would be impossible to apply pressure to the blood vessel. All of the other arteries listed can have pressure applied to them.

213.

B. A longitudinal fracture is a fracture or break in a bone that runs parallel with the bone. An intracapsular fracture is a bone broken inside a joint. In a spiral fracture the break coils around the bone. A compound (open) fracture is one in which there is an open wound.

214.

C. A type of fracture or break in a bone in which the broken bone is inside a joint is known as a/an intracapsular fracture. A compound (open) fracture is one where there is an open wound resulting from the fracture.

215.

B. When the temperature is taken with a standard oral thermometer, the thermometer should remain in place for 3 minutes. It is important that the thermometer have time to register accurately.

216.

D. The carotid artery is used if the pulse is taken at the side of the neck. The temporal pulse can be felt at the side of the head about even with the eyebrow.

217.

B. The popliteal pulse is taken back of the knee. It is easier to detect when the knee is slightly flexed.

218.

C. The apical pulse is always taken using a stethoscope. It has a strong beat and is more easily heard than all the other pulses. The apex is the pointed end of the heart.

219.

A. A patient having a Pap-smear should be placed in the lithotomy position. This position is sometimes called the stirrup position. This position is also used for cystoscopic examinations.

220.

C. In a physical examination, the art of observation used to detect significant physical features is known as inspection. The method ranges from the patient's general appearance to the more detailed observations including body contour, symmetry, rashes, color changes, to visible injuries and deformities. Gait and facial expression are also noted.

221.

A. The method of physical examination that uses the sense of touch is called palpation. The body is touched with the hand to determine the condition of the body and that of the underlying organ. It is used to perceive temperatures, vibrations, form, size, rigidity, elasticity, and texture. This process can be performed using one hand, both hands (bimanual), one finger (digital), the fingertips, or the palm of the hand.

Palpation should not be confused with palpitation, which means a heartbeat that is unusually rapid, strong, or irregular.

222.

B. The method of physical examination that uses a stethoscope to listen to sounds arising from the body is known as auscultation. Auscultation is hard to perform because the physician must distinguish between normal and abnormal sounds. This method is good for appraising sounds arising from the lungs, heart, and abdomen.

223.

D. The method of physical examination that involves the art of tapping or striking the body to elicit sounds or vibratory sensations is known as percussion. The fingers or a small hammer are utilized. Percussion helps the examiner to determine the position, size, and density of an underlying organ or cavity. The amount of air or solid matter present in the underlying organ or cavity can be determined by this method.

224.

B. A method of examination that involves measuring is known as mensuration. The length and diameter of an extremity, the extent of flexion or extension of an extremity, or the pressure of a grip are included in these measurements. Measurements are usually reported in centimeters.

225.

A. Manipulation is the forceful, passive movement of a joint to determine the range of motion of a part of the body. This procedure is utilized especially by the orthopedist and neurologist.

226.

B. Biaxin™ is classified as a broad-spectrum antibiotic. The generic name for this drug is clarithromycin and it belongs to a group of drugs known as macrolides. Macrolides are used to treat both Gram-positive microorganisms and Gram-negative cocci.

227.

D. Schedule II drugs under the Controlled Substances Act of 1970 requires that to have the prescription refilled the physician must write a *new prescription*. Schedule II drugs have a high potential for abuse due to severe physical and psychological dependence.

228.

D. The Z-track intramuscular injection is a method whereby the upper tissue is moved laterally before the needle is inserted at a 90-degree angle into the muscle. The skin is pulled to one side and held firmly in place as the needle is inserted. The needle is withdrawn and then the tissue is released. This method of injection prevents the medicine from leaking back through the needle track.

229.

B. The intradermal injection is given at a 5- to 15-degree angle to the skin. The subcutaneous injection is injected at a 45-degree or more angle and both the intramuscular and Z-track intramuscular are given at the 90-degree angle to the skin.

230.

A. Penicillin V potassium is the generic name for the drug Veetids. It is given PO (by mouth) and is used in the treatment of a large number of infections such as pneumonia and other respiratory diseases, urinary tract infections, septicemia, and meningitis plus others. It works by inhibiting bacterial cell wall synthesis.

231.

C. Tylenol w/codeine is an analgesic. It is used to relieve mild to moderate pain. Tylenol contains acetaminophen, which does not have anti-inflammatory action. It is a Schedule III drug on the Controlled Substances list, which requires a physician's prescription. Tylenol w/codeine is given without regard to meals and is moderately absorbed from the GI tract. It is metabolized by the liver and excreted in urine.

232.

B. Antiflatulents are drugs used to reduce gas in the stomach and intestines. Gas (flatulence) frequently accompanies indigestion. Simethicone is the major ingredient in these drugs. They facilitate the passage of gas by mildly stimulating intestinal motility. Examples of the products that contain simethicone are Phazyme, Gas-X, and Mylanta.

233.

D. Nitroglycerin is a vasodilator used in the treatment of angina pectoris. The classic vasodilators are nitrates. They dilate the walls of the arteries, therefore less force is needed to push blood through them. The most common vasodilator is sublingual nitroglycerin (Nitrostat). If taken at the beginning of an angina attack, it can take effect in 2–5 minutes and last from 30 to 60 minutes. Nitroglycerin can also be administered orally in time-release tablets or capsules, topically as an ointment, as a transdermal patch or by IV.

234.

B. Insulin is most commonly given by subcutaneous injection. It can also be given by intramuscular and intravenous injection. The IM and IV administration of regular insulin should only be used when rapid onset is desired. Two types of insulin may be mixed in the same syringe as long as one type is regular insulin. The sites utilized for subcutaneous injection are the fatty tissues on the outer upper arm, the front of the thigh, and the abdomen. Do not massage the site after injection because it may speed up the absorption of the insulin.

235.

D. The larger the gauge number, the smaller the needle lumen. A 26-gauge needle is very small and is used to perform a tuberculosis skin test by intradermal injection. Needles with gauges of 20 or 21 are used to draw blood by venipuncture.

Common needle gauges range from 16 to 30. Remember the gauge only refers to the lumen cavity size, not the length of the needle.

236.

C. To be sure that the correct drug (medicine) has been selected, one should read the label on three occasions. The label on the drug is checked when it is taken from the storage area; just before you draw up the injection; and then it is checked for the third time after injection when the drug is returned to storage or right before you discard the empty container.

237.

D. The four parts of a prescription include (1) superscription, (2) inscription, (3) subscription, and (4) signature. Superscription includes the patient's name, address, date, and the symbol Rx, which is Latin for recipe, meaning "to take."

238.

D. An induration of less than 5 mm is considered to be a negative reaction. Indurations of 10 mm or more constitute a positive reaction. A positive reaction should have further diagnostic procedures to determine whether active TB is present. The size of the induration is the only criterion used to determine a positive reaction—not the degree of redness.

239.

D. The abbreviation that means four times a day is qid. The abbreviation for every morning is qm.

240.

B. The abbreviation that means every other day is qod. The abbreviation that means every day is qd. The abbreviation that means every night is qn.

241.

B. A buccal tablet is formulated to be dissolved and absorbed when placed outside the teeth between the cheek and gums. They should not be chewed. Enteric-coated tablets will pass through the stomach without dissolving. Their special coating allows them to dissolve in the small intestine.

242.

C. The letter "C" denotes the category of the FDA pregnancy-rating system meaning that risk of this drug during pregnancy cannot be ruled out. "A" rating means that controlled studies show no risk. "B" ratings mean no evidence of risk in humans while the "D" rating means that positive evidence exists of risk in use during pregnancy.

243.

C. An anti-inflammatory agent used in treating rheumatoid arthritis, rheumatic fever, and other disorders is prednisone. Prednisone is an example of a corticosteroid drug that is used to treat more severe cases. Anti-inflammatory drugs act to diminish inflammation. NSAIDs such as aspirin and ibuprofen are used to treat milder symptoms.

244.

C. Triphasil 21 and 28 are oral contraceptives. Triphasil (levonorgestrel and ethinyl estradiol-triphasic regimen) is a combination oral contraceptive that acts by suppression of gonadotropins. Contraceptives hinder or prevent pregnancy. There are several means of preventing pregnancy: sterilization (vasectomy and tubal ligation), barrier devices (condoms and cervical caps), vaginal sponges, spermicide gels, oral contraceptives, and implantation devices. Contraceptive devices may also be classified as either temporary or permanent.

245.

A. Polymox and Trimox are trade names for amoxicillin. They are stable in the presence of gastric acid and are well absorbed from the gastrointestinal tract. They may be given with no regard to food. Amoxicillin is a semi-synthetic penicillin, an analogue of ampicillin. Trade names are names by which a company markets its own version of a drug. If more than one company markets the same drug, then drugs such as penicillin may have several trade names. Generic names are names officially designated as the name of a drug regardless of who markets it. When used with product or trade names that begin with capital letters, the generic name is placed in parentheses and is not capitalized. Drugs are also sometimes named by their action on the body. For example, amoxicillin is an antibiotic that destroys or controls bacterial growth. Warfarin sodium is an anticoagulant used to control the blood-clotting tendencies of patients with a history of stroke or heart attack.

246.

D. All of the reasons listed are true. The cuffs provide a means to put the sterile gloves on over the hands without contamination. While the hands are meticulously clean after surgical hand washing, they cannot be sterilized. Sterile gloves are an important part of maintaining sterility during surgery and other procedures that are especially vulnerable to infection.

All surfaces in and around the surgical or sterile procedural site should be as sterile as possible. Air currents and moisture can contaminate sterile fields. Other rules for maintaining sterility are (1) keep body motions and talking over a sterile field to a minimum since air currents carry microbes; (2) face each other when working over a sterile field; (3) keep the sterile field within eyesight and don't wander away; (4) do not allow nonsterile persons to contaminate a sterile field by reaching over it or breaching it in other ways. Sterile field techniques include (1) using fan folded drapes and towels so they can be unfolded easily; (2) when the entire setup is in one package and it is double wrapped, letting the underneath wrapping serve as the sterile table drape; (3) consider everything below your waist contaminated; (4) if an item is not known to be absolutely sterile, consider it contaminated; (5) keep a one inch strip around the sterile field, edges of wrappers, and sides of containers as a margin that is considered nonsterile; (6) regard any item touching moisture as contaminated. This includes sterile fields with spills on them.

247.

D. An employee of the doctor must not go outside the guidelines that have been established for the office. The basic rules that most medical offices follow are (1) keep telephone numbers of emergency assistance units, hospital emergency rooms and trauma centers, and fire and police stations prominently displayed by phones and on the emergency cart so they can be called at an instant's notice; (2) be prepared with a well-stocked set of supplies; and (3) have a good knowledge of first aid and CPR. A refresher course in first aid should be taken periodically.

248.

B. The Cheyne-Stokes breathing pattern frequently precedes death. It is characterized by slow, shallow breaths that increase in depth and frequency. This phase is followed by a period when the breaths are less frequent and shallow. Apnea is the next phase where the patient stops breathing a period of 10 to 20 seconds or longer. Then the whole process is repeated. This breathing pattern can occur with acute brain, heart, kidney, or lung damage or disease.

249.

C. Using Fried's Rule the medical assistant should substitute in the rule as follows: child's age in months over 150 month multiplied by adult dose equals pediatric dose.

$$25/150 \times 40.0 \text{ mg} = pediatric\ dose$$
$$1/6 \times 40.0 \text{ mg} = 6.7\ mg.$$

250.

B. Epilepsy is the chronic form of recurring seizures. Epileptics take medication to control seizures. In most cases this is effective. Most common causes are head injury, CNS infections, strokes, and familial tendencies toward epilepsy.

Acute seizures can be due to Reye's syndrome (a disease related to giving aspirin to children), high fever, and other causes. If they recur or are severe, medical help should be sought.

251.

D. "Did you have this problem last week?" is not an open-ended question. It can be answered with a simple yes or no. If the medical assistant is eliciting information about when the problem started, he or she should ask the question "When did this problem start?" Do not put words into the patient's mouth to repeat.

252.

C. All hinged instruments must be sterilized with the instrument open so that all parts are exposed. If they are autoclaved closed, you cannot be sure that all the instrument's parts are sterile.

253.

D. A 70% solution of alcohol is more effective than a 100%, 90%, or 80% solution. It is commonly used to cleanse the skin at injection and venipuncture sites. The 70% solutions of either ethyl or isopropyl alcohol are frequently used in the medical office as a disinfectant with other chemicals added.

254.

C. The autoclave is usually operated at approximately 15 pounds of pressure per square inch (psi) at a temperature of 250°F for at least 15 minutes. Pressure is used, not to kill organisms, but to raise the temperature above the boiling point of water, which is 212°F.

255.

A. The exposure time for disinfecting by boiling (moist heat) should not be less than 15 minutes. Boiling does not sterilize. It only disinfects. Boiling water will not get above a temperature of 212° F (unless pressurized). Instruments, such as nasal or ear specula that do not penetrate the body tissues, may be disinfected by this method.

256.

D. The timer for the desired time is not set until the gauges show that the proper temperature and pressure have been reached. These are usually 250°F with a 15 pound pressure.

257.

C. Because an article cannot be partially sterile, it is either sterile or nonsterile (contaminated). There is no in-between.

258.

D. When you are maintaining a sterile surgical environment always keep your gloved hands above waist level. Anything below waist level is considered nonsterile.

259.

B. The leads I, II, and III in the routine ECG or EKG require the use of two arms and one leg. The left leg along with the right and left arms make up the triangle, which is called the Einthoven's triangle. These leads are all bipolar. The right leg is used as a ground.

260.

A. A blood pressure is taken using a stethoscope and a sphygmomanometer. Medical office sphygmomanometers commonly have either of two types of pressure gauges. One is an aneroid dial, the other a mercury column. Units used in homes may have electonic or computerized systems.

261.

B. The lead designated as a VL is an augmented lead, which is also a unipolar lead. It records the electrical activity from the midpoint between the right arm and the left leg to the left arm.

262.

C. The position of the second standard chest lead V2 is the fourth intercostal space, left sternal margin. The V1, first standard chest lead, is at the fourth intercostal space, right sternal margin.

263.

C. A ventricular contraction that occurs prematurely is called a premature ventricular contraction (PVC). PAT stands for paroxysmal atrial tachycardia with a constant heart rate that usually falls between 150 and 250 beats per minute. APC stands for atrial premature contraction.

264.

B. The patient should stand 20 feet from the chart when taking a Snellen eye chart test. It is also important that the eye chart be well lighted with light positioned above the chart. The eyes are checked separately for visual acuity by covering one eye at a time with an eye occluder. The center of the chart should be at the patient's eye level. The medical assistant stands beside the chart during the test and indicates which line to read.

265.

A. A person who is nearsighted has a condition known as myopia. Hyperopia refers to farsightedness. Here the eyeball is too short from front to back. Presbyopia is a condition in older people that results in a decrease in ability to focus clearly on close-up objects. (The suffix -opia means vision. A related term used as a prefix is ophthalm-, which means eyes.)

266.

D. It is important always not to perform an ear irrigation if the tympanic membrane (eardrums) is perforated or ruptured. A perforated eardrum would permit fluid to flow into the middle ear. People with a perforated eardrum must not get water in that ear.

267.

B. One of the common symptoms that accompany otitis media is a temporary loss of hearing in the affected ear. Middle ear infections are commonly caused by a blocked eustachian tube. This causes a build-up of fluid that supports bacterial growth.

268.

A. Mammography, which uses low doses of x-rays, is an examination of the breasts used to detect different forms of breast disease. These include breast calcification, fibrocystic breasts, benign breast masses, and particularly breast cancer.

269.

B. Mammography can be used to detect a breast tumor when the growth is less than 1 cm in diameter. This is about the size of a pea. Remember there are 2.54 cm/1 inch. A tumor less than 1 cm cannot be detected by a breast palpation examination. The four clinical stages of carcinoma of the breast are as follows:

Stage I breast tumors less than 2 cm diameter

Stage II breast tumors 2–5 cm in diameter

Stage III breast tumors over 5 cm in diameter

Stage IV distant metastasis

270.

C. Triage comes from French and means to sort. It originated on the battlefield in wartime as a means to assess soldiers' injuries. Triage is a term also used in prioritizing the conditions of the injured, which follows a disaster. In the medical office it is important to have a written plan for both phone and face-to-face triages.

271.

D. A common temperature pattern in which the fever remains elevated, hovering slightly above 101°F for a period of two days, is called a constant fever or a continuous fever. This type of fever always remains above the patient's normal average range. It is seen with pneumococcal pneumonia.

272.

B. An intermittent fever is one that comes and goes, or it spikes and then returns into average range.

273.

A. A type of fever called remittent is one that has great fluctuations but never gets back into the average range. Because it is a constant fever with fluctuating levels, it is called remittent.

274.

B. A crisis fever is one that is quite elevated (maybe 102°F or more), then suddenly drops to normal or subnormal and remains at a subnormal temperature.

275.

D. Pulse deficit is the condition that refers to a difference in pulse rate between an apical pulse and radial pulse. Normally, these two sites will give the same pulse rate.

276.

B. The difference between the systolic and diastolic blood pressures is referred to as the pulse pressure. Blood pressure is recorded in millimeters. If this difference is greater than 30 mm or less than 50 mm, it is considered to be normal.

277.

D. The site where the pulse is taken should not make a difference in a normal pulse. If everything is normal, you should get the same results. The four characteristics to note when taking a pulse are rate, rhythm, volume of pulse, and condition of the arterial wall. These characteristics depend on size and elasticity of the artery, the strength of contractions of the heart, and the condition of the tissues surrounding the artery. Valuable information regarding abnormalities of the circulation of the heart can be learned from a patient's pulse.

278.

A. Therapeutic ultrasound uses high-frequency sound waves that are converted to heat. Therapeutic ultrasound treatments are recommended for the treatment of musculoskeletal disorders such as sprains, joint contractures, neuritis, arthritis, edema, synovitis, scar tissue, bursitis, fibrositis, strains, and dislocations. It should not be used directly over the spinal cord, over the heart or brain, over the ovaries or testes, or over areas of impaired sensation or inadequate circulation.

279.

C. The crutch length should allow the distance between the top of the crutch and the axilla to be approximately 1 1/2 to 2 inches. This is usually about two of your finger-widths.

The patient should stand erect, not bent, during the fitting. Place the crutches where the crutch tip is 4 to 6 inches to the side and 2 inches in front of each foot. The hand grips should be placed where the elbow will be flexed about 30 degrees. Use a goniometer to measure the elbow flexion.

280.

A. Pregnancy tests detect the presence of human chorionic gonadotropin (hCG) hormones in either urine or serum. This hormone is produced by the placenta during pregnancy.

281.

D. The specific gravity, one of the tests performed with a urinalysis, checks for the ability of the body to concentrate urine. The average range of specific gravity is 1.010 to 1.025.

282.

C. Clinitest is a test used to detect glucosuria. Clinitest will give a positive test for glucose; however, a more specific test for glucose is found as part of the Multistix® regime.

283.

C. When performing a venipuncture it is important for the medical assistant to not leave a tourniquet in place for more than 2 minutes. Longer periods of time increase discomfort to the patient and alter test results.

284.

B. Bacilli bacteria are found in the shape of rods. The two other shapes of bacteria are spiral, and cocci, which means round.

285.

D. When a medical assistant is performing a venipuncture the following steps should be followed. Have the patient hold the arm straight, apply the tourniquet above the elbow, and then have the patient open and close the fist. Have the patient hold the fist closed while you feel for the vein. Then clean the site with alcohol and insert the needle with the *bevel facing up*. Enter the skin about 1/2 inch below where you plan to enter the vein.

286.

A. The smallest microorganisms that cause disease in our bodies are the viruses. They do not contain all the cell parts needed to reproduce by themselves. Therefore, they must invade cells in our bodies, using some of our cell parts to reproduce.

287.

B. The federal regulations for the clinical laboratory that specified guidelines for quality control and quality assurance are from CLIA '88. CLIA '88 also establishes guidelines for adequate record keeping and qualified laboratory personnel.

Other federal agencies important to the medical clinic are (1) OSHA (Occupational Safety and Health Administration), which oversees safety and health issues; (2) CDC (Centers for Disease Control and Prevention), which investigates disease and recommends measures to prevent the spread of disease; (3) FDA (Food and Drug Administration), which oversees the testing and release of new drugs to the public; (4) DEA (Drug Enforcement Agency), which regulates controlled drugs; (5) ADA (Americans with Disabilities Act), which protects disabled persons from employment discrimination.

288.

D. A pathogenic fungus that can be seen in a physician's office is ringworm. The scientific name for this fungus is *Tinea capitis*. Athlete's foot and jock itch are closely related organisms. Urinary and vaginal yeast infections and thrush, a yeast infection of the mouth, are also types of fungal disease. Fungal diseases that attack the skin are known as dermatophytes.

289.

C. The centigrade or Celsius temperature scale is used in the medical laboratory. The freezing point for water on the centigrade scale is zero degrees while on the Fahrenheit this value is 32 degrees. The boiling point of water on the centigrade scale is 100 degrees while the Fahrenheit value is 212 degrees. These two illustrations show you why the centigrade scale is the scale of choice in the medical laboratory. The centigrade scale is easier to use in calculations.

290.

A. The stain most utilized in the medical laboratory to study bacteria is the Gram stain. Bacteria stained with Gram stain will be either purple or pink (red). If they are Gram positive, they will be viewed under the microscope as purple because the thicker cell walls absorb more dye. Gram negative will be pink or red because the thin cell walls absorb less dye.

The other answer choices are other types of stains. The acid-fast stain differentiates TB organisms from other bacteria. The Wright and Quick stain are used for blood smears to differentiate blood cell structures.

291.

D. A contrast media often used in radiographic diagnostic procedures when studying the gastric tract is barium sulfate. Gastric studies of both the upper and lower GI series require detailed preparatory instructions.

292.

B. Leukocytes in the urine are called pyuria. The term comes from the Greek word, pyon = pus, uria = urine condition. Leukocytes (white blood cells) in urine can be detected by either dipstick analysis or during microscopic examination of urine sediment. The other terms mentioned can also be analyzed for word roots, prefixes, or suffixes to reveal their meaning.

293.

C. The type of urine specimen that would be best to perform a pregnancy test with is a first morning specimen. The reason is that the first morning specimen is more concentrated than any other specimen. Therefore, the concentration of human chorionic gonadotropin (hCG) hormone, if present, would have a higher concentration.

294.

A. A glucose tolerance test (GTT) is used to diagnose diabetes mellitus. The test is performed while the patient is in a fasting state. The test checks to see how a person's metabolism responds to a highly concentrated solution of glucose. Both blood and urine specimens are collected at regular intervals.

295.

D. A cholecystogram is performed to examine the gallbladder for the presence of gallstones. The patient is given oral contrast medium, which is administered the evening before the examination.

296.

B. The metric system is the scientific measurement system that is utilized in the medical laboratory. It is based on the number 10 and the multiples and divisions often make it very easy to calculate. It has units to measure even incredibly small amounts making laboratory measurements more accurate.

297.

C. The normal range for a white blood cell count (WBC) for either men or women is 4,500 to 12,000 per cubic millimeter. An increase above 12,000 is known as leukocytosis. Smoking, because it decreases oxygen levels in the blood, can raise the WBC count by as much as 3,000 cells per cubic millimeter.

298.

D. To control or adjust the level of light when using a light microscope, the operator should use all three listed. The rheostat controls the light intensity. The condenser, also called the substage, controls the stream of light by raising or lowering it. The diaphragm, which controls the aperture of the condenser, can be opened or closed to adjust the amount of light.

299.

C. The best way to disinfect work surfaces and equipment in the medical laboratory is to use household bleach (sodium hypochlorite). It should be diluted to a 1:10 dilution. It is the recommended AIDS-related precaution.

300.

B. Glucose levels in a urine specimen without preservative will decrease when allowed to stand at room temperature for more than one hour. The reason is that bacteria will utilize the glucose in the urine as a food source.

You should make COPIES of this page to use with the 100-question test that you put together as you go through the entire review book. Refer to the Study Skills and Test-Taking Strategies section in the front of the book. It tells you how you might divide the book into short (100 question) tests. Also, note the correct way to mark the answer sheet.

Use the first blank to indicate the page number (P No.) where the question is given in the book and use the second blank for the question (Q No.). You will need to refer back to these pages and questions when you grade your test.

Example: P No. Q No.
     4   11   **1** Ⓐ Ⓑ Ⓒ Ⓓ Ⓔ
     4   12   **2** Ⓐ Ⓑ Ⓒ Ⓓ Ⓔ

P No.	Q No.		P No.	Q No.		P No.	Q No.	
___	___	**1** Ⓐ Ⓑ Ⓒ Ⓓ Ⓔ	___	___	**34** Ⓐ Ⓑ Ⓒ Ⓓ Ⓔ	___	___	**67** Ⓐ Ⓑ Ⓒ Ⓓ Ⓔ
___	___	**2** Ⓐ Ⓑ Ⓒ Ⓓ Ⓔ	___	___	**35** Ⓐ Ⓑ Ⓒ Ⓓ Ⓔ	___	___	**68** Ⓐ Ⓑ Ⓒ Ⓓ Ⓔ
___	___	**3** Ⓐ Ⓑ Ⓒ Ⓓ Ⓔ	___	___	**36** Ⓐ Ⓑ Ⓒ Ⓓ Ⓔ	___	___	**69** Ⓐ Ⓑ Ⓒ Ⓓ Ⓔ
___	___	**4** Ⓐ Ⓑ Ⓒ Ⓓ Ⓔ	___	___	**37** Ⓐ Ⓑ Ⓒ Ⓓ Ⓔ	___	___	**70** Ⓐ Ⓑ Ⓒ Ⓓ Ⓔ
___	___	**5** Ⓐ Ⓑ Ⓒ Ⓓ Ⓔ	___	___	**38** Ⓐ Ⓑ Ⓒ Ⓓ Ⓔ	___	___	**71** Ⓐ Ⓑ Ⓒ Ⓓ Ⓔ
___	___	**6** Ⓐ Ⓑ Ⓒ Ⓓ Ⓔ	___	___	**39** Ⓐ Ⓑ Ⓒ Ⓓ Ⓔ	___	___	**72** Ⓐ Ⓑ Ⓒ Ⓓ Ⓔ
___	___	**7** Ⓐ Ⓑ Ⓒ Ⓓ Ⓔ	___	___	**40** Ⓐ Ⓑ Ⓒ Ⓓ Ⓔ	___	___	**73** Ⓐ Ⓑ Ⓒ Ⓓ Ⓔ
___	___	**8** Ⓐ Ⓑ Ⓒ Ⓓ Ⓔ	___	___	**41** Ⓐ Ⓑ Ⓒ Ⓓ Ⓔ	___	___	**74** Ⓐ Ⓑ Ⓒ Ⓓ Ⓔ
___	___	**9** Ⓐ Ⓑ Ⓒ Ⓓ Ⓔ	___	___	**42** Ⓐ Ⓑ Ⓒ Ⓓ Ⓔ	___	___	**75** Ⓐ Ⓑ Ⓒ Ⓓ Ⓔ
___	___	**10** Ⓐ Ⓑ Ⓒ Ⓓ Ⓔ	___	___	**43** Ⓐ Ⓑ Ⓒ Ⓓ Ⓔ	___	___	**76** Ⓐ Ⓑ Ⓒ Ⓓ Ⓔ
___	___	**11** Ⓐ Ⓑ Ⓒ Ⓓ Ⓔ	___	___	**44** Ⓐ Ⓑ Ⓒ Ⓓ Ⓔ	___	___	**77** Ⓐ Ⓑ Ⓒ Ⓓ Ⓔ
___	___	**12** Ⓐ Ⓑ Ⓒ Ⓓ Ⓔ	___	___	**45** Ⓐ Ⓑ Ⓒ Ⓓ Ⓔ	___	___	**78** Ⓐ Ⓑ Ⓒ Ⓓ Ⓔ
___	___	**13** Ⓐ Ⓑ Ⓒ Ⓓ Ⓔ	___	___	**46** Ⓐ Ⓑ Ⓒ Ⓓ Ⓔ	___	___	**79** Ⓐ Ⓑ Ⓒ Ⓓ Ⓔ
___	___	**14** Ⓐ Ⓑ Ⓒ Ⓓ Ⓔ	___	___	**47** Ⓐ Ⓑ Ⓒ Ⓓ Ⓔ	___	___	**80** Ⓐ Ⓑ Ⓒ Ⓓ Ⓔ
___	___	**15** Ⓐ Ⓑ Ⓒ Ⓓ Ⓔ	___	___	**48** Ⓐ Ⓑ Ⓒ Ⓓ Ⓔ	___	___	**81** Ⓐ Ⓑ Ⓒ Ⓓ Ⓔ
___	___	**16** Ⓐ Ⓑ Ⓒ Ⓓ Ⓔ	___	___	**49** Ⓐ Ⓑ Ⓒ Ⓓ Ⓔ	___	___	**82** Ⓐ Ⓑ Ⓒ Ⓓ Ⓔ
___	___	**17** Ⓐ Ⓑ Ⓒ Ⓓ Ⓔ	___	___	**50** Ⓐ Ⓑ Ⓒ Ⓓ Ⓔ	___	___	**83** Ⓐ Ⓑ Ⓒ Ⓓ Ⓔ
___	___	**18** Ⓐ Ⓑ Ⓒ Ⓓ Ⓔ	___	___	**51** Ⓐ Ⓑ Ⓒ Ⓓ Ⓔ	___	___	**84** Ⓐ Ⓑ Ⓒ Ⓓ Ⓔ
___	___	**19** Ⓐ Ⓑ Ⓒ Ⓓ Ⓔ	___	___	**52** Ⓐ Ⓑ Ⓒ Ⓓ Ⓔ	___	___	**85** Ⓐ Ⓑ Ⓒ Ⓓ Ⓔ
___	___	**20** Ⓐ Ⓑ Ⓒ Ⓓ Ⓔ	___	___	**53** Ⓐ Ⓑ Ⓒ Ⓓ Ⓔ	___	___	**86** Ⓐ Ⓑ Ⓒ Ⓓ Ⓔ
___	___	**21** Ⓐ Ⓑ Ⓒ Ⓓ Ⓔ	___	___	**54** Ⓐ Ⓑ Ⓒ Ⓓ Ⓔ	___	___	**87** Ⓐ Ⓑ Ⓒ Ⓓ Ⓔ
___	___	**22** Ⓐ Ⓑ Ⓒ Ⓓ Ⓔ	___	___	**55** Ⓐ Ⓑ Ⓒ Ⓓ Ⓔ	___	___	**88** Ⓐ Ⓑ Ⓒ Ⓓ Ⓔ
___	___	**23** Ⓐ Ⓑ Ⓒ Ⓓ Ⓔ	___	___	**56** Ⓐ Ⓑ Ⓒ Ⓓ Ⓔ	___	___	**89** Ⓐ Ⓑ Ⓒ Ⓓ Ⓔ
___	___	**24** Ⓐ Ⓑ Ⓒ Ⓓ Ⓔ	___	___	**57** Ⓐ Ⓑ Ⓒ Ⓓ Ⓔ	___	___	**90** Ⓐ Ⓑ Ⓒ Ⓓ Ⓔ
___	___	**25** Ⓐ Ⓑ Ⓒ Ⓓ Ⓔ	___	___	**58** Ⓐ Ⓑ Ⓒ Ⓓ Ⓔ	___	___	**91** Ⓐ Ⓑ Ⓒ Ⓓ Ⓔ
___	___	**26** Ⓐ Ⓑ Ⓒ Ⓓ Ⓔ	___	___	**59** Ⓐ Ⓑ Ⓒ Ⓓ Ⓔ	___	___	**92** Ⓐ Ⓑ Ⓒ Ⓓ Ⓔ
___	___	**27** Ⓐ Ⓑ Ⓒ Ⓓ Ⓔ	___	___	**60** Ⓐ Ⓑ Ⓒ Ⓓ Ⓔ	___	___	**93** Ⓐ Ⓑ Ⓒ Ⓓ Ⓔ
___	___	**28** Ⓐ Ⓑ Ⓒ Ⓓ Ⓔ	___	___	**61** Ⓐ Ⓑ Ⓒ Ⓓ Ⓔ	___	___	**94** Ⓐ Ⓑ Ⓒ Ⓓ Ⓔ
___	___	**29** Ⓐ Ⓑ Ⓒ Ⓓ Ⓔ	___	___	**62** Ⓐ Ⓑ Ⓒ Ⓓ Ⓔ	___	___	**95** Ⓐ Ⓑ Ⓒ Ⓓ Ⓔ
___	___	**30** Ⓐ Ⓑ Ⓒ Ⓓ Ⓔ	___	___	**63** Ⓐ Ⓑ Ⓒ Ⓓ Ⓔ	___	___	**96** Ⓐ Ⓑ Ⓒ Ⓓ Ⓔ
___	___	**31** Ⓐ Ⓑ Ⓒ Ⓓ Ⓔ	___	___	**64** Ⓐ Ⓑ Ⓒ Ⓓ Ⓔ	___	___	**97** Ⓐ Ⓑ Ⓒ Ⓓ Ⓔ
___	___	**32** Ⓐ Ⓑ Ⓒ Ⓓ Ⓔ	___	___	**65** Ⓐ Ⓑ Ⓒ Ⓓ Ⓔ	___	___	**98** Ⓐ Ⓑ Ⓒ Ⓓ Ⓔ
___	___	**33** Ⓐ Ⓑ Ⓒ Ⓓ Ⓔ	___	___	**66** Ⓐ Ⓑ Ⓒ Ⓓ Ⓔ	___	___	**99** Ⓐ Ⓑ Ⓒ Ⓓ Ⓔ
						___	___	**100** Ⓐ Ⓑ Ⓒ Ⓓ Ⓔ

Reread the Study Skills and Test-Taking Strategies section in the front of this book BEFORE you take the 300-question practice test. Follow ALL of the suggestions such as (A) take all of the test at one time, (B) time yourself as you take the test, and (C) apply the check-on-five rule, and so on.

NOTE: On this answer sheet a mark is made after every fifth question to help you practice the check-on-five rule to pace yourself.

300-Question Practice Test
Answer Sheet 1–100
General Questions

1 Ⓐ Ⓑ Ⓒ Ⓓ Ⓔ	26 Ⓐ Ⓑ Ⓒ Ⓓ Ⓔ	51 Ⓐ Ⓑ Ⓒ Ⓓ Ⓔ	76 Ⓐ Ⓑ Ⓒ Ⓓ Ⓔ
2 Ⓐ Ⓑ Ⓒ Ⓓ Ⓔ	27 Ⓐ Ⓑ Ⓒ Ⓓ Ⓔ	52 Ⓐ Ⓑ Ⓒ Ⓓ Ⓔ	77 Ⓐ Ⓑ Ⓒ Ⓓ Ⓔ
3 Ⓐ Ⓑ Ⓒ Ⓓ Ⓔ	28 Ⓐ Ⓑ Ⓒ Ⓓ Ⓔ	53 Ⓐ Ⓑ Ⓒ Ⓓ Ⓔ	78 Ⓐ Ⓑ Ⓒ Ⓓ Ⓔ
4 Ⓐ Ⓑ Ⓒ Ⓓ Ⓔ	29 Ⓐ Ⓑ Ⓒ Ⓓ Ⓔ	54 Ⓐ Ⓑ Ⓒ Ⓓ Ⓔ	79 Ⓐ Ⓑ Ⓒ Ⓓ Ⓔ
___ 5 Ⓐ Ⓑ Ⓒ Ⓓ Ⓔ	___ 30 Ⓐ Ⓑ Ⓒ Ⓓ Ⓔ	___ 55 Ⓐ Ⓑ Ⓒ Ⓓ Ⓔ	___ 80 Ⓐ Ⓑ Ⓒ Ⓓ Ⓔ
6 Ⓐ Ⓑ Ⓒ Ⓓ Ⓔ	31 Ⓐ Ⓑ Ⓒ Ⓓ Ⓔ	56 Ⓐ Ⓑ Ⓒ Ⓓ Ⓔ	81 Ⓐ Ⓑ Ⓒ Ⓓ Ⓔ
7 Ⓐ Ⓑ Ⓒ Ⓓ Ⓔ	32 Ⓐ Ⓑ Ⓒ Ⓓ Ⓔ	57 Ⓐ Ⓑ Ⓒ Ⓓ Ⓔ	82 Ⓐ Ⓑ Ⓒ Ⓓ Ⓔ
8 Ⓐ Ⓑ Ⓒ Ⓓ Ⓔ	33 Ⓐ Ⓑ Ⓒ Ⓓ Ⓔ	58 Ⓐ Ⓑ Ⓒ Ⓓ Ⓔ	83 Ⓐ Ⓑ Ⓒ Ⓓ Ⓔ
9 Ⓐ Ⓑ Ⓒ Ⓓ Ⓔ	34 Ⓐ Ⓑ Ⓒ Ⓓ Ⓔ	59 Ⓐ Ⓑ Ⓒ Ⓓ Ⓔ	84 Ⓐ Ⓑ Ⓒ Ⓓ Ⓔ
___ 10 Ⓐ Ⓑ Ⓒ Ⓓ Ⓔ	___ 35 Ⓐ Ⓑ Ⓒ Ⓓ Ⓔ	___ 60 Ⓐ Ⓑ Ⓒ Ⓓ Ⓔ	___ 85 Ⓐ Ⓑ Ⓒ Ⓓ Ⓔ
11 Ⓐ Ⓑ Ⓒ Ⓓ Ⓔ	36 Ⓐ Ⓑ Ⓒ Ⓓ Ⓔ	61 Ⓐ Ⓑ Ⓒ Ⓓ Ⓔ	86 Ⓐ Ⓑ Ⓒ Ⓓ Ⓔ
12 Ⓐ Ⓑ Ⓒ Ⓓ Ⓔ	37 Ⓐ Ⓑ Ⓒ Ⓓ Ⓔ	62 Ⓐ Ⓑ Ⓒ Ⓓ Ⓔ	87 Ⓐ Ⓑ Ⓒ Ⓓ Ⓔ
13 Ⓐ Ⓑ Ⓒ Ⓓ Ⓔ	38 Ⓐ Ⓑ Ⓒ Ⓓ Ⓔ	63 Ⓐ Ⓑ Ⓒ Ⓓ Ⓔ	88 Ⓐ Ⓑ Ⓒ Ⓓ Ⓔ
14 Ⓐ Ⓑ Ⓒ Ⓓ Ⓔ	39 Ⓐ Ⓑ Ⓒ Ⓓ Ⓔ	64 Ⓐ Ⓑ Ⓒ Ⓓ Ⓔ	89 Ⓐ Ⓑ Ⓒ Ⓓ Ⓔ
___ 15 Ⓐ Ⓑ Ⓒ Ⓓ Ⓔ	___ 40 Ⓐ Ⓑ Ⓒ Ⓓ Ⓔ	___ 65 Ⓐ Ⓑ Ⓒ Ⓓ Ⓔ	___ 90 Ⓐ Ⓑ Ⓒ Ⓓ Ⓔ
16 Ⓐ Ⓑ Ⓒ Ⓓ Ⓔ	41 Ⓐ Ⓑ Ⓒ Ⓓ Ⓔ	66 Ⓐ Ⓑ Ⓒ Ⓓ Ⓔ	91 Ⓐ Ⓑ Ⓒ Ⓓ Ⓔ
17 Ⓐ Ⓑ Ⓒ Ⓓ Ⓔ	42 Ⓐ Ⓑ Ⓒ Ⓓ Ⓔ	67 Ⓐ Ⓑ Ⓒ Ⓓ Ⓔ	92 Ⓐ Ⓑ Ⓒ Ⓓ Ⓔ
18 Ⓐ Ⓑ Ⓒ Ⓓ Ⓔ	43 Ⓐ Ⓑ Ⓒ Ⓓ Ⓔ	68 Ⓐ Ⓑ Ⓒ Ⓓ Ⓔ	93 Ⓐ Ⓑ Ⓒ Ⓓ Ⓔ
19 Ⓐ Ⓑ Ⓒ Ⓓ Ⓔ	44 Ⓐ Ⓑ Ⓒ Ⓓ Ⓔ	69 Ⓐ Ⓑ Ⓒ Ⓓ Ⓔ	94 Ⓐ Ⓑ Ⓒ Ⓓ Ⓔ
___ 20 Ⓐ Ⓑ Ⓒ Ⓓ Ⓔ	___ 45 Ⓐ Ⓑ Ⓒ Ⓓ Ⓔ	___ 70 Ⓐ Ⓑ Ⓒ Ⓓ Ⓔ	___ 95 Ⓐ Ⓑ Ⓒ Ⓓ Ⓔ
21 Ⓐ Ⓑ Ⓒ Ⓓ Ⓔ	46 Ⓐ Ⓑ Ⓒ Ⓓ Ⓔ	71 Ⓐ Ⓑ Ⓒ Ⓓ Ⓔ	96 Ⓐ Ⓑ Ⓒ Ⓓ Ⓔ
22 Ⓐ Ⓑ Ⓒ Ⓓ Ⓔ	47 Ⓐ Ⓑ Ⓒ Ⓓ Ⓔ	72 Ⓐ Ⓑ Ⓒ Ⓓ Ⓔ	97 Ⓐ Ⓑ Ⓒ Ⓓ Ⓔ
23 Ⓐ Ⓑ Ⓒ Ⓓ Ⓔ	48 Ⓐ Ⓑ Ⓒ Ⓓ Ⓔ	73 Ⓐ Ⓑ Ⓒ Ⓓ Ⓔ	98 Ⓐ Ⓑ Ⓒ Ⓓ Ⓔ
24 Ⓐ Ⓑ Ⓒ Ⓓ Ⓔ	49 Ⓐ Ⓑ Ⓒ Ⓓ Ⓔ	74 Ⓐ Ⓑ Ⓒ Ⓓ Ⓔ	99 Ⓐ Ⓑ Ⓒ Ⓓ Ⓔ
___ 25 Ⓐ Ⓑ Ⓒ Ⓓ Ⓔ	___ 50 Ⓐ Ⓑ Ⓒ Ⓓ Ⓔ	___ 75 Ⓐ Ⓑ Ⓒ Ⓓ Ⓔ	___ 100 Ⓐ Ⓑ Ⓒ Ⓓ Ⓔ

300-Question Practice Test
Answer Sheet 101–200
Administrative Questions

101 Ⓐ Ⓑ Ⓒ Ⓓ Ⓔ	126 Ⓐ Ⓑ Ⓒ Ⓓ Ⓔ	151 Ⓐ Ⓑ Ⓒ Ⓓ Ⓔ	176 Ⓐ Ⓑ Ⓒ Ⓓ Ⓔ
102 Ⓐ Ⓑ Ⓒ Ⓓ Ⓔ	127 Ⓐ Ⓑ Ⓒ Ⓓ Ⓔ	152 Ⓐ Ⓑ Ⓒ Ⓓ Ⓔ	177 Ⓐ Ⓑ Ⓒ Ⓓ Ⓔ
103 Ⓐ Ⓑ Ⓒ Ⓓ Ⓔ	128 Ⓐ Ⓑ Ⓒ Ⓓ Ⓔ	153 Ⓐ Ⓑ Ⓒ Ⓓ Ⓔ	178 Ⓐ Ⓑ Ⓒ Ⓓ Ⓔ
104 Ⓐ Ⓑ Ⓒ Ⓓ Ⓔ	129 Ⓐ Ⓑ Ⓒ Ⓓ Ⓔ	154 Ⓐ Ⓑ Ⓒ Ⓓ Ⓔ	179 Ⓐ Ⓑ Ⓒ Ⓓ Ⓔ
105 Ⓐ Ⓑ Ⓒ Ⓓ Ⓔ	130 Ⓐ Ⓑ Ⓒ Ⓓ Ⓔ	155 Ⓐ Ⓑ Ⓒ Ⓓ Ⓔ	180 Ⓐ Ⓑ Ⓒ Ⓓ Ⓔ
106 Ⓐ Ⓑ Ⓒ Ⓓ Ⓔ	131 Ⓐ Ⓑ Ⓒ Ⓓ Ⓔ	156 Ⓐ Ⓑ Ⓒ Ⓓ Ⓔ	181 Ⓐ Ⓑ Ⓒ Ⓓ Ⓔ
107 Ⓐ Ⓑ Ⓒ Ⓓ Ⓔ	132 Ⓐ Ⓑ Ⓒ Ⓓ Ⓔ	157 Ⓐ Ⓑ Ⓒ Ⓓ Ⓔ	182 Ⓐ Ⓑ Ⓒ Ⓓ Ⓔ
108 Ⓐ Ⓑ Ⓒ Ⓓ Ⓔ	133 Ⓐ Ⓑ Ⓒ Ⓓ Ⓔ	158 Ⓐ Ⓑ Ⓒ Ⓓ Ⓔ	183 Ⓐ Ⓑ Ⓒ Ⓓ Ⓔ
109 Ⓐ Ⓑ Ⓒ Ⓓ Ⓔ	134 Ⓐ Ⓑ Ⓒ Ⓓ Ⓔ	159 Ⓐ Ⓑ Ⓒ Ⓓ Ⓔ	184 Ⓐ Ⓑ Ⓒ Ⓓ Ⓔ
110 Ⓐ Ⓑ Ⓒ Ⓓ Ⓔ	135 Ⓐ Ⓑ Ⓒ Ⓓ Ⓔ	160 Ⓐ Ⓑ Ⓒ Ⓓ Ⓔ	185 Ⓐ Ⓑ Ⓒ Ⓓ Ⓔ
111 Ⓐ Ⓑ Ⓒ Ⓓ Ⓔ	136 Ⓐ Ⓑ Ⓒ Ⓓ Ⓔ	161 Ⓐ Ⓑ Ⓒ Ⓓ Ⓔ	186 Ⓐ Ⓑ Ⓒ Ⓓ Ⓔ
112 Ⓐ Ⓑ Ⓒ Ⓓ Ⓔ	137 Ⓐ Ⓑ Ⓒ Ⓓ Ⓔ	162 Ⓐ Ⓑ Ⓒ Ⓓ Ⓔ	187 Ⓐ Ⓑ Ⓒ Ⓓ Ⓔ
113 Ⓐ Ⓑ Ⓒ Ⓓ Ⓔ	138 Ⓐ Ⓑ Ⓒ Ⓓ Ⓔ	163 Ⓐ Ⓑ Ⓒ Ⓓ Ⓔ	188 Ⓐ Ⓑ Ⓒ Ⓓ Ⓔ
114 Ⓐ Ⓑ Ⓒ Ⓓ Ⓔ	139 Ⓐ Ⓑ Ⓒ Ⓓ Ⓔ	164 Ⓐ Ⓑ Ⓒ Ⓓ Ⓔ	189 Ⓐ Ⓑ Ⓒ Ⓓ Ⓔ
115 Ⓐ Ⓑ Ⓒ Ⓓ Ⓔ	140 Ⓐ Ⓑ Ⓒ Ⓓ Ⓔ	165 Ⓐ Ⓑ Ⓒ Ⓓ Ⓔ	190 Ⓐ Ⓑ Ⓒ Ⓓ Ⓔ
116 Ⓐ Ⓑ Ⓒ Ⓓ Ⓔ	141 Ⓐ Ⓑ Ⓒ Ⓓ Ⓔ	166 Ⓐ Ⓑ Ⓒ Ⓓ Ⓔ	191 Ⓐ Ⓑ Ⓒ Ⓓ Ⓔ
117 Ⓐ Ⓑ Ⓒ Ⓓ Ⓔ	142 Ⓐ Ⓑ Ⓒ Ⓓ Ⓔ	167 Ⓐ Ⓑ Ⓒ Ⓓ Ⓔ	192 Ⓐ Ⓑ Ⓒ Ⓓ Ⓔ
118 Ⓐ Ⓑ Ⓒ Ⓓ Ⓔ	143 Ⓐ Ⓑ Ⓒ Ⓓ Ⓔ	168 Ⓐ Ⓑ Ⓒ Ⓓ Ⓔ	193 Ⓐ Ⓑ Ⓒ Ⓓ Ⓔ
119 Ⓐ Ⓑ Ⓒ Ⓓ Ⓔ	144 Ⓐ Ⓑ Ⓒ Ⓓ Ⓔ	169 Ⓐ Ⓑ Ⓒ Ⓓ Ⓔ	194 Ⓐ Ⓑ Ⓒ Ⓓ Ⓔ
120 Ⓐ Ⓑ Ⓒ Ⓓ Ⓔ	145 Ⓐ Ⓑ Ⓒ Ⓓ Ⓔ	170 Ⓐ Ⓑ Ⓒ Ⓓ Ⓔ	195 Ⓐ Ⓑ Ⓒ Ⓓ Ⓔ
121 Ⓐ Ⓑ Ⓒ Ⓓ Ⓔ	146 Ⓐ Ⓑ Ⓒ Ⓓ Ⓔ	171 Ⓐ Ⓑ Ⓒ Ⓓ Ⓔ	196 Ⓐ Ⓑ Ⓒ Ⓓ Ⓔ
122 Ⓐ Ⓑ Ⓒ Ⓓ Ⓔ	147 Ⓐ Ⓑ Ⓒ Ⓓ Ⓔ	172 Ⓐ Ⓑ Ⓒ Ⓓ Ⓔ	197 Ⓐ Ⓑ Ⓒ Ⓓ Ⓔ
123 Ⓐ Ⓑ Ⓒ Ⓓ Ⓔ	148 Ⓐ Ⓑ Ⓒ Ⓓ Ⓔ	173 Ⓐ Ⓑ Ⓒ Ⓓ Ⓔ	198 Ⓐ Ⓑ Ⓒ Ⓓ Ⓔ
124 Ⓐ Ⓑ Ⓒ Ⓓ Ⓔ	149 Ⓐ Ⓑ Ⓒ Ⓓ Ⓔ	174 Ⓐ Ⓑ Ⓒ Ⓓ Ⓔ	199 Ⓐ Ⓑ Ⓒ Ⓓ Ⓔ
125 Ⓐ Ⓑ Ⓒ Ⓓ Ⓔ	150 Ⓐ Ⓑ Ⓒ Ⓓ Ⓔ	175 Ⓐ Ⓑ Ⓒ Ⓓ Ⓔ	200 Ⓐ Ⓑ Ⓒ Ⓓ Ⓔ

300-Question Practice Test
Answer Sheet 201–300
Clinical Questions

201 Ⓐ Ⓑ Ⓒ Ⓓ Ⓔ   226 Ⓐ Ⓑ Ⓒ Ⓓ Ⓔ   251 Ⓐ Ⓑ Ⓒ Ⓓ Ⓔ   276 Ⓐ Ⓑ Ⓒ Ⓓ Ⓔ
202 Ⓐ Ⓑ Ⓒ Ⓓ Ⓔ   227 Ⓐ Ⓑ Ⓒ Ⓓ Ⓔ   252 Ⓐ Ⓑ Ⓒ Ⓓ Ⓔ   277 Ⓐ Ⓑ Ⓒ Ⓓ Ⓔ
203 Ⓐ Ⓑ Ⓒ Ⓓ Ⓔ   228 Ⓐ Ⓑ Ⓒ Ⓓ Ⓔ   253 Ⓐ Ⓑ Ⓒ Ⓓ Ⓔ   278 Ⓐ Ⓑ Ⓒ Ⓓ Ⓔ
204 Ⓐ Ⓑ Ⓒ Ⓓ Ⓔ   229 Ⓐ Ⓑ Ⓒ Ⓓ Ⓔ   254 Ⓐ Ⓑ Ⓒ Ⓓ Ⓔ   279 Ⓐ Ⓑ Ⓒ Ⓓ Ⓔ
205 Ⓐ Ⓑ Ⓒ Ⓓ Ⓔ   230 Ⓐ Ⓑ Ⓒ Ⓓ Ⓔ   255 Ⓐ Ⓑ Ⓒ Ⓓ Ⓔ   280 Ⓐ Ⓑ Ⓒ Ⓓ Ⓔ

206 Ⓐ Ⓑ Ⓒ Ⓓ Ⓔ   231 Ⓐ Ⓑ Ⓒ Ⓓ Ⓔ   256 Ⓐ Ⓑ Ⓒ Ⓓ Ⓔ   281 Ⓐ Ⓑ Ⓒ Ⓓ Ⓔ
207 Ⓐ Ⓑ Ⓒ Ⓓ Ⓔ   232 Ⓐ Ⓑ Ⓒ Ⓓ Ⓔ   257 Ⓐ Ⓑ Ⓒ Ⓓ Ⓔ   282 Ⓐ Ⓑ Ⓒ Ⓓ Ⓔ
208 Ⓐ Ⓑ Ⓒ Ⓓ Ⓔ   233 Ⓐ Ⓑ Ⓒ Ⓓ Ⓔ   258 Ⓐ Ⓑ Ⓒ Ⓓ Ⓔ   283 Ⓐ Ⓑ Ⓒ Ⓓ Ⓔ
209 Ⓐ Ⓑ Ⓒ Ⓓ Ⓔ   234 Ⓐ Ⓑ Ⓒ Ⓓ Ⓔ   259 Ⓐ Ⓑ Ⓒ Ⓓ Ⓔ   284 Ⓐ Ⓑ Ⓒ Ⓓ Ⓔ
210 Ⓐ Ⓑ Ⓒ Ⓓ Ⓔ   235 Ⓐ Ⓑ Ⓒ Ⓓ Ⓔ   260 Ⓐ Ⓑ Ⓒ Ⓓ Ⓔ   285 Ⓐ Ⓑ Ⓒ Ⓓ Ⓔ

211 Ⓐ Ⓑ Ⓒ Ⓓ Ⓔ   236 Ⓐ Ⓑ Ⓒ Ⓓ Ⓔ   261 Ⓐ Ⓑ Ⓒ Ⓓ Ⓔ   286 Ⓐ Ⓑ Ⓒ Ⓓ Ⓔ
212 Ⓐ Ⓑ Ⓒ Ⓓ Ⓔ   237 Ⓐ Ⓑ Ⓒ Ⓓ Ⓔ   262 Ⓐ Ⓑ Ⓒ Ⓓ Ⓔ   287 Ⓐ Ⓑ Ⓒ Ⓓ Ⓔ
213 Ⓐ Ⓑ Ⓒ Ⓓ Ⓔ   238 Ⓐ Ⓑ Ⓒ Ⓓ Ⓔ   263 Ⓐ Ⓑ Ⓒ Ⓓ Ⓔ   288 Ⓐ Ⓑ Ⓒ Ⓓ Ⓔ
214 Ⓐ Ⓑ Ⓒ Ⓓ Ⓔ   239 Ⓐ Ⓑ Ⓒ Ⓓ Ⓔ   264 Ⓐ Ⓑ Ⓒ Ⓓ Ⓔ   289 Ⓐ Ⓑ Ⓒ Ⓓ Ⓔ
215 Ⓐ Ⓑ Ⓒ Ⓓ Ⓔ   240 Ⓐ Ⓑ Ⓒ Ⓓ Ⓔ   265 Ⓐ Ⓑ Ⓒ Ⓓ Ⓔ   290 Ⓐ Ⓑ Ⓒ Ⓓ Ⓔ

216 Ⓐ Ⓑ Ⓒ Ⓓ Ⓔ   241 Ⓐ Ⓑ Ⓒ Ⓓ Ⓔ   266 Ⓐ Ⓑ Ⓒ Ⓓ Ⓔ   291 Ⓐ Ⓑ Ⓒ Ⓓ Ⓔ
217 Ⓐ Ⓑ Ⓒ Ⓓ Ⓔ   242 Ⓐ Ⓑ Ⓒ Ⓓ Ⓔ   267 Ⓐ Ⓑ Ⓒ Ⓓ Ⓔ   292 Ⓐ Ⓑ Ⓒ Ⓓ Ⓔ
218 Ⓐ Ⓑ Ⓒ Ⓓ Ⓔ   243 Ⓐ Ⓑ Ⓒ Ⓓ Ⓔ   268 Ⓐ Ⓑ Ⓒ Ⓓ Ⓔ   293 Ⓐ Ⓑ Ⓒ Ⓓ Ⓔ
219 Ⓐ Ⓑ Ⓒ Ⓓ Ⓔ   244 Ⓐ Ⓑ Ⓒ Ⓓ Ⓔ   269 Ⓐ Ⓑ Ⓒ Ⓓ Ⓔ   294 Ⓐ Ⓑ Ⓒ Ⓓ Ⓔ
220 Ⓐ Ⓑ Ⓒ Ⓓ Ⓔ   245 Ⓐ Ⓑ Ⓒ Ⓓ Ⓔ   270 Ⓐ Ⓑ Ⓒ Ⓓ Ⓔ   295 Ⓐ Ⓑ Ⓒ Ⓓ Ⓔ

221 Ⓐ Ⓑ Ⓒ Ⓓ Ⓔ   246 Ⓐ Ⓑ Ⓒ Ⓓ Ⓔ   271 Ⓐ Ⓑ Ⓒ Ⓓ Ⓔ   296 Ⓐ Ⓑ Ⓒ Ⓓ Ⓔ
222 Ⓐ Ⓑ Ⓒ Ⓓ Ⓔ   247 Ⓐ Ⓑ Ⓒ Ⓓ Ⓔ   272 Ⓐ Ⓑ Ⓒ Ⓓ Ⓔ   297 Ⓐ Ⓑ Ⓒ Ⓓ Ⓔ
223 Ⓐ Ⓑ Ⓒ Ⓓ Ⓔ   248 Ⓐ Ⓑ Ⓒ Ⓓ Ⓔ   273 Ⓐ Ⓑ Ⓒ Ⓓ Ⓔ   298 Ⓐ Ⓑ Ⓒ Ⓓ Ⓔ
224 Ⓐ Ⓑ Ⓒ Ⓓ Ⓔ   249 Ⓐ Ⓑ Ⓒ Ⓓ Ⓔ   274 Ⓐ Ⓑ Ⓒ Ⓓ Ⓔ   299 Ⓐ Ⓑ Ⓒ Ⓓ Ⓔ
225 Ⓐ Ⓑ Ⓒ Ⓓ Ⓔ   250 Ⓐ Ⓑ Ⓒ Ⓓ Ⓔ   275 Ⓐ Ⓑ Ⓒ Ⓓ Ⓔ   300 Ⓐ Ⓑ Ⓒ Ⓓ Ⓔ

Index

Page numbers in *italics* denote figures.

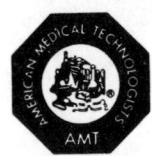

American Medical Technologists

REGISTERED MEDICAL ASSISTANT CERTIFICATION EXAMINATION
CONTENT SUMMARY

I. GENERAL MEDICAL ASSISTING KNOWLEDGE

  A. Anatomy and Physiology
    1. Body systems
    2. Disorders of the body
  B. Medical Terminology
    1. Word parts
    2. Definitions
    3. Common abbreviations and symbols
    4. Spelling
  C. Medical Law
    1. Medical law
    2. Licensure, certification, and registration
  D. Medical Ethics
    1. Principles of medical ethics
    2. Ethical conduct
  E. Human Relations
    1. Patient relations
    2. Other interpersonal relations
  F. Patient Education
    1. Patient instruction
    2. Patient resource materials

II. ADMINISTRATIVE MEDICAL ASSISTING

  A. Insurance
    1. Terminology
    2. Plans
    3. Claim forms
    4. Coding
    5. Financial aspects of medical insurance
  B. Financial Bookkeeping
    1. Terminology
    2. Patient billing
    3. Collections
    4. Fundamental medical office accounting procedures
    5. Banking
    6. Employee payroll
    7. Financial mathematics
  C. Medical Secretary-Receptionist
    1. Terminology
    2. Reception
    3. Scheduling
    4. Oral and written communications
    5. Records management
    6. Charts
    7. Transcription and dictation
    8. Supplies and equipment management
    9. Computers for medical office applications
    10. Office safety

III. CLINICAL MEDICAL ASSISTING

  A. Asepsis
    1. Terminology
    2. Universal blood and body fluid precautions
    3. Medical asepsis
    4. Surgical asepsis
  B. Sterilization
    1. Terminology
    2. Sanitization
    3. Disinfection
    4. Sterilization
    5. Record keeping
  C. Instruments
    1. Identification
    2. Usage
    3. Care and handling
  D. Vital Signs
    1. Blood pressure
    2. Pulse
    3. Respiration
    4. Height and weight
    5. Temperature
  E. Physical Examinations
    1. Problem oriented records
    2. Positions
    3. Methods of examination
    4. Specialty examinations
    5. Visual acuity
    6. Allergy testing
  F. Clinical Pharmacology
    1. Terminology
    2. Injections
    3. Prescriptions
    4. Drugs
  G. Minor Surgery
    1. Surgical supplies
    2. Surgical procedures
  H. Therapeutic Modalities
    1. Modalities
    2. Patient Instruction
  I. Laboratory Procedures
    1. Safety
    2. Quality control
    3. Laboratory equipment
    4. Urinalysis
    5. Blood
    6. Other specimens
    7. Specimen handling
    8. Records
    9. Microbiology
  J. Electrocardiography
    1. Standard, 12-lead ECG
    2. Mounting techniques
    3. Other ECG procedures
  K. First Aid
    1. First aid procedures
    2. Legal responsibilities

TASK INVENTORY NOTE

The tasks included in this inventory are considered by American Medical Technologists to be *representative* of the medical assisting job role. This document should be considered dynamic, to reflect the medical assistant's current role with respect to contemporary health care. Therefore, tasks may be added, removed, or modified on an ongoing basis.